Nursing in Haematological Oncology

This book is dedicated to all nurses caring for individuals with haematological cancers.

I hope it inspires you to provide excellent patient care while stimulating you to continually develop your practice for the benefit of patients and their families.

For Elsevier:

Senior Commissioning Editor: Ninette Premdas
Project Development Managers: Katrina Mather Gill Cloke
Project Manager: Frances Affleck
Design Direction: George Ajayi

Nursing in Haematological Oncology

SECOND EDITION

Edited by

Maggie Grundy

MSc RGN RM DipNursEd (Clinical Teaching) DipNurs (Lond) PGTC

Programme Director – Cancer Care, NHS Education for Scotland

Foreword by

Barry Quinn

MSc, PG Cert, BD, Bacc Phil, RN

President, European Group for Blood and Marrow Transplantation Nurses Group (EBMT-NG)

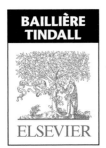

BAILLIÈRE TINDALL

ELSEVIER

EDINBURGH LONDON NEW YORK OXFORD PHILADELPHIA ST LOUIS SYDNEY TORONTO 2006

BAILLIÈRE
TINDALL
ELSEVIER

© Harcourt Publishers Limited 2000
© 2006, Elsevier Limited. All rights reserved.

The right of Maggie Grundy to be identified as editor of this work has been asserted by her in accordance with the Copyright, Designs and Patents Act 1988

First edition 2000
Second edition 2006

ISBN 10: 0 70202753 7
ISBN 13: 978-0-7020-2753-6

British Library Cataloguing in Publication Data
A catalogue record for this book is available from the British Library

Library of Congress Cataloging in Publication Data
A catalog record for this book is available from the Library of Congress

Note
Medical knowledge is constantly changing. Standard safety precautions must be followed, but as new research and clinical experience broaden our knowledge, changes in treatment and drug therapy may become necessary or appropriate. Readers are advised to check the most current product information provided by the manufacturer of each drug to be administered to verify the recommended dose, the method and duration of administration, and contraindications. It is the responsibility of the practitioner, relying on experience and knowledge of the patient, to determine dosages and the best treatment for each individual patient. Neither the Publisher nor the editor and contributors assume any liability for any injury and/or damage to persons or property arising from this publication.

The Publisher

Contents

Contributors

Gena Andrew RGN ENB Onc Dip Clin Teaching
Clinical Nurse Manager. Anchor Unit, Aberdeen Royal Infirmary, Aberdeen, UK

Joanne Atkinson RGN BA (Hons) DP HS PGDip Ed (RNT) MSc
Senior Lecturer Cancer and Palliative Care, Northumbria University, Newcastle upon Tyne, UK

Helen Balsdon BSc (Hons) ENB 237 N18 998 MSc
Senior Clinical Nurse for Oncology and Lead Nurse Cancer, Addenbrookes Hospital, Cambridge, UK

Marvelle Brown
Macmillan Senior Lecturer, Thames Valley University, School of Health & Science, Ealing, London, UK

Joyce Butters DCR (T) DCR (D) Dip Counselling
Macmillan Information and Support Radiographer, Radiotherapy Department, Velindre Hospital, Cardiff, Wales, UK

Linda Bywater MSc BA (Hons) RN
Independent Management Consultant, Kidlington, Oxon, UK

Sylvia Cole RGN RM BSc (Hons)
Haematology Nurse Specialist, Altnagelvin Area Hospital, Londonderry, Northern Ireland

Shirley Crofts MSc, BSc (Hons), RGN
Haematology Clinical Nurse Specialist, Royal South Hants Hospital, Southampton, UK

Carmen Cule DCR (T)
Deputy Radiotherapy Services Manager, Radiotherapy Department, Velindre Hospital, Cardiff, Wales, UK

Evelyn Dannie
Clinical Nurse Specialist, Department of Haematology, Hammersmith Hospital, London, UK

Lynne Dickinson RGN RM
Clinical Nurse Specialist, Clatterbridge Centre for Oncology, Wirral, UK

Shelley Dolan
Nurse Consultant, The Royal Marsden Hospital, Surrey, UK

Kathleen Dunne RGN RM RNT BEd (Hons) MSc DNSc
Nurse Lecturer, Altnagelvin Area Hospital, Londonderry, Northern Ireland

Mandy Ellis RGN ENB 998 934
Bone Marrow Transplant Coordinator, John Radcliffe Hospital, Oxford, UK

Janice Gabriel MPhil PgD BSc (Hons) RN FETC ONC CertMHS
Nurse Director, Central South Coast Cancer Network, Hampshire & Isle of Wight Strategic Health Authority, Southampton, UK

Alexandra Gray RGN BA (Hons) MSc (Ed)
Effective Use of Blood Project Manager, Scottish National Blood Transfusion Service, Edinburgh, UK

Jackie Green RGN ONC Cert Dip MSc
*Consultant Nurse Haematology/Lead Cancer Nurse,
Mayday NHS Trust, London, UK*

Jan Green RGN BA DipOnc
Transfusion Liaison Nurse, NBS Colindale, UK

Maggie Grundy MSC RGN RM DipNursEd (Clinical
Teaching) DipNurs (Lond) PGTC
*Programme Director – Cancer Care, NHS Education
for Scotland*

Sarah Hart MSc BSc (Hons) RGN FETC
*Clinical Nurse Specialist Infection Control, The Royal
Marsden Hospital, Surrey, UK*

Jan Hawthorn BSc PhD
Surrey, UK

Timothy Jackson MSc in Health Service Management,
SRN SCM RNMS Oncology Cert ENB 237 931 998 934
*Nurse Director, South East London Cancer Network,
London, UK*

Daniel Kelly PhD MSc BSc RGN NDN Cert ONC Cert
PGCE RNT
*Reader in Cancer and Palliative Care, Middlesex
University, London, UK*

Tracey King RGN ENB A27 N59 N37 998
*Support Services Manager, Myeloma Foundation of
Australia Inc, Sydney, Australia*

Ulu Mehmet SRD BSc PGDip PGCert
*Senior Dietitian, University Hospital of Wales,
Cardiff, Wales, UK*

Alexander Molassiotis RGN BSc MSc PhD
*Professor of Cancer and Supportive Care, University
of Manchester, School of Nursing, Manchester, UK*

Karen Phillips BSc (Hons) DipN CertEd
*Chemotherapy Nurse Specialist Trainer, University
Hospital of Wales, Cardiff, Wales, UK*

Helen Porter
*Director of Nursing, Clatterbridge Centre for
Oncology, Wirral, UK*

Elizabeth Rawlings RGN BSc
*Formerly Head Nurse, Haematology, Department of
Haematology, John Radcliffe Hospital, Oxford, UK*

Carol Richardson RGN BA (Hons) ENB Higher Award
Dip HE
*Matron Specialist Haematology, Newcastle upon
Tyne Hospitals Trust, Newcastle upon Tyne, UK*

Mike Tadman MSc PGDip (Education) BSc (Hons) RGN
*Senior Lecturer in Cancer Care, Oxford Brookes
University, Oxford, UK*

Shirley Tervit RGN Diploma Cancer Nursing
UK

Colin Thain MA (Hons) MSc MA PGDE RGN
*Senior Lecturer in Cancer Care, Department of
Nursing, University of Central Lancashire,
Preston, UK*

Deborah Tomlinson MN RSCN RGN Dip Cancer
Nursing
*Research Nurse, Program of Population Health
Sciences, Hospital for Sick Children, Toronto, Canada*

Breege Traynor MSc B Nurs RGN DN Cert ONC Cert
PGDip Pharmacovigilance
*Associate Director, AMGEN Limited,
Cambridge, UK*

Clare Woodcock BA (Hons) DipNS ENB 237 998 RGN
*Macmillan Clinical Nurse Specialist, East Berkshire
Palliative Care Team, King Edward VII Hospital,
Windsor, UK*

Foreword

When I began working with people undergoing treatment for cancer over twenty years ago in a hospice in Dublin I had no idea then that I would eventually find myself in this field of cancer care. Back then, I suspect, I did not even know what the word haematological oncology meant, and perhaps this is also true of many patients and their families when they first hear of their diagnosis. Hearing that you have been diagnosed with a disease that perhaps is difficult to pronounce or gives rise to much uncertainty can be very frightening. Many of the patients I have spoken to over the years describe the feeling of losing control in this unknown territory, surrounded by a variety of uniforms and badges, strange equipment and a new vocabulary. In this bewildering environment the well prepared nurse is an extremely important ally at this time.

This particular field of cancer care, which at first sight can appear very technical because of the nature of the disease and advances in treatment, is also an area of care where all the essential elements of nursing remain. As in other areas of health care the roles nurses perform, and will continue to develop are numerous. This is clearly demonstrated by the contributors to the second edition of this book. Ongoing advances include a greater understanding of the risk factors that may predispose people to these diseases; more specialised knowledge in diagnosing and staging of these malignant diseases; an increased understanding of how the treatments work; and an ability to deliver more targeted treatments with better results and less toxicity. These medical advances must be matched equally with our own advances in nursing care at the local, national and international level. Such developments will enable people to live longer while addressing quality of life issues. Treatments such as stem cell transplantation, which at one time would have been only available to a small percentage of patients, are now, because of advances in treatment regimens and supportive therapy, a viable option to many more people. This brings with it a demand for advancing nursing practice.

I often wonder what makes this field of health care so challenging. Is it the fact that we are dealing with diseases with uncertain outcomes?

Or, is it the fact that we must face the reality that some of the treatments we administer may also cause short and long-term morbidity and in some cases death? Is it because we are dealing with disease in which the cells that enable us to live and enjoy the normal pursuits of everyday life now cause severe problems to the body? Perhaps the truth lies in the fact that while we deal with a disease that forces us to understand and appreciate the cellular working of the body, we do so always mindful that we are caring for human beings. I have often said in the classroom and the clinical setting there is no 'them' and 'us' in cancer care. There is really no such thing as a nurse, doctor, therapist, pastor, patient, family member or friend because these are simply labels that describe one aspect of who we are. However, what we all share is our 'personhood', we share in common our humanity. I strongly believe, having spent time with people with cancer in many different settings, that we have much to learn from each other.

Over the last few years I have spent time listening to patients who have experience of the disease, treatments and care being discussed in this book, some of whom may have recently been diagnosed while others are living with advanced disease. Others recall their treatment and experience from many years ago. Always the conversation will come round to what has helped them through their experience and always they will mention the role of the nurse and the team. While each person may use different words and expressions they all agree that a good nurse has two key attributes: the knowledge and the clinical skills to deliver the required care; and more importantly, the ability to treat those they care for with dignity and respect. What can make a real difference in hearing a difficult piece of news or explaining a clinical procedure is the nurse who demonstrates understanding and care. I believe that each chapter of this second edition, while focusing on a particular key area of this specialty, demonstrates these attributes.

I enjoyed and indeed have recommended Maggie Grundy's first edition of 'Nursing in Haematological Oncology' to many of my nursing and allied health professional colleagues working in the clinical and academic settings. I am delighted to see this second edition which develops and advances the same standard of evidence based practice applied to practical clinical settings as in the first edition. Each chapter, while written with a focus on practice, enables the reader to reflect on the evidence, case scenarios, guided questions and suggested reading, and offers thought provoking insights into this field of care. Heamatological oncology is continually moving forward and this second edition, while addressing these new developments, also highlights the new and existing challenges these changes bring. It is mainly UK focused and addresses the knowledge and skills framework (KSF) and other relevant guidelines from the four UK health departments on patient care. However, this book will also be of great help to nurses working in other European countries.

The book is very credibly written by experts, fellow colleagues who continue to work in this field and clearly demonstrate their commitment to improving the quality of lives of patients and their families undergoing treatment for haematological malignant disease. Through the treatments discussed and the nursing support given, many more people now face the realities of survivorship and long-term recovery. We are reminded that palliative care, which should be present from diagnosis, is something each nurse has a responsibility to deliver. Sensitively and practically the book also addresses the reality that some of those we care for, including children, adolescents and adults, die of this disease. It helps us to reflect on this issue. While detailing the different dimensions of the field and recognising the individuality of each person undergoing treatment, we are reminded that we also need to care for ourselves, and one another. All of us, no matter in what role we work, are called to be leaders. While many good developments continue to happen in haematological oncology it is clearly recognised that much more research is required. Nurses working together with allied health professional and medical colleagues have a vital role to play in advancing clinical practice.

Patients are now cared for in a variety of settings – their homes, through their local general practice, their local hospital, a hospice and in settings specialising in these diseases. Wherever you work as a nurse delivering care you will find this book very helpful. I believe that nurses at all levels can benefit from this book whether they are new to haematological oncology, or are more advanced practitioners. While this book is aimed at nurses I believe it will be an excellent resource for any health care worker who is involved in supporting patients undergoing treatment for these malignant diseases.

I appreciate this book because, while it does address the essential knowledge and clinical skills required to deliver knowledgeable clinical care, it does so by being very conscious of the psychological dimension of care we deliver.

In addressing the diseases, the treatments and the nursing care issues in haematological oncology, this book is a valuable tool to complement clinical and academic practice. As the treatment for haematological oncology disease continues to develop, we as nurses may be asked to take on changing and exciting roles, however the challenge for nursing is that in whatever roles we deliver our clinical practice, the core of nursing must remain.

Barry Quinn MSc, BD, Bacc Phil, RN
President European Group for Blood and Marrow Transplantation
Nurses Group (2004–2006)
Acting Programme Leader/Lecturer Haemato-oncology Royal
Marsden School of Cancer Nursing & Rehabilitation Fulham Road
London
SW3 6JJ

Preface

Haemato-oncology is a rapidly advancing speciality and in recent years many changes have occurred in the organisation of services and nurses' roles. Supportive care and symptom management have improved and people with haematological cancers are living longer. The second edition of this book reflects these changes. The book contains eight new chapters: immune modulators and novel therapies, adolescents with cancer, sexuality and nursing practice, addressing the needs of families, fatigue, palliative care, leadership issues for specialist nurses and research priorities. Additionally, all existing chapters have been updated in light of contemporary changes in both patient care and nursing roles.

The book remains the only UK textbook addressing haemato-oncology written specifically for nurses. The first edition was primarily intended for qualified nurses working with or having an interest in haematological cancers. The second edition retains this focus but has been expanded to incorporate issues of interest to specialist nurses, many of whom are the current and future leaders in the specialty. The book will also be of interest to student nurses and those undertaking specialist courses.

The second edition retains the original format and is divided into three separate but complementary sections. The first section examines the diseases, the second, treatment and the third and largest section discusses nursing issues. The emphasis of the book is on the patient and nursing management but to manage patients effectively, knowledge of both normal and abnormal haematopoiesis and medical management is necessary. The first chapter therefore concentrates on the normal physiology of the blood followed by five chapters reviewing the differing haematological cancers and their related pathophysiology.

Many treatments such as chemotherapy and blood and marrow transplantation are common to a number of haematological cancers, as are many aspects of nursing care. Therefore to avoid repetition separate chapters have been devoted to individual treatment modalities and nursing issues are separated into a different section. Although the book deals mainly with adults, it would not be complete without making some reference to the special problems of children and adolescents and separate chapters are included.

Considerable expertise is required to support individuals with haematological cancers and the nursing issues section provides essential information. Venous access is a particular problem for patients as veins tend to fibrose owing to the huge number of venepunctures and the enormous quantity of drugs that require intravenous delivery. A chapter therefore outlines the particular issues associated with the differing vascular devices available and guidelines for their care. Further chapters discuss the potentially life-threatening issues of infection and haemorrhage and other important aspects of care including oral care, nutrition, fatigue, sexuality and fertility issues and the reduction of nausea and vomiting. The immunosuppression experienced by patients results in prolonged periods of isolation and this, combined with the life-threatening nature of the disease and the aggressive chemotherapy regimens, means that psychological care is an important aspect of care and issues such as reaction to and adaptation to diagnosis, treatment and relapse are also included.

Advances in the treatment of haematological cancers have resulted in an increased life expectancy for many patients, which in turn may lead to discrimination in employment and financial problems. Social issues, quality of life and survivorship are therefore addressed. For others, their disease will prove to be ultimately incurable, although they may live for many years with their disease. Symptom management, supportive care and quality of life are therefore of paramount importance and a chapter is devoted to palliative care. The family plays an increasingly important part in supporting patients throughout their cancer experience, whatever the final outcome, and their needs are sometimes forgotten. The needs of families are therefore also included. Furthermore, many ethical dilemmas may arise when nursing patients with haematological cancers and these issues are also explored.

Nurses working with individuals with a life-threatening illness may suffer from stress and burnout. This may be especially so in haemato-oncology as patients are frequently hospitalised for prolonged periods of time, on numerous occasions. Nurses therefore get to know patients and their families extremely well and may become emotionally attached to them, nursing them through one or more relapses and episodes of acute illness. When a patient dies, nurses may experience a grief-like reaction and eventually this may lead to stress and dissatisfaction with the job. Staff support strategies may help to reduce stress, improve staff retention and prevent burnout. A further chapter therefore deals with the issues of staff support and retention.

In today's rapidly changing health service, leaders are required within every specialty and development of leadership skills is discussed. Those who take up the leadership challenge must ensure that their lead demonstrates care based on the best available evidence, necessitating a knowledge of current research and the gaps in the evidence base and perhaps more importantly an understanding of how to disseminate and utilise this knowledge in practice. The penultimate chapter explores the research priorities identified by practitioners in the specialty. To conclude, the final chapter explores future developments in this rapidly evolving specialty.

The division of the book into three separate sections should allow nurses to easily find a specific area of interest. There are many areas of overlap between the different disorders and consequently much cross-referencing between chapters. This should enable readers to dip into the book at different points to find the information they require without having to read the book sequentially. Reflection points, case studies and discussion questions are included to stimulate reflection on practice and encourage readers to discuss with colleagues issues within their own practice. The chapters are all relatively short and readers may want to explore issues in greater depth. To facilitate this, suggested reading is also included at the end of each chapter.

A number of different authors have contributed their knowledge and clinical expertise to this book, building on the knowledge and expertise provided by those who contributed to the first edition of this text. We hope that others caring for individuals with haematological cancers will benefit from this accumulated knowledge and expertise.

Maggie Grundy
Aberdeen 2006

Acknowledgements

Grateful thanks to the many colleagues and friends who have provided help, support, advice, expertise and encouragement and in doing so have contributed, in their own unique ways, to the publication of this book. Especial thanks to those authors who contributed to the first edition and in doing so provided such an excellent foundation for this second edition.

SECTION 1

The diseases

Chapter **1**

Haematopoiesis

Breege Traynor

KEY POINTS

- Although disseminated throughout many skeletal cavities, the bone marrow acts as a single organ system as a result of stem cell migration via the peripheral blood.
- Haematopoiesis – blood cell production – is a diverse and productive process.
- The bone marrow gives rise to all the cells that an individual requires for an intact immune system, coagulation and oxygenation.
- Haematopoiesis is a hierarchical system and pluripotent stem cells are the origin of all mature myeloid and lymphoid cells.
- The framework on which haematopoietic cells grow is the stromal layer, comprised of endothelial cells, macrophages, fibroblasts, adventitial reticular cells, adipocytes and T cells.

INTRODUCTION

The bone marrow is a complex and sophisticated organ and haematopoiesis – blood cell production – is a diverse and productive process. The marrow gives rise to all the cells that an individual requires for an intact immune system, coagulation and oxygenation. Haematopoiesis is controlled by a set of autocrine and paracrine loops. A series of progenitor cells and a complex array of haematopoietic growth factors, cytokines and chemokines maintain haematopoiesis and allow a measured production of cells under 'steady-state' conditions. Furthermore, increasing understanding of cytogenetics and the regulatory mechanisms that control blood cell production is helping to piece together both normal and abnormal haematopoiesis (Janowska-Wieczorek et al 2001). This chapter describes how myeloid and lymphoid cells are formed, how haematopoiesis is positively and negatively controlled, and highlights some of the known genetic aberrations that may contribute to myelo- or lymphoproliferative disorders.

HAEMATOPOIESIS

Blood is a fluid tissue that constitutes approximately 7% of adult body weight (Abboud & Lichtman 2001). Total volume is around 5.5 litres in adult humans and some 2.5 litres of blood cells – erythrocytes, leucocytes, platelets – circulate in 3 litres of protein-rich plasma. One of the largest organs of the body, blood supports the activities of all other tissues and provides nutrients, oxygen, hormones, cleansing of waste and body defence.

Blood cells each have varying specialised functions and a finite lifespan. The number of circulating cells is maintained within extremely narrow limits and cells are replaced at a rate equal to their loss. Erythrocytes are subjected to mechanical and oxidant stress, leucocytes are destroyed during the process of dealing with microorganisms, and platelets are consumed during coagulation. As a result, some 5×10^{11} myeloid cells need to be manufactured daily to account only for cells lost through the normal ageing process (Molineux & Dexter 1998). In times of need, however, erythropoiesis can be increased 20–30-fold, granulopoiesis at least 20-fold and thrombopoiesis at least 3-fold (Emerson et al 2000).

FETAL HAEMATOPOIESIS

Fetal haematopoiesis, in particular erythropoiesis, begins extra-embryonically in the walls of the yolk sac after the second week of gestation. Leucopoiesis and thrombopoiesis commence at approximately 6 weeks' gestation. After approximately 12 weeks the yolk sac ceases to produce blood cells and the liver becomes the major site of blood cell production until the 24th week of gestation, feeding fetal bone marrow stroma with stem cells (Segel & Palis 2001, Marshall & Thrasher 2001). Cavities within bone appear around the fifth month of gestation and the marrow becomes the exclusive site of granulopoiesis and thrombopoiesis from week 24 onwards. Hepatic haematopoiesis gradually wanes until only a small amount of erythropoiesis (~10%) remains (Abboud & Lichtman 2001).

BONE MARROW

At birth haematopoietic cells occupy all the bone marrow space – a volume so large that it is nearly equivalent to the marrow space occupied by haematopoietic cells in adults. By the fourth year of childhood yellow, fatty marrow begins to replace the haematopoietic elements in bone marrow until red marrow is confined to the pelvis, sternum, ribs, vertebrae, cranium and the proximal epiphyses of the femora and humeri by age 18 (Abboud & Lichtman 2001). However, the absolute amount of haematopoietic tissue is constant in both adult and child (Babior & Stossel 1994) and, if the need for haematopoiesis increases, marrow throughout the body can become reactivated. The amount of active bone marrow amounts to about 2600 g, representing approximately 5% of total adult body weight and producing approximately 6 billion cells per kilogram of body weight per day (Fliedner 1998, Abboud & Lichtman 2001). The marrow is perfused with blood every 6 minutes and 5% of the cardiac output circulates directly there. This ensures an adequate supply of nutrients and oxygen and the removal of mitotic metabolites (Emerson et al 2000). Although disseminated throughout many skeletal cavities, the bone marrow acts as a single organ system as a result of stem cell migration via the peripheral blood (Fliedner 1998).

STEM CELLS

A stem cell is defined as: 'a single cell [with the ability] to repopulate long-term hematopoiesis in the whole animal'

(Quesenberry & Colvin 2001)

Haematopoietic tissue can be broadly divided into three cell populations: stem cells, committed progenitor cells and maturing/mature cells. Stem cells comprise approximately 4% of the total number of haematopoietic cells, while committed progenitors account for 3% and maturing cells for 95%. Haematopoiesis is a largely hierarchical system and pluripotent stem cells are the origin of all mature myeloid and lymphoid cells. These stem cells are ultimately responsible for the maintenance of haematopoiesis, although their number relative to the total marrow cellularity is very small; they represent only about 1 in 100,000 bone marrow mononuclear cells (Kvalheim & Smeland 1998) and cannot be identified morphologically. The process of differentiation from immature haematopoietic stem cells to the various haematopoietic lineages is defined by the patterns of surface antigens expressed (Yasui et al 2003). Attempts to measure numbers of stem cells have focused on measuring a membrane glycoprotein – Cluster of Differentiation 34 or CD34. CD34$^+$ expression is highest in early progenitors and progressively reduces with maturation. Using monoclonal anti-CD34$^+$ antibodies, CD34$^+$ cells can be identified using cytofluorimetric analysis. More recently, research has indicated that a different marker – AC133 – may also be a useful candidate for isolation of a more primitive haematopoietic stem cell (Yasui et al 2003).

The characteristics that define a haematopoietic stem cell are (Bianco et al 2001, Summers et al 2001):

- self-renewal
- extensive proliferative capacity
- ability to sustain long-term lymphomyeloid haematopoiesis.

Self-replication is necessary to maintain the stem cell pool and extensive proliferation and differentiation give rise to the wide variety of blood cells that the body requires. The regulation of the balance between self-renewal and lineage commitment is an issue central to the understanding of haematopoiesis (Molineux & Dexter 1998).

For all practical purposes stem cells can be considered 'immortal' and they give rise to multiple lines of progeny in an ordered, structured manner. The pluripotent stem cell gives rise to the myeloid stem cell, the Colony-Forming Unit-Granulocyte, Erythrocyte, Monocyte, Megakaryocyte (CFU-GEMM) or to the lymphoid stem cell. Further differentiation produces a variety of progenitor cells, each committed to a single cell pathway. The exception to this rule is in the case of neutrophils and monocytes which share a progenitor cell – the Colony-Forming Unit-Granulocyte, Monocyte (CFU-GM) (Fig. 1.1).

Committed progenitor cells have less capacity for self-replication but are normally in a state of cell division. They are primarily responsible for the generation of mature cells and their mitotic rate reflects the balance between replication, differentiation and cell death. True stem cells are proliferatively quiescent and reside in the G_0/G_1 phase of the cell cycle (Summers et al 2001) (see Chapter 9). In the clinical situation, for example after myelotoxic chemo- or radiotherapy, stem cells are ultimately responsible for regenerating long-term haematopoiesis while the developmentally restricted progenitor cells facilitate short-term recovery (Fig. 1.2) (Dexter 1990, Chan & Watt 2001, Quesenberry & Colvin 2001). Greater maturity leads to a loss of self-replication ability.

Figure 1.1
Haematopoietic stem cells.

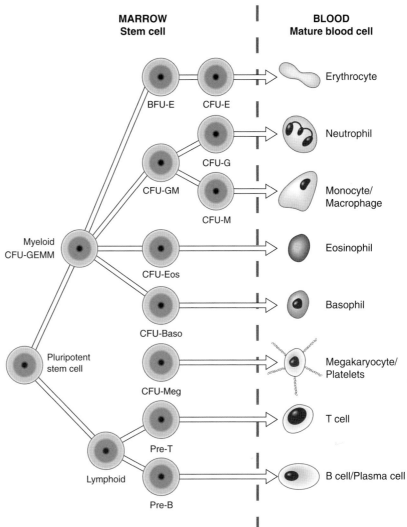

Key:
CFU-GEMM: colony-forming unit-granulocyte, erythrocyte, monocyte, megakaryocyte
BFU-E: burst-forming unit-erythroid
CFU-GM: colony-forming unit-granulocyte, monocyte
CFU-Eos: colony-forming unit-eosinophil
CFU-Baso: colony-forming unit-basophil
CFU-Meg: colony-forming unit-megakaryocyte
Pre-T: pre-T cell
Pre-B: pre-B cell
CFU-E: colony-forming unit-erythroid
CFU-G: colony-forming unit-granulocyte
CFU-M: colony-forming unit-monocyte

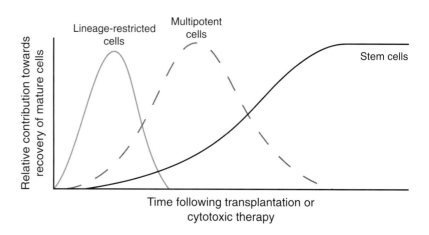

Figure 1.2
Relative contribution of progenitor cells towards the recovery of mature blood cells (reproduced with the kind permission of Professor T. M. Dexter).

BONE MARROW MICROENVIRONMENT

STROMAL LAYER

The bone marrow has cells from two lineages – haematopoietic tissue and the supporting stromal layer. Recent research has indicated that marrow stromal cells are progenitors of skeletal tissue components such as bone, cartilage, the haematopoietic-supporting stroma and adipocytes. Thus, in addition to supporting blood cell development, the stromal layer may also be of interest as a source of post-natal non-haematopoietic stem cells for therapeutic use (Bianco et al 2001). In humans the stromal matrix becomes established in the clavicle from 6 to 8 weeks' gestation and stem cells migrate to the developing marrow spaces to seed blood cell development, reaching a peak at weeks 16–18, when all marrow spaces are available for seeding (Fliedner 1998).

Blood cells develop in niches and the bone marrow is a rich mixture of all types of cells at all stages of development (Chan & Watt 2001). Each lineage occupies a specific marrow location. Megakaryocytes develop next to the venous sinus with their cytoplasmic projections extending directly into the lumen. Budding platelets form at the tips of the projections and are 'washed away' into the circulation. Red cell precursors lie adjacent to the venous sinus in erythroblastic islands and each is associated with a macrophage. Granulocyte and monocyte precursors lie deeper within the medullary cavity but become motile as they mature and are able to migrate towards the venous sinus to be released into the circulation (Pallister 1994).

The framework on which haematopoietic cells grow is the stromal layer. The layer is comprised of endothelial cells, macrophages, fibroblasts, adventitial reticular cells, adipocytes and T cells (Taichman &

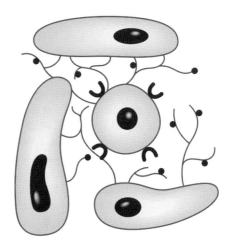

Figure 1.3
Stromal layer. Stromal cells provide a specialised adhesive microenvironment in which endogenous growth factors are presented to developing stem cells.

Emerson 1998, Chan & Watt 2001). It provides a structural scaffolding for haematopoiesis and induces locally the generation of a complex mesenchymal tissue, including vessels and bone, that is required to support cell development (Bianco et al 2001, Dennis & Charbord 2002). Close physical contact between the stem cell and the bone marrow stromal layer is required in order for haematopoietic stem cells to proliferate (Kronenwett et al 2000).

Stromal cells provide a specialised adhesive microenvironment in which stem and progenitor cells are embedded (Fig. 1.3) and the survival, quiescence, proliferation, commitment, differentiation, migration and death of stem cells and their progeny are controlled by external cues provided by this microenvironment (Chan & Watt 2001). This control is exerted via a specific set of molecules that determine or regulate the fate of stem cells.

INTRINSIC HAEMATOPOIETIC GROWTH FACTORS

Intricate cytokine interactions are employed in haematopoietic cell growth, differentiation and maturation (Chan & Watt 2001). Several growth factors, cytokines and chemokines are expressed and secreted by both early and differentiated human haematopoietic cells and thus may regulate haematopoiesis in an autocrine/paracrine manner. Janowska-Wieczorek et al (2001) have identified eight possible sources of autocrine or paracrine growth factors that control haematopoiesis:

- stromal fibroblasts
- endothelium
- cytokines derived from other organs – liver, kidney – arriving via the bloodstream
- accessory cells
- differentiating haematopoietic cells
- osteoblasts

- early haematopoietic cells
- interactions between haematopoietic cells and adhesion receptors.

Therefore 'crosstalk' between haematopoietic cells and their environment is evident in normal human haematopoiesis (Janowska-Wieczorek et al 2001) and, as molecular biology advances and understanding of protein signalling continues, additional regulators are becoming elucidated (Heath et al 2004).

Studies in the 1960s demonstrated that the production of colonies of mature blood cells in vitro rested absolutely with the availability of haematopoietic growth factors. Growth factors are a family of glycoproteins that play a pivotal, but complex, role in controlling haematopoiesis and overlapping combinations regulate the growth and differentiation of progenitor cells.

The factors that determine whether pluripotent stem cells differentiate or self-replicate still remain relatively unclear but stem cell factor, the ligand for the c-kit tyrosine kinase receptor (also known as steel factor, kit ligand, or mast cell growth factor), is one of the proteins involved (Antonchuk et al 2004). Administration of stem cell factor appears to stimulate expansion of the most primitive haematopoietic subsets and to mobilise clonogenic progenitor cells into the circulation (Demetri & Anderson 2000). Regulation of the later stages of mature cell development is better understood with factors such as granulocyte-colony stimulating factor, erythropoietin, and thrombopoietin stimulating more mature, committed precursor cells: neutrophils, erythrocytes, and platelets respectively (Molineux & Dexter 1998, Beutler 2001, Kuter et al 2001). Growth factors exert their cellular activities by attaching themselves to distinct high-affinity receptor sites (Crawford & Lee 2000, Ghalie & Tallman 2000). Receptor expression is generally (but not exclusively) restricted to the particular cell lineage. As a growth factor binds to its receptor it becomes internalised, triggering the expression of cellular genes. This initiates cell cycling and shortens the G_1 stage of the cell cycle (for further detail of the cell cycle see Chapter 9). The production of mature cells and the time required for that production are both influenced by the concentration of growth factor available to the dividing progenitor (Metcalf 1990).

STEM CELL CIRCULATION

Haematopoietic stem cells are present in bone marrow, umbilical cord blood and mobilised peripheral blood (Summers et al 2001). While the normal stem cell 'home' may be the marrow space, small numbers (<0.1% of all nucleated cells) can be found in the peripheral blood where they circulate in the mononuclear cell fraction (Cutler & Antin 2001). In normal individuals steady-state peripheral blood contains between several hundred and several thousand stem cells per millilitre.

In fetal life this balance is dramatically different. There is a very high concentration of stem cells in embryonic blood (>65,000 Colony forming unit-culture (CFU-C) per mL in weeks 16–18) as haematopoietic and lymphopoietic tissue are established (Fliedner 1998). The stem cells seen in the neonate seem to be the tail-end of this dramatic stem cell mobility and studies have demonstrated that cord blood stem cells in the G_0 and G_1 phases of the cell cycle can be expanded ex vivo, with potential applications for autologous or allogeneic transplantation or gene therapy (Summers et al 2001). Stem cell movement continues throughout life and allows the bone marrow to act as one unique organ system, although distributed through many bones of the skeleton. As with cord blood cells, bone marrow stem cells capable of long-term repopulation of the marrow are mainly in the G_0/G_1 phases of the cell cycle rather than S/G_2 or M phases (Summers et al 2001). It is due to stem cell migration via the peripheral blood that all active bone marrow sites can maintain a sufficient population of stem cells (Fliedner 1998). Circulating progenitors form part of haematopoietic cell renewal systems and depleted bone marrow sites are repopulated by endogenous stem cell seeding. Thus circulation of stem cells can be considered as an ongoing, natural process that is used day-to-day to ensure haematopoietic functional integrity (Fliedner 1998).

Recognition of this natural phenomenon has led to developments in transplant medicine with mobilisation and collection of peripheral blood stem cells (see Chapter 13). In transplantation, the kinetics of haematopoietic recovery have been shown to be dependent on the source and quantity of CD34$^+$ cells reinfused, with faster recovery following infusion of mobilised peripheral blood stem cells (Pecora 2000). Administration of colony stimulating factors has been demonstrated to increase the concentration of CD34$^+$ cells from $3.8 \pm 0.8 \times 10^3$ to $61.9 \pm 11.3 \times 10^3$/mL blood. A leucopheresis is then capable of collecting 5×10^8 CD34$^+$cells, which is about 26 times the number of cells normally found and sufficient for transplantation (Fliedner 1998). The threshold of stem cells required for successful transplantation is thought to be 2.5–5.0×10^6 cells/kg body weight (Kronenwett et al 2000, Vogel et al 2000). Further, positive selection of CD34$^+$ cells prior to transplantation may have additional benefits to patients because of tumour cell purging and lymphocyte depletion (Vogel et al 2000).

Following mobilisation, there is a selective release of stem cells from the marrow into the blood but such a perturbance is temporary and the system returns to normal within a few days. Collection of stem cells for transplantation thus relies on making best use of this window of opportunity after mobilisation. Adhesive interactions between stem cells and the stromal layer play a central role in migration, circulation and proliferation of stem cells and circulation of stem cells may be related to the expression level of adhesion molecules (Kronenwett et al 2000).

MATURE BLOOD CELLS

MEGAKARYOCYTES/PLATELETS

The marrow precursor for platelets is the Colony-Forming Unit-Megakaryocyte (CFU-Meg). From this cell thrombopoiesis proceeds to

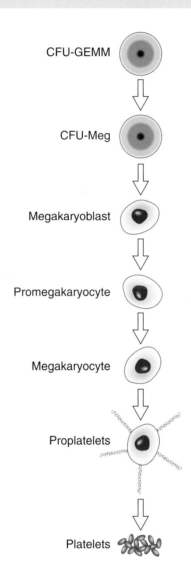

Figure 1.4
Thrombopoiesis.

give rise to the megakaryoblast, a cell that is difficult to detect morphologically but which can be detected by staining. The megakaryoblast gives rise to the megakaryocyte, a large distinctive cell and the source of platelets (Fig. 1.4). Each megakaryocyte can produce between 1000 and 3000 platelets. Platelets are disc-shaped enucleated fragments which survive approximately 7–10 days in the peripheral circulation and account for less than 1% of the total blood volume. Approximately one-third of the platelet population is concentrated in the spleen, which acts as a reservoir pool (Kuter 1997).

The production of megakaryocytes and platelets is regulated by the amount of thrombopoietin in the circulation. Thrombopoietin is produced at a constant rate by liver parenchymal cells and its level is determined primarily by the rate of clearance by platelets as there does not appear to be a sensor of platelet mass (Kaser et al 2001). Upon binding to the thrombopoietin receptor – C-Mpl – thrombopoietin increases the growth of early marrow precursors of all lineages but only stimulates the maturation of late precursors in the megakaryocyte line, thereby increasing platelet production (Wagemaker et al 1998, Kuter 2001). Thrombopoietin is not an absolute requirement for thrombopoiesis and is not required for the shedding of platelets from megakaryocytes. The role of thrombopoietin is to amplify differentiated megakaryocytes from the CFU-Meg to the mature megakaryocyte (Kuter 1997).

The usual platelet count is $150–400 \times 10^9/L$. There is a wide variation in platelet counts between individuals although, within an individual, the platelet count is stable unless altered by disease (Kuter 2001). There is no diurnal variation in platelets and only modest changes occur with menstruation (Kuter 1997). Platelets are essential in preventing haemorrhage by adhering to injured blood vessel walls and aggregating to form a platelet plug. They form an integral part of haemostasis by maintaining the competence of the vascular endothelium. In cases of thrombocytopenia, fine blood vessels lose their competence, leading to haemorrhage.

ERYTHROCYTES

Erythrocytes account for approximately 45% of total blood volume and their function is oxygen/carbon dioxide exchange. This exchange is made possible by the presence of haemoglobin and the biconcave shape of the erythrocyte, increasing O_2/CO_2 efficiency by making the interior of the cell more accessible. Red blood cells, like platelets, function entirely within the bloodstream and normally live for around 120 days.

Erythropoiesis (Fig. 1.5) is stimulated in response to the degree of oxygen perfusion. When blood oxygenation decreases, the level of erythropoietin in plasma rises, accelerating the commitment of erythroid precursor cells into erythroid development. The first identifiable erythroid progenitor cell is the Burst-Forming Unit-Erythroid (BFU-E), which expresses $CD34^+$ and has receptors for a number of growth factors and cytokines. From BFU-E, the Colony-Forming Unit-Erythroid (CFU-E) develops. CFU-E cells express numerous erythropoietin receptors and in the absence of erythropoietin, CFU-E cells undergo apoptosis (Beutler 2001). Adherence of erythropoietin to its receptor is essential for transformation to the pronormoblast where the cell develops increasing amounts of haemoglobin. As further differentiation into the normoblast takes place, the nucleus is lost and the cell reaches the reticulocyte stage. Reticulocytes remain in the bone marrow for about 2 days as they accumulate haemoglobin and lose some of their ribonucleic acid (RNA). They subsequently enter the circulation where, after a further day, any

Figure 1.5
Erythropoiesis.

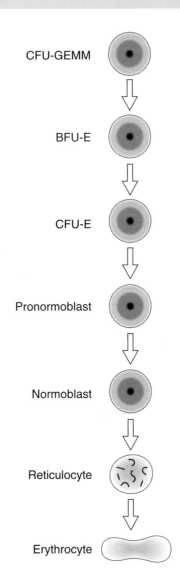

CFU-GEMM

BFU-E

CFU-E

Pronormoblast

Normoblast

Reticulocyte

Erythrocyte

Key:
CFU-GEMM: colony-forming unit-granulocyte,
erythrocyte, monocyte, megakaryocyte
BFU-E: burst-forming unit-erythroid
CFU-E: colony-forming unit-erythroid

residual RNA is lost and they become adult erythrocytes. The transit time from the pronormoblast to the reticulocyte entering the peripheral blood is approximately 5 days. Increased numbers of circulating reticulocytes are indicative of increased erythropoiesis and conversely reticulocytopenia is indicative of red cell aplasia. After red cells age, they are destroyed by macrophages in the liver, spleen and marrow (Beutler 2001).

Table 1.1
Leucocytes

	Classification	$\times 10^9$/L	% Total WBC
Neutrophil	Granulocytes	2.5–7.5	40–75%
Eosinophil		0.015–0.1	1–6%
Basophil		0.04–0.44	<1%
Monocyte	Mononuclear cells	0.2–0.8	2–10%
Lymphocyte		1.5–3.5	20–50%

LEUCOCYTES

The primary function of the white blood system is host defence. Leuco-cytes function extravascularly and the blood vessels merely serve as avenues that a white cell uses to get from one place to another. Within the leucocyte family are subpopulations of cells, each of which has a distinct but related function (Table 1.1).

Neutrophils

Neutrophils develop from the CFU-GM – a common committed pro-genitor cell that they share with the monocyte line (Fig. 1.6). Derived from the CFU-GEMM, the CFU-GM gives rise to the Colony-Forming Unit-Granulocyte (CFU-G) and the Colony-Forming Unit-Monocyte (CFU-M), granulocyte and monocyte progenitor cells respectively. The myeloblast is the earliest recognisable granulocyte precursor. It is a large cell with a high ratio of nucleus to cytoplasm. Over a series of cell divi-sions from promyelocyte, to myelocyte, to metamyelocyte, the cytoplasm is lost, the nucleus attenuates and the neutrophilic granules develop. The metamyelocyte and band neutrophil (with a kidney-shaped nucleus) are non-proliferating cells that precede the development of the mature neu-trophil (Bainton 2001). These latter stages represent the maturation-storage compartment of neutrophil production (Babior & Golde 2001). The nucleus of the mature circulating neutrophil is segmented into 2–4 lobes that are joined by a thin chromatin strand. This segmentation is indicative of a fully mature cell but the purpose of nuclear segmentation is unknown (Bainton 2001). The myelocyte to blood transit time is 5–7 days but during infections this may decrease to approximately 48 hours (Babior & Golde 2001).

Neutrophils have a limited lifespan and thus put a continuous replace-ment demand on the marrow. The normal human neutrophil production rate is $0.85–1.6 \times 10^9$ cells/kg/day (Babior & Golde 2001). The marrow holds approximately 11 days' supply of banded and segmented neu-trophils in a large storage pool to ensure that a reserve of cells is avail-able and release of neutrophils from the marrow is a function of their rate of loss from the blood.

Granulocytes spend their lives in three environments – marrow, blood and tissues (Bainton 2001). On entering the blood, neutrophils divide equally into circulating and marginated pools. This maintains a further reserve of neutrophils ready to migrate into the tissues in

Figure 1.6
Neutrophil and monocyte
development.

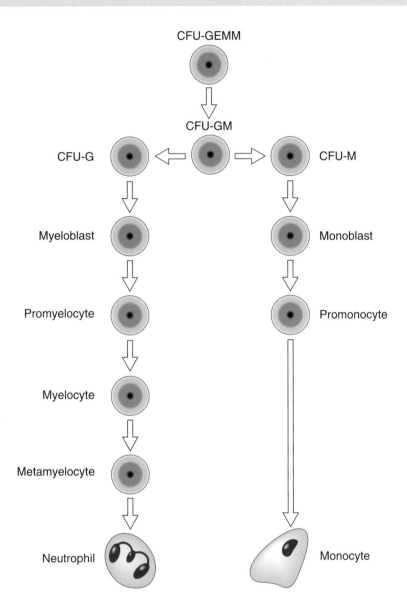

Key:
CFU-GEMM: colony-forming unit-granulocyte, erythrocyte,
monocyte, megakaryocyte
CFU-GM: colony-forming unit-granulocyte, monocyte
CFU-G: colony-forming unit-granulocyte
CFU-M: colony-forming unit-monocyte

response to infection or inflammation. Neutrophils can move from the marginated to the circulating pool in response to exercise, epinephrine injections and stress. The mature neutrophil circulates for approximately 7–10 hours before entering the tissues where it may survive for another 2 days. However, this flow is unidirectional – once they have entered the tissues, neutrophils do not reappear in the blood (Babior & Golde 2001).

Neutrophils are small, highly phagocytic, granulocytes that play a vital role in host defence mechanisms. They become motile in response to a variety of chemotactic factors derived from bacteria, damaged tissues and the C5, C6 and C7 parts of complement (see later section on immunity). Chemotaxis helps them to locate and move towards a site of infection. Following phagocytosis, neutrophils degranulate and hydrogen peroxide is produced by glucose oxidation, playing an important part in bacterial killing.

Steroids can increase neutrophil counts by increasing the inflow of neutrophils and decreasing the rate of egress from the circulation. Endotoxin causes neutropenia as a result of margination and sequestration, followed by neutrophilia as the marrow responds (Babior & Golde 2001).

Eosinophils

Eosinophils descend from the eosinophil committed progenitor cell, the Colony-Forming Unit – Eosinophil (CFU-Eos), which matures into the first recognisable cell – the eosinophilic myeloblast. This differentiates into the eosinophilic promyelocyte and from there through the stages of myelocyte and metamyelocyte, finally becoming a mature cell. Eosinophils are distinguishable morphologically by their large cytoplasmic granules that stain reddish-orange. Once released into the blood less than 1% of eosinophils circulate. Approximately half are marginated and the remainder migrate to areas exposed to the external environment:

- skin epithelium
- bronchial mucosa
- gastrointestinal tract
- vaginal and uterine walls
- lactating mammary gland.

Eosinophils are primarily tissue-dwelling cells and their lifespan in the tissues is approximately 12 days (Wardlaw & Kay 2001).

Eosinophils have a variety of roles. They participate in modulating and regulating the inflammatory response. By degranulation they release factors that degrade the vasoactive amines released by basophils and mast cells. They can neutralise histamine and hydroxytryptamine. Eosinophils play an important role in defending against parasitic infections and are able to phagocytose, although their ability to do so is much less than that of neutrophils or macrophages (Kircher & Marquardt 2002). Eosinophils can cause severe tissue damage in some situations and the observation that eosinophil proteins are toxic to airway epithelium has led to the consensus that eosinophils are a major contributor to tissue damage in asthma (Wardlaw & Kay 2001, Kircher & Marquardt 2002).

Eosinophils have a diurnal variation. They are highest at night during sleep, lowest in the morning and begin to rise again by mid-afternoon. Eosinophil counts also vary with age, exercise, and environmental stimuli, particularly allergen exposure.

Basophils

Basophils, the least common of the granulocytes, descend from the committed progenitor cell Colony Forming Unit – Basophil (CFU-Baso). This matures into the first recognisable cell – the basophilic myeloblast. Further differentiation leads to the basophilic promyelocyte, the myelocyte, the metamyelocyte and finally to a mature cell. Basophils are distinguishable morphologically by their large blue cytoplasmic granules.

Basophils synthesise and store histamine as well as a heparin-like substance and differ from other granulocytes in that they have no ability to phagocytose. Basophil degranulation is stimulated primarily by the binding of IgE to the basophil cell surface. This may be localised to the skin or lungs (as in asthma) or it may be widespread and severe as in anaphylactic shock (Galli et al 2001).

Basophils have a lifespan of a few days in the circulation and can be recruited into the tissues during immune or inflammatory responses. Basophils are found in small numbers in blood (0.5%) and can be found in tissues in situations of inflammation, for example, hypersensitivity, contact allergy or skin allograft rejection (Bainton 2001).

MONOCYTES/MACROPHAGES

Monocytes/macrophages also arise from the CFU-GM (Fig. 1.6), which gives rise to the Colony-Forming Unit-Monocyte (CFU-M) – the monocyte precursor cell. The first recognisable cell in the bone marrow is the monoblast. This differentiates into the promonocyte and finally to the monocyte. Monocytes account for 2–10% of leucocyte numbers and $0.2–0.8 \times 10^9$/L cells in peripheral blood. They are the largest circulatory cells and have a blood transit time of some 14 hours.

Monocytes, however, are still immature cells and mature further in the tissues to become macrophages (Kircher & Marquardt 2002). Macrophages are long-lived phagocytic cells that have some capacity for cell division. Thus the macrophage, like the lymphocyte, may be able to act as its own stem cell. Macrophages may be wandering or fixed in strategic locations:

- lungs   alveolar macrophages
- liver   Kupffer cells
- kidneys   glomerulus mesangial cells
- brain   microglia
- bone   osteoclasts
- spleen   sinusoids
- lymph nodes   medullary sinuses.

Macrophages provide nonspecific immune defence and play a crucial role in initiating and regulating the immune response. Macrophages trap and concentrate antigens ready for presentation to T lymphocytes in association with Class I major histocompatibility complex (MHC) molecules and they trap antigen–antibody complexes to stimulate B cell memory. They can also secrete an array of powerful chemical substances – monokines – including interferon and interleukin-1 (Kircher & Marquardt 2002).

DOWN-REGULATION OF HAEMATOPOIESIS

It would be logical to maintain a population of stem cells in a quiescent state during normal haematopoiesis to preserve resources and prevent marrow 'wear out'. Thus both positive and negative regulatory factors are required to maintain haemostasis. While the positive stimulation of growth factor proteins has been widely evaluated, Quesenberry & Colvin (2001) suggest a number of factors that may help to down-regulate haematopoiesis. These include:

- macrophage inflammatory protein-1 α (MIP-1α)
- transforming growth factor-β (TGF-β)
- tumour necrosis factor-α (TNF-α)
- activin
- inhibin
- interferon – alpha, beta and gamma
- prostaglandin E
- leukaemia inhibitory factor.

MIP-1α reversibly inhibits the cell cycling of early progenitor cell populations either by blocking entry of the stem cell into S phase of the cell cycle, removing cells from S phase, or both, resulting in inhibition of early multipotent colony formation. TGF-β has also been shown to inhibit early stem cells (Molineux & Dexter 1998, Quesenberry & Colvin 2001). Negative regulatory factors maintain haematopoiesis at a constant size by inhibiting cells from undergoing mitosis and by preventing stem cell loss through apoptosis (programmed cell death and fragmentation). In times of stress, perhaps in addition to the increases in positive growth factors (e.g. G-CSF), a decrease in negative growth factors would allow quiescent stem cells to enter the cycling pool and thus be recruited for a needed haematological response (Testa et al 1993).

IMMUNITY

The immune system is the body's defence mechanism and has several major functions (Kircher & Marquardt 2002):

- distinguish self from non-self
- protect the organism from exogenous factors such as microorganisms or toxins

- prevent attack by endogenous factors such as tumours or autoimmune phenomena (immune surveillance).

Immune mechanisms can be grouped into acquired and innate. Acquired immunity usually requires prior exposure to a particular stimulus. For example, a vast range of antibodies can be made against a specific antigen and memory B cells retain the ability to manufacture these same antibodies again should a future need arise.

Innate mechanisms are those that are present from birth. The fetus is capable of synthesising IgM antibody by 10.5 weeks' gestation, and IgG and IgA by weeks 12 and 30, respectively, although neonatal IgG is also derived from maternal transfer across the placenta. Monocytes first appear in spleen and lymph nodes at 4–5 months' gestation, with gradual maturation of macrophage function with advancing fetal age. Synthesis of complement components also appears early around the time of immunoglobulin synthesis (Kircher & Marquardt 2002). Additional innate mechanisms include physical barriers such as the skin and mucous membranes and chemical barriers such as the body secretions, e.g. gastric acid, saliva, proteolytic enzymes, etc. (Pallister 1994). Paradoxically too, the colonisation of the body by commensal organisms forms part of the body's intrinsic immunity, helping to protect against colonisation by more virulent pathogens. Indeed, despite the complexity and versatility of the immune system, host defence is still highly dependent on such barriers.

MAJOR HISTOCOMPATIBILITY COMPLEX/HUMAN LEUCOCYTE ANTIGEN SYSTEM

At the core of the immune system is the ability to distinguish between 'self' and 'non-self' and the mechanisms that control immunity are complex. Immune responses involve interactions between macrophages and lymphocytes, based on specific recognition of foreign antigens. This means that the cells involved in immunity must be able to recognise not only foreign antigens but also each other. This recognition process centres around the products of the major histocompatibility complex (MHC). The MHC directs the synthesis of three different types of protein – MHC classes I, II and III. MHC III proteins are complement components while the proteins of MHC classes I and II are designated as human leucocyte antigens (HLA) (Kircher & Marquardt 2002). Class I antigens (HLA-A, HLA-B and HLA-C) are expressed on the surface membrane of all nucleated cells of the body and hence the term human leucocyte antigen is not strictly speaking correct. Class II antigens (HLA-D, HLA-Dr, HLA-Dp and HLA-Dq) are restricted to cells of the immune system and are thus expressed only on monocytes, macrophages, B cells and, under certain circumstances, activated T cells.

The immune system can deal with foreign antigens effectively and efficiently if they are presented in close association with an appropriate MHC molecule and the function of both class I and II MHC molecules is to present antigen to T cells, thus initiating the immune response. Class I molecules regulate interactions between CD8[+] cells and target cells and class II molecules regulate interactions between CD4[+] cells and antigen-presenting cells (Smyth et al 2001, Kircher & Marquardt 2002, Maher & Davies 2004). Cytotoxic T cells recognise antigen in association with class I MHC molecules and have the potential to respond to any infected host cell (Kircher & Marquardt 2002, Maher & Davies 2004, Papamichail et al 2004).

The HLA/MHC system is important in marrow, stem cell and tissue transplantation and in transfusions of platelets and white cells. The major histocompatibility complex is controlled by genes on a region of chromosome 6. Each individual derives three genes from each parent and thus carries a total of six MHC antigens, a pair from each of HLA-A, HLA-B and HLA-C. These vary widely from one individual to the next, with the exception of identical twins, and this diversity will result in tissue rejection unless an 'identical' donor can be found.

The ABO blood group system is another major histocompatibility complex that must be matched (see Chapter 12). Red cells carry ABO antigens but not HLA antigens. Neutrophils carry HLA antigens and a neutrophil-specific antigen, while platelets carry HLA antigens and a platelet-specific antigen.

THE COMPLEMENT CASCADE

The complement system is a family of plasma proteins that plays an important part in the inflammatory response and microbial killing. Complement proteins (C1–C9) are sequentially activated by the presence of specific antigens in the body and the formation of antigen–antibody complexes. Three groups of complement proteins are involved in:

- antigen recognition – C1 and its subunits
- immune activation – C2–C4
- cell membrane lysis – C5–C9.

Complement can also be stimulated by a variety of substances present in microbial infection, e.g. bacterial endotoxin. C5a, a fragment of C5 is the most potent chemotactic factor for neutrophils and can also act as an anaphylotoxin, stimulating the release of histamine from tissue mast cells in anaphylaxis (Kircher & Marquardt 2002).

LYMPHOCYTES

Cells of the lymphoid system start life in the bone marrow and are derived from the lymphoid stem cell. Like the CFU-GEMM, the lymphoid stem cell is multipotent. It can either self-replicate or differentiate to produce B or T lymphocytes. Lymphoid cells, unlike myeloid cells, do not necessarily follow a unidirectional development flow from mitotic stem cell to mature cell. They can oscillate between mitotic forms and dormant memory cells capable of recruitment into a mitotic pool on demand. Lymphocytes also migrate back and forth between the blood, lymphatic system and tissues seeking out antigen (Maher & Davies 2004).

Shortly after birth lymphocytes number approximately $3.5–8.5 \times 10^9/L$ while by the end of the first week of life they have increased to about $12 \times 10^9/L$. The normal adult range of $1.5–3.5 \times 10^9/L$ is reached by about the age of 12 years. It is not possible to distinguish between B and T lymphocytes based on morphological characteristics only. Distinction between the two relies on cell membrane markers and gene rearrangements (Kircher & Marquardt 2002). Full blood counts therefore generally report a total lymphocyte count as part of a white cell differential. Lymphocytes display a diurnal variation. They are lowest at 9 am and highest at 9 pm, which is the inverse of the plasma cortisol concentration.

T lymphocytes

T lymphocytes originate in the bone marrow from the PRE-T progenitor cell but migrate to the thymus gland where they are processed by thymosin and become immunologically competent. Cells pass through the developmental phases of prothymocyte and T lymphoblast into mature T cell. T lymphocytes make up approximately 70–80% of the circulating lymphocyte population and can migrate rapidly in response to stimuli. They are responsible for cellular immunity, including resistance against intracellular organisms which evade humoral immunity (Kircher & Marquardt 2002).

There are several subpopulations of T cell. Regulatory T cells orchestrate the immune system to ensure a consistent, coordinated response. Helper T cells assist B lymphocytes to differentiate into plasma cells and to produce IgG immunoglobulin (antibodies). Suppressor T cells turn off the immune system and suppress the responses of other lymphocytes. A number of effector T cells are also present. Cytotoxic T cells rid the body of infected or malignant cells but are also responsible for tissue rejection and organ graft failure. Natural killer (NK) cells are another form of T lymphocyte. They are called 'natural' killer cells because, unlike cytotoxic T cells, they do not need to recognise a specific antigen or MHC molecule before acting (Papamichail et al 2004).

Both cytotoxic T cells and NK cells kill on contact. When a T cell meets an antigen it undergoes blast transformation. Activated T lymphocytes are produced which bind to the target cell and secrete a lethal burst of substances known as cytokines or, more specifically, lymphokines. Lymphokines, such as Interleukin-2, are potent chemicals that can both attract macrophages and have a direct cytotoxic effect by causing cellular lysis (Smyth et al 2001, Papamichail et al 2004).

T cells carry various different glycoproteins on their surface membrane. All mature peripheral-blood T cells express T1 and T3 antigens. Helper T cells (about 65%) express T4. Cytotoxic and suppressor T cells (about 35%) express T8. However, the relationship between the presence of phenotypic markers and functional activities is not so clear-cut. The defining characteristic of the T4 and T8 subpopulations is the nature of the MHC molecule with which they interact. T4 cells recognise antigen in association with class II MHC molecules (HLA-D, HLA-Dr) while T8 cells recognise antigen in association with class I MHC antigen (HLA-A, -B or -C) (Kircher & Marquardt 2002, Maher & Davies 2004).

B lymphocytes

The B cell population is a very heterogeneous pool of clonal cells, each of which displays antigen specificity and can produce only a single antibody. B cells originate in the marrow and, unlike T cells, mature there too. They originate from the PRE-B progenitor cell that passes through the developmental phases of prothymocyte and B lymphoblast into mature B cell. B cells have surface immunoglobulin and complement receptors and are responsible for the mediation of humoral immunity and immune 'memory'. On exposure to foreign antigens they synthesise RNA and differentiate into plasma cells. Plasma cells manufacture and contain antibodies – IgG, IgA, IgM, IgE and IgD – but there is normally only one immunoglobulin in a cell. Antibodies can interact with foreign particles such as toxins or bacteria but are unable to penetrate living cells (Kircher & Marquardt 2002).

B cells make up about 10–20% of circulating lymphocytes and have a lifespan of days to weeks. They too are migratory, which facilitates their meeting with antigens, but some leave the blood to reside in the lymphoid tissues:

- lymph nodes
- spleen
- appendix
- tonsils
- marrow.

GENETICS

Tumour formation involves the accumulation of several cellular mutations that allow a cell to proliferate autonomously (Kalderon 2000) and tumour growth is then a balance between this uncontrolled cellular proliferation and reduced apoptosis (programmed cell death) (Archer et al 2000). The marrow has the most active cell division of any organ and therefore it is predictable that some genetic mutations will occur. Indeed, as progress has been made in understanding the molecular basis of malignant transformation, it has become apparent that cancer has many aspects of a genetic disease, either as an entirely somatic cell gene deregulation or as a specific genetic susceptibility. The latter genetic susceptibility is estimated to occur in approximately 8–10% of patients with cancer (Birindelli et al 2000). While many mutated cells will undergo apoptosis, others will develop into abnormal clones that the immune system may or may not be able to control (Maher & Davies 2004).

Some of the genetic aberrations involve the translocation of chromosomal regions and result in the juxtaposition of genes that would normally be apart. This can activate cellular oncogenes – genes whose activation is associated with the initial and continuing conversion of normal cells to tumour cells – and may provide growth stimulation to the abnormal clone. A growing number of genetic rearrangements are now recognised as associated with marrow diseases (Table 1.2).

The Philadelphia (Ph) chromosome is characteristic of chronic myeloid leukaemia and is seen in more than 90% of cases (see Chapter 4). The Philadelphia chromosome is a translocation between chromosomes 9 and 22. This brings together, on chromosome 22, the breakpoint cluster region (bcr) gene and the cellular proto-oncogene Abelson (c-abl) from chromosome 9. The newly formed bcr/abl gene has tyrosine kinase activity, which leads to an increase in granulopoiesis (Kabarowski & Witte 2000).

C-myc is a proto-oncogene involved in normal cell growth that is expressed continually in cycling cells, increasing as cells enter S phase and expressed at very low levels in G_0 cells. However, its functions also include inhibition of terminal differentiation and apoptosis. Deregulated c-myc is part of a multi-step process of oncogenesis that involves mutations of other proto-oncogenes. C-myc is inappropriately expressed in a wide range of human tumours, including Burkitt's lymphoma (Archer et al 2000).

About 60% of individuals with acute myeloid leukaemia have some form of genetic defect, and some of these are specific for the leukaemia subtype (Table 1.2) (for a fuller explanation of AML subtypes see Chapter 4). Some of the known genetic aberrations associated with myeloid and lymphoid malignancies are outlined in Table 1.2.

The genetics of endogenous growth factors may also be influential. The chromosomal locations of the cytokine genes are clustered in the human genome. The gene for erythropoietin rests on chromosome 7(q11–22) (Coze 1994). The genes for interleukin-3 (IL-3), interleukin-4 (IL-4), interleukin-5 (IL-5), granulocyte-macrophage colony stimulating factor (GM-CSF) and macrophage colony stimulating factor (M-CSF) have all been located on the long arm of chromosome 5 (Ghalie & Tallman 2000) and deletions involving chromosome 5 have been described in various haematopoietic diseases. The granulocyte colony stimulating factor (G-CSF) gene is located on the long arm of chromosome 17(q11.2–21) near the t(15;17) translocation breakpoint which is characteristic of acute promyelocytic leukaemia (Crawford & Lee 2000). However, while growth factor autocrine loops have been described in patients with AML, experiments in transgenic mice expressing IL-3, GM-CSF, and IL-6 have indicated that autocrine/paracrine expression of these factors results in a hyperproliferative state but not acute neoplastic transformation (Janowska-Wieczorek et al 2001).

CONCLUSION

Haematopoiesis is a complex hierarchical system. The immune and blood systems both develop from a single common pluripotent stem cell. This stem cell divides infrequently but gives rise to the myeloid and lymphoid progenitor cells from which mature cells are derived. Endogenous

Table 1.2
Genetic rearrangement in marrow disease

Disease	Genetic mutation	Comments
Chronic myeloproliferative diseases		
Chronic myeloid leukaemia	t(9;22)(q34; q11) BCR/ABL oncogene	Philadelphia chromosome: associated with >90% cases CML.
Acute myeloid leukaemias		
AML with recurrent genetic abnormalities / AML with maturation	t(8;21)(q22; q22) Acute Myeloid Leukaemia (AML) / ETO gene	AML-ETO: associated with ~5–12% cases of AML and ~one-third cases AML with maturation. Usually conveys a favourable outcome.
AML with abnormal bone marrow eosinophils	Inv 16(p13; q22) or t(16;16)(p13;q22)	Inversion of chromosome 16 generally indicates a favourable prognosis. Occurs primarily in younger individuals.
Acute promyelocytic leukaemia	t(15;17)(q22; q21) Promyelocytic Leukaemia – (PML) / Retinoic Acid Receptor Alpha (RARα) gene	PML/RARα: associated with almost 100% cases APM. Used as a tumour-specific marker.
AML with multilineage dysplasia	Monosomy 7 or 5 Trisomy 8, 9 or 11	
B-cell neoplasms		
Precursor B cell lymphoblastic leukaemia/lymphoma	t(1;19)(q23; p13) or t(9;22)(q34;q11) BCR/ABL	
Follicular lymphoma	t(14;18)(q32;q21) B-Cell Leukaemia/lymphoma 2 (BCL2) gene	Associated with 60–80% of follicular lymphomas and ~10% of Hodgkin's lymphomas.
Burkitt's lymphoma	t(8;14)(q24; q32) c-myc oncogene	Located on chromosome 8q24. Observed in almost all cases.
Mantle cell lymphoma (MCL)	t(11;14)(q13; q32) BCL1 gene	Molecular hallmark of MCL. Also found in B-CLL and multiple myeloma.
Diffuse large B-cell lymphoma (LBCL)	t(3; 14)(q27; q32) BCL6 gene	Located on chromosome 3q27. Observed in 50% of LBCL cases and 10% follicular lymphomas.
T-cell neoplasms		
Precursor T-cell lymphoblastic leukaemia/lymphoma	t(1;14)(p32; q11) TAL1 (T-Cell leukaemia) / SCL (stem cell leukaemia haematopoietic transcription factor) gene	Located on chromosome 1p32. Observed in ~25% T-ALL cases.
Anaplastic large cell lymphoma (ALCL)	t(2;5)(p23;q35) Nucleolar phosphoprotein gene-Anaplastic lymphoma kinase (NPM-ALK) gene	NPM – Located on chromosome 5q35 / ALK – Located on chromosome 2p23. Observed in 50–60% of CD30-positive ALCL cases.
T-cell prolymphocytic leukaemia	t(14;14)(q11;q32) Trisomy 8	Seen in ~80% of cases.
Hodgkin's lymphoma		
Hodgkin's lymphoma	t(14;18)(q32;q21) B-Cell Leukaemia/lymphoma 2 (BCL2) gene	Associated with ~10% of Hodgkin's lymphomas.

Information compiled from Birindelli et al 2000, Jaffe et al 2001, Kabarowski & Witte 2000, Douer 2004, Fruchtman 2004, Radich 2004, Winton & Langston 2004.

regulatory factors – both positive and negative – ensure a balanced system that is neither over- nor under-productive. In any cell undergoing multiple mitoses the potential for genetic aberrations exists. A number of these are associated with myeloid and lymphoid disease.

DISCUSSION QUESTIONS

1. What is the importance of stem cell self-regulation in haematopoiesis?

2. What role do growth factors play in haematopoiesis?

3. What is the role of apoptosis in normal and abnormal haematopoiesis?

4. Each of the leucocytes has a distinct function. What are their distinct functions?

5. What is the importance of the HLA system in bone marrow transplantation and blood transfusion?

6. What are the most well-documented genetic abnormalities in haematological cancers?

ACKNOWLEDGEMENT

The author is deeply indebted to Mrs Debbie Lorimer for her original illustrations.

References

Abboud C N, Lichtman M A 2001 Structure of the marrow and the hematopoietic microenvironment. In: Beutler E, Lichtman M A, Coller B S, Kipps T J, Seligsohn U (eds) Williams Hematology, 6th edn. McGraw-Hill, New York, pp 29–58

Antonchuk J, Hyland C D, Hilton D J, Alexander W S 2004 Synergistic effects on erythropoiesis, thrombopoiesis, and stem cell competitiveness in mice deficient in thrombopoietin and steel factor receptors. Blood 104(5):1306–1313

Archer C, Trott P, Dowsett M 2000 Apoptosis pathways. In: Bronchud M H, Foote M, Peters W P, Robinson M O (eds) Principles of molecular oncology. Humana Press, New Jersey, pp 237–255

Babior B M, Golde D W 2001 Production, distribution, and fate of neutrophils. In: Beutler E, Lichtman M A, Coller B S, Kipps T J, Seligsohn U (eds) Williams Hematology, 6th edn. McGraw-Hill, New York, pp 753–759

Babior B M, Stossel T P 1994 Hematology: a pathophysiological approach, 3rd edn. Churchill Livingstone, New York

Bainton DF 2001 Morphology of neutrophils, eosinophils, and basophils. In: Beutler E, Lichtman M A, Coller B S, Kipps T J, Seligsohn U (eds) Williams Hematology, 6th edn. McGraw-Hill, New York, pp 729–743

Bianco P, Riminucci M, Gronthos S, Gehron Robey P 2001 Bone marrow stromal stem cells: nature, biology, and potential applications. Stem Cells 19:180–192

Beutler E 2001 Production and destruction of erythrocytes. In: Beutler E, Lichtman M A, Coller B S, Kipps T J, Seligsohn U (eds) Williams Hematology, 6th edn. McGraw-Hill, New York, pp 355–368

Birindelli S, Aillo A, Lavarino C, Sozzi G, Pilotti S, Pierotti M A 2000 Genetic markers in sporadic tumors. In: Bronchud M H, Foote M, Peters W P, Robinson M O (eds) Principles of molecular oncology. Humana Press, New Jersey, pp 45–93

Chan J Y, Watt S M 2001 Adhesion receptors on haematopoietic progenitor cells. British Journal of Haematology 112:541–557

Coze CM 1994 Glossary of cytokines. In: Brenner M (ed) Clinical haematology: cytokines and growth factors. Baillière Tindall, Edinburgh, pp 1–15

Crawford J, Lee M E 2000 Recombinant human granulocyte colony-stimulating factor support of the cancer patient. In: Armitage J O, Antman K H (eds) High-dose cancer therapy. Pharmacology, hematopoietins, stem cells, 3rd edn. Williams and Wilkins, Baltimore, pp 411–436

Cutler C, Antin J H 2001 Peripheral blood stem cells for allogeneic transplantation: a review. Stem Cells 19:108–117

Demetri G D, Anderson K C 2000 Blood bank support for patients undergoing high-dose chemotherapy. In: Armitage J O, Antman K H (eds) High-dose cancer therapy. Pharmacology, hematopoietins, stem cells, 3rd edn. Williams and Wilkins, Baltimore, pp 511–534

Dennis J E, Charbord P 2002 Origin and differentiation of human and murine stroma. Stem Cells 20:205–214

Dexter T M 1990 Haematopoietic growth factors. Review of biology and clinical potential. Gardiner-Caldwell Communications, Macclesfield

Douer D 2004 Acute promyelocytic leukaemia: a target for pre-emptive strike? Blood 104(7):1913–1914

Emerson S G, Adams S, Taichman R 2000 The hematopoietic microenvironment. In: Armitage J O, Antman K H (eds) High-dose cancer therapy. Pharmacology, hematopoietins, stem cells, 3rd edn. Williams and Wilkins, Baltimore, pp 185–192

Fliedner T M 1998 The role of blood stem cells in hematopoietic cell renewal. Stem Cells 16:361–374

Fruchtman S M 2004 Treatment paradigms in the management of myeloproliferative disorders. Seminars in Oncology 41(2), Suppl 3:18–22

Galli S J, Metcalfe D D, Dvorak A M 2001 Basophils and mast cells and their disorders. In: Beutler E, Lichtman M A, Coller B S, Kipps T J, Seligsohn U (eds) Williams Hematology, 6th edn. McGraw-Hill, New York, pp 801–815

Ghalie R G, Tallman M S 2000 Granulocyte-macrophage colony-stimulating factor. In: Armitage J O, Antman K H (eds) High-dose cancer therapy. Pharmacology, hematopoietins, stem cells, 3rd edn. Williams and Wilkins, Baltimore, pp 393–410

Heath V, Suh H S, Holman M et al 2004 C/EBPα deficiency results in hyperproliferation of hematopoietic progenitor cells and disrupts macrophage development in vitro and in vivo. Blood 104(6):1639–1647

Jaffe E S, Harris N L, Stein H, Vardiman J W (eds) 2001 Pathology and genetics of tumours of haematopoietic and lymphoid tissues. IACR Press, Lyon

Janowska-Wieczorek A, Majka M, Ratajczak J, Ratajczak M Z 2001 Autocrine/paracrine mechanisms in human hematopoiesis. Stem Cells 19:99–107

Kabarowski J H S, Witte O N 2000 Consequences of BCR-ABL expression within the hematopoietic stem cells in chronic myeloid leukemia. Stem Cells 18:399–408

Kalderon D 2000 Growth factor-signaling pathways in cancer. In: Bronchud M H, Foote M, Peters W P, Robinson M O (eds) Principles of molecular oncology. Humana Press, New Jersey, pp 127–167

Kaser A, Brandacher G, Steurer W et al 2001 Interleukin-6 stimulates thrombopoiesis through thrombopoietin: role in inflammatory thrombocytosis. Blood 98(9):2720–2725

Kircher S, Marquardt D 2002 Introduction to the immune system. In: Adelman D C, Casale T B, Corren J (eds) Manual of allergy and immunology, 4th edn. Williams and Wilkins, Baltimore, pp 1–24

Kronenwett R, Martin S, Haas R 2000 The role of cytokines and adhesion molecules for mobilization of peripheral blood stem cells. Stem Cells 18:320–330

Kuter D J 1997 The regulation of platelet production in vivo. In: Kuter D J, Hunt P, Sheridan W, Zuker-Franklin T (eds) Thrombopoiesis and thrombopoietins. Humana Press, New Jersey, pp 377–395

Kuter D J 2001 Megakaryopoiesis and thrombopoiesis In: Beutler E, Lichtman M A, Coller B S, Kipps T J, Seligsohn U (eds) Williams Hematology, 6th edn. McGraw-Hill, New York, pp 1339–1355

Kvalheim G, Smeland E B 1998 Characterization of blood stem cells In: Reiffers J, Goldman J M, Armitage J O (eds) Blood stem cell transplantation. Martin Dunitz, London, pp 19–36

Maher J, Davies E T 2004 Targeting cytotoxic T lymphocytes for cancer immunotherapy. British Journal of Cancer 91:817–821

Marshall C J, Thrasher A J 2001 The embryonic origins of human haematopoiesis. British Journal of Haematology 112:838–850

Metcalf D 1990 The colony stimulating factors: discovery, development and clinical applications. Cancer 65(10):2185–2195

Molineux G, Dexter T M 1998 Biology of G-CSF. In: Morstyn G, Dexter T M, Foote M (eds) Filgrastim in clinical practice, 2nd edn. Marcel Dekker, New York, pp 1–39

Pallister C 1994 Blood. Physiology and pathophysiology. Butterworth Heinemann, Oxford

Papamichail M, Perez S A, Gritzapis A D, Baxevanis C N 2004 Natural killer lymphocytes: biology, development and function. Cancer Immunology Immunotherapy 53:176–186

Pecora A 2000 CD34+ cell selection and ex vivo expansion in autologous and allogeneic transplantation. In: Rowe J M, Lazarus H M, Carella A M (eds) Handbook of bone marrow transplantation. Martin Dunitz, London, pp 1–19

Quesenberry P J, Colvin G A 2001 Hematopoietic stem cells, progenitor cells, and cytokines. In: Beutler E, Lichtman M A, Coller B S, Kipps T J, Seligsohn U (eds) Williams Hematology, 6th edn. McGraw-Hill, New York, pp 153–174

Radich J P 2004 Targeting ALL leukemia. Blood 104(5):1235–1236

Segel G B, Palis J 2001 Hematology of the newborn In: Beutler E, Lichtman M A, Coller B S, Kipps T J, Seligsohn U (eds) Williams Hematology, 6th edn. McGraw-Hill, New York, pp 77–92

Smyth M J, Godfrey D I, Trapani J A 2001 A fresh look at tumor immunosurveillance and immunotherapy. Nature Immunology 2(4):293–299

Summers V J, Heyworth C M, De Wynter E A, Chang J, Testa N G 2001 Cord blood G_0 CD34+ cells have a thousand fold higher capacity for generating progenitors in vitro than G_1 CD34+ cells. Stem Cells 19:505–513

Taichman R S, Emerson S G 1998 The role of osteoblasts in the hematopoietic microenvironment. Stem Cells 16:7–15

Testa N G, Coutinho L H, Radford J A, Will A 1993 Growth factors and the microenvironment. In: van Furth R (ed) Hemopoietic growth factors and mononuclear phagocytes. Karger, Basel, pp 36–43

Vogel W, Scheding S, Kanz L, Brugger W 2000 Clinical applications of CD34+ peripheral blood stem cells. Stem Cells 18: 87–92

Wagemaker G, Neelis K J, Hartong S C C et al 1998 The efficacy of recombinant thrombopoietin in murine and nonhuman primate models for radiation-induced myelosuppression and stem cell transplantation. Stem Cells 16:375–386

Wardlaw A J, Kay A B 2001 Eosinophils and their disorders. In: Beutler E, Lichtman M A, Coller B S, Kipps T J, Seligsohn U (eds) Williams Hematology, 6th edn. McGraw-Hill, New York, pp 785–799

Winton E F, Langston A A 2004 Update in acute leukemia 2003: A risk adapted approach to acute myeloblastic leukemia in adults. Seminars in Oncology 31(2) Suppl 4:80–86

Yasui K, Matsumoto Y, Hirayama F, Tani Y, Nakano T 2003 Differences between peripheral blood and cord blood in the kinetics of lineage-restricted hematopoietic cells: Implications for delayed platelet recovery following cord blood transplantation. Stem Cells 21:143–151

Further reading

Metcalf D 2000 Summon up the blood – in dogged pursuit of the blood cell regulators. AlphaMed Press, Ohio

An interesting account of the search for the haematopoietic growth factors that control blood cell development. A history of the science as seen through the eyes of one of the key contributors.

Chapter 2

Myelodysplastic syndromes

Jackie Green

KEY POINTS
- The myelodysplastic syndromes (MDS) are a group of haematopoietic disorders.
- MDS affects predominately elderly adults.
- Clinical progression of the disease and prognosis is extremely variable.
- Supportive care is an important part of treatment.

INTRODUCTION

The myelodysplastic syndromes (MDS) are a group of haematological disorders characterised by disruption in the production of effective blood cells. Bone marrow, blood cell morphology and the number, structure and functional ability of all blood cells may be abnormal, resulting in anaemia, leucopenia and thrombocytopenia.

Myelodysplastic syndromes have the potential to transform into acute myeloid leukaemia (AML) although not all individuals diagnosed with MDS will develop AML. MDS will transform in about 30% of patients although the time interval from diagnosis to transformation varies tremendously (Gyger et al 1988). However, MDS is frequently a chronic progressive disease, requiring a gradual increase in supportive care and treatment. This chapter examines MDS: the diseases, diagnosis, classification, treatment and specific nursing issues.

MDS: THE DISEASES

MDS are a group of disorders characterised by one or more peripheral blood cytopenias secondary to bone marrow dysfunction. Anaemia is common and usually dysplastic changes are present in more than one blood cell lineage. Bone marrow cellularity may be normal or become hypercellular. Both cell division and numbers of blast cells may be increased. MDS is associated with impaired maturation of blood cells and increased apoptosis (programmed cell death). Blood cells may have functional deficits predisposing to infection or bleeding (Heaney & Golde 1999). MDS may arise de novo and be considered an idiopathic disease, or secondarily after treatment with chemotherapy or radiation therapy for another disease. MDS is sometimes referred to as a 'pre-leukaemic' condition. However, not all patients progress to AML and many die from the effects of cytopenias or other co-morbid conditions common in an elderly population (Albitar et al 2002, Greenberg et al 2002). Accurate estimation of the incidence of MDS is difficult, because it may be asymptomatic and remain undetected for several years.

The causes of MDS remain unclear although exposure to radiation, chemicals, cytotoxic drugs and benzene has been implicated (Heaney & Golde 1999). MDS predominately affects the elderly (median age 70 years), although patients as young as 2 years old have been reported (Tuncer et al 1992). MDS has a non-age incidence of 3/100,000 rising to 20/100,000 in those over 70 years. Secondary MDS can arise as a result of chemotherapy/radiation for other malignancies. The incidence is not known but may represent as many as 10–15% of all cases of MDS diagnosed annually.

Clinical progression and prognosis of the disease is extremely variable. It may remain stable for many years or progress rapidly to AML. Secondary myelodysplasia usually has a poorer prognosis than de novo MDS (Cheson 1992). Survival and prognosis is directly related to the disease classification and prognostic indicators, including percentage of bone marrow blast cells, degree of peripheral blood cytopenias and cytogenetic abnormalities.

DIAGNOSIS

Those affected by MDS frequently present with the features of bone marrow failure: symptoms of anaemia, repeated infections, and bleeding and/or bruising. Approximately 10% of patients diagnosed with MDS present with splenomegaly (Mufti & Galton 1992).

The myelodysplastic syndromes are diagnosed primarily on the basis of characteristic full blood count assays, morphological abnormalities on the peripheral blood film, and characteristic bone marrow appearances. Although MDS may sometimes be diagnosed on the basis of a blood film alone, a bone marrow aspirate and trephine are needed to confidently diagnose and assess the severity of the disease (Bowen et al 2003).

Diagnosis is easily made if morphological abnormalities are found in the three major blood cell lineages: erythroid (red cells), myeloid cells (granulocytes, including neutrophils), and megakaryocytes (platelets) (Oscier & Oscier 1997). However, morphological dysplasia is not necessarily indicative of MDS, as some similar morphological abnormalities to those found in early MDS may be seen in vitamin B12 deficiency, alcohol excess, after chemotherapy and HIV infection. Cytogenetic analysis is also recommended for all those who have bone marrow examination (Bowen et al 2003).

CLASSIFICATION OF MYELODYSPLASTIC SYNDROME

MDS has classically been subdivided into five categories according to the abnormalities found within the bone marrow. This classification is known as the French-American-British (FAB) system after the French, American and British haematologists who designed the system (Bennett et al 1982) (Table 2.1). The FAB classification has been used as a prognostic indicator depending on the percentage of blast cells, ringed sideroblasts, monocytes and presence of Auer rods. Survival times and the prognosis of the disease vary significantly.

More recently the World Health Organization (WHO) (Harris et al 1999) has published a new classification system intended to supersede the FAB system (Box 2.1). However, the WHO system is still being evaluated and has not yet been universally accepted (Greenberg et al 2002, Bowen et al 2003). The FAB classification therefore remains widely used.

Survival times and the prognosis of the disease vary significantly even among patients of the same subgroup (Mufti & Galton 1992). The above

Table 2.1
French–American–British
(FAB) classification of MDS
(Bennett et al 1982)

FAB type	% of blasts	% of blasts in peripheral blood
1: Refractory anaemia (RA)	<5	<1
2: RA with ringed sideroblasts (RARS)	<5 ringed sideroblasts >15 of total erythrocytes	<1
3: RA with excess blasts (RAEB)	5–20	>5
4: RAEB in transformation (RAEB-t)	20–30 or presence of Auer rods	>5
5: Chronic myelomonocytic leukaemia	5–20 monocyte count >1.0 × 10^9/L	>5

Box 2.1   WHO classification of myelodysplastic syndromes (Harris et al 1999)

- Refractory anaemia (RA)
- Refractory anaemia with ringed sideroblasts (RARS)
- Refractory cytopenia with multilineage dysplasia (RCMD)
- Refractory anaemia with excess blasts – 1 (RAEB-1)
- Refractory anaemia with excess blasts – 2 (RAEB-2)
- Myelodysplastic syndrome unclassified (MDS-U)
- Myelodysplastic syndrome associated with isolated del(5q) chromosome abnormality

Figure 2.1
International Prognostic
Scoring System (IPSS) for MDS
(Greenberg et al 1997)

Survival and AML evolution score value					
Prognostic variable	**0**	**0.5**	**1.0**	**1.5**	**2.5**
Bone marrow blasts %	<5	5–10	–	11–20	21–30
Karyotype	Good	Intermediate	Poor		
Cytopenias	0/1	2/3			

Scores for Risk Groups	
Risk category	**Combined score**
Low	0
Intermediate 1 (Int-1)	0.5–1.0
Intermediate 2 (Int-2)	1.5–2.0
High	≥2.5

Karyotype: Good = normal, -Y, del(5q), del(20q);
Poor = complex (≥ 3 abnormalities) or chromosome 7 abnormalities
Intermediate = other abnormalities
Cytopenias: haemoglobin concentrate <10g/dL, neutrophils <1.5 x 10^9/L and platelets <100 x 10^9/L

classification systems are used in conjunction with additional prognostic scoring systems such at the International Prognostic Scoring System (IPSS) (Greenberg et al 1997) (Fig. 2.1). The IPSS considers three parameters: bone marrow blast percentage, bone marrow cytogenetics and the number of blood lineages with cytopenia. The IPSS identifies four risk groups: low risk, intermediate 1, intermediate 2 and high risk. The higher the risk score the poorer the prognosis (Table 2.2). Other prognostic

Table 2.2
Mean survival in relation to
risk score (Greenberg et al
1997)

Risk & score		Median survival (years)		
		Under 60	Over 60	Over 70
Low	0	11.8	4.8	3.9
Int 1	0.5–1.0	5.2	2.7	2.4
Int 2	1.5–2.0	1.8	1.1	1.2
High	>2.5	0.3	0.5	0.4

factors include age and gender with males having slightly poorer survival than females (Greenberg et al 1997, Verburgh et al 2003).

Although it is recommended that management of MDS should be based on the IPSS score (Bowen et al 2003), it is important to remember that this scoring system is only an indicator of prognosis. All patients with MDS have a reduced life expectancy, although patients react to their illness and treatment differently. An individual patient's prognosis will depend on their own specific circumstances and many patients live beyond their predicted survival time. The classification relates to adults as the disease follows a very different pattern in children.

TREATMENT AND MANAGEMENT OF MYELODYSPLASTIC SYNDROMES

There is no consistently effective treatment that provides long-term improvements in haemopoiesis. Therefore, it is recommended that, where appropriate, management decisions are based on the patient's IPSS score and patient choice (Cheson et al 2000, Bowen et al 2003). Quality of life is important in decisions about treatment. Management decisions should be taken with the informed involvement of the patient. In order to facilitate patient involvement, the proposed management of MDS should be explained to the patient and supported with written information related to guidelines.

SUPPORTIVE CARE

Supportive care remains the most important aspect of management for all patients with MDS. The aim is to reduce morbidity and mortality and to provide an acceptable quality of life (Bowen et al 2003). Management of the various cytopenias is therefore essential.

Anaemia

At presentation, approximately two-thirds of patients will be anaemic and virtually all will experience anaemia at some point in their illness, due to ineffective erythropoiesis and other disease- and treatment-related influences, e.g. chemotherapy, haemorrhage (Casadevall et al 2004). Anaemia may cause fatigue and breathlessness affecting the individual's quality of life. Red cell transfusion is used to correct anaemia. It is not possible to identify a single optimal haemoglobin level below which a red cell transfusion should be given, as it is dependent on the individual. However, in clinical practice transfusion is used if the individual is symptomatic. Guidelines also suggest haemoglobin is maintained >8 g/dL (Murphy et al 2001). Disease progression may require an increasing number of red cell transfusions due to a chronic anaemia state. This may cause an increase in body iron stores and iron overload, as the body has no means of increasing iron excretion (Hughes-Jones & Wickramasinghe 1996). If iron stores become greatly increased, damage may occur to the heart, liver and endocrine organs. In order to monitor iron stores ferritin levels should be monitored and a target ferritin level of <1000 µg/L is recommended (Franchini & Gandini 2000).

To prevent iron overload it is recommended that once a patient has received 5 g iron (approximately 25 units of red cells), iron chelation should be considered for those patients who are likely to require long-term red cell transfusion (Bowen et al 2003). However, iron chelation treatment in MDS is based on limited evidence. It is recommended that desferrioxamine (an iron-chelating compound) 20–40 mg/kg should be administered to patients who are likely to need long-term blood component transfusions. Desferrioxamine is usually administered subcutaneously over 8–12 hours, three times a week. Desferrioxamine (up to 2 g per unit of blood) can also be administered intravenously at the same time as the blood transfusion, provided it is not added to or given through the same line (British National Formulary 2004). Auditory and ophthalmic review are essential prior to commencing desferrioxamine because it is known to produce visual and hearing disturbances.

Erythropoietin (EPO), a colony stimulating factor (which promotes the growth and differentiation of blood cells), may increase haemoglobin concentration and reduce the need for red cell transfusion in selected MDS patients, reducing the risk of iron overload (Box 2.2). Studies using EPO have been small, involving less than 120 patients, and suggest that patients with refractory anaemia (RA) or RA with excess blasts (RAEB) are more likely to respond to EPO (Estey et al 1997). It is recommended that patients with RA and RAEB who have minimal blood transfusion requirement (<2 units a month) and an EPO level <200 U/L should be considered for EPO (Hellstrom Lindberg et al 1998).

A combination of G-CSF (granulocyte-colony stimulating factor) and EPO has been shown to have a synergistic effect and is recommended to

---

Box 2.2   Colony stimulating factors

1. *Granulocyte-macrophage colony stimulating factor (GM-CSF)* – promotes growth & differentiation of granulocyte and macrophage progenitors
2. *Granulocyte-colony stimulating factor (G-CSF)* – stimulates neutrophil precursors to produce large amounts of circulating neutrophils
3. *Erythropoietin (EPO)* – promotes erythrocyte production

> **Box 2.3**   Guidelines for the management of symptomatic anaemia (Bowen et al 2003)
>
> - RARS + serum EPO <500 U/L   Consider EPO + G-CSF
>   + low or no transfusion
>
> - RA/RAEB + serum EPO <200 U/L   Consider EPO
>   + low or no transfusion
>
> - Other + high EPO serum   1. Consider immunosuppression
>   + high transfusion dependence   2. Supportive care

improve anaemia for some individuals (Bowen et al 2003). For patients with RARS, symptomatic anaemia, EPO serum levels <500 U/L and a transfusion requirement of less than two units of blood a month EPO + G-CSF is recommended (Hellstrom Lindberg et al 1998). However, not all patients with anaemia secondary to MDS respond to growth factors and clinical trials investigating their use continue. There is an assumption that improving anaemia will improve quality of life, although there are few data to support this. One randomised trial comparing EPO and G-CSF with supportive care found that the combination was expensive and did not improve quality of life (Casadevall et al 2004). A summary of recommended management of anaemia in MDS can be seen in Box 2.3.

Thrombocytopenia

Spontaneous bleeding is a potentially serious complication of MDS and it is suggested that treatment is based on symptoms (Ancliff & Machin 1998). Patients may experience unexplained bruising, nosebleeds (epistaxis), a petechial rash or gum bleeding. Patients who experience spontaneous bleeding should be advised to seek medical and/or nursing advice and support immediately. Platelet transfusion may be required to both stop bleeding and reduce the risk of further bleeding. Treatment of thrombocytopenia is outlined in Chapter 16.

Management of infection

White cell count, and in particular the neutrophil count, can be significantly lowered in MDS, increasing the risk of developing a life-threatening infection. The lower the neutrophil count the higher the risk of infection – the risk of infection rises as the neutrophil count falls. Immunosuppressed patients can become infected with pathogenic and opportunistic organisms (Mimms 1993) (see Chapter 15).

The evidence-base for symptomatic management of infection in MDS is limited. The use of prophylactic antibiotic therapy has not been proven and individuals with MDS may require hospital admission for intravenous antibiotic therapy. The use of colony-stimulating factors (CSF) may be considered in the cases of severe neutropenia in order to maintain a neutrophil count $>1 \times 10^9$/L (Negrin et al 1996). CSFs may improve the supportive therapy of patients with MDS by minimising the risk of infection as fewer infections have been reported with their use (Ganser et al 1989). Intermittent use of CSFs for patients with severe neutropenia and recurrent infections has been found to be beneficial (Ozer et al 2000). However, prolonged use of CSFs is not recommended in MDS (Pagliuca et al 2003).

STEM CELL TRANSPLANTATION

A small percentage of patients with MDS may be eligible for bone marrow transplantation. It is suggested that allogeneic stem cell transplantation results in long-term survival in 30–55% of patients and has the best chance of cure (Anderson et al 1996, Deeg et al 2000). Eligibility for stem cell transplantation is dependent on several factors:

- stage and duration of the disease
- the individual's general health (including previous medical history, lung, renal and cardiac status) and physical ability to tolerate treatment
- availability of a histocompatible sibling or unrelated donor
- psychological state
- age.

Good risk factors for transplant for the individual with MDS are considered to be <10% blasts and good cytogenetics (Anderson et al 1993, Sutton et al 1996). An example of good cytogenetics is chromosomal abnormality 5q, where there is a deletion of the long arm (q) of chromosome 5. This is associated with macrocytic anaemia in elderly women and has a low risk of transformation to AML. However, loss of the short arm (p) of chromosome 17 is found in advanced disease and associated with drug resistance and short-term survival.

It is also suggested that autologous stem cell transplant may prolong survival (De Witte et al 1997). Factors associated with improved outcome are: shorter disease duration, age, primary MDS with <10% blasts in the bone marrow (Deeg et al 2000). The type of transplant is usually determined by the likely survival outcome, donor availability and wellbeing of the individual requiring a transplant.

INTENSIVE CHEMOTHERAPY

Individuals with MDS aged over 65 and those under 65 who are not eligible for stem cell transplantation should be considered for intensive chemotherapy (Bowen et al 2003). Prospective studies have compared supportive therapy versus intensive chemotherapy (Hellstrom Lindberg et al 1992, Miller et al 1993). Such studies suggest that of all high-risk MDS patients (IPSS >2), those with RAEB in transformation and lacking independent adverse risk factors may respond to intensive chemotherapy. Independent adverse risk factors can be considered as karyotype, age, performance status and duration of disease (Estey et al 1997). There does not appear to be any superior chemotherapy combination. However, a combination such as that used in AML treatment is commonly used. Estey et al (2001) suggest that regimens containing cytosine arabinoside, idarubicin, +/– fludarabine are likely to produce the best outcome at present. If MDS transforms to AML, the treatment is that of AML, usually high-intensity combination chemotherapy +/– bone marrow transplantation (see Chapter 4). This is again dependent on the individual's wishes, physical and mental well-being (Estey et al 1997).

SPECIFIC NURSING ISSUES

The nursing care of an individual with MDS requires specific skills in order to maximise their quality of life whilst living with the disease. As MDS may significantly reduce life expectancy, great emphasis needs to be placed on quality of life. Good symptom management is therefore imperative to achieve and improve outcomes for patients. It is essential that nurses caring for these patients understand the disease process, treatment options and side effects. Psychological and social factors and education are also important nursing considerations due to the unpredictability of the disease process and reduced life expectancy. Nurses need to provide the individual and their families with specific information and education related to bone marrow depression and living with MDS.

SPECIFIC EDUCATION AND INFORMATION NEEDS

Nurses should observe for signs of anaemia, such as fatigue, shortness of breath, pallor and reduction in activity due to excessive tiredness. Expert nursing care can help the individual to prioritise activities in order to ensure that they have sufficient energy for the activities that are most valuable to them (see Chapter 22). For individuals who require blood transfusion it is essential that the British Committee for Standards in Haematology (BCSH) guidelines (1999) and local hospital policy are followed to ensure the transfusion is administered safely (see Chapter 12). Individuals require information and understanding of the need for transfusion as well as the associated risks. It is recommended that written information is given to support verbal information and consent is obtained (Department of Health 2001). It is also important for patients to be aware of how they can help themselves to cope with anaemia. Information and education about appropriate diet, fluid intake and managing their breathlessness and lethargy should be provided.

Nurses must also be aware of signs and symptoms of thrombocytopenia (see Chapter 16). Bleeding can be a frightening experience. Patients and their families require explicit information about what to do if bleeding occurs. Emergency contact numbers of the ward or the day care unit are generally very helpful and provide reassurance. Verbal and written information outlining what to do during office hours and out of hours is important. Education is extremely important and individuals should be made aware of risk factors associated with bleeding and bruising. Advice should be given about activities that increase the risk of bleeding and bruising such as contact sports, climbing at high altitudes, flying in aeroplanes, avoiding cuts and scratches whilst gardening. It is acknowledged that not all those with MDS will participate in such activities, and advice should be adapted to the individual's needs. If any surgical intervention or dental work is required, the haematology team caring for the individual should be notified prior to such an event so that the risks of bleeding can be reduced and clotting factors and platelet levels are maintained at a safe volume.

The individual with MDS requires education to understand the infection risks associated with the disease. Being able to identify early signs of infection is significant and can help to reduce the risk of severe infection. Infection may have a significant impact on an individual's lifestyle such as hospital admissions due to septic episodes, the need to avoid crowded places, antibiotic therapy and potentially time off work due to infection. Individuals therefore require support both from the haematology team and in the social setting from employers, family and any social organisations they may attend.

Nurses have an important role in educating individuals about what to do in the event of an infection and measures to minimise the risk of an infective process. Patients should be informed both verbally and in written format of the actions they should take if they become unwell, have hot and cold episodes, shivers or a high temperature (>38°C). Information should include who to contact and what to do. The need to act promptly and not ignore these signs should be emphasised.

REFLECTION POINT   Patients with MDS may have a reduced life expectancy. How can nurse help facilitate self-care that may improve the individual's quality of life?

PSYCHOLOGICAL IMPACT

A diagnosis of MDS potentially has a great psychological impact on individuals. The unpredictability of the disease, frequent hospital attendance and potentially frequent hospital admissions can have an enormous impact on an individual's life and psychological needs should be considered at all times. Some individuals and their carers will require professional counselling to help them to live with the disease. Others may benefit from the support and understanding provided by the multidisciplinary team. Nurses can help considerably by ensuring that treatments and hospital appointments, as far as possible, are made flexible in order to minimise the disruption to the individual's lifestyle and particularly the working environment. It is possible that the individual may require medical information to be given to employers in order to assist them in retaining employment. Other individuals may wish to give up work and may need some assistance with financial support.

The psychological impact of living with this group of diseases should not be underestimated. In order to identify what living with MDS means to the patient the nurse requires excellent communication skills and the ability to actively listen. It is important that nurses recognise the need to refer appropriately to other colleagues. Seeking advice from multidisciplinary team members and recognising when referral to a counsellor is appropriate is an essential aspect of care (psychological issues are discussed further in Chapter 23).

REFLECTION POINT   Treatment of MDS will invariably require frequent hospital attendances. Consider what psychological impact this may have on the individual and their family.

SOCIAL IMPLICATIONS

The diseases also have significant social implications and nurses must be aware of these. Although the nurse may not be the most appropriate person to deal with some of the issues, such as completing forms for financial support or advising on writing a will, they are in an ideal position to act as a coordinator and refer the individual to appropriate personnel (social needs are discussed further in Chapter 25).

Case study 2.1

Ron, a 72-year-old male, presented at his GP practice for a wellman health check. On examination the GP noted he had a petechial rash on his lower limbs. Ron also explained that his exercise tolerance had significantly reduced recently. The GP arranged for a full blood count to be taken, which indicated a haemoglobin of 8.4 g/dl, a platelet count of 84×10^9/L and a white blood cell count of 1.8×10^9/L.

Ron was referred to the consultant haematologist who performed a bone marrow aspirate and trephine. A diagnosis of refractory anaemia with excess blasts was confirmed. The biopsy confirmed 15% blasts in the bone marrow.

Treatment options were discussed with Ron and in view of his age supportive care was considered the most appropriate treatment. Two units of blood were transfused in the haematology day care unit to try and aid his exercise tolerance. Ron achieved a good response to the blood transfusion and was able to walk to the local shops. He felt his exercise tolerance was back to normal. Ron later required two hospital admissions with infective episodes and therefore GCSF was prescribed. Following this he required no further admissions for infective episodes.

At one hospital visit the clinic nurse noted that Ron was very quiet and on further discussion he admitted that he considered his quality of life to be significantly reduced as he could only think that he was going to die soon. He could not see the value in maintaining friendships at his local golf club. In fact the only visitors he would see were his immediate family. The nurse referred him to the counsellor.

At the next hospital visit three weeks later Ron was discussing his latest golf club luncheon and planning a weekend away. He is supported by blood components monthly and continues to plan short breaks away.

CONCLUSION

MDS varies in its manifestations, disease classification, treatment options and life expectancy. It is essential that individuals with MDS are fully informed about their disease. Nurses have a very specialist role in supporting individuals with MDS to live their lives to the full within the constraints placed upon them by the disease.

Clearly there are differing treatment options available, ranging from supportive therapy to intensive chemotherapy and stem cell transplantation. Nursing care aims to meet individual needs at all stages in the disease pathway. This demands experienced/expert nurses with the skills and knowledge to meet these needs.

DISCUSSION QUESTIONS

1. How are myelodysplastic disorders diagnosed?

2. What is the relevance of the International Prognostic Scoring System for patients and nurses?

3. Why is intensive chemotherapy not always the appropriate treatment of choice for individuals diagnosed with MDS?

4. What information and support does the individual with MDS and their family require?

References

Albitar M, Manshouri T, Shen Y et al 2002 Myelodysplastic syndrome is not merely 'preleukaemia'. Blood 100(3):791–798

Ancliff P, Machin S 1998 Trigger factors for the prophylactic platelet transfusion. Blood Reviews 12:234–238

Anderson J E, Appelbaum F R, Fischer L D et al 1993 Allogeneic bone marrow transplantation for 93 patients with myelodysplastic syndrome. Blood 82:677–681

Anderson J E, Appelbaum F R, Schoch G et al 1996 Allogeneic bone marrow transplantation for refractory anaemia: a comparison of two preparative regimes and analysis of prognostic factors. Blood 87:51–58

Bennett J M, Catousky D, Daniel M T et al 1982 Proposals for the classification of the myelodysplastic syndromes. British Journal of Haematology 51(2):189–199

Bowen D, Culligan D, Jowitt S et al of the UK MDS Guidelines Group 2003 Guidelines for the diagnosis and therapy of adult myelodysplastic syndrome. British Journal of Haematology 120:187–200

British Committee for Standards in Haematology 1999 Guidelines for the administration of blood and blood components in the management of transfused patients. Transfusion Medicine 9:227–238

British National Formulary 2004 BNF 48. British Medical Association, London

Casadevall N, Durieux P, Dubois S et al 2004 Health, economic and quality of life effects of erythropoietin and granulocyte colony-stimulating factor for the treatment of myelodysplastic syndromes: a randomised controlled trial. Blood 104(2):321–327

Cheson B D 1992 Chemotherapy and bone marrow transplantation for myelodysplastic syndromes. Seminars in Oncology 19(1):85–94

Cheson B D, Bennett J M, Kantarjian H et al 2000 Report of an international working group to standardise criteria for myelodysplastic syndromes. Blood 96: 3671–3674

Deeg H, Shulman H M, Anderson J E et al 2000 Allogeneic and syngeneic marrow transplantation for myelodysplastic syndromes in patients 55–66 years of age. Blood 95(10):1188–1194

Department of Health 2001 Good practice in consent: achieving the NHS Plan commitment to patient centred consent practice. Health Service Circular (HSC) 2001/023

De Witte T, Van Biezen A, Hermans J et al 1997 Autologous bone marrow transplantation for patients with myelodysplastic syndromes (MDS) or acute myeloid leukaemia following MDS. Chronic or acute leukaemia working parties of the European Group for Blood and Marrow Transplantation. Blood 90(10):3853–3857

Estey E, Thall P, Beran M 1997 Effect of diagnosis (refractory anaemia with excess blasts, refractory anaemia with excess blasts in transformation or AML) on outcome of AML type chemotherapy. Blood 90(8):2969–2977

Estey E, Thall P F, Cortes J E et al 2001 Comparison of idarubicin + ara-C, fludarabine + ara-C and topetocan + ara-C based regimes in treatment of newly diagnosed acute myeloid leukaemia, refractory anaemia with excess blasts in transformation, or refractory anaemia with excess blasts. Blood 98:3575–3583

Franchini M, Gandini G 2000 Safety and efficacy of subcutaneous bolus injection of desferrioxamine in adult patients with iron overload. Blood 95:2776–2779

Ganser A, Volkers B, Greher J et al 1989 Recombinant human granulocyte macrophage colony stimulating factor in patients with myelodysplastic syndromes – a phase I/II trial. Blood 73:31–37

Greenberg P, Cox C, Le Beau M et al 1997 International scoring system for evaluating prognosis in myelodysplastic syndromes. Blood 89(6):2079–2088

Greenberg P L, Young N S, Gattermann N 2002 Myelodysplastic syndromes. Hematology 1:136–161

Gyger M, Infante-Rivard C, D'Angelo G 1988 Prognostic value or clonal chromosomal abnormalities in patients with myelodysplastic syndromes. American Journal of Hematology 28(1):13–20

Harris N L, Jaffe E S, Diebold J et al 1999 World Health Organization classification of neoplastic diseases of the haematopoietic and lymphoid tissue: report of the Clinical Advisory Committee meeting (1997), Airline House, Virginia. Journal of Clinical Oncology 17:3835–3849

Heaney M L, Golde D W 1999 Medical progress: myelodysplasia. New England Journal of Medicine 340(21):1649–1660

Hellstrom Lindberg E, Robert K H, Gahrton G et al 1992 A predictive model for clinical response to low dose ara-C: a study of 102 patients with myelodysplastic syndromes or acute leukaemia. British Journal of Haematology 81:503–511

Hellstrom Lindberg E, Ahlgren T, Beguin T et al 1998 Treatment of anaemia in myelodysplastic syndromes with granulocyte stimulating factor plus erythropoietin: results from a randomised phase II study and long-term follow up of 71 patients. Blood 92:68–75

Hughes-Jones N, Wickramasinghe E 1996 Lecture notes on haematology, 6th edn. Blackwell Science, London

Miller K B, Head D R, Cassileth P A et al 1993 The evaluation of low-dose cytarabine in treatment of myelodysplastic syndromes: a phase-III international group study. Annals of Hematology 65:162–168

Mimms C, Playfair J, Roitt I, Wakelin D, Williams R 1993 Medical microbiology. Mosby, St Louis

Mufti G, Galton D 1992 The myelodysplastic syndromes. Churchill Livingstone, Edinburgh

Murphy M F, Wallington T B, Kelsey P et al 2001 British Committee for Standards in Haematology, Blood Transfusion Task Force. Guidelines for clinical use of red cell transfusions. British Journal of Haematology 113(1):24–31

Negrin R, Stein R, Doherty K 1996 Maintenance treatment of the anaemia of myelodysplastic syndromes with recombinant human granulocyte colony stimulatory factor and in vitro surgery. Blood 87(10):4076–4081

Oscier C, Oscier D 1997 ABC of haematology, the myelodysplastic syndromes. British Journal of Medicine 314:883–886

Ozer H, Armitage J O, Bennett C L et al 2000 2000 update of recommendations for the use of hematopoietic colony stimulating factors: evidence-based, clinical practice guidelines. American Society of Clinical Oncology Growth Factors Expert Panel. Journal of Clinical Oncology 18:3558–3585

Pagliuca A, Carrington P A, Pettingell R et al 2003 Guidelines on the use of colony-stimulating factors in haematological malignancies. British Journal of Haematology 123:22–33

Sutton L, Chastang C, Ribaud P 1996 Factors influencing outcomes in de novo MDS treated by allogenic BMT. Blood 88:358–365

Tuncer M, Pagliuca A, Hicsonmez G 1992 Primary myelodysplastic syndrome in children: the clinical experience in 33 cases. British Journal of Haematology 82(2):347–353

Verburgh E, Achten R, Maes B et al 2003 Additional prognostic value of bone marrow histology in patients subclassified according to the international prognostic scoring system for myelodysplastic syndromes. Journal of Clinical Oncology 21(2):273–282

Further reading

Bowen D, Culligan D, Jowitt S et al of the UK MDS Guidelines Group 2003 Guidelines for the diagnosis and therapy of adult myelodysplastic syndrome. British Journal of Haematology 120:187–200
This is a very detailed outline of recommended guidelines by the British Committee for Standards in Haematology (BCSH) for the management and diagnosis of myeloproliferable disorders. It discusses differing prognostic scoring systems. The article gives clear evidence-based guidance on the treatment of this group of diseases.

Heaney M, Golde D 1999 Medical progress: myelodysplasia. New England Journal of Medicine 340(21):1649–1660
This is a very useful article that outlines the history and classification of myelodysplasia. The article describes the diagnostic tests and discusses current prognostic scoring systems and treatments for this group of diseases.

Chapter 3

Aplastic anaemia

Evelyn Dannie

KEY POINTS
- Aplastic anaemia is a frequently fatal disease.
- Aplastic anaemia may be inherited or acquired.
- Treatment options include supportive care, bone marrow transplant and immunosuppressive therapy.

INTRODUCTION

Aplastic anaemia (AA) was first described by Paul Ehrlich in 1888 in a pregnant young woman who died following a short illness consisting of severe anaemia, bleeding and a high fever. At post-mortem, nucleated red cells were absent from the bone marrow, having been replaced by fat cells (Plates 1 and 2).

Today AA is still frequently fatal and although certain subsets are curable it remains a disease of poor prognosis. AA can be divided into two main groups: 'inherited' and 'acquired'. The pathophysiology and treatment options for both groups of the disease are reviewed within this chapter. Patient education strategies and specific nursing issues are also addressed.

THE DISEASE

DEFINITION OF APLASTIC ANAEMIA

AA is characterised by pancytopenia (reduced red cells, white cells and platelets) associated with a 'hypocellular' bone marrow in which haemopoietic cells are replaced by fat cells. The prognosis of the disease is directly related to the severity of bone marrow depression (Gordon-Smith 1989, Dokal 2001).

Severe AA is defined by the Camitta criteria with two out of three of the following criteria being present:

- neutrophils $<0.5 \times 10^9/L$
- platelets $<20 \times 10^9/L$
- reticulocytes $<40 \times 10^9/L$ (<1%).

In severe AA the marrow shows severe hypocellularity with <25% of the marrow being normal or populated by cells (Lewis 1965, Camitta et al 1975).

EPIDEMIOLOGY

The incidence of AA in developed countries is probably in the order of 2–4 per million of the population per year (Szklo et al 1985, Heimpel 2000). These data are only estimates and there is substantial geographic variation in incidence with up to 30 cases per million in some parts of Asia. In the Far East the incidence appears to be higher than in the West. This may be due in part to the high incidence of hepatitis, the widespread use of chloramphenicol as an effective and cheap antibiotic, and the extensive use of and exposure to insecticides (Young & Issaragrasil 1986, Young 2000).

There is a male predominance in AA, with two peaks in age distribution, between the ages of 10 and 25 and over 60 years. However, the incidence in the older age group can be confused with the myelodysplastic syndromes and the small peak in childhood is due to the inclusion of inherited cases such as Fanconi's anaemia.

The majority of patients fall into the acquired AA category. Occasionally in acquired AA it is possible to identify a factor which may have acted as a trigger to initiation of the disease. However, in the majority of cases (~70%) there is no obvious aetiological factor and the disease is referred to as idiopathic (Table 3.1).

ACQUIRED APLASTIC ANAEMIA

Pathophysiology

The pathophysiology of acquired AA is poorly understood. Studies over the past few decades have demonstrated that AA arises because of damage to haemopoietic stem cells. Patients with AA have a reduced number of haemopoietic progenitors and cluster of differentiation

Table 3.1
Classification of the aplastic
anaemias

Inherited	Acquired		
	Idiopathic	Secondary to other diseases	Inevitable
Fanconi's anaemia	Drug induced	Systemic lupus erythematosus (SLE)	Ionising radiation
Dyskeratosis congenita	Viral	Acute lymphoblastic leukaemia (ALL)	Cytotoxic drugs
Others	Toxins		

(CD) 34$^+$ cells compared to normal controls. Immunological abnormalities in AA combined with response, in the majority of cases, to immunotherapy suggest that abnormalities in immune function must play a role in its pathophysiology. These abnormalities include cytotoxic T-lymphocyte activation and increased expression of gamma interferon and tumour necrosis factor alpha (TNFα). The increased levels of lymphocytes and cytokines indicate that AA is an immune attack on the haemopoietic system, which induces programmed cell death. However, it is likely that the primary triggers of these abnormalities are diverse and may include drugs, chemicals and viruses which may act as nonspecific trigger factors, although in the majority of cases the primary aetiology is unclear (Knospe & Crosby 1971, Kurtzman & Young 1989, Nissen-Druey 1989, Dokal 1996a, Heimpel 2000, Marin 2000, Young 2000, Dokal 2001).

Triggers of acquired aplastic anaemia

Drugs and chemicals

A wide variety of drugs have been implicated as causative agents in AA (Heimpel & Heit 1980, Baumelou et al 1993). The risk of developing AA is small (International Agranulocytosis and Aplastic Anaemia Study 1986). Chloramphenicol is perhaps the best documented and most notorious of all drugs with the potential to cause AA. It produces what is termed an idiosyncratic response with AA occurring weeks or months after discontinuation of the drug. Chloramphenicol contains a nitrobenzene ring and is similar to amidopyrine, a drug known to cause agranulocytosis. Toxicity is dose-related and has been ascribed to mitochondrial damage inhibiting the growth of both granulocyte, macrophage colony-forming units (CFU-GM) and erythrocyte colony-forming units (CFU-E) (see Chapter 1) (Yunis et al 1980, Alter & Young 1993, Wilholm et al 1998). It has also been shown to induce an autoimmune reaction (Nagro & Maver 1969). A variety of other drugs have the potential to cause AA and are detailed in Box 3.1.

Idiosyncratic AA has also been associated with a number of chemicals (Jick 1977, Smith 1996). In particular, the effects of benzene, commonly found in organic solvents, coal tar derivatives and petroleum products are well studied. Long-term exposure to benzene leads to decreased blood cell progenitors and DNA damage. Other chemicals associated with AA include insecticides and pesticides, toluene and acetanilide.

Box 3.1   Trigger factors associated with aplastic anaemia

Drugs

- Antibiotics (e.g. chloramphenicol)
- Anti-inflammatory (e.g. phenylbutazone, indometacin, gold)
- Antithyroid (e.g. carbimazole)
- Antimalarial (e.g. chloroquine)
- Anticonvulsant (e.g. phenytoin)

Infective agents

- Viruses (e.g. hepatitis A, B and C)
- Bacterial (e.g. mycobacteria)

Toxins

- Commercial solvents
- Insecticides

Systemic disease

- Systemic lupus erythematosus

These substances have been shown to inhibit haematopoietic colony formation (Gallicchio et al 1987, Yin et al 1987, 1996, Fleming & Timmeny 1993). Marrow aplasia may also result following exposure to radiation. Bone marrow cells are affected by high-energy rays, with the greatest damage being to the actively dividing pool of blood cell precursor and progenitor cells (Kirshbaum et al 1971, Gale 1987).

Viruses and infection   Some viruses are well-documented trigger factors, with AA often occurring during or early after viral hepatitis (both A and B and non-A and non-B) or exposure to other viruses such as Epstein–Barr, B19 parvovirus, and retroviruses such as the human immunodeficiency virus (HIV). No single pathological phenomenon explains AA.

Bacterial and fungal infections depress bone marrow function (Alter & Young 1993, Young 2000, Heimpel 2000, Hoffbrand et al 2001). These infections are often treated with antibiotics and it is often unclear whether an ensuing AA is caused by the infection, the drug or a combination of both, or whether the infection is a result of the illness and not the cause of the AA.

Only a minority of infected patients develop bone marrow failure, and infection appears to act as a trigger rather than the cause of AA. It is conceivable that an immune imbalance of any origin can act as a trigger to AA (Kurtzman & Young 1989, Dokal 2001). Viral infections and drugs can act synergistically, increasing their potential as risk factors, and the incidence of AA rises sharply after exposure to a virus such as hepatitis and a drug such as chloramphenicol (Hagler et al 1975, Wilholm 1998, Heimpel 2000, Young 2000).

Clinical features

Clinical manifestations are related to the severity of the disease. Reduction of platelets leads to bruising and bleeding from mucous membranes. Neutropenia and red cell depletion tend to occur later in the disease trajectory, resulting in susceptibility to infection and anaemia. The bone marrow shows hypoplasia with loss of haematopoietic tissue and marked decreases in all cell lines (Gordon-Smith 1989, Hoffbrand et al 2001).

REFLECTION POINT

Fatigue is a common experience for patients with severe aplastic anaemia. There are a number of reasons for this but a low haemoglobin level is a major contributing factor. The sheer frustration of not being able to pursue a normal lifestyle can cause individuals added anxiety. Identify strategies which could be developed through participative nurse/patient relationships to help individuals to minimise the effects of fatigue.

TREATMENT

The main aim of treatment is to improve blood counts to prevent dependency on transfusions of blood and blood components and reduce the risk from opportunist infections and haemorrhage (Gordon-Smith 1989, Ball 2000). The pathophysiology of the disease suggests two approaches to treatment:

- replacement of the deficient stem cells by bone marrow transplantation (BMT), or
- immunosuppressive therapy to stop the immunological process (Young & Barrett 1995, Dokal 2001, British Committee for Standards in Haematology (BCSH) 2003).

In both cases a relatively long period of intensive supportive treatment is necessary until the choice of specific therapy is made and during treatment until self-supporting peripheral blood counts are obtained. Figure 3.1 outlines treatment options.

SUPPORTIVE CARE

Blood and blood components

Supportive therapy has improved considerably over the last 30 years. The major supportive measures are the provision of blood components and both prophylactic and therapeutic antibiotic therapy. One of the first treatment decisions is eligibility for BMT. Blood components must be used sparingly if the individual is eligible for BMT and blood components from family members must be avoided to minimise sensitisation (see Chapter 12). Blood component support consists mainly of packed red cells and platelet transfusions and is based on clinical need. In non-bleeding patients 3–4 units of red cells are transfused every 3–4 weeks to maintain haemoglobin at a level that allows the patient to be

Figure 3.1
Treatment options for patients
with severe aplastic anaemia
and inherited aplastic anaemia

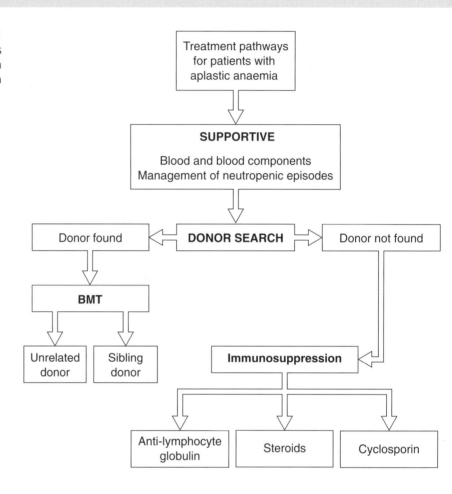

asymptomatic. To delay and prevent the development of human leuco-cyte antigen (HLA) antibodies leuco-depleted blood components should be used from the onset. For patients who are cytomegalovirus (CMV) antibody negative, CMV negative blood components should be used as this will reduce the risk of severe CMV infection should haemopoietic stem cell transplant become a treatment option (Dokal 2001). In severe AA, prophylactic platelet transfusions should be given to reduce the risk of fatal haemorrhage (Gordon-Smith & Lewis 1990, Dokal 2001).

Infection

Patients with AA are at risk from infections, which progress rapidly in the presence of neutropenia, and protective measures are designed to avoid acquired bacterial or fungal infections (see Chapter 15). Whilst there is still debate about the appropriateness of prophylactic antimicro-bials it is reasonable to give these to patients with a low neutrophil count and to those who are receiving immunosuppressive therapy. All patients will need prompt therapy with broad-spectrum intravenous antibiotics if they develop pyrexia.

HAEMOPOIETIC STEM CELL TRANSPLANTATION (HSCT/BMT)

Irrespective of the underlying pathophysiology, haemopoietic stem cell transplantation (HSCT/BMT) has become the treatment of choice for the young person with severe AA when an identical HLA donor is available (Storb et al 1974, Dokal 1996a, Bacigalupo et al 2000a, Dokal 2001). HSCT is fully discussed in Chapter 13, but a brief discussion is included here in relation to the management of AA.

HSCT has been shown to have a clear survival advantage over no treatment or other treatment options (Camitta et al 1982, Bacigalupo et al 2000a). The 5-year disease-free survival rate from sibling donors is in the range 75–90%. Transplants from unrelated donors are less successful but should be considered in patients who are relatively young and have not responded to immunosuppressive therapy (Sullivan & Witherspoon 1988, Dokal 2001). Improved survival has been attributed to many factors, including intensified conditioning regimens to prevent graft rejection, the use of ciclosporin to prevent graft rejection and graft versus host disease (GvHD), better blood component preparation to reduce allosensitisation and prompt use of antimicrobials. However, graft rejection, GvHD and infection remain limiting factors to the success of transplant (Young & Barrett 1995, Locatelli et al 2000).

The indication for transplant is considered in two parts: first, relating to the disease and second, to the transplant itself. In the first instance, concerns may arise as to whether the disease can be treated successfully with alternative therapy, and in the second considerations relate to the recipient's age, general health and the availability of a suitable donor.

The main conditioning regimen used includes cyclophosphamide 200 mg/kg with ciclosporin and methotrexate for GvHD prophylaxis. For patients >30 years old conditioning regimens including cyclophosphamide and antithymocyte globulin (ATG) appear to have a higher survival rate for sibling donors, 90% at 3 years, compared with regimens employing irradiation programmes, 60–70% at 3 years (Paquetto et al 1995, Bacigalupo et al 2000a, BCSH 2003).

An analysis of 993 evaluable BMT patients (Hows et al 1996) showed that actual survival after sibling BMT was 65% at 10 years compared with only 20% transplanted from partially mismatched family donors and HLA-matched unrelated donors. The incidence of graft rejection has fallen from 30% before 1980 to approximately 5–10% (Passweg et al 1997) but GvHD remains a problem. The probability of acute GvHD is 18% and chronic GvHD 26% as reported to the International Bone Marrow Transplant Registry (IBMTR) (Passweg et al 1997).

IMMUNOSUPPRESSIVE THERAPY

Antilymphocyte globulin and antithymocyte globulin

The use of antilymphocyte globulin (ALG) and antithymocyte globulin (ATG) as immunosuppressive therapy has become an accepted form of treatment in AA (Bacigalupo 1989, Ball 2000, Gordon-Smith & Marsh

2000). ALG and ATG are the sera produced by the immunisation of horses or rabbits with human thymocytes (ATG) or thoracic duct lymphocytes (ALG). They are lymphotoxic reagents with activity against all blood and marrow cells, including progenitors, and are used to decrease rejection of transplanted HLA-matched bone marrow.

The mechanism of action of ALG is almost certainly immunosuppressive: it is cytolytic of T cells and inhibits T-cell function. ALG rapidly reduces circulating lymphocytes, usually to less than 10% of starting values, and when total blood counts return to pretreatment values months later, activated lymphocyte numbers in recovered patients remain decreased (Lopez-Karpovitch et al 1989).

A review of the results in the 1980s suggested that about 45% of patients with severe AA responded to ALG (Young & Speck 1984). Early protocols used 10–28 daily intravenous infusions but a short course of 40 mg/kg/day for 4 days is effective and less toxic, especially for induction of serum sickness (Bielory et al 1988). ALG has not proved very useful in children with AA or in patients with severe neutropenia (Locasciulli et al 1990). Immediate allergic reactions are rare but a test dose is recommended. Serum sickness due to immune complex deposition is seen in all patients. This is manifested in a number of distressing symptoms, which can be treated effectively with corticosteroids (Ball 2000).

Manifestation of serum sickness following ALG and ATG

- fever
- rash
- joint pains
- arthralgia
- myalgia
- lassitude
- renal toxicity.

Response to ALG and ATG is usually seen within 3–6 months after commencing treatment. If no response is observed after 6 months, a second dose from a different source may be given. Approximately 50–60% of patients will respond to ALG. The marrow does not return entirely to normal and some degree of cytopenia may persist for several years without requiring support. Relapse occurs in 10–15% of responders. There are no criteria for determining response to ALG and it is recommended as a first-line treatment for candidates ineligible for BMT (Marsh & Gordon-Smith 1988, Gordon-Smith & Lewis 1990, Alter & Young 1993, Marsh et al 1999).

Case study 3.1

Kathleen was found to be anaemic when volunteering to donate blood. Her GP prescribed iron supplements. She noticed her motions were black, she bruised easily, suffered nosebleeds and was always tired. Five months later she presented with symptoms of anaemia and being generally unwell.

On examination, she was pale, with clinical symptoms of anaemia, no lymphadenopathy or hepatosplenomegaly. Her blood count was: Hb

Case study 3.1 – Cont'd

4.6 g/L, WCC 2×10^9/L, platelets 13×10^9/L. All other indices were within normal limits. A bone marrow examination showed hypoplasia with markedly decreased erythropoiesis. She was supported with blood, platelets and antimicrobials. Her siblings were HLA typed and her older sister was a perfect match. As Kathleen was well, immunosuppressive therapy using ALG was proposed. She received two courses three months apart and responded well, maintaining her blood counts with no support. She remained reasonably well for 5 years, when her blood counts began a downward trend with marrow hypocellularity. The decision to treat her by allogeneic BMT was made

and this was planned to occur within 3 months of relapse.

Her conditioning regimen was cyclophosphamide and total body irradiation. GvHD prophylaxis consisted of ciclosporin and methotrexate. She received healthy marrow from her sister following her conditioning and made a fairly uneventful recovery with minimal GvHD. Kathleen has recovered well and continues to be followed up at yearly intervals at the late effects clinic with minimal problems. Her current medications are Prempack C, penicillin and thyroxine.

Corticosteroids

Very high doses of corticosteroids have been used as an alternative to ALG. In some patients they can stimulate erythropoiesis and produce a trilineage response. Corticosteroids are administered intravenously, with a starting dose of 20 mg/kg/day for 3 days, gradually reducing over the next month. The response rate has been reported to be similar to that with ALG, and combination therapy using prednisolone and ciclosporin has produced responses such as a reduction in blood component requirements (Bacigalupo et al 1993). However, toxicity is high. Commonly observed toxicities include hypertension, hyperglycaemia, fluid retention and aseptic necrosis of the femur or humerus. The period of hospitalisation for patients receiving corticosteroids is often longer, due to masking of fevers and increased episodes of fungal infections (Bitencourt et al 1995, Young & Barrett 1995, Dokal 1996a, Ball 2000, Gordon-Smith & Marsh 2000).

Ciclosporin

Ciclosporin is an effective immunosuppressive agent used both as a first-line treatment of AA and as GvHD prophylaxis in BMT. It is a specific T-cell inhibitor that prevents the production of interleukin-2 and interferon while continuing to allow production of colony-stimulating factors (Kahan 1989). Initial reports of its use in the treatment of AA suggested a 50% response rate in individuals refractory to ALG (Hinterberger-Fischer et al 1989). The recommended oral dose is 12 mg/kg/day in adults and 5–10 mg/kg/day in children, in order to maintain adequate blood levels (Alter & Young 1993). These regimens require regular monitoring of blood levels. Toxicities are not insignificant and are mostly dose-related (Young & Barrett 1995, BCSH 2003).

Commonly reported side effects associated with ciclosporin

- hypertension
- seizures
- hirsutism
- immunodeficiency
- raised creatinine levels
- *Pneumocystis carinii* pneumonia.

Recently, combination therapy consisting of ALG, ATG and ciclosporin has been shown to produce useful haematological response in 75% of cases (Rosenfeld et al 1995). This response is enhanced if granulocyte-colony stimulating factor (G-CSF) is added to the above combination, with 82% of patients showing haematological reconstitution of the three main blood cell lines. This appears to be an alternative treatment for patients with severe AA who lack an HLA identical donor (Bacigalupo et al 1995, 2000b).

INHERITED OR FAMILIAL APLASTIC ANAEMIA

A number of inherited disorders are associated with AA. Among these, Fanconi's anaemia (FA) and dyskeratosis congenita (DC) are the most common (Young & Alter 1994, Dokal 1996a,b).

FANCONI'S ANAEMIA

Fanconi's anaemia was first described in 1927 in a family in which three brothers developed AA. The brothers also had microencephaly, abnormal skin pigmentation, internal strabismus and genital hypoplasia. Further families and cases were described and it was later suggested that the condition be named Fanconi's anaemia. Since 1982 more than 700 cases have been reported, in varying detail, to the International Fanconi Anaemia Registry (IFAR) at the Rockefeller Institute in the USA with males more commonly affected than females (ratio 2:1) (Auerbach et al 1989, Auerbach & Allen 1991).

Pathophysiology

Fanconi's anaemia (FA) is inherited as a recessive trait (e.g. resulting from the marrying of first cousins) and is often associated with other congenital abnormalities. Cells from patients characteristically show a high frequency of chromosomal breakage. These increased chromosomal abnormalities are thought to be caused by a defect in the processing of DNA repair, and underline the increased predisposition to malignancies seen in these patients (Gordon-Smith & Rutherford 1989, Dokal 1996a, 2000a).

The underlying defect in FA is unknown and the relationship between birth defects, haematopoietic failure, and the characteristic abnormally high frequency of spontaneous chromosomal breakage in this malignancy is elusive. The variability in expression of the disease makes firm diagnosis of FA on clinical grounds difficult and unreliable, and cytogenetic analysis is necessary to confirm diagnosis. The haematopoietic defect in FA is evident at the progenitor cell level: colonies derived from bone marrow CFU-GM, CFU-E, erythroid burst forming unit (BFU-E), as well as blood BFU-E, are all decreased in FA patients with AA. Within the last decade research has identified four FA genes that appear to be involved in a novel pathway important in maintaining chromosome stability. It is hoped that clarification of the functional role of these genes may help to tailor new treatments for individual patients (Alter & Young 1993, Garcia-Higuera et al 1999, Dokal 2003a).

Clinical features

The typical clinical features of FA, while characteristic, are not present in all patients. Children are usually of low birth weight at term and do not grow normally. Microcephaly, microphthalmia, broad nasal base and a small mouth and jaw give a classical appearance. The skin shows a general hyperpigmentation with increased patches of pigment (café-au-lait patches) and other areas of depigmentation. Internal strabismus is common. Males often have undescended testes and horseshoe or pelvic kidney are common. Skeletal abnormalities with hypoplastic veins may be present (Gordon-Smith & Rutherford 1989, Gordon-Smith & Lewis 1990, Dokal 2003a).

The blood count is usually normal at birth and common features such as anaemia, bruising or nosebleeds associated with bone marrow failure do not present until age 5–10 years. A low platelet count is usually the most common presenting haematological finding; anaemia then becomes apparent, granulocytes being the last affected cell line. In typical cases the bone marrow becomes hypoplastic with replacement of haematopoietic tissue by fat cells. There is progressive bone marrow failure, probably due to chromosomal instability, leading to progressive depletion of stem cells. Reduction in CFU-GM and BFU-E is evident prior to the occurrence of pancytopenia and there is a high incidence of acute leukaemic transformation in these children (Gordon-Smith & Lewis 1990, Alter & Young 1993, 1998, Young & Alter 1994, Joenje & Patel 2001). Presentation is usually in the first decade of life and patients die young from complications of bone marrow failure or leukaemia (Smith et al 1989, Dokal 1996a).

Treatment of Fanconi's anaemia

The treatment of FA remains the same as for acquired AA (see Fig 3.1). Specific treatment usually consists of blood and blood-component support; anabolic steroids, which are known to cause a number of side effects (Young & Barrett 1995); and BMT, which is now a well-established treatment for inherited AA and offers the only possibility of a cure (Gluckman et al 1995, Davis et al 1996, Guardiola et al 1998).

However, the poor results seen following non-sibling donor transplants suggest that alternative strategies are necessary. The identification of the FA genes has led to in-vitro gene transfer studies; however,

Figure 3.2
Treatment options in familial
aplastic anaemia (Fanconi's
anaemia and dyskeratosis
congenita)

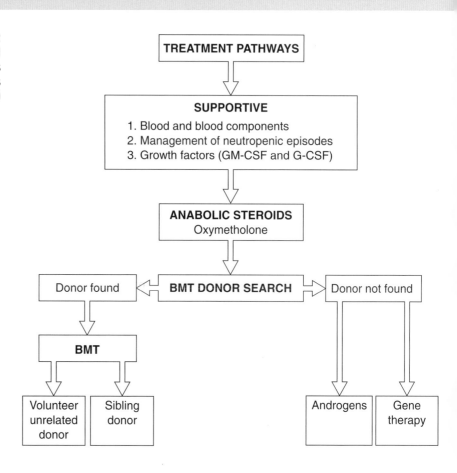

such research protocols are still in their infancy and currently being evaluated (Fu et al 1997). Treatment options in familial AA are shown in Figure 3.2.

DYSKERATOSIS CONGENITA

Dyskeratosis congenita (DC) is a rare inherited disorder characterised by reticulate skin pigmentation, mucosal leucoplakia and nail dystrophy. Aplasia occurs in 50% of cases. The disease presents usually within the first 10 years of life, and has a predisposition to malignancy (Drachtman & Alter 1992). Most patients die from complications of AA, pulmonary disease and malignancy (Sirinavin & Trowbridge 1975, Alter & Young 1993, Dokal 1996b, 2003b). In the majority of families the pattern of inheritance is compatible to an X-linked recessive trait and approximately 85% out of 200 published cases are male. DC shares many features with FA, for example, bone marrow failure, a predisposition to malignancy and chromosomal instability. In DC the precise pathophysiology of bone marrow failure remains unclear but it is possible that the chromosomal instability is caused by mutations in the nucleolar protein dyskeratin leading to progressive depletion of the stem cell pool, which manifests as pancytopenia towards the first decade of life or mid-teens (March et al 1992, Dokal 1996b, 2003b, Vulliamy et al 2002).

Clinical features

In DC, cutaneous features are the most common clinical feature. The reticulated skin pigmentation involves the face, neck, shoulders and trunk. Nail dystrophy (Plate 3) involves both hands and feet, and nail plates are small with longitudinal ridging. Leucoplakia involves the oral mucosa, but is also seen in the conjunctiva, and anal, urethral and genital mucosa (Alter & Young 1993, Dokal 1996b, 2000b). Characteristically, a number of other important features are also observed: these are shown in Box 3.2 (Chambers & Salinas 1982, Kelly & Stelling 1982, Brown et al 1993, Knight et al 1998).

Clinical manifestations often occur during childhood; skin and nail changes usually appear by the age of 10 years, mucosal leucoplakia later, and by mid-teens serious progressive bone marrow failure is seen in 50% of affected individuals; 10% develop a malignancy. Seventy per cent of deaths are related to bone marrow failure and 30% are due to bleeding or opportunist infections such as CMV. Mean age at death is approximately 30 years (Forni et al 1993, Dokal 1996b, 2000b).

Treatment for DC

Treatment for patients with DC is similar to that in FA and is currently unsatisfactory. For those presenting with bone marrow failure, anabolic steroids and growth factors granulocyte-monocyte-colony stimulating factor (GM-CSF) and G-CSF may provide transient improvement in marrow function (Oehler et al 1994). BMT has been used successfully

---

Box 3.2 Abnormalities seen in dyskeratosis congenita (adapted from Drachtman & Alter 1995)

Part of body affected	Abnormality
Skin	Pigmentation of face, neck, shoulders and trunk
Nails	Dystrophy involving hands and feet
Eyes	Conjunctivitis, blepharitis, glaucoma, cataracts, strabismus, loss of eyelashes, optic nerve dystrophy
Teeth	Dental decay, early loss of teeth
Tongue	Leucoplakia
Hair	Early hair loss
Skeleton	Osteoporosis, fractures, aseptic necrosis, scoliosis and mandibular hypoplasia, short stature
Genitourinary tract	Hypoplastic testes, phimosis, urethral stenosis, and horseshoe kidney
Gastrointestinal tract	Oesophageal strictures, hepatomegaly, cirrhosis of liver

in only a few children with DC. Unfortunately, there is a high incidence of early and late fatality, mainly due to interstitial pulmonary complications (Dokal 1996b, Yabe et al 1997, Lau et al 1999). Therefore, even with an identical HLA-matched sibling donor, the results are poor; thus, there is a great need to develop alternative treatment strategies such as gene therapy. DC patients may be good candidates for gene therapy, as it is a single-gene disorder and the main cause of mortality relates to bone marrow failure with no satisfactory treatment (Dokal 1996a, 2003b).

SPECIFIC NURSING ISSUES

Nursing management of patients with AA requires expert skills and knowledge. The nurse plays an active role by providing appropriate therapeutic psychosocial and supportive care. Treatment is usually delivered in specialist centres and nurses must be well versed in potential and expected complications such as life-threatening infections and haemorrhage (BCSH 1995, 2003).

While the development of day care units and high-quality outpatient services enables supportive treatment to be administered, hospitalisation becomes necessary in neutropenic episodes, when ALG is initiated and for BMT.

Information, education and support of the patient and family are important aspects of care (Walker et al 1994, Whedon & Wujcik 1997). Nurses must be able to provide information on support for both patient and carers outwith the hospital environment such as AA support groups. Provision of information and education should be ongoing from diagnosis and encompassed in the individual's care plan. Equally important is nurse education, with emphasis on research-based practice, to ensure the delivery of quality care to this group of patients

REFLECTION POINT

Nursing challenges in this field are numerous and offer a wide range of issues for nursing research. Consider the importance of research-based practice. What areas would you like to see further researched? Consider how you and your colleagues could undertake a research project.

CONCLUSION

In spite of improved means of support and treatment and advances in nursing care, AA remains a devastating and frustrating disease from which a proportion of patients still die. For patients with severe AA, BMT from a sibling donor is the treatment of choice. For those lacking donors, treatment is still unsatisfactory. Despite years of research the primary pathology remains unclear, highlighting the need for new research strategies. However, as acquired AA and FA have several features in common, new research findings such as the recent identification and clarification of the functional role of the FA genes may indicate gene therapy as a viable treatment option for AA, and further studies may lead to a better understanding of the pathophysiology of acquired AA and the possibility of new treatment options tailored to the individual.

DISCUSSION QUESTIONS

1. How would you explain the main criticisms, difficulties and limitations of the differing treatment approaches to a more junior nurse?

2. Assess critically your current patient education programme. Are there any improvements which could be made to this programme?

3. What physical, emotional and psychosocial problems may the individual with aplastic anaemia and their significant others experience?

4. What support services available both within and outwith your own organisation could be employed to minimise distress and enhance individuals' coping mechanisms?

References

Alter B P, Young N S 1993 The bone marrow failure syndromes. In: Nathan D G, Oski F A (eds) Bone marrow failures in infancy and childhood. W B Saunders, Philadelphia, p 216–316

Alter B P, Young N S 1998 The bone marrow failure syndromes. In: Nathan D G, Oski F A (eds) Bone marrow failures in infancy and childhood, 2nd edn. W B Saunders, Philadelphia, pp 237–335

Auerbach A D, Allen R G 1991 Leukaemia and preleukaemia in Fanconi anaemia patients: a review of the literature and report of the International Fanconi Registry. Cancer Genetics and Cytogenetics 51:1–12

Auerbach A D, Rogatko A, Schroeder-Kurth T M 1989 International Fanconi Register First Report. In: Schroeder-Kurth T M, Auerbach A D, Obe G (eds) Fanconi's anaemia: clinical, cytogenetic and experimental aspects. Springer-Verlag, Heidelberg

Bacigalupo A 1989 Treatment of severe aplastic anaemia. Baillière's Clinical Haematology 2(1):19–35

Bacigalupo A, Brocoiag Acress W, Caroluneto M et al 1995 Antilymphocyte globulin, ciclosporin, granulocyte colony stimulating factor in patients with acquired aplastic anaemia. A pilot study of the EBMT SAA Working Party. Blood 85:1348–1353

Bacigalupo A, Brand R, Oneto R, Bruno B, Socie G 2000a Treatment of acquired severe aplastic anaemia BMT compared with immunosuppressive therapy. The European group for blood and marrow transplantation experience. Seminars in Haematology 37:69–80

Bacigalupo A, Bruno B, Saraccop C 2000b Antilymphocytic globulin, ciclosporin, prednisolone and GCSF for severe aplastic anaemia: an update of the GITMO/EBMT study on 100 patients. Blood 95:1931–1934

Bacigalupo A, Chaple M, Hows J, Van Lint E T, Korthof E, Comotti B 1993 Treatment of aplastic anaemia with antilymphocytic globulin and methylprednisolone with or without androgens: a randomized study from the EBMT SAA Working Party. British Journal of Haematology 83:145–151

Ball S E 2000 The modern management of severe aplastic anaemia. British Journal of Haematology 110:41–43

Baumelou E, Guiguet M, Mary Y M and the French cooperative group for epidemiology study of aplastic anaemia 1993 Epidemiology of aplastic anaemia in France: a case control study. Medical history and medication use. Blood 81:1471–1478

Bielory L, Gascon P, Lawlet T, Nienhuis A W, Young N S, Frank M 1988 Human serum sickness. A prospective clinical analysis of 35 patients treated with equine antithymocyte globulin for bone marrow failure. Medicine 67:40–57

Bitencourt M A, Medeiroe C R, Zanis-Neto J et al 1995 Prednisolone and ciclosporin for severe acquired aplastic anaemia. 101 cases treated in a single institution. Blood 86(Suppl. 1):476a(abstr)

British Committee for Standards in Haematology 2003 Guidelines for the diagnosis and management of acquired aplastic anaemia British Journal of Haematology 123:782–801

British Committee for Standards in Haematology Clinical Haematology Task Force 1995 Guidelines on the provision of facilities for care of adult patients with haematological malignancies (including leukaemia and lymphoma and severe bone marrow failure). Clinical and Laboratory Haematology 17(1):3–10

Brown K E, Kelly T E, Myers B M 1993 Gastro-intestinal involvement in a woman with dyskeratosis congenita. Digestive Diseases and Sciences 38:181–184

Camitta B M, Rapeport J M, Parkman R, Nathan D G 1975 Selection of patients for bone marrow transplantation in severe aplastic anaemia. Blood 45: 355–363

Camitta B M, Storb R, Thomas E D 1982 Aplastic anaemia: pathogenesis, diagnosis, treatment and progress. New England Journal of Medicine 306:645–652

Chambers J K, Salinas C F 1982 Ocular findings in dyskeratosis congenita. Birth Defects 18:167–174

Davis S M, Khan S, Wagner J E et al 1996 Unrelated bone marrow transplantation for Fanconi's anaemia. Bone Marrow Transplantation 17:43–47

Dokal I 1996a Severe aplastic anaemia including Fanconi's anaemia and dyskeratosis congenita. Current Opinion in Haematology 3:453–460

Dokal I 1996b Dyskeratosis congenita: an inherited bone marrow failure syndrome. British Journal of Haematology 92:775–779

Dokal I 2000a The genetics of Fanconi's anaemia. Baillière's Clinical Haematology 13(3):407–425

Dokal I 2000b Dyskeratosis congenita in all its forms British Journal of Haematology 110:768–799

Dokal I 2001 Management of aplastic anaemia. Post Graduate Doctor Caribbean 17(4):110–115

Dokal I 2003a Inherited aplastic anaemia. The Haematology Journal 4:3–9

Dokal I 2003b Dyskeratosis congenita: its link to telomerase and aplastic anaemia. Blood Reviews 17:217–225

Drachtman R A, Alter B P 1992 Dyskeratosis congenita clinical and genetic heterogeneity. American Journal of Paediatric Haematology/Oncology 14:297–304

Drachtman R A, Alter B P 1995 Dyskeratosis congenita. Dermatology Clinics 13:33–39

Ehrlich P I 1888 In: Nathan D G, Oski F A (eds) 1993 Bone marrow failures in infancy and childhood. W B Saunders, Philadelphia

Fleming L E, Timmeny W 1993 Aplastic anaemia and pesticides: an etiologic association Occupational Medicine 35:1106–1116

Forni G L, Melevendi C, Jappelli S, Rasore-Quadino A 1993 Dyskeratosis congenita unusual presenting features within a kindred. Paediatric Haematology and Oncology 10:145–149

Fu K L, Ten Foe J R, Joenje H et al 1997 Functional correction of Fanconi anaemia group A hematopoietic cells by retroviral gene transfer. Blood 90:3296–3303

Gale R P 1987 The role of bone marrow transplantation following nuclear accidents. Bone Marrow Transplantation 2:1–6

Gallicchio V S, Casale G P, Watts T 1987 T inhibition of human bone marrow-derived stem cell colony formation (CFU-E, BFU-E and CFU-GM) following in vitro exposure to organophosphates. Experimental Haematology 15:1099–2007

Garcia-Higuera I, Kuang Y, D'Andrea A D 1999 The molecular and cellular biology of Fanconi's anaemia. Current Opinion in Haematology 2:83–88

Gluckman E, Auerbach A D, Horwitz M M et al 1995 Bone marrow transplantation for Fanconi's anaemia. Blood 96:2856–2862

Gordon-Smith E C 1989 Aplastic anaemia aetiology and clinical features. Baillière's Clinical Haematology 2(1):1–18

Gordon-Smith E C , Rutherford T R 1989 Fanconi's anaemia constitutional familial aplastic anaemia. Baillière's Clinical Haematology 2(1):139–152

Gordon-Smith E C, Lewis S M 1990 Aplastic anaemia and other types of bone marrow failure. In: Hoffbrand V V, Lewis S M (eds) Post-graduate haematology. Heinemann Medical Books, London, pp 83–120

Gordon-Smith E C. Marsh J 2000 Management of acquired aplastic anaemia. Reviews in Clinical Experimental Haematology 4:260–280

Guardiola P, Socie G, Pasquinin R et al 1998 Allogeneic stem cell transplantation for Fanconi Anaemia. Severe Aplastic Anaemia Working Party of the EBMT and EUFAR. European Group for Blood and Marrow Transplantation. Bone Marrow Transplantation 21(Suppl 2):S24–27

Hagler L, Pastore B, Bergin J J, Wresch M R 1975 Aplastic anaemia following viral hepatitis. Reports of two fatal cases and literature review. Medicine (Baltimore) 54:139–163

Heimpel H 2000 Epidemiology and aetiology of aplastic anaemia. In: Schrezenmeier H, Bacigalupo A (eds) Aplastic anaemia pathophysiology and treatment. Cambridge University Press, Cambridge, pp 97–116

Heimpel H, Heit W 1980 Drug-induced aplastic anaemia clinical aspects. Clinics in Haematology 9:641–662

Hinterberger-Fischer F M, Hocker P, Lechner K, Seewann H, Hinterberger W 1989 Oral ciclosporin A is effective treatment for untreated and also for previous immunosuppressed patients with severe bone marrow failure. European Journal of Haematology 43:136–142

Hoffbrand V, Pettit J E, Moss P A 2001 Essential haematology, 4th edn. Blackwell Scientific Publications, Oxford

Hows J, Bacigalupo A, Downis T, Brand R 1996 Alternative donor (ALT/BMT) for SAA in Europe. Blood 86(Suppl 1):290A

International Agranulocytosis and Aplastic Anaemia Study 1986 Risks of aplastic anaemia. A first report of their relation to drug use with special reference to analgesics. Journal of the American Medical Association 256:1749–1759

Jick H 1977 The discovery of drug-induced illness. New England Journal of Medicine 296:481–485

Joenje H, Patel J K 2001 The emerging genetic and molecular basis of Fanconi's anaemia. National Reviews in Genetics 2:446–457

Kahan B D 1989 Ciclosporin. New England Journal of Medicine 321:1725–1738

Kelly T E, Stelling C B 1982 Dyskeratosis congenita: radiological features. Paediatric Radiology 12:31–36

Kirshbaum J D, Matsuo T, Sato K, Ichimura M, Tsuchimoto T, Ishimura T 1971 A study of aplastic anaemia in an autopsy series with special reference to atomic bomb survivors in Hiroshima and Nagasaki. Blood 38(1):17–26

Knight S, Vulliamy T, Copplestone A 1998 Dyskeratosis congenital registry identification of new features of DC. British Journal of Haematology 103:990–996

Knospe Y M, Crosby Y M 1971 A disorder of the bone marrow sinusoidal microcirculation rather than stem cell failure. Lancet 1:20–25

Kurtzman G, Young N 1989 Viruses and bone marrow failure. Baillière's Clinical Haematology 2(1):51–67

Lau Y L, Ha Sy, Chan C 1999 Bone marrow transplant for dyskeratosis congenita. British Journal of Haematology 105:571

Lewis S M 1965 Course and prognosis in aplastic anaemia. British Medical Journal 1:1027–1030

Locasciulli A, Vant Veer L, Bacigalupo A et al 1990 Treatment with marrow transplantation or immunosuppression of childhood acquired aplastic anaemia. A report from the EBMT SAA Working Party. Bone Marrow Transplantation 6:211–217

Locatelli F, Bruno B, Zecca M 2000 Ciclosporin A and short term methotrexate versus ciclosporin A as GVHD prophylaxis in patients with severe aplastic anaemia given allogeneic bone marrow transplantation from an HLA identical sibling. Results of the GITMO/EBMT randomized trial. Blood 96:1690–1697

Lopez-Karpovitch X, Zarzosa M E, Cardenas M R, Piedras J 1989 Changes in peripheral blood mononuclear cell subpopulations during antithymocyte globulin therapy in aplastic anaemia. Acta Haematologica 81:176–180

March C W, Will A J, Hows J H et al 1992 Stem cell origin of the haematopoietic defect in dyskeratosis congenita. Blood 79:3138–3144

Marin P 2000 Clinical presentation natural course and prognostic factors. In: Schrezenmeier H, Bacigalupo A (eds) Aplastic anaemia: pathophysiology and treatment. Cambridge University Press, Cambridge, pp 117–133

Marsh J C, Gordon-Smith E C 1988 The role of antilymphocyte globulin in the treatment of chronic acquired bone marrow failure. Blood Reviews 2(4):141–148

Marsh J, Schrezenmeier H, Marin P, Liham O, Ljungman P, McCann S 1999 A prospective randomized multicentre study comparing ciclosporin alone versus the combination of antilymphocytic globulin and ciclosporin for treatment of patients with non-severe aplastic anaemia. A report from the European Blood and Marrow Transplant severe aplastic working party. Blood 93:2191–2195

Nagro T, Maver A M 1969 Concordance for drug-induced aplastic anaemia in identical twins. New England Journal of Medicine 281:11–17

Nissen-Druey C 1989 Pathophysiology of aplastic anaemia. Baillière's Clinical Haematology, 2(1):37–39

Oehler L, Reiter E, Freidl J et al 1994 Effective stimulation of neutrophils with RH G-CSF in dyskeratosis congenita. Annals of Haematology 69:325–327

Paquetto A T, Tobynl N, Frane M et al 1995 Long-term outcome of aplastic anaemia in adults treated with antilymphocyte globulin comparison with bone marrow transplantation. Blood 85:283–290

Passweg J R, Socie G, Hinterberger W, Bacigalupo A, Biggs J, Camitta B 1997 Bone marrow transplantation for severe aplastic anaemia: has outcome improved? Blood 90:858–864

Rosenfeld S J, Kimball J, Vining D, Young N S 1995 Intensive immunosuppression with antithymocyte globulin and ciclosporin as treatment for severe aplastic anaemia. Blood 85:3058–3065

Sirinavin C, Trowbridge A A 1975 Dyskeratosis congenita, clinical features and genetic aspects. Report of a family and review of the literature. Journal of Medical Genetics 12:339–354

Smith M T 1996 Overview of benzene-induced aplastic anaemia European Journal of Haematology 57(Suppl):107–111

Smith S, Marx N W, Jordon C J, Van Niekerk C H 1989 Clinical aspects of a cluster of 42 patients in South Africa with Fanconi's anaemia. In: Schreoder-Kurth T M, Auerbach A, Obe G (eds) Fanconi anaemia: clinical, cytogenetic and experimental aspects. Springer-Verlag, Heidelberg

Storb R, Thomas E D, Weiden P L et al 1974 Allogeneic marrow grafting for treatment of aplastic anaemia. Blood 43:157–180

Sullivan K M, Witherspoon R P 1988 Long-term results of allogeneic bone marrow transplantation. Transplant Proceedings 21:2926–2928

Szklo M, Sensenbrenner L, Markowitz J, Weida S, Warm S, Linett M 1985 Incidence of aplastic anaemia in metropolitan Baltimore, a population based study. Blood 66:115–119

Vulliamy T, Marrone A, Dokal I, Mason P 2002 Association between aplastic anaemia and mutations in telomerase RNA. Lancet 359:2168–2170

Walker F, Roethke S K, Martin G 1994 An overview of the rationale, process and nursing implications of peripheral blood stem cell transplantation. Cancer Nursing 17(2):141–148

Whedon M B, Wujcik D 1997 Blood and marrow stem cell transplantation. Principles, practice and nursing insights, 2nd edn. Jones and Bartlett, Boston

Wilholm B-E, Kelly J, Kaufmann D et al 1998 Relation of aplastic anaemia to use of chloramphenicol eye drops in two international case studies. British Medical Journal 316:666

Yabe M, Yabe H, Hattori J et al 1997 Fatal interstitial pulmonary disease in a patient with dyskeratosis congenita after allogeneic bone marrow transplantation. Bone Marrow Transplantation 19:389–392

Yin S, Li Y, Tian F, Jin C 1987 Occupational exposure to benzene in China. British Journal of Industrial Medicine 44:192–195

Yin S, Hayes R, Linet M, Li G, Domeseci M, Travis L, Tian F 1996 An expanded cohort study of cancer among benzene-exposed workers in China. Environmental Health Perspectives 104(Suppl 6):1339–1341

Young N, Barrett J A 1995 The treatment of severe acquired aplastic anaemia. Blood 85(12):3367–3377

Young N S 2000 The aetiology of acquired aplastic anaemia. Reviews in Clinical Experimental Haematology 4:236–259

Young N S, Alter B P 1994 Aplastic anaemia, acquired and inherited. W B Saunders, Philadelphia

Young N S, Issaragrasil S 1986 Aplastic anaemia in the orient. British Journal of Haematology 62:1–6

Young N S, Speck B 1984 Antithymocyte and antilymphocyte globulins: clinical trials and mechanism of action. In: Young N S, Levine A, Humphries R K (eds) Aplastic anaemia stem cell biology and advances in treatment. Alan R Liss, New York, pp 221–226

Yunis A A, Miller A M, Salem Z, Arimura G K 1980 Chloramphenicol toxicity, pathogenic mechanisms and the role of p-NO2 in aplastic anaemia. Clinical Toxicology 17(3):359–373

Further reading

Ball S E 2000 The modern management of severe aplastic anaemia. British Journal of Haematology 110:41–43
Excellent overview for disease management in this group of patients.

British Committee for Standards in Haematology 2003 Guidelines for the diagnosis and management of acquired aplastic anaemia. British Journal of Haematology 123:782–801
Recently updated guidelines produced by specialists in the field. Excellently written in simple, easily understood language. Well referenced.

Dokal I 2003a Inherited aplastic anaemia. The Haematology Journal 4:3–9
This review, though somewhat scientific, highlights recent advances in the genetics of AA with a view to unravelling the pathophysiology and helping with accurate diagnosis and treatment.

Dokal I 2003b Dyskeratosis congenital: its link to telomerase and aplastic anaemia. Blood Reviews 17:217–225
This article helps to increase understanding of the possible link of AA to dyskeratosis congenita. Clear description of normal haemopoiesis and how it becomes defective in patients presenting with AA.

Gordon-Smith E C (ed) 1989 Aplastic anaemia. Baillière's Clinical Haematology 2(1). Baillière Tindall, London
Several chapters in this are written by the editor, who is a leader in the field of AA. A very wel-written book with short, concise chapters covering all aspects of aplastic anaemia with contributions by different professionals. A small, easily read and understood book.

Hoffbrand V, Pettit J E, Moss P A 2001 Essential haematology, 4th edn. Blackwell Scientific Publications, Oxford
A good handbook for nurses.

Chapter 4

The leukaemias

Joanne Atkinson and Carol Richardson

KEY POINTS
- Leukaemia is an unregulated proliferation of immature blood cells.
- There are a number of different subtypes of leukaemia.
- Advances in leukaemia treatment have improved the chance of potential cure.
- Specialist care is required to support the patient and their family.

INTRODUCTION

The leukaemias are a heterogeneous group of malignant blood disorders, a type of cancer caused by the unregulated proliferation of immature blood cells. Malignant cells arise as a result of abnormal blood cell maturation at an early stage of differentiation. Howard &

Figure 4.1
The origin of white blood cells
in relation to the major types
of leukaemia (originally
published in Leukaemia Stats
CRUK 2003; reproduced with
permission).

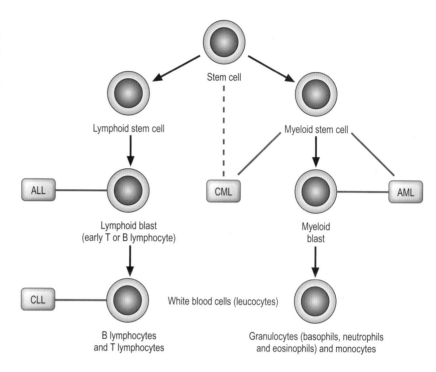

Hamilton (2002) suggest that these leukaemic cells are often considered to be fast growing and aggressive, when in fact this is an over-simplification. The cell cycle of leukaemic cells is in fact slower than that of normal cells hence the repopulation of the bone marrow with normal haematopoietic cells following cytotoxic therapy. However leukaemic cells are indifferent to normal biological feedback signals and therefore over-proliferate and overpopulate the bone marrow, inhibiting the function of normal haematopoietic cells, resulting in marrow failure and, if untreated, death.

The four most common types of leukaemia are:

- acute myeloid leukaemia (AML)
- acute lymphoblastic leukaemia (ALL)
- chronic myeloid leukaemia (CML)
- chronic lymphoblastic leukaemia (CLL).

Figure 4.1 illustrates a simplified version of the origin of white blood cells in relation to the major types of leukaemia (Cancer Research UK (CRUK) 2003).

EPIDEMIOLOGY

The various types of leukaemia are substantially different in their cellular origin and clinical behaviour. It is important to recognise this when interpreting statistics on incidence and mortality of leukaemia as a set of diseases. Leukaemia represents 2.5% of all cancers in the United Kingdom with around 6647 cases diagnosed in 1999 (Forman et al 2003). Overall leukaemia is slightly more common in men than women, with a male to female incidence ratio of 1.3:1.0. Leukaemias represent the ninth most common malignancy in men with 3700 cases diagnosed in 1999 and the twelfth most common malignancy in women with 2950 new cases diagnosed in 1999 (Forman et al 2003).

Leukaemia is the commonest cancer in children (0–14 years), accounting for almost one-third of all malignancies. Around 370 cases are diagnosed each year in the UK, accounting for around 25% of childhood malignancies. Most of the childhood leukaemias are of the acute lymphoblastic type, with the highest incidence occurring in the 0–4 years age group (Cancer Research Campaign (CRC) 1995, CRUK 2003).

The lifetime risk of developing leukaemia is 1:94 for males and 1:127 for females (Quinn et al 2000). The prevalence of all leukaemias in the UK is estimated at 10,830 for males and 9350 for females (Forman et al 2003). Incidence trends in the UK and other developed countries are either stable or increasing slowly. It can be argued that some of the increase may be due to better diagnostic tools (especially in the elderly) and better registration.

There are some interesting observations to be made when considering the incidence of leukaemia in the UK. Data suggest that the disease incidence is marginally higher in more affluent societal groups (Quinn et al 2001). However, there is little if any geographical variation across the UK. This is echoed when analysing data from an international perspective as geographical variation for leukaemia is less marked than for any other cancer. When geographical variation is evident it can be accounted for by considering proven and suspected risk factors (Groves et al 1995, Petridou & Trichopoulos 2002), e.g. the exposure of the individual to ionising radiation in certain geographical areas.

The mortality rate in children has halved between the 1950s and the present day (CRC 1995). However, in adults the picture is not as favourable. In 1992 there were around 4000 deaths from all types of leukaemia in the UK (CRC 1995). For adults there has been little variation in these trends, in fact CRUK (2003) identifies that the mortality rate for all leukaemias remains at 4000. Such statistics must be interpreted with caution as mortality trends rely heavily on diagnosis and death certification, both of which have improved in accuracy over the past 10 years.

AETIOLOGY

Many patients with leukaemia have no recognisable aetiological factors; this makes it difficult to consider prevention and early detection, which is contrary to the situation in some solid tumours where health promotion is a key issue for practitioners. However, there is a body of knowledge available that identifies known and suspected aetiological factors.

GENETIC PREDISPOSITION

Most cases of leukaemia are sporadic. Leukaemic cells can carry a variety of abnormalities, including chromosomal gain or loss or structural changes, such as deletions, duplications, inversions and translocations. Some chromosomal rearrangements are extremely complex; however, it is essential that any cytogenetic rearrangements are established as they play an important part in diagnosis, prognosis and treatment choice (National Institute for Clinical Excellence (NICE) 2002). Chromosomal rearrangements can activate proto-oncogenes or inactivate tumour suppressor genes, leading to the loss of growth control (proliferation) in blood cell precursors. Chromosomal changes have been a key area of leukaemia research since the discovery of the Philadelphia chromosome (resulting from a rearrangement between chromosome 9 and 22) in chronic myeloid leukaemia.

In adults familial clustering has been observed in all types of leukaemia. Some clustering might be explained by low-risk inherited gene variants although a small proportion of leukaemias involve a strong inherited susceptibility (Houlston et al 2002, Wiley et al 2002). Furthermore, some genetically determined disorders, for example Down's syndrome, carry a predisposition towards developing leukaemia (Horwitz 1997). Other syndromes that have demonstrated such a predisposition are Bloom's syndrome, Fanconi's anaemia and diseases such as ataxia telangiectasia. Although such predispositions account for only a small number of leukaemia cases, they can offer valuable insights into its pathophysiology (Bratt-Wyton 2000).

RADIATION

There is conclusive evidence that links exposure to ionising radiation to the development of leukaemia. Marked increased incidence has been found in survivors of the atomic bombs in Japan and survivors of the Chernobyl nuclear disaster. However, there are still active debates about the risk of exposure to low levels of radiation.

Numerous epidemiological studies have been undertaken to establish causal links between nuclear power stations and an increase in leukaemia incidence. Early studies suggested an increase in the incidence of childhood leukaemia around Seascale, which lies adjacent to the Sellafield nuclear facility in Cumbria (Gardner et al 1990, Drapper et al 1993). Although the causal link remains inconclusive, some authors suggest the increase in incidence may be due to population mixing in the area rather than the nuclear installations (Kinlen et al 1995, Dickinson & Parker 2002).

Electromagnetic fields and low-dose radiation have also been identified as potential causes of leukaemia; however, there is much conflicting information (Boyle et al 2003). Results are inconclusive because overall the empirical evidence is weak – this is an area identified for intensive research (World Health Organization (WHO) 2003).

CHEMICALS

Exposure to certain types of chemicals has been proven to increase the incidence of leukaemia. Exposure to benzene, a hydrocarbon used commonly in the petrochemical industry, is a known risk factor. Employees in the painting, printing and chemical manufacturing industries are also at risk to exposure, as shown in a number of studies (Hayes et al 1997). As a result of these findings occupational exposure to benzene in the UK is very strictly regulated.

Agricultural chemicals have been linked with an increase in incidence in some types of leukaemia and further studies are suggested in this area (Morrison et al 1992).

The smoke from cigarettes can be considered as a chemical toxin and there is a causal relationship between cigarette smoking and the incidence of myeloid leukaemia where there has been as much as a two-fold increase in incidence reported (Kane et al 1999).

CHEMOTHERAPY AND RADIATION THERAPY

Various chemotherapy agents have been proven to increase the risk of secondary acute myeloid leukaemia. This is especially true of the alkylating agents such as busulphan and cyclophosphamide. The risk is greater with combination chemotherapy and radiation therapy (Howard & Hamilton 2002).

VIRUSES AND INFECTIONS

Although no causative agent has been identified, there is evidence that infection has a role in the aetiology of leukaemia in children. Migration of populations and population mixing has been identified in some studies to increase the risk of childhood leukaemia (Kinlen et al 1995). On the contrary, there is some evidence to suggest that lack of exposure to infections in infancy is responsible for an abnormal response to common infections when the exposure occurs later in childhood (Greaves 2002).

Viruses are known to be the main cause of leukaemia in animals; however, in humans the only well-proven association is with the human T-cell leukaemia virus (HTLV1), this is linked to a rare form of adult leukaemia known as adult T-cell leukaemia/lymphoma. This virus is endemic in southwest Japan, the Caribbean and some parts of Africa.

THE ACUTE LEUKAEMIAS

In the past 40 years advances in the treatment of acute leukaemia have improved the chance of potential cure. This may largely be a result of clinical trials (a pivotal part of haematology practice) and the development and continued improvements in bone marrow transplantation. However, perhaps some of the greatest strides have been in the supportive therapy given to very dependent patients in order to preserve quality of life. The specialist nature of supportive care requires insight and knowledge not only into disease processes, but also appropriate therapeutic interventions and their impact.

Differentiation between acute myeloid leukaemia (AML) and acute lymphoblastic leukaemia (ALL) is essential because treatment and prognosis differ. The basic physiological knowledge that underpins practice in this area is that of haematopoiesis, commonly known as the formation of blood (see Chapter 1). This group of patients is very vulnerable and requires expert and intensive care. Practitioners should be cognisant of the impact an altered blood picture has on the patient as a result of the disease process and treatment. This is essential knowledge on which to base care delivery and appropriate patient assessment. All practitioners should demonstrate a clear understanding of the dynamics of haematopoiesis in order to facilitate quality care delivery and adequately support the patient and their family (Atkinson 2004).

ACUTE MYELOID LEUKAEMIA

Acute myeloid leukaemia (AML) is rare in childhood and the incidence increases with age. Cases may present as de novo or secondary to other predisposing factors, for example myelodysplastic syndrome and previous chemotherapy. Survival statistics in AML should not be considered in isolation from the patient, there are many different perspectives to be examined and individual prognostic factors are an essential part of this process. Morphological and cytochemical analysis of the blood and bone marrow from patients with AML allows categorisation of the disease into subtypes; this is the most important factor in assigning the appropriate therapy and predicting outcome (Table 4.1).

Clinical features

Patients with AML usually present with symptoms generally associated with bone marrow failure. Infections resulting from neutropenia are common and may arise from bacteria, fungi or viruses. An abnormally low platelet count (thrombocytopenia) can result in purpuric rashes, spontaneous bruising, menorrhagia, gingival bleeding and epistaxis. Bleeding may be life-threatening (see Chapter 16). The patient with AML may be anaemic presenting with pallor and lethargy. In practice there is little uniformity in presentation (Howard & Hamilton 2002). Some patients are remarkably asymptomatic whilst others are seriously ill. Tissue infiltration by leukaemic cells and clotting problems may occur in any case of AML but are characteristic of specific French-American-British (FAB) subtypes.

Classification

AML has historically been classified into subtypes using the FAB system (Table 4.1). However, an increasing recognition of the need to consider

Table 4.1
French–American–British
(FAB) classification system

Leukaemia	Incidence	Chromosomal abnormalities	Specific clinical features
M0 (Undifferentiated)	5%		Poorer prognosis.
M1 (Minimal myeloid differentiation)	15%	Inversion (Inv) (3)	
M2	25%	Translocation (t) (8:21)	Younger adults favourable prognosis with t(8:21).
M3 (Acute promyelocytic leukaemia APML)	10%	t(15:17)	Younger adults. Best prognosis. Disseminated intravascular coagulation (DIC) common.
M4 (Acute myelomonocytic leukaemia)	25%		Similar to M1 and M2 but more frequent extra-medullary disease.
M4 eo (as above with eosinophilia)		Inv (16) and other 16 abnormalities	As M4. Good prognosis.
M5 (Acute monocytic leukaemia AMOL)	10%	Abnormal 11 Q23	Poorer prognosis – older adults, extra-medullary involvement common.
M6 (Erythroid leukaemia)	5%	Deletion (Del) 5 Del 7	Poorer prognosis in older adults, may have prolonged onset period.
M7 (Acute megakaryoblastic leukaemia)	10%	Occasional Inv 3, t(3:3) Trisomy21: t(9:22): t(1:22) (In infants)	Poor prognosis, high blood blast counts and organ infiltration are rare. Markedly elevated serum lactate dehydrogenase levels. Marrow aspirates are usually dry taps, because of myelofibrosis.

genetic events in the classification of all haemopoietic and lymphoid malignancies has resulted in the development of the World Health Organization classification system (Jaffe et al 2001), which is superceding the FAB classification system in AML. The WHO classification incorporates and interrelates morphology, cytogenetics, molecular genetics and immunologic markers in an attempt to structure a classification that is universally applicable and prognostically relevant. The WHO histological classification of acute myeloid leukaemia identifies four major classification categories:

1. Acute myeloid leukaemia with recurrent genetic abnormalities
2. Acute myeloid leukaemia with multilineage dysplasia
3. Acute myeloid leukaemia, therapy related
4. Acute myeloid leukaemia not otherwise categorised.

These categories are further broken down to acknowledge the importance of factors that predict the biology of the leukaemic process, some cytogenetic predispositions and specific molecular ramifications that predict response to therapy (Jaffe et al 2001).

Diagnosis

A diagnosis of AML may be suspected due to a combination of clinical features and blood tests. Diagnosis depends on a logical sequence of tests. Peripheral blood count and film may demonstrate an elevated white cell count but equally it may also be normal and low. Anaemia and thrombocytopenia may also be demonstrated and usually leukaemic blast cells (primitive haemopoietic cells) are present.

Examination of the bone marrow will confirm diagnosis; this will include cell morphology, cytochemical, immunological and cytogenetic phenotyping in order to confirm the type, subtype and stage of the disease. Bone marrow samples are usually taken from the posterior iliac crest and it is usual to take a core of bone (a trephine biopsy) in addition to aspirating marrow. The trephine biopsy is particularly useful in the case of a 'dry tap' where no marrow can be sucked out, or a 'blood tap' where a sample of blood is sucked out (Spence & Johnston 2001).

Treatment

The treatment for AML is cytotoxic therapy. The first objective of treatment is to achieve a complete remission (CR), defined as less than 5% blasts in a normacellular bone marrow (Howard & Hamilton 2002). Given that the blood count is frequently abnormal at the start of antileukaemic treatment, the two to three weeks after treatment can be a very stormy time as the systemic therapy impacts upon the patient's bone marrow. Patients are vulnerable to infection and frequently develop septicaemia and bleeding. Initial chemotherapy is known as the induction phase; it is administered in pulses allowing time for recovery. There are several pulses of chemotherapy in the induction phase after which time a sequence of chemotherapy is given known as the consolidation phase (see Chapter 9). Treatment lasts for several months.

The impact of treatment cannot be under-estimated. Patients will often be admitted for extended periods of time and will require intensive supportive care and isolation in order to protect against catastrophic infection. Nurses should also never under-estimate the impact that the whole experience has on the patient's family who throughout this period will require support, information and reassurance (see Chapter 24).

Chemotherapy regimens are constantly changing and at diagnosis most patients will be entered into a clinical trial. Information gained from clinical trials contributes to the continuing improvement of treatment for future patients with AML whilst also ensuring that patients receive equitable treatment. At any point patients can opt to withdraw from a trial without prejudice. The consultant is also free to give alternative

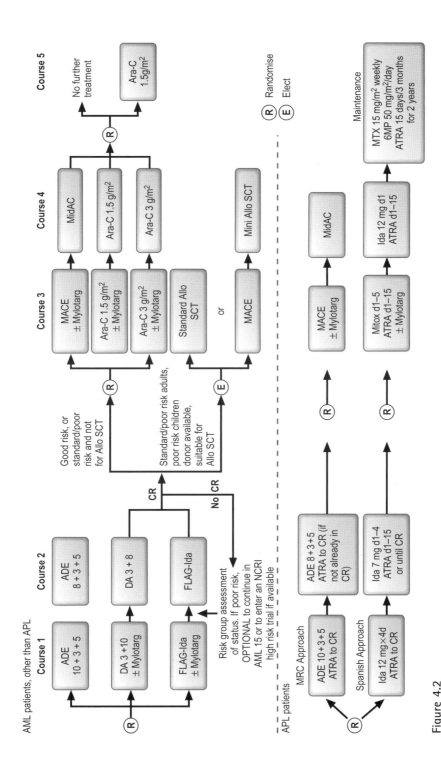

Figure 4.2
Medical Research Council AML-15 trial (reproduced with permission – Medical Research Council Working Parties on Leukaemia in Adults and Children. Protocol for Patients aged under 60).

treatment to that specified in the trial protocol (at any stage) if it is felt to be in the patient's best interest.

AML is largely treated according to established protocols or current Medical Research Council trials. Figure 4.2 illustrates the AML-15 trial overview, this should be considered within the context of all clinical features and the patient's performance status before treatment is commenced. Chemotherapy drugs commonly used in AML include fludarabine, cytarabine, mitoxantrone, gemtuzumab (Mylotarg) and idarubicin. Patient understanding and consent is essential throughout this process.

Stem cell transplantation is used in AML, although studies examining the therapeutic impact of autologous transplantation demonstrate little benefit to survival (Soutar & King 1995). However, allogeneic transplantation is considered in suitable patients who are under the age of 50 years, with minimal co-morbidity. There is much debate about patient suitability for transplant, e.g. age, disease and cytogenetics. Very much depends upon the patient, the availability of a donor, the transplant team and existing guidelines.

Recent years have seen the evolution of 'mini grafting.' This procedure utilises a non-ablative schedule with which it is possible to achieve a high level of donor engraftment, thereby exerting a graft versus leukaemia effect. Mini grafting has allowed allogeneic transplantation to be used for patients who would otherwise have been excluded because of age or co-existing medical conditions (NICE 2003). The utilisation and impact of transplantation is considered in Chapter 13.

ACUTE PROMYELOCYTIC LEUKAEMIA (APML) (FAB M3, WHO AML WITH RECURRENT GENETIC ABNORMALITIES)

Patients with this condition constitute an acute medical emergency as granules in the promyelocytes release thromboplastin, causing disseminated intravascular coagulation (DIC), which can lead to life-threatening haemorrhage (see Chapter 16). A specific chromosomal translocation (t:15:17) is identified in this disease subtype involving the retinoic acid receptor on chromosome 17 (Spence & Johnston 2001). As a result APML is particularly sensitive to treatment with the differentiation agent all-trans retinoic acid (ATRA), which is administered in conjunction with an anthracycline. ATRA induces promyelocytic blasts to differentiate into mature granulocytes, this is accompanied by haemopoietic remission and disappearance of the altered retinoic acid receptor. The prognosis of this combination therapy is relatively favourable (Jaffe et al 2001) as it reduces the risk of relapse and early death from bleeding and also improves long-term survival.

Prognosis

The main issues to be considered when assessing the prognosis of the patient with AML are related to age, initial response to treatment and genetic abnormalities. Approximately 80–90% of younger patients will achieve a complete remission with conventional chemotherapy, however many will relapse and longer-term survival rates are around 35%

(Howard & Hamilton 2002). Allogeneic transplant can increase these statistics; however this is not without risk. Older patients over the age of 55–60 years have much more difficulty tolerating chemotherapy and longer-term survival rates are significantly lower. The older patient usually presents with a less favourable performance status and considerable co-morbidity. This is an important consideration in AML as 70% of patients are over 60 years of age and outcomes in this group are poor, with treatment-related deaths of around 25% (NICE 2003). Overall prognosis has improved over the last decade through the evolution of treatment, and improved clinical tests and assessment. This is particularly evident when examining the case of APML as overall prognosis was poor prior to the introduction of ATRA as an effective treatment in combination with chemotherapy. Recently, arsenic trioxide has been used with good effect for patients who have relapsed or are resistant to conventional treatment (Shen et al 1997). Further studies are ongoing.

ACUTE LYMPHOBLASTIC LEUKAEMIA

Acute lymphoblastic leukaemia (ALL) has a peak incidence in childhood between the ages of 4 and 7 years and a further gradual rise in incidence in later years over the age of 40. The characteristics of the disease differ greatly in children and adults. In children ALL is often curable with chemotherapy whereas in adults cure may prove much more difficult. This is thought to be due to the involvement of a more immature precursor cell in most cases of adult ALL (Howard & Hamilton 2002).

Classification   FAB classification is based on the morphological appearance of the cell. ALL has three subtypes – L1, L2 and L3 – under this specific classification. However, since immunophenotyping strategies have been refined, WHO classification identifies precursor T- and B-cell leukaemia. The WHO classification outlined by Jaffe et al (2001) identifies two major classification categories:

- precursor B-lymphoblastic leukaemia/lymphoblastic lymphoma (precursor B-cell acute lymphoblastic leukaemia)
- precursor T-lymphoblastic leukaemia/lymphoblastic lymphoma (precursor T-cell acute lymphoblastic leukaemia).

Cytogenetics and cell markers are helpful prognostically. For example Philadelphia positivity (the cytogenetic translocation of chromosome 9 and 22) leads to an unfavourable prognosis. Classification of the disease must also be viewed in the context of the patient's clinical features.

Clinical features   Presenting features of the patient with ALL are variable as a result of bone marrow failure or the organ infiltration by lymphoblasts commonly occurring in this disease. The patient with ALL will have an accumulation of malignant lymphoblasts in the bone marrow leading to a reduction in normal cells in the peripheral blood. As a result of this, and similar to AML, the patient may present with symptoms of anaemia, haemorrhage and infection. However, in ALL the patient may well have bone and joint pain. This is largely due to marrow expansion as a result of an over-production of blast cells; however, in some atypical cases there may be bone involvement resulting in severe pain. Patients with ALL may also present with superficial lymphadenopathy, abdominal distension due to abdominal lymphadenopathy and hepatosplenomegaly, which in turn could lead to anorexia and nausea. T-cell ALL is also associated with a large mediastinal nodal mass leading to respiratory embarrassment. Central nervous system involvement is more often seen in ALL, resulting in meningeal syndrome where patients present with headaches, nausea and vomiting, cranial nerve palsies and other symptoms of raised intracranial pressure. The meninges and the testes are considered as sanctuary sites in ALL – disease may manifest or relapse in these areas and once established this complication is very difficult to treat. Patients are therefore routinely treated with prophylactic intrathecal chemotherapy and cranial irradiation may be indicated for some patients. In males the testes should be examined as a matter of course for disease involvement (Liesner & Goldstone 1997).

Diagnosis

ALL may be suspected due to a combination of clinical features and blood tests. Blood count and film may demonstrate an elevated white cell count; however, the count may also be low or normal. Only 20% of patients will have a white cell count in excess of $50 \times 10^9/L$ (Howard & Hamilton 2002). Anaemia and thrombocytopenia are common; blast cells will be evident in the peripheral blood to varying degrees. A suspected diagnosis of ALL can be confirmed by bone marrow aspirate and trephine biopsy. Cytochemistry, immunophenotyping and cytogenetics play an important part in the diagnostic process, and are key to establishing classification, treatment, response and prognosis. They are also essential in order to distinguish between B-ALL and T-ALL.

Treatment

The mainstay of treatment is cytotoxic therapy with the principles being similar to those of AML. However, drug schedules vary depending on protocol. Frequently used drugs include steroids, vincristine, L-asparaginase and cytarabine. A common example of current therapy for adults is shown in Figure 4.3. Research has shown that the use of intrathecal chemotherapy and high-dose systemic chemotherapy is effective CNS prophylaxis in adults (Cortes & Kantarjian 1995). Prophylaxis with cranial radiation is therefore reserved for those patients at high risk of CNS relapse (Bratt-Wyton 2000).

Transplantation will be considered for the patient with ALL. Allogeneic transplant from an HLA-matched donor performed in first remission can result in long-term survival of around 40% (Howard & Hamilton 2002). Technological strategies surrounding transplantation have improved – with specialised supportive care, quality of life for the transplant patient can be maintained. In ALL, as in AML, there is no clear evidence that autologous transplantation produces higher survival rates than chemotherapy without transplantation (NICE 2003); however, autologous transplantation is currently used as a convenient and

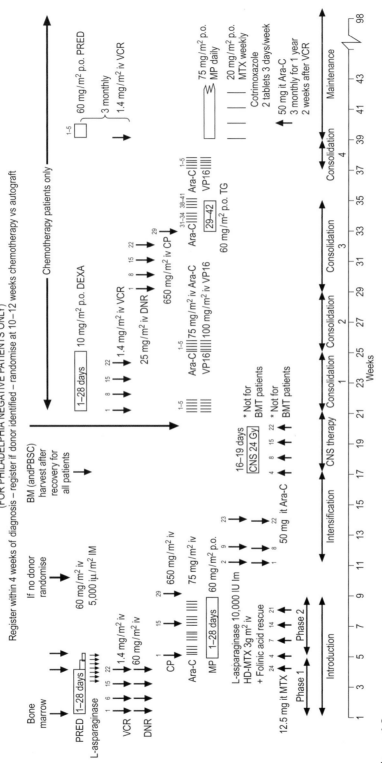

Figure 4.3
Medical Research Council ALL-12 trial (reproduced with permission – Medical Research Council Working Parties on Leukaemia in Adults and Children. Protocol for Philadelphia Negative Patients Only).

relatively safe method of escalating the chemotherapy dose (Howard & Hamilton 2002).

Prognosis

The majority of adult patients achieve remission; however, they are not curable with chemotherapy alone. With chemotherapy alone only 30% will be long-term survivors (Howard & Hamilton 2002). Most patients that achieve long-term remission with chemotherapy alone are in the young-adult population with good prognostic features. For many other adults with ALL long-term remission is dependent on allogeneic transplantation.

TREATMENT OF RELAPSE

Patients who relapse after induction and consolidation chemotherapy may well be offered further treatment in the hope of achieving a second remission. This is dependent on the individual, the disease process and the patient's wishes. Some patients who become refractory to first-line induction therapy, relapse early or develop systemic complications may well have to carefully consider their treatment options (Booth & Bruera 2003)

SUPPORTIVE CARE AND MANAGEMENT OF THE PATIENT WITH ACUTE LEUKAEMIA

The successful treatment of acute leukaemia is a challenge for clinicians and is a highly specialised field of care. Prognosis has improved markedly for patients with acute leukaemia and this in part can be attributed to the improved support and management available.

Specialist care should be evident throughout the disease trajectory to support the patient and their family. The consultation at which patients learn they have a haematological cancer can be described as a crucial event. A sensitive and compassionate approach is essential as this is literally a life-changing experience for patients. The way bad news is broken is always remembered with clarity and colours later relationships with health-care professionals, establishing a culture of trust or deep resentment (NICE 2003).

Patients with acute leukaemia will need periods of intensive inpatient treatment lasting over many months. Most will be re-admitted many times over a period of months. A range of different levels of service corresponding with a variety of forms of leukaemia is required to effectively manage patients. These levels of care, identified by the British Committee for Standards in Haematology (BCSH 1995) and further clarified in the Improving Outcomes in Haematological Cancers document (NICE 2003) offer a template for service delivery and development. Whilst the directives identified in the Improving Outcomes document are admirable and have highlighted haematology as a central priority, revenue is limited and implementation of the recommendations is resource dependent.

CHEMOTHERAPY AND ITS SIDE EFFECTS

As a result of the aggressive nature of treatment for leukaemia, patients tend to have severe chemotherapy-related side effects (see Chapter 9). Clinicians often regard suppression of the bone marrow as being the major dose-limiting toxicity of chemotherapy (Spence & Johnston 2001). However for patients nausea and vomiting is more likely to be reported as the most distressing side effect (Atkinson & Virdee 2001). Successful treatment relies upon a careful history of the symptoms combined with recent research about the mechanisms of nausea and vomiting being applied to clinical practice (Regnard & Hockley 1995). It is essential that a $5HT_3$ antagonist such as ondansetron is given as prophylaxis before and during chemotherapy due to the vomiting stimulus involved (see Chapter 17). However, assumptions should not be made, especially that delayed emesis can be managed using $5HT_3$ antagonists – a logical approach to assessment and treatment should be used.

As a result of treatment many patients suffer from anorexia. Specialist dietetic and nutritional support should be available and is essential in both the inpatient and the outpatient settings (see Chapter 19). For many patients eating and drinking is a pleasure they are unable to participate in due to stomatitis. The relevance and importance of identifying and managing oral symptoms post-chemotherapy and the associated distress has been highlighted in many studies (Field et al 1995). Despite these studies, mouth care remains problematic; it is a key issue that requires expert assessment and treatment (see Chapter 18).

Neutropenic sepsis

Infection is a major problem for patients with leukaemia; because they are severely immunocompromised even a small infection can very quickly escalate into life-threatening septicaemic shock. The key to good management of infection lies with prompt recognition of the early signs followed by immediate action. Neutropenic protocols should be utilised at a local and national level; however, this should not replace nursing expertise. Early recognition of infection requires the highest level of nursing skill. Symptoms may well be subtle and appear inconsequential. Listening to the patient and careful assessment of vital signs, haemodynamic changes, full blood count, blood cultures and a rising C-reactive protein (CRP) are very important, as well as an understanding of the disease process (see Chapter 15).

A key aspect of supportive care should include the involvement of the microbiology team to ensure prompt and appropriate treatment is delivered in response to infection. The evolution of antibiotic therapy has transformed survival and prophylaxis has reduced significantly the risk of opportunistic infection. However, the increasing incidence of fungal infections in the hospital setting is a challenge for haematology health-

care professionals. Prophylaxis, vigilance and strict infection control policies are essential in order to protect this vulnerable group of patients.

The use of growth factors in acute leukaemia remains an area of
debate. Granulocyte-colony stimulating factor (G-CSF) or granulocyte-
macrophage colony stimulating factor (GM-CSF) are used in research
trials. These growth factors can help to prevent overwhelming sepsis and
are given post-chemotherapy to increase the neutrophil count, but also
as part of the treatment regime. However, the resources and revenue
required to ensure consistent usage of growth factors can often be considered to be restrictive.

Blood component support

Transfusion of blood and platelets is an integral part of the care of the
leukaemic patient. Transfusion of blood components is not without risk
and safety issues should be paramount. Local and national guidelines
are in place to ensure patient safety. Individuals with leukaemia are particularly susceptible to transfusion-related complications because of the
need for multiple transfusions and their immunocompromised status
(see Chapter 12).

The nurse's role in caring for patients at risk of bleeding requires scientific knowledge and understanding of the disease. Platelet counts may
be abnormal due to accelerated disease or bone marrow suppression following chemotherapy (see Chapter 16).

Alopecia

Our hair is an important part of the way we view ourselves and others
view us. Alopecia can seriously impact upon the individual's perception
of themselves and their body image. The change in body image as a
result of alopecia is often sudden and as such can provoke feelings of
anxiety. It has been reported that hair loss for some patients is catastrophic and can impact upon treatment consent and compliance
(Dougherty & Bailey 2001). Nurses have a responsibility to support the
patient at this very difficult time and should not make assumptions about
the impact of alopecia on the patient irrespective of their sex or age (see
Chapters 21 & 23).

Venous access

All individuals with acute leukaemia will require venous access at
some time during their disease experience. Treatment schedules are often
protracted and venous access is required for blood products, blood sampling, antibiotic therapy, chemotherapy and other supportive treatment.
Frequent venepuncture is uncomfortable and often distressing for the
patient, therefore ideally the patient should be assessed for central
venous access (see Chapter 14).

Fertility issues

The use of high-dose chemotherapy and radiotherapy in the treatment
of leukaemia can result in numerous side effects that impact upon the
individual's fertility. Historically the issues surrounding this side effect
of treatment have been afforded a low priority – this may have been due
to lower long-term survival (Dannie 2000). As survival has improved,

quality of life post-treatment has become increasingly important and fertility is a major concern for patients and their partners. It is essential that fertility specialists are integrated into the multidisciplinary team and that discussions surrounding sexuality and fertility issues are not uninvited guests into the nurse–patient relationship (see Chapters 20 & 21).

Case study 4.1

Brenda is a 54-year-old female with no relevant past medical history other than hypertension. She presented to her GP with flu-like symptoms and a productive cough and a lump in her right groin. A course of antibiotics was given with little effect and the lump became painful to touch. A second appointment with the GP was arranged and a full blood count taken, revealing anaemia, an elevated white cell count and platelets within normal limits. A referral was made to a haematologist where a diagnosis of acute myeloid leukaemia was confirmed following a bone marrow aspiration and trephine. Cytogenetic analysis revealed no poor prognostic factors. Informed consent was obtained and Brenda was entered into the AML15 protocol. Brenda went into remission after her first course of treatment and following successful completion of the planned four courses of intensive chemotherapy a further bone marrow biopsy revealed continuing remission. Brenda is now well and looking forward to becoming a grandmother again.

THE CHRONIC LEUKAEMIAS

The chronic leukaemias, although labelled with the same name, are very different from the acute leukaemias with the term chronic attributed to these diseases as a result of the longer survival times.

CHRONIC MYELOID LEUKAEMIA

Chronic myeloid leukaemia (CML) is a clonal malignant myeloproliferative disorder (Goldman 1997) that arises from an acquired genetic change in a pluripotential stem cell. By the time this leukaemia is diagnosed the number of leucocytes is greatly increased in the peripheral blood, and normal blood cell production is almost completely replaced by leukaemic cells, which, however, still function almost normally (Goldman 1997). The annual incidence of CML is 1–1.5 per 100,000 (Goldman 1997, Howard & Hamilton 2002) with presentation most common in the fifth and sixth decades.

Clinical features

Patients normally present in the chronic phase and have characteristic symptoms of fatigue, weight loss, sweating, anorexia and pallor. On clinical examination the most common finding is splenomegaly, which can cause nausea and bloating. Chronic leukaemia is often detected as a result of a routine blood test performed for unrelated reasons; 20% of patients may be totally asymptomatic prior to diagnosis (Goldman 1997).

Classification

The WHO classification of chronic myleoproliferative diseases identifies chronic myeloid leukaemia (CML). However, CML is unusual in that it has three distinct clinical phases – a relatively indolent chronic phase, followed by an ominous accelerated phase where patients are sicker and require more intensive support, and finally, and almost invariably fatal, an acute leukaemic phase termed 'blastic crisis'.

Diagnosis

The major diagnostic tool is a full blood count. Peripheral blood film will point to a diagnosis of CML but bone marrow is usually examined as confirmation. Cytogenetic study of the marrow shows the presence of the Philadelphia or Ph chromosome. Over 95% of cases of CML are Philadelphia positive, with the chromosomal translocation normally referred to as t(9:22) (q34:q11). The Philadelphia chromosome carries a specific fusion gene known as bcr-abl resulting from juxtaposition of the abl proto-oncogene (from chromosome 9) with part of the bcr gene on chromosome 22 (Goldman 1997). This is important when considering treatment options.

Treatment

Treatment for CML varies according to the phases of the illness and other prognostic indicators, e.g. the presence or absence of the Philadelphia chromosome. Traditionally interferon or conventional chemotherapy such as hydroxyurea and busulfan were the treatments of choice and were largely successful in controlling the disease during the chronic phase. However, problems arose from the debilitating side effects of the treatment and the relatively recent emergence of the drug imatinib (Glivec) (a tyrosine kinase inhibitor) has revolutionised treatment for CML. Imatinib directly targets the product of the bcr-abl fusion gene on the Philadelphia chromosome reducing the amount of abnormal protein produced by the chromosomal translocation, thereby controlling disease progression. NICE (2003) recommends that imatinib should be offered to patients with chronic phase Philadelphia positive CML if treatment with interferon fails to control the disease or produces unacceptable side effects. It is also recommended as an option for the treatment of adults with Philadelphia positive CML in accelerated phase or blast crisis provided they have not received imatinib before. Long-term effects of imatinib are as yet unknown.

Currently the only proven chance for cure of CML is through allogeneic bone marrow transplantation. This results in the ablation of the Philadelphia positive clone of cells, so arresting the disease.

Patients may experience a period of stability in chronic phase and may become Philadelphia negative at this stage; however, those in blast crisis demonstrate symptoms of acute leukaemia. Between chronic phase and blast crisis there may be an intervening period of disease acceleration. This accelerated phase is poorly defined and is usually associated with an insidious deterioration in the patient's health, increasing splenic size and raised white cell count. Cytogenetic studies will reflect an increase in Philadelphia positivity.

Prognosis

Any form of treatment that reduces the white cell count and the size of the spleen has a clinical benefit for the patient. Average survival is wide-ranging – figures of 3–7 years are quoted, although there are wide variances. The new therapeutics may have an impact on survival but there is insufficient mature data to confirm this. Only allogeneic transplant is a proven curative treatment however only 15% of CML patients are eligible as the disease tends to occur in the older person. When patients enter the accelerated phase, treatment options are limited and prognosis poor.

CHRONIC LYMPHOCYTIC LEUKAEMIA

Chronic lymphocytic leukaemia (CLL) is a disease characterised by a clonal proliferation of B lymphocytes, which are arrested at an early stage of development. It is the commonest type of leukaemia in the western world and is a disease of the elderly; most patients are over the age of 50.

Clinical features

CLL is a highly variable disease and many patients have no symptoms. Presenting features include fatigue, anaemia, infection, weight loss, night sweats, lymphadenopathy and hepatosplenomegaly.

Diagnosis

Diagnosis is often incidental and is suggested by a high lymphocyte count. Clinicians treating these patients should take into account a detailed history, which must include staging of the disease, age, and other factors such as thrombocytopenia and anaemia.

Staging

Staging is important in CLL as it helps in making decisions as to whether to institute treatment as well as offering prognostic information (Howard & Hamilton 2002). The easiest method of staging this disease is the Binet adaptation of the previous Rai system; this is simple to apply and correlates to survival.

- Stage A – No anaemia or thrombocytopenia; fewer than three lymphoid areas enlarged
- Stage B – No anaemia or thrombocytopenia; three or more lymphoid areas enlarged
- Stage C – Anaemia and thrombocytopenia, indicating impaired bone marrow function.

Treatment

Patients who are well with stable or controlled disease may be watched without treatment, for others treatment may ultimately become necessary. Intermittent chlorambucil and steroids are the drugs of choice, although trials are underway to assess the efficacy of fludarabine chemotherapy and campath immunotherapy in the treatment of CLL. Patients with CLL may also have impaired immune systems requiring antibiotic, antifungal and antiviral support. Immunoglobulins may be given as supportive therapy in order to bolster the immune system and prevent infection.

Prognosis

None of the aforementioned treatments will cure CLL – the emphasis is on control of symptoms and possible prolongation of life. Prognosis is as variable as the disease itself. Relapse is inevitable; some patients will live a relatively normal life whilst others may die rapidly from marrow failure. Long-term cures are rare. The median overall survival in most CLL patients is 5–8 years (Mead 1997).

SUPPORTIVE CARE AND MANAGEMENT OF THE PATIENT WITH CHRONIC LEUKAEMIA

Many of the patients with chronic leukaemia suffering from accelerated or advanced disease require the same degree and complexity of care as patients with acute leukaemia. The challenge when caring for these patients is related to support. There is no potential cure and patients are subjected to a 'waiting game' anticipating transformation of their disease. Patients report that they feel unable to continue with their normal activities and are unable to consider their future (Spence & Johnston 2001). The treatment of these patients is largely delivered in the outpatient setting and support mechanisms need to be in-built to respond to their changing needs.

REFLECTION POINT

Care of the leukaemic patient requires insight and knowledge into disease processes, the appropriate therapeutic interventions and their impact. This group of patients is very vulnerable and requires expert and intensive care. Practitioners working in this area should be cognisant of the impact that an altered blood picture has on the patient as a result of the disease process and treatment. Consider this issue in the context of your professional practice.

CHALLENGES FOR CARE

Within the specialism of haematology it is easy to allow care to be driven by the medical model. Haematology nurses are the patients' advocates and it is vital that the patient remains central in all care delivery. The nature of leukaemia means that treatment is frequently delivered before the patient has had time to come to terms with the diagnosis. Timely and relevant information as well as support for the patient and family is required from the point of admission to enable them to take control of the management of their disease. This can be achieved through education, providing the patient with information suitable to their needs and being cognisant of patient anxieties, and is the role of every haematology nurse.

Service delivery and development are high on the UK National Health Service agenda; never before have nurses had such opportunities to develop services to suit the needs of the patients and enhance the profile of the multidisciplinary team. However, resources remain a challenge.

CONCLUSION

Leukaemia as a disease has no respect for age, gender or ethnicity. Expert care underpinned by specialist knowledge is essential in order to provide care that meets the needs of the patients and their families throughout the disease trajectory. In specialist haematology clinical practice is significantly expanded from generic nurse training and as such it can be overwhelming and stressful for the health-care professional caring for the patient (Atkinson 2004). Investing in staff and enhancing knowledge through education and training is vitally important to meet the needs of patients and their families.

DISCUSSION QUESTIONS

1. How could palliative care services for this patient group be integrated in your clinical practice?

2. What is the psychosocial impact of the disease on the family unit?

3. What role does the nurse play in the multidisciplinary haematology team?

ACKNOWLEDGEMENT

The authors would like to give their heartfelt thanks to Brenda for her help – her unselfish endeavour, courage and fortitude have been inspirational.

References

Atkinson J 2004 How does specialist education in the physiology of haemopoiesis impact upon the care delivery in haematology? MSc Dissertation, Northumbria University, Unpublished

Atkinson J, Virdee A 2001 Promoting comfort for patients with symptoms other than pain. In: Kinghorn S, Gamlin R (eds) Palliative nursing bringing comfort and hope. Baillière Tindall, Edinburgh

Booth S, Bruera E 2003 Palliative care consultations in haemato-oncology. Oxford University Press, Oxford

Boyle P, Autier P, Bartelink H et al 2003 European code against cancer and scientific justification. Annals of Oncology 14:973–1005

Bratt-Wyton R 2000 The leukaemias. In: Grundy M. Nursing in haematological oncology. Baillière Tindall, Edinburgh, pp 44–59

British Committee for Standards in Haematology 1995 Guidelines on the provision of facilities for the care of adult patients with haematological malignancies. Clinical and Laboratory Haematology 17:3–10

Cancer Research Campaign 1995 Leukaemia – UK Factsheet 23.1. Cancer Research Campaign, London

Cancer Research UK 2003 Cancer Stats – Leukaemia – UK. CRUK, London

Cortes J, Kantarjian H M 1995 Acute lymphoblastic leukaemia: a comprehensive review with emphasis on biology and therapy. Cancer 76(12):2392–2417

Dannie E 2000 Fertility issues. In: Grundy M (ed) Nursing in haematological oncology. Baillière Tindall, Edinburgh, pp 236–249

Dickinson H O, Parker L 2002 Leukaemia and non-Hodgkin's lymphoma in children of male Sellafield radiation workers. International Journal of Cancer 99:437–444

Dougherty L, Bailey C 2001 Chemotherapy. In: Corner J, Bailey C (eds) Cancer nursing: care in context. Blackwell Science, Oxford, pp 179–221

Drapper C J, Stiller C A, Cartwright R A et al 1993 Cancer in Cumbria and in the vicinity of the Sellafield nuclear installation, 1963–1990. British Medical Journal 306:89–94

Field D, Douglas C, Jagger C et al 1995 Terminal illness: views of patients and their lay carers. Palliative Medicine 9:45–54

Forman D, Stockton D, Moller H et al 2003 Cancer prevalence in the UK: results from the EUROPREVAL study. Annals of Oncology 14:648–654

Gardner M J, Hall A J, Snee M P et al 1990 Results of case control study of leukaemia and lymphoma among young people near Sellafield nuclear plant in West Cumbria. British Medical Journal 300:423–429

Goldman J 1997 ABC of clinical haematology: chronic myeloid leukaemia. British Medical Journal 314:657–667

Greaves M 2002 Childhood leukaemia. British Medical Journal 324:263–297

Groves F D, Linet M S, Devesa S S 1995 Patterns of occurrence of the leukaemias. European Journal of Cancer 31a:941–949

Hayes R B, Yin S N, Dosemeci M et al 1997 Benzene and the dose related incidence of haematological neoplasms in China. National Cancer Institute Benzene Study Group. Journal of the National Cancer Institute 89:1065–1071

Horwitz M 1997 The genetics of familial leukaemia. Leukaemia 11:1347–1359

Houlston R S, Catovsky D, Yuille M R 2002 Genetic susceptibility to chronic lymphocytic leukaemia. Leukaemia 16:1008–1014

Howard M R, Hamilton P J 2002 Haematology: an illustrated colour text, 2nd edn. Churchill Livingstone, Edinburgh

Jaffe E S, Harris N L, Stein H et al 2001 Pathology and genetics of tumours of haematopoietic and lymphoid tissues. IARC Press, Lyon

Kane E V, Roman E, Cartwright R et al 1999 Tobacco and the risk of acute leukaemia in adults. British Journal of Cancer 81:1228–1233

Kinlen L J, Dixon M, Stiller C A 1995 Childhood leukaemia and non-Hodgkin's lymphoma near large rural construction sites, with a comparison with Sellafield nuclear site. British Medical Journal 10:763–768

Liesner R J, Goldstone A H 1997 ABC of clinical haematology: the acute leukaemias. British Medical Journal 314:733–745

Mead G M 1997 ABC of clinical haematology: malignant lymphomas and chronic lymphocytic leukaemia. British Medical Journal 314:1103–1113

Morrison H L, Wilkins K, Semenciw R 1992 Herbicides and cancer. Journal of the National Cancer Institute 84:1866–1874

National Institute for Clinical Excellence 2002 Technology appraisal: leukaemia (chronic myeloid – Imatinib) No. 50. www.nice.org. Updated Oct 2004. Accessed 12 July 2004

National Institute for Clinical Excellence 2003 Improving outcomes in haematological cancers: the manual. NICE, London

Petridou E, Trichopolous D 2002 Leukaemias. In: Trichopolous D (ed) Textbook of cancer epidemiology. Oxford University Press, New York

Quinn M, Babb P, Kirby L et al 2000 Registrations of cancer diagnosed in 1994–1997. England and Wales Health Statistics Quarterly 07 Autumn. Office for National Statistics, London, pp 71–82

Quinn M, Babb P, Brock A et al 2001 Cancer trends in England and Wales 1950–1999. Vol. SMPS No. 66. TSO, London

Regnard C F B, Hockley J 1995 Flow diagrams in advanced cancer and other diseases. Edward Arnold, London

Shen Z X, Chen G K, Ni J H 1997 Use of arsenic trioxide (as203) in the treatment of acute promyelocytic leukaemia: clinical efficacy and pharmacokinetics in relapsed patients. Blood 89:3354–3360

Soutar R L, King D J 1995 Fortnightly review: bone marrow transplantation. British Medical Journal 310:31–36

Spence R A J, Johnston P G 2001 Oncology. Oxford University Press, Oxford

Wiley J S, Dao-Ung L P, Gu B J 2002 A loss of function polymorphic mutation in the p2x7 receptor gene and chronic lymphocytic leukaemia: a molecular study. Lancet 359:1114–1119

World Health Organization 2003 Electro-magnetic fields project. WHO Press, Albany

Further reading

Booth S, Bruera E 2003 Palliative care consultations in haemato-oncology. Oxford University Press, Oxford
A key aspect of care delivery in haematology is the integration of palliative care services. This text addresses some of the contentious issues that arise, whilst also considering key symptoms and their management. The authors adopt a disease-specific approach. Communication and supporting the family make interesting reading.

Howard M R, Hamilton P J 2002 Haematology: an illustrated colour text. Churchill Livingstone, Edinburgh
A useful introductory text, a concise summary of the haematological diseases.

Hoffbrand A V, Pettit J E, Moss P A H 2001 Essential haematology, 4th edn. Blackwell Science, Oxford
A very useful reference book that identifies clearly the pathophysiology of the diseases and clinical features. The text adopts a medical model; however, this can be easily translated into the clinical area.

Chapter **5**

Myeloma

Tracey King

CHAPTER CONTENTS

INTRODUCTION

This chapter reviews myeloma, its management and related nursing issues. Myeloma is a complex and highly individual disease. Although there are many common characteristics that help to define the disease, clinical manifestations can vary between individuals. Myeloma was first reported in London in 1844 when the treatment was orange peel, rhubarb pills and morphine. Thankfully the management of myeloma has moved on since 1844 and although not yet curable, the disease is progressively more treatable.

THE DISEASE

Myeloma (also referred to as myelomatosis) is a complex malignant plasma cell disorder characterised by an excess of plasma cells in the bone marrow, the presence of a monoclonal paraprotein (an immunoglobulin or fragment of) in the serum and/or urine, and lytic bone disease (lytic describes the punched-out holes seen in bones affected by myeloma). The disease is often referred to as 'multiple' myeloma as it is usually present in several areas of the body at diagnosis. Bone pain is a major cause of morbidity in myeloma and 75–80% of patients will present with bone pain as a predominant symptom (Bataille & Harrousseau 1997).

EPIDEMIOLOGY

Myeloma accounts for 1% of all cancers and 15% of haematological cancers (Durie 1999). The annual United Kingdom incidence is 4.0 (females) and 5.8 (males) per 100,000 with 3669 people being diagnosed with myeloma in 1999 (Office for National Statistics 2002). Between 10,000–15,000 people are living with myeloma at any one time in the UK (UK Myeloma Forum (UKMF) 2001). Median age at diagnosis is 60–65 with 2% of cases under 40 and 5% under 50 years of age. Incidence is slightly higher in Afro-Caribbean ethnic groups than in Caucasians although it is not understood why (UKMF 2001). With modern treatment median survival is approximately four years.

AETIOLOGY

The causes of myeloma are uncertain although exposure to pesticides is thought to be a potential trigger factor. Exposure to radiation and benzene have traditionally been linked to myeloma but evidence is inconclusive (Joshua & Gibson 2002). Human herpes virus-8 (HHV-8) has been implicated in the pathogenesis of myeloma, but further investigation is needed to confirm this relationship (Kelleher & Chapel 2002).

PATHOPHYSIOLOGY

PLASMA CELL GROWTH

Plasma cells are mature B lymphocytes that normally comprise <5% of cells within the bone marrow. In myeloma, monoclonal plasma cells (myeloma cells) proliferate uncontrollably and increase to more than 10% in the bone marrow. Accumulation of myeloma cells within the bone marrow disrupts normal marrow function resulting in anaemia, lowered resistance to infection and thrombocytopenia. Myeloma cells also have an affinity to bone and disrupt the normal mechanism of bone turnover (Durie 1999).

Plasma cells produce various cytokines with interleukin-6 (IL-6) being the major proliferative cytokine for malignant plasma cells (Yi 2002). Elevated IL-6 serum levels in myeloma correlate with tumour burden and serve as prognostic markers (Raje & Anderson 2002). Plasma cells also secrete a variety of other cytokines including vascular endothelial growth factor (VEGF), important for angiogenesis and blood supply to myeloma cells. Increased angiogenesis occurs in the bone marrow environment in myeloma and seems to both increase the proliferative rate and decrease the apoptotic rate of malignant plasma cells (Raje & Anderson 2002). These cytokines help to adapt the microenvironment surrounding myeloma cells, ensuring their continued growth (Fig. 5.1).

SECRETION OF IMMUNOGLOBULINS

Normal plasma cells produce immunoglobulins (antibodies) that play a vital role in the body's defence against bacterial and viral infections. The five main groups of immunoglobulins are IgG, IgM, IgA, IgD and IgE. Each immunoglobulin is made up of two light and two heavy polypeptide chains. The type of heavy chain determines the immunoglobulin isotype, i.e. G, M, A, D and E. The light chain portions are of two classes, lamda (λ) or kappa (κ).

Myeloma cells produce abnormal immunoglobulin, usually of one type only, which is secreted in excessive amounts (a paraprotein). Myeloma is often classified according to the immunoglobulin type, e.g. IgG myeloma (Table 5.1). In about 30% of cases more light chain portions

Figure 5.1
Myeloma cell interaction with
microenvironment (reproduced
with permission of Dr Paul
Richardson).

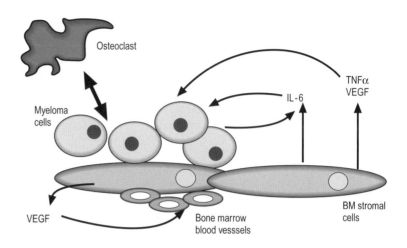

Table 5.1
Percentages of different types
of myeloma

Types of monoclonal protein	Percentage of patients
IgG	52%
IgA	21%
IgD	2%
IgE	<0.01%
IgM	12% (0.01% of myeloma cases) (rarely myeloma, typically associated with Waldenstrom's macroglobulinaemia)
Light chain	11%
No paraprotein (non-secretory)	1%
2 or more paraproteins	<1%
Heavy chains (G or A) only	<1%

From IMF (UK) Concise review of the disease and treatment options 1999, reproduced with permission.

are produced than can bind to heavy chain portions. These free light chains are known as Bence-Jones proteins (after Henry Bence-Jones, who first described them in 1850) and are excreted via the kidney into the urine.

The presence of the abnormal paraprotein in the serum or urine is the most characteristic biological marker of myeloma. Paraproteins are also known as M-protein, myeloma protein or monoclonal component. Measurement of paraprotein is the most commonly used means of monitoring the course of the disease (San Miguel et al 2002). Abnormal paraproteins can be measured both in the serum by electrophoresis and in the urine by measurement of Bence-Jones proteinuria (San Miguel et al 2002). In 1% of cases, no paraprotein is detectable; this is known as non-secretory disease.

Abnormal paraproteins can adhere to:

- each other
- blood cells and blood vessel walls, causing hyperviscosity
- blood clotting factors, causing increased bleeding or clotting tendency
- hormones, causing metabolic or endocrine dysfunction.

Some types of myeloma are more susceptible to hyperviscosity than others (e.g. IgM and IgA myeloma) (Durie 1999). Paraproteins can also cause cast nephropathy (myeloma kidney). Damage to the proximal tubules is caused by an accumulation of protein casts causing obstruction and dilation (Shaver-Lewis & Shah 2002). Normal immune function is suppressed owing to reduced levels of normal immunoglobulins (hypogammaglobulinemia).

BONE DISEASE

The precise mechanism involved in myeloma bone disease remains unclear, but several factors are known to play a part. Bone resorption and formation is controlled by the action of osteoclasts (bone resorption) and osteoblasts (bone formation). In healthy individuals this process remains in equilibrium. Myeloma cells disrupt this equilibrium by stimulating the activity of osteoclasts, causing increased bone resorption, whilst impairing the function of osteoblasts and reducing new bone formation (Bataille et al 1990). Cytokines produced by myeloma cells influence the development of bone disease: potent osteoclast-activating factors (OAF), IL-1β and tumour necrosis factor (TNFα and TNFβ) are involved in increasing the number and activity of osteoclasts, resulting in bone loss and the development of lytic bone lesions (Souhami & Tobias 1995, Torcia et al 1996).

More recently, a cytokine known as receptor activator of nuclear factor kappa B (RANKL) and its decoy receptor osteoprotegerin (OPG) have been found to be central to the regulation of normal bone resorption. RANKL (expressed by bone marrow stromal cells) supports osteoclast differentiation and OPG binds to RANKL and therefore inhibits osteoclast formation. Myeloma cells disrupt the activity of RANKL and OPG in favour of increased bone resorption (Berenson 2002).

A vicious circle of dependency is formed between the myeloma and bone cells resulting in bone loss; the resultant lytic lesions present on x-ray (Fig. 5.2). The bone loss can be diffuse (osteopenia) but more commonly appears as lytic lesions occurring at the site of deposits of myeloma cells (Bataille et al 1995, Oyajobi & Mundy 2004). Once a lesion has developed it is very rare for re-calcification to occur (Oyajobi & Mundy 2004). Common sites of lytic lesions include the vertebrae, ribs, skull, long bones, sternum and pelvis. Loss of height due to vertebral collapse is a common complication with patients losing 5 cm in height on average by the time of diagnosis (Kuehl & Bergsagel 2002). Spinal cord compression (SCC) can also occur due to plasma cell infiltration of the vertebrae and/or vertebral destruction.

Figure 5.2
X-ray of myeloma bone disease
of skull (reproduced with
permission of Miasoft).

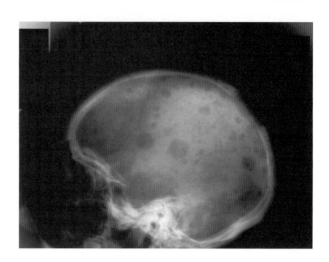

CYTOGENETICS

Cytogenetic aberrations found in myeloma and other plasma cell disorders are not as well characterised as those seen in most other haematological cancers (Sawyer & Singhal 2002). Individuals with abnormal karyotypes are thought to have a poorer prognosis than those with normal karyotypes (Seong et al 1998). Chromosomal abnormalities are usually quite complex and more recently complete or partial deletion of chromosome 13 has been identified as an adverse prognostic indicator in myeloma (Barlogie et al 1998, Seong et al 1998, Facon et al 2001).

PLASMA CELL DISORDERS RELATED TO MYELOMA

A variety of disorders are related to myeloma. Some disorders can precede myeloma (e.g. monoclonal gammopathy of uncertain significance – MGUS, smouldering myeloma), whilst others may occur separately or simultaneously with myeloma (e.g. AL amyloidosis, plasmacytoma, plasma cell leukaemia and Waldenstrom's macroglobulinaemia). Plasma cell disorders related to myeloma are shown in Table 5.2.

MONOCLONAL GAMMOPATHY OF UNCERTAIN SIGNIFICANCE

MGUS is an indolent disorder characterised by the accumulation of <10% plasma cells within the bone marrow and the presence of a serum monoclonal protein without evidence of myeloma (Kyle & Rajkumar

Table 5.2
Plasma cell disorders related
to myeloma

Disorder	Description
MGUS (monoclonal gammopathy of uncertain significance)	<10% plasma cells in BM No organ damage IgG usually <20 g/L IgA usually <10 g/L
Smouldering myeloma	Between MGUS and myeloma Stage 1A myeloma Asymptomatic
Plasmacytoma	Localised tumours Single or multiple Confined within bone – solitary lesion Outside bone – extramedullary
Plasma cell leukaemia	Aggressive disorder >20% myeloma cells in peripheral blood Liver and spleen often affected
Waldenstrom's macroglobulinaemia	Low-grade lymphoproliferative disorder Produces IgM Infiltration of bone marrow, spleen, liver, lymph nodes No bone disease

2002). Two percent of cases per year progress to myeloma or another plasma cell disorder (Leif Bergsagel 2004).

AL AMYLOIDOSIS

There are many different types of amyloidosis, each with its own precursor to the production of amyloid protein in fibrillular form. Amyloid protein appears as aggregated fibrils and occurs as extracellular deposits in various tissues and organs. In immunoglobulin light chain (AL) amyloidosis the light chain portions of monoclonal immunoglobulin form the amyloid fibrils. These are deposited in tissue around the body, e.g. kidney, nerves and heart tissue. Most patients have AL amyloidosis alone, but up to 10–15% of patients with myeloma will also have amyloid deposited in tissues or organs.

CLINICAL MANIFESTATIONS OF MYELOMA

Clinical presentation is varied; nonetheless there are a number of characteristic features that occur as a consequence of uncontrolled growth of plasma cells and the presence of a paraprotein.

SKELETAL INVOLVEMENT

The major clinical manifestations of myeloma are related to bone disease (Berenson 2002) and include:

- bone pain
- hypercalcaemia
- pathological fractures
- spinal cord compression.

Bone pain and bone disease

Bone pain is one of the most distressing symptoms of myeloma, with about 70% of patients presenting at diagnosis with pain of varying intensity, often of the lower back and ribs (Durie 2003). Fractures of bone weakened by myeloma lesions are common and contribute to bone pain. Common sites for pathological fractures include ribs and vertebrae. The great majority of patients with myeloma will develop bone disease and resultant complications. The extent of bone disease is an important prognostic factor (Oyajobi & Mundy 2004). Assessment of bone disease is important in determining the extent of disease and detection of lesions at risk of fracture or nerve compression. The gold standard to date has been a skeletal survey using standard x-ray imaging. Magnetic resonance imaging (MRI) is useful for patients with suspected spinal cord compression. Computerised tomography (CT) scanning is useful for imaging extramedullary disease. However, MRI or CT imaging is not routinely indicated for assessing myeloma bone disease (UKMF 2001). Positron emission tomography (PET) scan (a sensitive whole-body scanning technique using a radioactive sugar to show disease activity) may be useful for disease monitoring, especially in non-secretory disease where the lack of secreted paraprotein makes monitoring of disease difficult (Samson 2003).

HYPERCALCAEMIA

Hypercalcaemia caused by the release of calcium from the bone is present in 30% of patients at diagnosis (Durie 2003). It results from increased bone resorption and may be aggravated by reduced calcium excretion via the kidneys in those with renal impairment (Ludwig & Fritz 2002). Dehydration and renal impairment will exacerbate hypercalcaemia. Characteristic symptoms of hypercalcaemia include nausea, vomiting, constipation, thirst, fatigue, confusion and polyuria (Ludwig & Fritz 2002).

RENAL DISEASE

Impaired renal function is a common complication of myeloma (Shaver-Lewis & Shah 2002). Up to 20% of patients present with renal failure and 50% have a degree of impairment at some stage of their disease (UKMF

2001). Renal failure is more frequent in light-chain and IgD disease (Shaver-Lewis & Shah 2002). Advanced renal failure requiring major intervention occurs in 3–12% of patients (Clarke et al 1999). Most commonly renal disease consists of cast nephropathy. Tubular dysfunction, amyloidosis, and light-chain deposition may also occur (Lokhurst 2002). The cause of renal failure in myeloma is often multifactorial. Causes include:

- the presence of the paraprotein as it passes through the renal tubules
- deposition of light chain portions of immunoglobulins
- amyloid deposits
- use of nephrotoxic drugs (e.g. non-steroidal anti-inflammatory drugs, cytotoxic therapy, antimicrobial agents)
- dehydration
- hypercalcaemia
- infection
- hyperviscosity.

Hypercalcaemia, dehydration and infection are the most important precipitating factors (Lokhorst 2002).

With modern supportive therapy, the survival of those with myeloma and renal failure is not dramatically changed. Overall prognosis is determined by the response of the underlying disease to therapy, rather than renal function (Shaver-Lewis & Shah 2002).

HYPERVISCOSITY

An increased concentration of paraprotein in the blood gives rise to increased blood viscosity and expansion of plasma volume; circulation becomes sluggish and can result in hyperviscosity syndrome (Dimopoulos 2002). Hyperviscosity is present in <10% of patients and is more common in IgM and IgA myeloma and Waldenstrom's macroglobulinaemia. Symptoms include visual disturbances, headaches, ataxia bleeding tendencies and somnolence. Blood transfusion can aggravate the problem by further increasing blood volume (Dimopoulos 2002).

BONE MARROW INFILTRATION

The increased numbers of myeloma cells within the bone marrow compromise normal bone marrow function and resultant blood cell production, resulting in anaemia and increased susceptibility to infection.

Infection The predisposition to infection is probably the single most characteristic feature of myeloma besides bone disease (Durie 2003); 5–14% of patients will present with infection (Savage et al 1982, Marcelin et al 1997). Individuals with myeloma are particularly susceptible to viral and pneumococcal infections, but any bacterial, fungal and opportunistic infections can occur. Principal sites of infection are the respiratory and urinary tracts and the skin (Kelleher & Chapel 2002). The timing of serious infection varies with phase of disease. The infection risk is greater in the induction phase of treatment, when first-line therapy is commenced, at relapse or in progressive disease (Kelleher & Chapel 2002). Bacterial infection is the cause of death in approximately one-third of patients with myeloma (Kelleher & Chapel 2002).

Anaemia

Anaemia is present in two-thirds of patients at presentation and becomes more common with recurrent or progressive disease (UKMF 2001). Symptoms of anaemia include tachycardia, dyspnoea, decreased libido and fatigue. Anaemia is also associated with depressed erythropoietin (EPO) levels and as a consequence of chemotherapy or radiation given to treat the myeloma. Depressed EPO levels are due to an impaired availability of stored iron and overproduction of cytokines that inhibit erythropoiesis (Lokhorst 2002). Almost all those with anaemia suffer with symptoms of fatigue, which is often associated with depression, emotional disturbances, or impaired cognitive function (Ludwig & Fritz 2002) (see Chapter 22).

NEUROLOGICAL EFFECTS

Nerve tissue damage can be caused by the direct effect of the paraprotein against nerve tissue or the deposition of amyloid fibrils on nerves (carpal tunnel syndrome). These effects result in peripheral neuropathies (Durie 2003), which can be compounded by therapies that cause nerve damage. Increased susceptibility to infection can result in varicella zoster (shingles) and Bell's palsy, which affect the nervous system (Durie 2003).

DIAGNOSIS AND INVESTIGATIONS

One-third of patients will be diagnosed from a routine full blood count and are referred straight to a haematologist. The remaining two-thirds of patients are diagnosed following referral to other specialities such as renal, orthopaedic and rheumatology (National Institute for Clinical Excellence (NICE) 2003). Diagnosis is usually confirmed by demonstration of a paraprotein in the serum or urine and/or lytic lesions on x-ray, together with bone marrow aspirate demonstrating over 10% plasma cells in the bone marrow (Greipp 1992).

STAGING AND PROGNOSTIC FACTORS

The Durie/Salmon staging system is used for myeloma (Durie & Salmon 1975) (Table 5.3). It brings together the major clinical parameters in correlation with measured myeloma cell mass.

Table 5.3
Durie/Salmon myeloma
staging system

Stage	Criteria	Myeloma cell mass billions/m^2

I	Haemoglobin >10g/dL
	Serum calcium normal or
	   <10.5 mg/dL
	Bone x-ray normal bone
	   structure or solitary bone
	   plasmacytoma
	Low M-component production
	   rates
	IgG value <50 g/L
	IgA value <30 g/L
	Urine light chain M-component
	On electrophoresis <4g/24 hr
		600 (low)

II	Fitting neither stage I nor stage II	600–1200
III	One or more of the following:	>1200

Sub classification
   (either A or B)
A: relatively normal
   renal function
   (serum creatinine)
   <170 μmol/L
B: abnormal renal
   function (serum
   creatinine)
   ≥170 μmol/L
	Haemoglobin value 8.5 g/dL
	Serum calcium value
	   ≥3.0 mmol/L
	Advanced lytic bone lesions
	High M-component
	   production rates
	IgG value >70 g/L
	IgA value >50 g/L
	Urine light chain M-component
	On electrophoresis >12 g/24 hr	

Table 5.4
Proposed International
Prognostic Index (IPI)

Stage I	Serum beta-2-microglobulin (β2M) <3.5 μg/mL Serum albumin ≥35 g/L
Stage II	β2M < 3.5 μg/mL Serum albumin <35 g/L or β2M 3.5–5.5 μg/mL
Stage III	β2M > 5.5 μg/mL

Recently an International Prognostic Index (IPI) (Greipp et al 2003) (Table 5.4) has been proposed using serum β2-microglobulin and serum albumin measurements to stratify patient risk. Pre-treatment serum β2-microglobulin (β2M) is the most powerful single prognostic factor for predicting length of survival (Greipp et al 2003). Accurate staging of the disease and identification of prognostic factors allows risk groups to be identified. This information is used to categorise patients and select optimal therapies (Durie 1999).

TREATMENT

New developments in molecular biology, immunology, cytogenetics and imaging studies have changed understanding of plasma cell disorders considerably over the last few years (Zomas & Dimopoulos 2002). This has resulted in a refinement of clinical approach, an increased number of active treatment options and improvements in symptom control.

The aim of treatment is to extend disease-free survival, provide lasting relief of pain and other symptoms, and preserve normal performance and quality of life for as long as possible (UKMF 2001).

DEFINITION OF CLINICAL RESPONSE

An objective response to therapy is generally defined as >50% reduction in paraprotein levels (UKMF 2001). Response duration is the most consistent indicator of subsequent survival (Myeloma Trialists' Collaborative Group 1998). The therapeutic approach has been aimed at achieving a stable disease phase or plateau (defined as a stable paraprotein for a period of 3 months, associated stability and freedom from evidence of active end-organ damage such as anaemia and active bone disease) (UKMF 2001).

TREATMENT OPTIONS

Figure 5.3
Disease phases (reproduced with permission from IMF (UK) Concise Review of the Disease and Treatment Options 1999).

Chemotherapy with or without high-dose therapy (HDT) and haemopoietic stem cell rescue, and more recently immunomodulatory therapies, are used in the management of myeloma. The disease course usually follows periods of active disease and remission (Fig. 5.3). Treatment pathways are planned for each individual patient taking into account disease profile, general health and personal choices. Some patients may choose a pathway of active treatment at all costs, whilst others may choose more passive treatment options and supportive therapies. A summary of potential treatment pathways can be seen in Figure 5.4

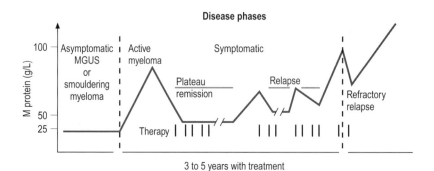

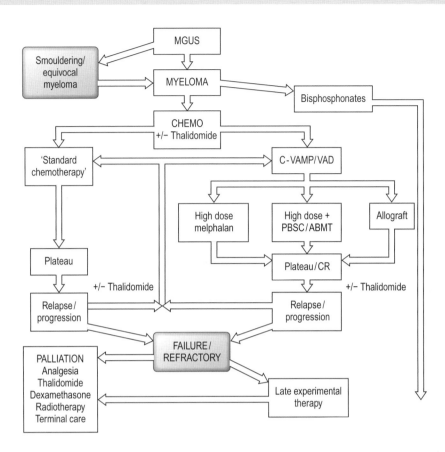

In planning initial treatment, future therapy options also need to be considered, most importantly, the potential for high-dose therapy (HDT) and stem cell transplantation. Some treatment choices may preclude patients from other therapies later in the course of their disease. For example, treatment with melphalan causes severe myelosuppression and damages stem cells and can lead to difficulties in mobilisation and subsequent harvesting of cells prior to transplant (Tricot et al 1995). Treatment with melphalan is therefore avoided if HDT and transplantation is planned.

REFLECTION POINT

Consider the nurse's role in ensuring the patient is fully informed and supported to make informed decisions about their treatment pathway.

INDICATIONS FOR TREATMENT

Chemotherapy induction

Current chemotherapy options include the alkylating agent melphalan, which was first used to treat myeloma in the late 1950s. The addition of prednisolone was found to improve response and intermittent courses of melphalan and prednisolone (M&P) have been standard therapy for myeloma for the last 30 years (Alexanian et al 1969). Response rates with M&P are 50–60% (Zomas & Dimopoulos 2002). Combination chemotherapy was introduced in the early 1970s with various alkylating agent combinations being used. Infusional regimens such as VAD (vincristine, adriamycin (doxorubicin), dexamethasone) were developed in the early 1980s and have been used successfully with reported response rates in chemotherapy-naive patients between 60–80% (Zomas & Dimopoulos 2002).

Infusional regimens produce rapid reduction of paraprotein levels and may be the preferred treatment for those in whom rapid tumour control is desirable, for example those with symptomatic disease (Zomas & Dimopoulos 2002). Regimens such as VAD are particularly useful for those with renal impairment as its components are not excreted renally. VAD and similar regimens are usually followed by HDT and stem cell transplantation and have the added benefit of stimulating mobilisation of stem cells (UKMF 2001), which is essential if the patient is to progress to transplantation.

Reports have suggested that high-dose dexamethasone (HDD) alone is responsible for much of the efficacy of VAD (Alexanian et al 1986). HDD alone has also been found to induce responses in 43% of newly diagnosed patients (Alexanian et al 1992). Intermittent oral HDD (plus dexamethasone) is therefore recommended as initial therapy in those for whom cytotoxic therapy is contraindicated, e.g. those presenting with severe pancytopenia (UKMF 2001).

UKMF guidelines (2001) recommend:

- M +/– P as initial treatment of choice for patients for whom HDT is not planned
- Cyclophosphamide regimen for patients not suitable for melphalan
- VAD-type regimen as primary treatment for patients intended for HDT.

Current regimens for up-front therapy regimens (first therapy given to treat the disease) are shown in Table 5.5. New up-front therapy regimens being studied include the use of novel treatments, alone or in combination with steroids and chemotherapy and include the use of drugs such as thalidomide and bortezomib (Velcade) (see Chapter 11).

High–dose therapy and stem cell transplantation in myeloma

Autologous stem cell transplantation

HDT and autologous stem cell transplantation have been used to treat myeloma since the 1980s with an increased use in the past decade. Data from the British Society of Blood and Marrow Transplantation (BSBMT) registry shows that more patients were transplanted for myeloma in 2002 than any other haematological malignancy (Fig. 5.5)

The use of HDT and stem cell transplantation has enabled an escalation of the dose of melphalan in conditioning regimens with an increase in overall survival. Conditioning regimens usually comprise VAD-like

Table 5.5
Current regimens for up-front
therapy

Abbreviation	Drugs
MP	Melphalan and prednisolone
C Weekly	Cyclophosphamide +/– prednisolone
ABCM	Doxorubicin (adriamycin), BCNU (carmustine), cyclophosphamide, melphalan
VAD	Vincristine, doxorubicin (adriamycin), dexamethasone
C-VAMP	Cyclophosphamide, vincristine, doxorubicin (adriamycin), prednisolone
CTD	Cyclophosphamide, thalidomide, dexamethasone
Z-Dex	Oral idarubicin and dexamethasone

Table 5.5
Current regimens for up-front
therapy

Figure 5.5
Number of transplants
undergone in UK per disease
category (data adapted from
BSBMT Data Registry 2002).

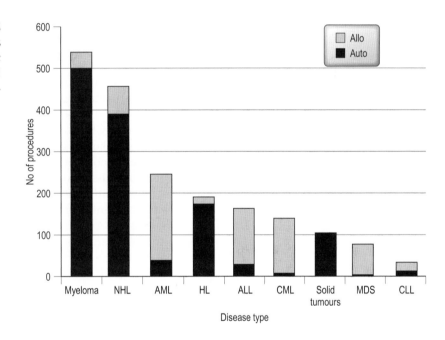

regimens to reduce tumour load and melphalan at a dose of 200 mg/m². HDT has been shown to result in improved survival over conventional chemotherapy regimens with a median survival of 54.8 months versus 42.3 months respectively (Child et al 2003). As first-line therapy HDT is associated with complete remission (CR) (100% reduction in paraprotein and <5% plasma cells in bone marrow) in 24–75% of individuals with a low treatment-related mortality (TRM) of <5% (Bladé et al 1998, UKMF 2001). HDT and stem cell transplantation is therefore recommended as standard treatment for patients with myeloma up to the age of 60 years (UKMF 2001). In practice, autograft procedures are being offered to those who are biologically fit for the procedure irrespective of age. HDT may be considered in those with severe renal impairment, but requires to be carried out in centres with special expertise (UKMF 2001).

Although HDT and stem cell transplantation improve CR rates and survival in myeloma, the majority of patients will relapse (Singhal 2002).

The role of tandem autograft procedures (two transplants planned at the onset, usually within 2–6 months of each other) is being explored in clinical trials to establish any survival benefit. Further evidence of efficacy is required. Many patients will have enough stem cells collected at the time of their first transplant to enable them to undergo a second or even third autograft procedure at time of relapse. As the benefits of tandem transplants are as yet unproven, delaying transplantation until relapse or a second transplant at relapse is a viable option (Durie et al 2003), especially if a first remission was of at least one, and preferably more than two, years (Fermand et al 1998).

Allogeneic transplantation

The role of allogeneic transplantation in myeloma has also been explored with the aim of improving complete remission rates and prolonging survival. Due to the increased toxicity and median age at diagnosis allogeneic transplantation is not a suitable therapy for the majority of patients. TRM, although improving, remains high at 21% (Gahrton et al 2001). Allogeneic transplantation is most effective when carried out early in the course of the disease. Patients transplanted in first response have a 60% chance of entering CR (Corradini et al 1999). An autograft procedure usually pre-empts the allograft, the aim being to reduce tumour load. Hence the patient undergoes two transplant procedures.

Current research is focussing on reduced intensity conditioning (RIC) allogeneic transplants (mini or non-myeloablative transplants) followed by donor T-lymphocyte infusions (DLI) to eradicate residual disease. This approach uses a less toxic conditioning regimen whilst harnessing the potentially curable graft-versus-myeloma (GvM) effect mediated by DLI (Kroger et al 2001). The RIC transplant also allows for an increase in the upper age limit for allogeneic transplant. With appropriate patient selection and early treatment in tandem with an autograft, RIC allografts appear to offer the best chance of long-term disease control for a small group of patients who are both young and fit enough.

Radiotherapy

Myeloma cells are particularly sensitive to radiotherapy (Rowell & Tobias 1991). Radiotherapy plays an important role in the treatment of those with myeloma with most patients requiring radiotherapy at some time in the course of their disease (Berenson 2002). The most common indication for radiotherapy is for palliation of painful bone lesions (Berenson 2002), but it is also used in the following ways (Shrieve 2002):

- curative treatment of solitary plasmacytoma
- part of conditioning for stem cell transplant in the form of total-body irradiation (TBI)
- treatment of spinal cord compression
- treatment of structural instability from focal disease.

Radiotherapy can reduce stem cell yield and should be restricted to patients with an absolute indication (Shrieve 2002).

Maintenance treatment

Once disease control has been established and a plateau reached, the aim of maintenance treatment is to maintain this period of stable disease. Traditionally interferon alpha (IFN-α) has been used as maintenance treatment, but has been shown to provide only marginal benefit (Berenson et al 2002) with no statistically significant impact on overall survival (Durie et al 2003). As potential benefits must be balanced against possible toxicity and quality of life, interferon is not the treatment of choice for many patients (UKMF 2001).

The role of thalidomide

Thalidomide is arguably the most significant advance in the treatment of myeloma in the last 30 years (Cavenagh 2003). It is an immunomodulatory drug with multiple mechanisms of action including inhibition of tumour necrosis factor α (TNF-α) production, a wide range of stimulatory and inhibitory effects on the immune system and the ability to inhibit the growth and survival of myeloma cells and blood vessel formation (angiogenesis) (Cavenagh et al 2003). Thalidomide has been also shown to be synergistic with other anti-myeloma agents, particularly dexamethasone. Initial use in refractory disease showed response rates in the region of 30–40%, rising to 65% when used in combination with steroids +/− chemotherapy (Cavenagh et al 2003). These findings have prompted further investigations and emerging evidence suggests that thalidomide may be of benefit as first-line therapy alone or in combination and/or for maintenance following conventional and HDT and stem cell transplant. Its role in the treatment of myeloma continues to be explored in ongoing clinical trials.

Risks to the unborn child exposed to thalidomide are well documented. It is essential that all patients prescribed thalidomide are made aware of these risks before commencing treatment.

Treatment for refractory and relapsed disease

As almost all patients with myeloma will relapse, the overall management strategy should include plans to treat relapse (UKMF 2001). Early relapse carries a poor prognosis and is unlikely to respond well to most chemotherapy treatments (UKMF 2001). Patients who relapse or progress after a long stable plateau phase are more likely to respond well to further treatment (UKMF 2001).

Conventional treatment options following relapse include further chemotherapy, HDT plus stem cell transplant, high-dose dexamethasone, thalidomide +/− steroids and hemi-body radiotherapy. A variety of new therapies are also emerging including derivatives of thalidomide, proteasome inhibitors, skeletal targeted radiotherapy, immune vaccines and monoclonal antibodies (see Chapter 11). Where they may fit with current management remains to be seen.

SUPPORTIVE TREATMENT

Treatment of the disease importantly includes supportive care of those complications associated with myeloma. Improvements in supportive treatment and care have improved survival and quality of life of patients with myeloma in recent years.

TREATMENT OF BONE DISEASE

The underlying cause of bone disease should be treated and the anti-myeloma therapies discussed earlier play an important role in disease control (Durie et al 2003).

Bisphosphonates

This group of drugs has been shown to substantially inhibit new bone destruction by inhibiting osteoclast activity. They are recommended as long-term therapy for all patients requiring treatment (Kyle 2000, UKMF 2001). Bisphosphonates have helped to revolutionise control of bone disease by reducing pain and skeletal events and improving quality of life (Djulbegovic et al 2002). The possible direct anti-myeloma activity of bisphosphonates is currently being investigated within clinical trials (Ludwig & Fritz 2002). Measures to improve bone health include regular evaluation of skeletal disease and radiation therapy and/or orthopaedic surgery to restore the structural integrity of bones (Durie et al 2003).

Bone pain

Pain is mainly due to bone lesions or pathological fractures caused by active disease (Ludwig & Fritz 2002). Persistent pain or sudden sharp pain may indicate a pathological fracture (Lokhorst 2002). Effective pain control is a priority and possible in almost all myeloma patients using medications administered regularly (Ludwig & Fritz 2002). Although non-steroidal anti-inflammatory drugs (NSAIDs) are often more effective in the treatment of bone pain, their use has been associated with renal impairment. As those with myeloma have an increased risk of renal dysfunction, NSAIDs should be avoided (UKMF 2001).

Opiate analgesia is often required for the control of myeloma bone pain and used with good effect, alone or in combination with adjuvant methods. Local radiotherapy to the site of a painful lytic lesion is also effective, with most patients achieving pain control (Berenson 2002).

A relatively novel procedure beginning to be used for the relief of pain caused by myeloma bone disease is percutaneous vertebroplasty. This involves the injection of bone cement into the vertebral body to relieve pain and stabilise the fractured vertebrae (NICE 2003).

Sensory pain in the form of peripheral neuropathy is increasingly being recognised. It is usually associated with administration of vincristine, thalidomide and bortezomib (Velcade) and can be progressive. Severity tends to be dose-related.

Spinal cord compression

About 10–20% of patients will develop spinal cord compression during the course of their disease as a result of tumour infiltration (Berenson 2002, Lokhorst 2002). Immediate treatment with systemic steroids and radiotherapy is important to prevent the development of a permanent neurological deficit (Berenson 2002).

Hypercalcaemia

Hypercalcaemia is the most frequent metabolic complication of myeloma (Ludwig & Fritz 2002). Successful treatment of myeloma and resultant bone disease is the best therapy (Ludwig & Fritz 2002). Those requiring immediate therapy should be well hydrated and treated with additional bisphosphonates (Berenson 2002).

REFLECTION POINT

Consider how bone disease affects those with myeloma. What advice should nurses offer to help prevent the complications associated with bone disease?

BONE MARROW FAILURE

Anaemia

Symptomatic anaemia should always be treated to maintain an optimal quality of life (Ludwig & Fritz 2002). Traditionally, symptomatic anaemia has been managed by red cell transfusion, but there is growing evidence to support the use of recombinant human erythropoietin (rh-EPO) in the treatment of chemotherapy-related anaemia (UKMF 2001). Rh-EPO is indicated in patients with myeloma who have chronic renal failure (UKMF 2001). Caution should be used when treating patients with a high paraprotein level with red cell transfusion, due to the risk of exacerbating hyperviscosity (UKMF 2001). Anaemia usually improves with response to treatment for the myeloma (UKMF 2001).

Infection

Infections are a common and recurrent problem. Antibiotic therapy should be initiated promptly if active infection is suspected (Durie 2003). The use of prophylactic antibiotics with recurrent infection is controversial due to the risk of developing antibiotic resistance (Kelleher & Chapel 2002). Replacement immunoglobulin therapy with high-dose gammaglobulin may be required in patients with recurrent infections (Durie 2003). Haematopoietic growth factors such as granulocyte-colony stimulating factor (G-CSF) may be used to increase white blood cell levels in an effort to overcome the infectious complications of high-dose therapy (Durie 2003).

Active immunisation with pneumococcal vaccination is recommended (UKMF 2001), although in general, patients with myeloma mount an impaired antibody response to vaccination (Kelleher & Chapel 2002).

HYPERVISCOSITY SYNDROME

Treatment for hyperviscosity involves treating the underlying plasma cell disorder to reduce the blood paraprotein levels. In acute cases, therapeutic plasmapheresis may be required to prevent neurological and cardiac complications associated with hyperviscosity.

RENAL IMPAIRMENT

Everyone presenting with renal failure should be carefully evaluated for potentially reversible factors (Shaver-Lewis & Shah 2002). With appropriate rehydration, reversal of hypercalcaemia and chemotherapy to treat myeloma, renal function will normalise in about 50% of patients (Lokhurst 2002). As light-chain deposition is associated with renal damage, one of the primary goals of therapy is a rapid reduction in the paraprotein level. Plasmapheresis is sometimes used as a means of rapidly lowering paraprotein concentrations and improving acute renal failure (Shaver-Lewis & Shah 2002).

For a small proportion of patients (3–12%) (Clarke et al 1999), long-term renal replacement therapy in the form of peritoneal dialysis or haemodialysis, will be required (Shaver-Lewis & Shah 2002). Treatment regimes may need to be altered in line with renal function.

Case study 5.1

Ron is 65 years old and almost due to retire. He had been feeling pain in his lower back, tiredness and lethargy for about 3 months, which he assumed was work- and stress-related. After reaching for a book on a high shelf, Ron felt sudden acute pain in his right side. On visiting his GP Ron had a chest x-ray that showed a pathological fracture of one of his ribs. He was also found to be anaemic with a haemoglobin of 9 g/dL. He was referred to a haematologist for investigations and a diagnosis of myeloma was confirmed by bone marrow biopsy. Ron was immediately started on regular bisphosphonate treatment and discussed the potential treatment options with his haematologist. To support the verbal information given, the nurse in the clinic gave Ron a booklet and contact numbers for information and support organisations. His son also obtained further information from the International Myeloma Foundation UK website. Ron went on to have a course of VAD chemotherapy with a plan to having his stem cells collected and stored after three cycles before going on to receive high-dose therapy and stem cell transplantation.

SPECIFIC NURSING ISSUES

Nurses have a unique opportunity to contribute to all aspects of care for patients and their families. They contribute at every level and often provide the essential continuity and coordination necessary for the efficient management and care of any patient. Prevention, detection and management of specific complications are of particular importance in the nursing care of those with myeloma.

MANAGEMENT OF PAIN

Bone pain is the most debilitating symptom of the disease and effective pain control is a priority. Pain is a multidimensional experience, encompassing physical, psychological and spiritual aspects. Assessment of all these aspects is the first step in effective pain management. Pain assessment tools are widely used and assist in achieving accurate and objective assessment. Visual analogue scales (VAS) and numerical rating scales (NRS) are simple and quick ways to assess pain and evaluate the effectiveness of an intervention (Carr & Mann 2000). Methods of pain relief vary but often opiate analgesia is required. The World Health Organization analgesic ladder (WHO 1990) provides an effective tool in the use of appropriate analgesics.

Non-pharmacological interventions, such as massage, application of hot and cold packs to the site of pain, and relaxation methods, are also widely used with some success. Despite the lack of evidence to support the effectiveness of non-pharmacological techniques, their benefits should not be underestimated. These interventions should be used in conjunction with, rather than in place of, pharmacological therapies. Although the treatment of pain is a multidisciplinary team effort, nurses play a vital role in optimum pain management.

IMPROVING BONE HEALTH

General measures to improve bone health include adequate pain control, exercise and avoidance of activities that increase the likelihood of falls/trauma. Low impact exercise such as walking and swimming are helpful to enhance bone strength and remodelling (Durie et al 2003).

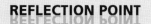

REFLECTION POINT   What are the potential difficulties in pain management for an individual with myeloma?

SPINAL CORD COMPRESSION

Early recognition of the signs and symptoms of spinal cord compression (SCC) and awareness of the importance of prompt treatment to prevent permanent damage is an essential nursing role. The resulting signs and symptoms depend on the spinal tracts involved. Most common signs include pain in the back or neck experienced by 90% of patients (Held & Peahota 1993). Other symptoms include limb weakness and sensory changes with numbness or tingling in the limbs. Sphincter disturbance, including urinary hesitancy and retention, incontinence and constipation are late occurring symptoms (Kay 1992). SCC is always a neurological and oncological emergency (Dougherty & Lister 2004). Patients should be educated as to the risk of SCC and the signs that may require immediate action. Professionals also have a responsibility to ensure their own awareness of SCC and to take prompt and appropriate action as required (British Association of Surgical Oncology 1999).

PREVENTION OF INFECTION

Nurses need to be aware of this and recognise and report early signs and symptoms (see Chapter 15). Patients and carers also need to be educated to recognise signs of infection increasing the chance of early intervention.

PREVENTION OF HYPERCALCAEMIA

Nurses should be aware of the signs and symptoms of hypercalcaemia and the need for patients to be adequately hydrated in order to help to prevent this complication and its consequences, such as renal failure. The frequency and intensity of symptoms depend upon the degree of hypercalcaemia. Nursing care includes early detection and support through treatment.

PREVENTION OF RENAL IMPAIRMENT

The importance of a 2–3-litre daily fluid intake cannot be overstated. Good hydration helps to prevent renal impairment in a variety of ways, e.g. by preventing volume depletion, reducing concentration of paraproteins in distal tubules, reducing precipitation of uric acid crystals and helping to prevent hypercalcaemia (Shaver-Lewis & Shah 2002).

Careful monitoring and education of patients, especially those at high risk, about the need for a high fluid intake is an essential nursing role. Patients may require intravenous fluids at times when oral hydration is difficult, e.g. if pyrexial, nil by mouth or experiencing nausea and vomiting. For those with chronic renal failure open communication and liaison with the specialist renal team is required to optimise the care and outcome for the patient with chronic renal failure (UKMF 2001).

PREVENTION OF CONSTIPATION

Constipation is commonly experienced by individuals with myeloma and is associated with a combination of factors including side effects of treatments such as chemotherapy, thalidomide and opiate analgesia or as a result of hypercalcaemia, dehydration or reduced mobility. Prevention and early detection is an essential part of care and nurses should be aware of the potential for constipation. Prophylactic measures such as stool softeners and stimulant laxatives may be necessary, especially for individuals receiving opiate analgesia (Curtiss 1996) or thalidomide. Monitoring elimination will allow early detection of a change in bowel habit and prompt intervention. Normal bowel movement has been defined as ranging between three times a day and three times a week (Nazarko 1996). It is therefore important to establish the patient's usual bowel habit. Education and support as to the benefits of a balanced diet with plenty of fruit, fibre and fluid along with gentle exercise, can help to reduce the risk of constipation.

PALLIATIVE AND SUPPORTIVE CARE

As myeloma remains an incurable disease, supportive and palliative care are important aspects of care. Patients with myeloma are usually older at diagnosis and often have co-morbidities. Both patients and their families need to be helped to understand that although treatment is not aimed at a cure, it will relieve symptoms of their disease and prolong survival and its quality (UKMF 2001). A positive, enthusiastic and realistic approach to the management of myeloma is an essential element of good care. Key attributes for effective care include:

- a specialised understanding of the nature of myeloma and range of treatment options available
- early detection, recognition and support of the main complications of myeloma
- providing a specialist resource for information, education and support for patients and their families.

The introduction of the palliative care team should be considered at all stages of the disease, preferably from the point of diagnosis. Optimum symptom management is essential as myeloma is often a chronic, painful and debilitating illness. With comprehensive symptom management and support from diagnosis, nurses can help patients with myeloma to live life to the full.

Provision of information is a key part of the nurse's role. Research has consistently shown that cancer patients want to receive detailed high-quality information about their condition and possible treatment, given in an honest, timely and sensitive manner at all stages of the patient pathway (NICE 2004). Full and clear information improves knowledge and understanding, reduces anxiety, increases the patient's sense of control and increases both acceptance of treatment and satisfaction with it (NICE 2004).

CONCLUSION

Myeloma is a complex and individual disease, not yet considered curable but highly treatable. Treatment options available to those with myeloma have never been more abundant than in the last few years. Increased understanding of cytogenetics and immunotherapy has increased interest in the field of myeloma. With new agents and combinations of therapies being explored it is hoped that in time myeloma will become more of a chronic illness than an incurable malignancy. Nurses have a significant role to play in the education and care of patients and can help to significantly improve the quality of life of the increasing number of patients living with myeloma.

DISCUSSION QUESTIONS

1. What is the role of the nurse in caring for individuals with myeloma?

2. What information do individuals with myeloma require for decision-making on treatment choices?

References

Alexanian R, Haut A, Khan A U et al 1969 Treatment for multiple myeloma: combination chemotherapy with different melphalan dose regimens. Journal of the American Medical Association 208: 1680–1685

Alexanian R, Barlogie B, Dixon D 1986 High-dose glucocorticoid treatment in resistant myeloma. Annals of Internal Medicine 105:8–11

Alexanian R, Dimopopoulos M A, Delasalle K, Barlogie B 1992 Primary dexamethasone treatment in multiple myeloma. Blood 80:887–890

Barlogie B, Sawyer J, Ayers D et al 1998 Chromosome 13 myeloma is a distinct entity with poor prognosis despite tandem autotransplants. Blood 92:259A

Bataille R, Harrousseau J L 1997 Multiple myeloma. New England Journal of Medicine 336:1657–1664

Bataille R, Chappard D, Basle M 1995 Excessive bone resorption in human plasmacytomas: direct induction by tumor cells in vivo. British Journal of Haematology 90:721–724

Bataille R, Delmas P D, Chappard D, Sany J 1990 Abnormal serum bone GLA protein levels in multiple myeloma: crucial role of bone formation and prognostic implications. Cancer 66:67–72

Berenson J R 2002 Bone disease in myeloma. In: Mehta J, Singhal S (eds) Myeloma. Martin Dunitz, London, pp 97–117

Berenson J R, Crowley J J, Grogan T M et al 2002 Maintenance therapy with alternate day prednisone improves survival in multiple myeloma patients. Blood 99(9):3465–3467

Bladé J, Samson D, Reece D et al 1998 Criteria for evaluating disease response and progression in patients with multiple myeloma treated by high-dose therapy and haemopoietic stem cell transplantation. Myeloma Subcommittee of the EBMT, European Group for Blood and Marrow Transplant. British Journal of Haematology 102(5):1115–1123

British Association of Surgical Oncology 1999 The management of metastatic bone disease in the United Kingdom In: Dougherty L, Lister S (eds) The Royal Marsden Hospital manual of clinical nursing procedures, 6th edn. Blackwell, Oxford

British Society for Blood and Marrow Transplantation (BSBMT) 2002 Data registry. BSBMT, London

Carr E, Mann E 2000 Pain: creative approaches to effective management. Macmillan, Basingstoke

Cavenagh J 2003. Thalidomide an update. Myeloma Today UK 15(1):3–4

Cavenagh J D, Oakervee H, UK Myeloma Forum and the BCSH Haematology/Oncology Task Force 2003 Thalidomide in multiple myeloma: current status and future prospects. British Journal of Haematology 120(1):18–26

Child J A, Morgan G J, Davies F E et al 2003 High dose chemotherapy with haematopoietic stem cell rescue for multiple myeloma. New England Journal of Medicine 348:1875–1883

Clarke A D, Shetty A, Soutar R 1999 Renal failure and multiple myeloma: pathogenesis and treatment of renal failure and management of underlying myeloma. Blood Reviews 13:79–90

Corradini P, Voena C, Tarella C et al 1999. Molecular and clinical remissions in multiple myeloma: role of autologous and allogeneic transplantation of hematopoietic cells. Journal of Clinical Oncology 17:208–215

Curtiss C 1996 Constipation. In: Groenwald S, Hansen Frogge M, Goodman M, Henke Yarbo C (eds) Cancer symptom management, 4th edn. Jones and Bartlett, Boston

Dimopoulos M A 2002 Waldenstrom's macroglobulinaemia. In: Mehta J, Singhal S (eds) Myeloma. Martin Dunitz, London, pp 465–480

Djulbegovic B, Wheatley K, Ross J et al 2002 Bisphosphonates in multiple myeloma. Cochrane Database Systematic Reviews 3:CD003188

Dougherty L, Lister S 2004 The Royal Marsden Hospital manual of clinical nursing procedures, 6th edn. Blackwell, Oxford

Durie B G M 1999 A concise review of the disease and treatment options. International Myeloma Foundation (UK), Edinburgh

Durie B G M 2003 A concise review of the disease and treatment options. International Myeloma Foundation, Los Angeles

Durie B G M, Salmon S E 1975 A clinical staging system for multiple myeloma. Cancer 36:842–854

Durie B G M, Kyle R, Belch A et al 2003. Myeloma management guidelines: a consensus report from the scientific advisors of the International Myeloma Foundation. Hematology Journal 4(6):379–398

Facon T, Avet-Loiseau H, Guillerm G et al Intergroupe Francophone du Myelome 2001 Chromosome 13 abnormalities identified by FISH analysis and serum β2-microglobulin produce a powerful myeloma staging system for patients receiving high-dose therapy. Blood 97:1566–1571

Fermand J P, Ravaud P, Chevret S et al 1998 High dose therapy and autologous peripheral blood stem cell transplantation in multiple myeloma: up front or rescue treatment? Results of a multicentre sequential randomised clinical trial. Blood 92:3131–3136

Gahrton G, Svensson H, Cavo M et al for the European Group for Blood and Marrow Transplantation 2001 Progress in allogenic bone marrow and peripheral blood stem cell transplantation for multiple myeloma: a comparison between transplants performed 1983–93 and 1994–98 at European Group for Blood and Marrow Transplantation centres. British Journal of Haematology 113:209–216

Greipp P R 1992 Advances in the diagnosis and management of myeloma. Seminars in Haematology 29:24–45

Greipp P R, San Miguel J F, Fonseca R et al 2003 Development of an International Prognostic Index (IPI) for myeloma: report of the International Myeloma Working Group. Hematology Journal 4(Suppl 1):S42

Held J L, Peahota A 1993 Nursing care of the patient with spinal cord compression. Oncology Nursing Forum 20(10):1507–1516

Joshua D E, Gibson J 2002 Epidemiology of plasma cell disorders. In: Mehta J, Singhal S (eds) Myeloma. Martin Dunitz, London, pp 140–150

Kay P 1992 A–Z of hospice care and palliative medicine. EPL Publications, Northampton

Kelleher P, Chapel H 2002. Infections: principles of prevention and therapy. In: Mehta J, Singhal S (eds) Myeloma. Martin Dunitz, London, pp 223–239

Keuhl M W, Bergsagel P L 2002 Multiple myeloma: evolving genetic events and host interactions. Nature Reviews Cancer 2:175–187

Kroger N, Kruger W, Renges H et al 2001 Donor lymphocyte infusion enhances remission status in patients with persistent disease after allografting for multiple myeloma. British Journal of Haematology 112:421–423

Kyle R A 2000 The role of bisphosphonates in multiple myeloma. Annals of Internal Medicine 132:734–736

Kyle R A, Rajkumar S V 2002 Monoclonal gammopathies of undetermined significance. In: Mehta J, Singhal S (eds) Myeloma. Martin Dunitz, London, pp 415–432

Leif Bergsagel P 2004 Epidemiology, aetiology and molecular pathogenesis, In: Richardson P G, Anderson K C (eds) Multiple myeloma. Remedica Publishing, London, pp 1–24

Lokhurst H 2002 Clinical features and diagnostic criteria. In: Mehta J, Singhal S (eds) Myeloma. Martin Dunitz, London, pp 151–168

Ludwig H, Fritz E 2002 Supportive therapy. In: Mehta J, Singhal S (eds) Myeloma. Martin Dunitz, London, pp 397–412

Marcelin A G, Dupin N, Bouscary D et al 1997 HHV-8 and multiple myeloma in France. Lancet 350:1144.

Myeloma Trialists' Collaborative Group 1998 Combination chemotherapy versus melphalan plus prednisone as treatment for multiple myeloma: an overview of 6,633 patients from 27 randomized trials. Journal of Clinical Oncology 16(12):3832–3842

National Institute for Clinical Excellence 2003 Improving outcomes in haematological cancers: the manual. NICE, London

National Institute for Clinical Excellence 2004 Improving supportive and palliative care for adults with cancer. NICE, London

Nazarko L 1996 Preventing constipation in older people. Professional Nurse 11(12):816–818

Office for National Statistics 2002 Cancer Statistics Registrations: Registrations of Cancer Diagnosed in 1999, England. Series MB1, No. 30. HMSO, London

Oyajobi B O, Mundy G R 2004 Pathophysiology of myeloma bone disease. In: Gahrton G, Durie B G M, Samson D (eds) Multiple myeloma and related disorders. Arnold, London, pp 74–88

Raje N, Anderson K C 2002. Cytokine abnormalities in plasma cell disorders. In: Mehta J, Singhal S (eds) Myeloma. Martin Dunitz, London, pp 53–64

Rowell N P, Tobias J S 1991 The role of radiotherapy in the management of multiple myeloma. Blood Reviews 5:84–89

Samson D 2003 Myeloma bone disease and imaging techniques. Myeloma Today UK 17:4–5

San Miguel J, Almeida J, Orfao A 2002 Laboratory investigations. In: Mehta J, Singhal S (eds) Myeloma. Martin Dunitz, London, pp 243–268

Savage D G, Lindenbaum J, Garrett T J 1982 Biphasic pattern of infection in multiple myeloma. Annals of Internal Medicine 96:47–50

Sawyer J R, Singhal S 2002 Cytogenetics in plasma cell disorders. In: Mehta J, Singhal S (eds) Myeloma. Martin Dunitz, London, pp 65–80

Seong C, Delasallie K, Hayes K et al 1998 Prognostic value of cytogenetics in multiple myeloma. British Journal of Haematology 101:189–195

Shaver-Lewis M J, Shah S V 2002 The kidney in plasma cell disorders. In: Mehta J, Singhal S (eds) Myeloma. Martin Dunitz, London, pp 203–221

Shrieve D C 2002 The role of radiotherapy. In: Mehta J, Singhal S (eds) Myeloma. Martin Dunitz, London, pp 367–381

Singhal S 2002 High-dose therapy and autologous transplantation. In: Mehta J, Singhal S (eds) Myeloma. Martin Dunitz, London, pp 328–347

Souhami R, Tobias S 1995 Cancer and its management, 2nd edn. Blackwell Science, Oxford

Tricot G, Jagannath S, Vesole D et al 1995 Peripheral blood stem cell transplant for multiple myeloma: identification of favourable variables for rapid engraftment in 225 patients. Blood 85:588–596

Torcia M, Lucibello M, Vannier E et al 1996 Modulation of osteoclast-activating factor activity of multiple myeloma bone marrow cells by different interleukin-1 inhibitors. Experimental Hematology 24:868–874

UK Myeloma Forum 2001 Guidelines on the diagnosis and management of multiple myeloma. British Journal of Haematology 115:522–540

World Health Organization 1990 Cancer pain relief and palliative care: report of a WHO expert panel. WHO Technical Report 804. WHO, Geneva

Yi Q 2002 Immunoregulatory mechanisms and immunotherapy. In: Mehta J, Singhal S (eds) Myeloma. Martin Dunitz, London, pp 81–96

Zomas A, Dimopoulos M A 2002 Conventional treatment of myeloma. In: Mehta J, Singhal S (eds) Myeloma. Martin Dunitz, London, pp 313–326

Further reading

The following web sites provide a useful resource for information on myeloma the disease, treatment options, medical research, patient information guides and educational events.

- The UK Myeloma Forum *www.ukmf.org.uk*
- International Myeloma Foundation UK *www.myeloma.org.uk*
- International Myeloma Foundation *www.myeloma.org*
- Multiple Myeloma Research Foundation *www.multiplemyeloma.org*

The following publications provide a comprehensive resource on all aspects of myeloma and related disorders.

Gahrton G, Durie B G M, Samson D (eds) 2004 Multiple myeloma and related disorders. Arnold, London

Malpas J S, Bergsagel D E, Kyle R A (eds) 1995 Myeloma biology and management, 2nd edn. Oxford Medical Publications, Oxford

Mehta J, Singhal S (eds) 2002 Myeloma. Martin Dunitz, London

National Institute for Clinical Excellence 2003 Improving outcomes in haematological cancers – the manual. NICE, London

Richardson P G, Anderson K C (eds) 2004 Multiple myeloma. Remedica Publishing, London

Chapter 6

The lymphomas

Maggie Grundy and Gena Andrews

KEY POINTS

- The lymphomas are a diverse group of cancers arising from lymphoid tissue.
- Lymphomas comprise two distinct groups: Hodgkin's lymphoma and non-Hodgkin's lymphoma.
- Accurate classification and staging of the disease are important in ensuring optimum treatment and management.
- Many lymphomas are potentially curable.

INTRODUCTION

The lymphomas are a diverse group of cancers arising from lymphoid tissue and comprise two distinct groups: Hodgkin's lymphoma (HL) and non-Hodgkin's lymphoma (NHL). Both these groups contain a number of disease subtypes. Accurate identification of the specific subtype is important in determining prognosis and the most effective treatment and management. This chapter illustrates the similarities and differences between HL and NHL and outlines their treatment and specific nursing management.

THE DISEASES

Hodgkin's disease was first described by Thomas Hodgkin in 1832 and originally thought to be an infectious condition rather than a malignant one. Hodgkin's disease is now more commonly called Hodgkin's lymphoma and has two main types: nodular lymphocyte-predominant Hodgkin's lymphoma accounting for approximately 5% of cases and classical Hodgkin's lymphoma. Classical HL is further divided into four subtypes:

- nodular sclerosis (most common form of HL)
- mixed cellularity
- lymphocyte-rich
- lymphocyte-depleted (Jaffe et al 2001).

The term non-Hodgkin's lymphoma encompasses all lymphomas which are not Hodgkin's lymphoma. The NHL's are a diverse group of diseases and their classification is more complex. Historically, a number of different classification systems have been used for NHL. The Revised European-American Lymphoma (REAL)/World Health Organization (WHO) classification system is now accepted (Harris et al 1999). This system classifies all lymphoid malignancies (including HL). Lymphomas and lymphoid leukaemias of the same cell type are considered to be the same disease with differing clinical presentations or stages. Those presenting with peripheral blood involvement are considered to be leukaemias and those with lymphoid tissue involvement lymphomas (Harris et al 2000). Accurate classification is important in determining optimum treatment and management. The most commonly occurring NHLs are diffuse large B-cell lymphoma (33%) and follicular lymphoma (22%); all other NHLs represent less than 10% of the total number of cases (Evans & Hancock 2003). The different subtypes of NHL are shown in Table 6.1.

INCIDENCE

Hodgkin's lymphoma represents less than 1% of all cancers (Pileri et al 2002). It is the 23rd most common cancer in the UK with an incidence of 3 per 100,000 (Leukaemia Research Fund (LRF) 2003a, Cancer Research UK (CRUK) 2005a). Incidence rates have remained relatively stable over the past 20 years (Mackie 2001). Two age-related peaks in incidence are apparent, the first in young adults between the ages of 15–25 and the second in those over 65 years of age (Sweetenham 1998). HL is more common in white people and less common among Asians (Vose et al 2002, Argiris & Kaklamani 2004). In Western Europe and the USA, mortality rates have decreased by two-thirds since the 1960s and it is now

Table 6.1
The Revised European–American Lymphoma/World Health Organization (REAL/WHO) classification of lymphoid neoplasms (Jaffe et al 2001)

B-cell neoplasms	T- and natural killer (NK)-cell neoplasms
Precursor B-cell neoplasm – Precursor B-lymphoblastic leukaemia/lymphoma	**Precursor T-cell neoplasm** – Precursor T-lymphoblastic leukaemia/lymphoma – Blastoid NK-cell lymphoma
Mature (peripheral) B-cell neoplasms – Chronic lymphocytic leukaemia/B-cell small lymphocytic lymphoma – B-cell promyelocytic leukaemia – Lymphoplasmacytic lymphoma – Splenic marginal zone B-cell lymphoma – Hairy cell leukaemia – Plasma cell myeloma/plasmacytoma – Extranodal marginal zone B-cell lymphoma (MALT lymphoma) – Nodal marginal zone B-cell lymphoma – Follicular lymphoma – Mantle cell lymphoma – Diffuse large B-cell lymphoma – Burkitt's lymphoma	**Mature (peripheral) T-cell neoplasms** – T-cell prolymphocytic leukaemia–T-cell large granular lymphocytic leukaemia – Aggressive NK-cell leukaemia – Adult T-cell lymphoma/leukaemia (HTLV1+) – Extranodal NK/T-cell lymphoma, nasal type – Enteropathy-type T-cell lymphoma – Hepatosplenic T-cell lymphoma – Mycosis fungoides/Sézary syndrome – Primary cutaneous anaplastic large cell lymphoma – Peripheral T-cell lymphoma, not otherwise specified – Angioimmunoblastic T-cell lymphoma – Primary systemic anaplastic large cell lymphoma

one of the most curable cancers (Swerdlow et al 2001, Yung & Lynch 2003). However, survival rates differ depending on age and stage of disease. For those under 60, 5-year survival is 80% whereas for patients over 60 years, 5-year survival is 23% (Mackie 2001).

Non-Hodgkin's lymphoma occurs mainly in the elderly. Incidence increases over the age of 50 and most people are over 60 (CRUK 2005b). NHL is the 6th most common cancer in the UK (CRUK 2005a) and the 5th most common cancer in the USA (Baris & Zahm 2000). The age standardised incidence rate in the UK was calculated as 12.9 per 100,000 per year in 2001 (CRUK 2005b).

In the UK, NHL is approximately four times more common than HL (Cancer Research Campaign 1998). Incidence rates for NHL are higher in Western Europe and the USA than in South America and Asia. However, incidence has increased consistently worldwide over the last 30–40 years by 3–5% per year (Quinn et al 2001, Ries et al 2002). In the UK, the greatest increases have been in older people (CRUK 2005b). The reasons for this increasing incidence remain unclear. Human immunodeficiency virus (HIV)-related lymphomas, improved diagnostic techniques and newer classification systems are all suggested as contributory factors. However, the increase is thought to be too great to be attributed to these factors alone and the figures are thought to represent a real rise in incidence (Baris & Zahm 2000, Quinn et al 2001).

NHL is the 8th most common cause of cancer death in the UK (CRUK 2004). Age standardised mortality rates are cited as 5.8 per 100,000 in 2003 (CRUK 2005b). However, mortality statistics are considered somewhat unreliable as other causes of death, e.g. infection, are often recorded.

Survival rates differ significantly with age and gender. Five-year survival rates range from 65% in those under the age of 44 to 13% in those over 80 and are higher in women (CRUK 2005b). Overall both NHL and HL are commoner in men than women (Baris & Zahm 2000, LRF 2003a,b). The causes of NL and NHL remain unclear although a number of risk factors have been established and are outlined in Table 6.2.

PATHOPHYSIOLOGY

Lymphomas arise from the uncontrolled growth of a group of lymphocytes. The majority of lymphomas are derived from B lymphocytes (approximately 85%) although a minority arise from T lymphocytes (approximately 15%). The different subtypes of lymphomas arise from B and T cells at different stages of differentiation (Harris et al 2001). Normal B and T lymphocytes are involved in cellular and humoral immunity and therefore immune function may be abnormal in lymphoma, increasing the risk of infection.

Classical HL is characterised by the abnormal giant multinucleated Reed–Sternberg cells and Hodgkin's cells which correspond to a specific subtype of HL (Pileri et al 2002). These characteristic giant cells are absent in nodular lymphocyte-predominant HL and abnormal lymphocytic and histiocytic cells (popcorn cells) are present (Thomas et al 2004).

HL is peculiar amongst malignant diseases as the abnormal Reed–Sternberg and Hodgkin's cells are few in number in the tumour (the opposite of most cancers where large amounts of malignant cells are found) and surrounded by an inflammatory infiltrate composed of T cells, histiocytes, eosinophils, fibroblasts and plasma cells and sustained by the production of cytokines including tumour necrosis factor α, interleukins and gamma interferon (Skinnider & Mak 2000, Pileri et al 2002, Thomas et al 2004). It is thought that cytokines produced by cells of the inflammatory infiltrate contribute to the development and survival of Reed–Sternberg cells. Reed–Sternberg cells also produce cytokines which initiate and sustain the inflammatory infiltrate. Most of the cytokines identified are associated with either a humoral or cell-mediated immune response (Skinnider & Mak 2000).

In nodular lymphocyte-predominant HL tumour cells, normal B-cell antigens are usually present and immunoglobulin is expressed (Yung & Linch 2003), whereas in classical HL most tumour cells do not express antigens specific to normal B or T lymphocytes but acquire a number of other antigens not usually expressed by normal cells (Diehl et al 2003). Tumour cells also fail to express immunoglobulin normally expressed by B cells. Normal B lymphocytes would be expected to die through

Table 6.2
Risk factors

Hodgkin's lymphoma	Non–Hodgkin's lymphoma
The Epstein–Barr virus is associated with HL particularly in children and the elderly. HL in young adults has the lowest rates of Epstein–Barr-associated disease (Jarrett et al 1996) Risk is increased in several immunodeficient states, e.g. HIV infection, although not as commonly as with NHL (Swerdlow 2003) Genetic susceptibility demonstrated in studies of twins (Mack et al 1995) Occupational exposure – woodworkers have the most consistent association with HL (McCunney 1999)	Both congenital and acquired immunodeficiency or suppression is associated with an increased incidence of NHL including: – Primary immune deficiency states, e.g. ataxia telangiectasia, Fanconi's anaemia and Wiskott–Aldrich syndrome – Acquired immune deficiency states, e.g. HIV (Dal Maso & Franceschi 2003) – Therapeutic immunosuppression, e.g. following organ/haemopoietic stem cell transplant (Opelz & Henderson 1993, Curtis et al 1999, Swerdlow et al 2000) – Autoimmune disorders, e.g. rheumatoid arthritis, systemic lupus erythematosus (Swerdlow 2003) A family history of lymphoma or other haematological cancer is thought to increase the risk of developing NHL (Zhu et al 1998) Infectious agents such as the Epstein–Barr virus (Hsu & Glaser 2000) and the human T-cell lymphotrophic virus-1 (HTLV-1) have also been associated with the development of NHL (Manns et al 1999) *Helicobacter pylori* infection has been identified as a risk factor in gastric mucosa-associated tissue lymphoid (MALT) lymphoma (Bouzourene et al 1999) Hepatitis C virus has been associated with NHL. However, findings are inconsistent Occupational exposure to pesticides, solvents, hair-dye and sunlight have all been implicated but their impact as causative agents remains unproven (Adami et al 1995, Rego 1998, Schroeder et al 2001, La Vecchia & Tavani 2002)

normal cell death (apoptosis) mechanisms if they do not express immunoglobulin. This lack of susceptibility to apoptosis is thought to be a contributory factor in the development of HL (Straus et al 2001, Meyer et al 2004).

In NHL, chromosomal translocations are thought to represent the main mechanism for the activation of proto-oncogenes and the suppression of tumour suppressor genes which promote tumour growth. A number of chromosomal translocations have been noted, e.g. t(8;14) in Burkitt's lymphoma, t(14;18) in follicular lymphoma, t(11;14) in mantle-cell lymphoma (De Vita & Canellos 1999, Evans & Hancock 2003). These translocations are not thought to be of great enough magnitude to cause NHL but they do help to define distinct subtypes of disease (Harris et al 2001).

Lymphoma cells spread by the lymphatic and haemopoietic systems and can infiltrate tissue, destroying normal structure and lymphatic tissue. Organs such as the spleen and bone marrow may be infiltrated. Lymph nodes are often the primary site of involvement although other lymphatic tissue may also be affected. The most common presentation is a painless swelling of one group of lymph nodes. In HL the cervical nodes are most frequently affected first, although the mediastinal, axillary and inguinal nodes may also be the primary site (Plates 4 & 5). HL tends to follow a predictable course with the disease progressing from one group of lymph nodes to adjacent groups and is likely to be diagnosed at an early stage. Progression of NHL is less predictable and many patients have widespread extranodal disease or leukaemic symptoms on diagnosis (Hoffbrand et al 2001).

CLINICAL FEATURES

Painless, localised lymphadenopathy is frequently the only manifestation of HL. The nodes are often described as rubbery and may increase and decrease in size (Hoffbrand et al 2001). Mediastinal masses frequently occur and individuals may have a cough, dyspnoea or chest discomfort (Yung & Linch 2003). However, if the disease is more extensive, generalised lymphadenopathy and/or systemic symptoms such as fatigue, fever, night sweats, unexplained weight loss and pruritis may be present. These symptoms are thought to be caused by the release of cytokines (Skinnider & Mak 2000). Pain in affected lymph nodes with alcohol consumption has also been reported (Hoffbrand et al 2001).

NHL may also present as painless, localised or generalised lymphadenopathy. Systemic symptoms are less likely to occur in NHL than in HL but extranodal involvement is more likely, with the spleen and liver often being enlarged. However, approximately 15–20% of NHL initially occurs extranodally and can occur virtually anywhere in the body (CRUK 2005b). The gastrointestinal system is the commonest primary extranodal site and individuals may present with indigestion and other abdominal symptoms. Occasionally, individuals may present with symptoms of metabolic disturbance such as hypercalcaemia.

Clinical features depend on the extent and site of the disease. Enlarged lymph nodes may cause pressure on other organs resulting in pain or dysfunction. Obstruction of lymph drainage due to enlarged inguinal or axillary nodes may result in lymphoedema in upper or lower limbs, whereas pressure on the superior vena cava may result in oedema of the neck and face, obstructing the airways and causing dyspnoea (superior vena cava syndrome). Anaemia or pancytopenia may be present if the bone marrow is involved. Hypogammaglobulinaemia may also occur, substantially increasing infection risk.

DIAGNOSIS

Lymph node biopsy is required for diagnosis and to determine the histology and classification of the lymphoma. Immunophenotyping and cytogenetic studies are used to determine cell surface antigens and chromosomal rearrangements.

STAGING

Extensive clinical examination and a variety of investigations are undertaken to stage the disease (Table 6.3). Staging establishes the extent of the disease and is a further determinant of prognosis and treatment. The Ann Arbor Staging System was originally devised for HL based on the predictable progression of the disease (Carbone et al 1971) and subsequently modified slightly (Lister et al 1989). This staging system is also used in NHL but because of the more unpredictable nature of these diseases it is less reliable. The Ann Arbor Staging System consists of four stages with stage I representing localised disease and stage IV representing advanced disease (Fig. 6.1):

- Stage I: One lymph node region or lymphoid structure such as the spleen or thymus involved.
- Stage II: Two or more lymph node regions on the same side of the diaphragm involved.
- Stage III: One or more lymph node regions or lymphoid structures on both sides of the diaphragm involved. Stage III is further subdivided:
  - III_1 involvement limited to spleen, splenic hilar nodes, coeliac nodes or mesenteric nodes (splenic involvement is frequently a precursor to widespread haematological spread).
  - III_2 para-aortic, mesenteric, iliac nodes and upper abdominal nodes involved.
- Stage IV: Extranodal disease which is widespread and disseminated.

Additionally, localised extranodal involvement confined to a single site is indicated by the subscript$_E$. A nodal mass of >10 cm in diameter, or widening of the mediastinum by more than one-third is classed as bulky disease and indicated by the subscript$_x$.

Table 6.3
Staging investigations

Investigation	HL	NHL
Full blood count	Normocytic, normochromic anaemia is common in both HL and NHL Reduced numbers of erythrocytes, leucocytes and platelets may occur if the bone marrow is involved	
	Eosinophilia common Leucocytosis present in approximately one-third of individuals Lymphopenia and loss of cell-mediated immunity may occur in advanced disease	
Erythrocyte sedimentation rate (ESR)	Frequently raised especially if 'B' symptoms present	
Biochemistry	C-reactive protein increased Serum lactate dehydrogenase increased (raised levels indicate a poor prognosis)	Serum uric acid levels may be raised
	Liver function may be abnormal if the liver is involved	
Serum protein electrophoresis		Excess immunoglobulins may be secreted by some lymphomas
Chest x-ray	May show mediastinal involvement	
Computerised tomography (CT) or magnetic resonance imaging (MRI) scans of chest, abdomen and pelvis	Provides information on presence and extent of organ involvement	
Positive emission tomography (PET) scans are increasingly being advocated for staging investigations. However, currently PET scanners are not always available and their cost and effectiveness have yet to be fully evaluated (NICE 2003).		
Bone marrow aspiration and trephine biopsy	Detects bone marrow involvement	

The four stages are also suffixed A or B. If an individual is asymptomatic, the suffix A is added. Systemic symptoms of night sweats, fever of over 38°C during the previous month, and weight loss >10% of body weight in the previous 6 months are indicated by the suffix B. The presence of B symptoms indicates more advanced disease.

REFLECTION POINT
REFLECTION POINT

Consider what support an individual undergoing staging investigations and their relatives/friends might require.

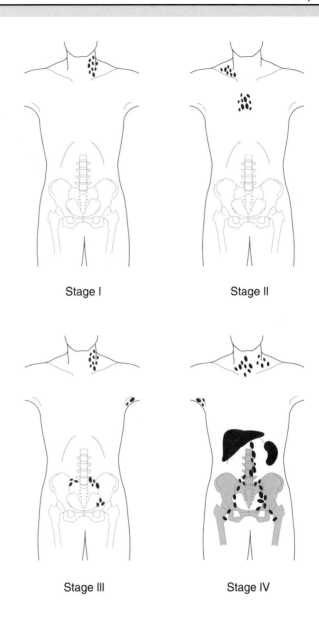

Figure 6.1
Ann Arbor Staging System
(from Hoffbrand et al 2001,
reproduced with permission)

Stage I   Stage II

Stage III   Stage IV

PROGNOSTIC INDICATORS

In HL, staging and the presence of bulky disease remain the major prognostic factors (Diehl et al 2004). However, factors indicative of a poor prognosis have been identified. Factors considered indicative of a less favourable prognosis in stage I and II disease are shown in Table 6.4

For advanced HL a seven-factor prognostic scoring system has been identified (Hasenclever & Diehl 1998). This system predicts 5-year rates of freedom from disease and overall survival. Prognosis is determined by the number of adverse factors present at diagnosis. The presence of

European Organisation for Research and Treatment of Cancer (EORTC 1999)	German Hodgkin's Lymphoma Study Group 2003 (cited in Diehl et al 2004)
Stage II with involvement of ≥4 nodal regions Stage I–II with ≥1 risk factors Age ≥50 years Raised ESR ≥50 mm/h if asymptomatic or ≥30 mm/h if 'B' symptoms present Mediastinal/thoracic ratio >0.35	≥3 involved nodal regions Extranodal disease Raised ESR ≥50 mm/h if asymptomatic or ≥30 mm/h if 'B' symptoms present Large mediastinal mass Stage I–II with ≥1 risk factors Stage IIB with raised ESR and ≥3 involved nodal regions but without a large mediastinal mass or extranodal disease

each factor reduces the 5-year failure-free survival by approximately 8%. Adverse prognostic factors are identified as:

- Hb <10.5 g/L
- male
- stage IV disease
- age 45 or over
- white cell count $>15 \times 10^9$/L
- lymphocytopenia $<0.6 \times 10^9$/L or <8% of total white cell count
- albumin <4 g/L.

For NHL it is recognised that staging is insufficient to determine prognosis and other factors have been identified as having an influence on response to treatment and survival. The International Prognostic Index incorporates five factors identified as predictors of an adverse outcome (Shipp et al 1993):

- age >60
- performance status >2
- serum lactic dehydrogenase (LDH) levels >1 times normal
- stage of disease – Ann Arbor III or IV
- number of extranodal sites involved >1.

Based on the number of adverse factors present at diagnosis individuals are assigned to one of four risk groups:

- low – score of 0 or 1
- low intermediate – score of 2
- high intermediate – score of 3
- high – score of 4 or 5.

Low-risk patients have a 5-year survival rate of 73% whereas in the high-risk group survival rates drop to 26% (Marcus 2003). Higher risk groups have an increased risk of death owing to a lower complete remission rate and a higher relapse rate (Coiffier 2001). Prognostic indicators are used as a basis for treatment decisions for individuals. However, although these indicators are significantly more accurate predictors of prognosis than the Ann Arbor staging system, initial response to treatment is the best indicator of outcome (Marcus 2003).

TREATMENT

HODGKIN'S LYMPHOMA

Both radiotherapy and chemotherapy are used in the treatment of HL and a high incidence of long-term disease-free survival has been achieved. Both treatment modalities can be used either alone or in combination depending on the stage of the disease.

Early stage (localised) disease

For several decades radiotherapy alone has been used as a curative treatment for stage I and II disease. Extended field radiotherapy techniques have been used to ensure treatment to all obviously diseased lymph nodes and adjacent, apparently normal lymph nodes at risk of containing subclinical disease. The 'mantle' technique includes all lymph node groups above the diaphragm and the 'inverted-Y' technique includes all lymph node groups below the diaphragm (see Chapter 10 for further information on the mantle and inverted-Y techniques).

The disadvantages of using these techniques are now recognised and include relapse outside the treatment field and an increased risk of secondary malignancies especially leukaemia, non-Hodgkin's lymphoma, breast cancer (particularly in women who have had mantle radiotherapy) and lung cancer (Linch et al 2000). Other long-term effects such as pulmonary fibrosis and cardiac disease are also common. Combinations of radiotherapy and chemotherapy are therefore now advocated. Doxorubicin, bleomycin, vinblastine and dacarbazine (ABVD) is considered to be the standard regimen for localised disease. Two to three cycles are given followed by reduced-dose radiotherapy to decrease the risk of long-term effects (Yung & Linch 2003, Diehl et al 2004, Meyer et al 2004).

Optimum treatment combinations continue to be researched. Recent research has focused on reducing the long-term toxicities of treatment while maintaining cure rates; clinical trials are ongoing. The use of chemotherapy alone is also being investigated.

Advanced disease

Advanced stage disease includes stages III and IV, the presence of bulky disease or B symptoms (Cheson 2004). The original, successful drug combination for HL was mechlorethamine, vincristine, procarbazine and prednisolone (MOPP). However, approximately one-fifth of patients either did not achieve complete remission with this regimen or relapsed shortly after completion of treatment (DeVita & Hubbard 1993). This was thought to be due to development of drug resistance. Treatment with MOPP also carries a high risk of developing secondary leukaemias and myelodysplasia. ABVD (doxorubicin, bleomycin, vinblastine and dacarbazine) has now replaced MOPP as the standard chemotherapy regimen against which all other drug combinations are compared. ABVD has a lower risk of secondary malignancies and less toxic effects, particularly on fertility (Diehl et al 2004). Six to eight cycles of ABVD are given over 6–8 months (Diehl et al 2003).

Clinical trials have compared ABVD with other drug regimens and they have shown similar results. Alternative regimens are therefore in use for advanced disease including:

- CHIVPP/PABLOE (chlorambucil, vinblastine, procarbazine, prednisolone, doxorubicin, bleomycin, vincristine, etoposide)
- CHIVPP/EVA (chlorambucil, vinblastine, procarbazine, prednisolone, etoposide, vincristine, doxorubicin)
- PVACE-BOP (procarbazine, vinblastine, doxorubicin, chlorambucil, etoposide, bleomycin, vincristine, prednisolone).

Other regimens currently being investigated in an attempt to improve efficacy of treatment include:

- Stanford V (mechlorethamine, doxorubicin, vinblastine, vincristine, bleomycin, etoposide, prednisolone, granulocyte-colony stimulating factor)
- BEACOPP (bleomycin, etoposide, doxorubicin, cyclophosphamide, vincristine, procarbazine).

Radiotherapy may be used in combination with chemotherapy for bulky disease and as consolidation treatment.

Relapsed disease

Some individuals will relapse and the length of initial remission is related to the success of subsequent chemotherapy. Those who have an initial remission of over a year may well achieve a second lengthy remission with further chemotherapy, whereas high-dose chemotherapy and autologous haemopoietic stem cell transplant (HSCT) are likely to be the treatment of choice for those individuals who relapse in under a year or only have a partial response to initial chemotherapy. HSCT may also be considered for patients at high risk of relapse as part of their initial treatment regimen (Mink & Armitage 2001).

Novel treatments

A variety of novel treatments are currently being investigated for HL including:

- gemcitabine
- anti-CD30 monoclonal antibodies
- rituximab anti-CD20 monoclonal antibody
- radioimmunoconjugates.

See Chapter 11 for further information on novel therapies.

NON-HODGKIN'S LYMPHOMA

Treatment of NHL is largely determined by histology and clinical aggressiveness.

Low-grade lymphomas

Generally low-grade lymphomas (of which follicular lymphomas are the most common) grow slowly, tend to follow a chronic course and inevitably relapse. The majority of low-grade lymphomas affect the elderly, are at an advanced stage when diagnosed and are generally regarded as incurable (McLaughlin 2002, Evans & Hancock 2003). Median overall survival for advanced disease is 8–10 years (Coiffier 2001).

A small group of patients present with localised disease (stage I–II). Radiotherapy results in complete remission in 95% and relapse-free 10-year survival in 50% of individuals (Coiffier 2001).

Individuals with advanced disease may be asymptomatic for several years and there currently appears to be no survival benefit from commencing curative chemotherapy at diagnosis. A period of observation, 'watch and wait', is usually initiated where progression of the disease is monitored but treatment is not commenced until symptoms occur. When symptoms occur, single-agent or combination chemotherapy may be commenced. Combination chemotherapy may induce remission more often, faster and for longer than with single-agent therapy but overall survival is not affected. Durable remissions are rare and most patients relapse within 2–3 years following standard therapy (McLaughlin 2002). Single-agent chemotherapy uses chlorambucil or fludarabine. Commonly used combination regimens include:

- CHVP (cyclophosphamide, doxorubicin, tenoposide, prednisolone)
- CVP (cyclophosphamide, vincristine, prednisolone) may be used for the elderly
- CHOP (cyclophosphamide, doxorubicin, vincristine, prednisolone)
- Fludarabine combined with either mitoxantrone or cyclophosphamide.

Interferon-alpha (INF-α) has also been investigated both alone and in combination with chemotherapy in the treatment of low-grade NHL. Although found to prolong remission in some individuals, overall survival is not affected (Fisher et al 2000).

More recently rituximab, an anti-CD20 monoclonal antibody which specifically targets B lymphocytes, has shown promise in clinical trials. Rituximab does not affect other cells in the body and therefore many of the side effects associated with other cancer therapies are avoided. As a single agent it has been shown to induce remission rates of 40–50% in follicular lymphoma and has now been approved by the National Institute for Clinical Excellence (NICE 2002) for use in relapsed stage III or IV when standard chemotherapy has failed. Use of rituximab continues to be investigated in combination with CHOP (R-CHOP) and fludarabine as first-line treatment for low-grade lymphoma and is showing high response rates and increased time to disease progression (Winter et al 2004).

High-dose chemotherapy and HSCT may prolong disease-free survival. However, the use of HSCT in low-grade lymphoma remains controversial. Individuals may survive for lengthy periods of time without transplantation and the toxicities of transplant and associated morbidity need to be balanced against the slow progression of this form of lymphoma. The optimal time for HSCT in low-grade lymphoma has yet to be established. Non-myeloablative allogeneic transplant regimens are also being investigated for low-grade lymphoma with some promising results (Winter et al 2004) (see Chapter 13 for further information on HSCT).

Case study 6.1

Elizabeth was diagnosed with stage IVB low-grade non-Hodgkin's lymphoma involving her kidneys, at the age of 74. She was treated with R-CVP and after her sixth course had a CT scan of her chest, abdomen and pelvis to check the response of her disease. Results showed a very good response and she received two final courses of treatment. She has now completed eight courses and is disease free.

REFLECTION POINT   Individuals with lymphoma face an uncertain future. Consider what help an individual may need to cope with this uncertainty.

Gastric mucosa-associated lymphoid tissue (MALT) lymphoma

MALT lymphomas are unusual low-grade lymphomas associated with *Helicobacter pylori* infection. Treatment of *H. pylori* alone with antibiotics can induce complete lymphoma regression in 60–70% of cases (Bayerdörffer et al 1995, Roggeroet al 1995). For those individuals who do not respond to antibiotic therapy, conventional chemotherapy and radiotherapy are used.

Aggressive lymphomas

Aggressive tumours are rapidly fatal unless treated promptly. However, high-grade lymphomas are also extremely susceptible to chemotherapy and potentially curable. Most individuals have advanced disease at diagnosis but a minority present with localised stage I or II disease, for which treatment consists of either chemotherapy alone (e.g. CHOP) or a shortened course of chemotherapy followed by involved field radiotherapy (Evans & Hancock 2003).

For advanced disease intensive combination chemotherapy is used with approximately 80% of individuals achieving a remission. However, approximately 50% will relapse in the first 5 years (Johnson 1995). The CHOP drug regimen has been used since the mid-1970s and despite numerous clinical trials of other chemotherapy regimens no survival advantage over CHOP has been shown (Marcus 2003). However, recently the addition of rituximab to the CHOP regimen has resulted in increased overall survival in patients with diffuse large B-cell lymphoma (Coiffier et al 2002).

The optimal use of HSCT in initial therapy for aggressive lymphomas is conflicting (Marcus 2003). However, a recent clinical trial found that individuals with a high intermediate international prognostic index score had a significantly higher 5-year survival than those treated with CHOP alone (Milpied et al 2004). These authors recommend that patients under the age of 60 with a high intermediate risk of death should receive high-dose therapy and autologous HSCT as initial therapy.

If aggressive lymphomas relapse or there is an incomplete response to initial chemotherapy, prognosis is generally poor and high-dose chemotherapy, e.g. IVE (ifosfamide, epirubicin, etoposide) and HSCT, may result in long-term remission (Philip et al 1995, Vose et al 2001). Allogeneic transplants may also be suitable for young patients with a matched donor (see Chapter 13).

Highly aggressive Burkitt's lymphomas and lymphoblastic lymphomas are treated with similar chemotherapy regimes to those for lymphoblastic leukaemia (see Chapter 4).

Palliative treatment

Both radiotherapy and chemotherapy may be used as palliative treatment for both HL and NHL if organomegaly or lymphadenopathy are causing pain or dysfunction.

Surgery

Surgery has a small role in the treatment of NHL. Gastric lymphomas frequently present with acute abdominal pain and are frequently diagnosed at exploratory laparotomy and surgically excised.

Newer treatments

Clinical trials are also examining the use of monoclonal antibodies, vaccines and radioimmunoconjugates (anti-CD20 antibodies conjugated with radioactive isotopes Y-90 ibritumomab tiuxetan or I-131-tositumomab) in the treatment of NHL (see Chapter 11 for further discussion of these novel agents).

COMPLICATIONS ASSOCIATED WITH HL AND NHL

Tumour lysis syndrome

Tumour lysis syndrome (TLS) can occur spontaneously, or following chemotherapy or radiotherapy for large bulky tumours or conditions with high numbers of rapidly proliferating cells, e.g. aggressive lymphomas (particularly Burkitt's lymphoma). Specific chemotherapeutic or biological agents have also been associated with TLS, e.g. intrathecal methotrexate and rituximab (Simmons & Somberg 1991, Yang et al 1999). Following chemotherapy, rapid cell lysis results in a large circulating volume of the breakdown products of cell metabolism (particularly nucleic acids, potassium and phosphate) leading to hyperuricaemia, hyperkalaemia, hyperphosphataemia and hypocalcaemia. Raised levels of cellular metabolites increase the demands on the kidneys and may result in acute renal failure.

The cardiovascular and nervous systems may also be affected as a result of altered metabolite levels. Clinical manifestations of increased metabolite levels include nausea and vomiting, diarrhoea, lethargy and weakness, loin pain, haematuria, oliguria progressing to anuria, muscle cramps, parasthesia, muscle twitching, carpopedal spasm, tetany, convulsions, hypotension, cardiac arrhythmias and cardiac arrest.

For those most at risk of TLS, serum electrolytes and renal function tests should be monitored before and after treatment is commenced. Preventative measures should be implemented before chemotherapy is commenced. Oral allopurinol prevents synthesis of uric acid and is usually commenced 24 hours prior to the start of chemotherapy. Allopurinol does not, however, break down existing uric acid crystals and recently the enzyme urate-oxidase has been investigated for treating hyperuricaemia (Pui et al 2001, Patte et al 2002). Diuretics may also be administered to aid in the dilution and excretion of urine. Intravenous hydration is commenced 24–48 hours before chemotherapy commences to prevent renal failure (Flombaum 2000). Uric acid is more soluble in an alkaline environment and sodium bicarbonate may be added to the fluid regimen to alkalinise urine, helping to increase uric acid excretion. Urinary pH should be maintained at ≥ 7 rather than normal urinary pH of 5–6.

Nursing management consists of close observation of the individual's condition. Accurate records of fluid balance should be maintained to ensure hydration and prevent fluid overload.

Superior vena cava syndrome

Enlarged lymph nodes caused by a growing lymphoma may result in obstruction or compression of the superior vena cava which is surrounded by several lymph node chains (Haapoja & Blendowski 1999). Clinical features depend on the degree of obstruction and include dyspnoea, cough, cyanosis with distention of the upper chest and neck veins and oedema of the neck and face. Raised intracranial pressure may result in dizziness, a feeling of fullness in the head, headache and visual disturbances. Superior vena cava syndrome (SVCS) is potentially life-threatening and an oncological emergency if it develops rapidly with respiratory distress caused by laryngeal oedema and cerebral oedema causing stupor, coma and seizures. Treatment of SVCS is with diuretics and steroids to reduce inflammation and swelling. Radiotherapy or chemotherapy are used to reduce the size of the lymphoma. Elevating the head of the bed and oxygen therapy help to reduce dyspnoea. SVCS is extremely frightening for the patient and their relatives and high levels of supportive care are required.

Spinal cord compression

Spinal cord compression (SCC) is also an oncological emergency and occurs due to pressure on the spinal cord by the lymphoma. Compression causes interruption of the blood flow, oedema of affected tissues and nerves, eventually leading to ischaemia and death of nerve cells. Nurses should be alert to warning signs of this condition. Complaints of back pain, motor weakness, numbness or paraesthesia in the legs should be acted upon immediately. Prompt treatment with radiotherapy is required to prevent paralysis and irreversible damage.

Lymphoedema

Lymphadenopathy in the axillae or groins can cause obstruction and reduced lymph drainage. Steroids and radiotherapy may help to reduce to the size of the lymph nodes and improve oedema. However, lymphoedema, a chronic and progressive form of oedema resulting from the inability of the lymphatic system to drain normal amounts of fluid from interstitial spaces, may develop (Mortimer 1995). Pain, swelling, numbness, stiffness and loss of limb function can occur. Lymphoedema can adversely affect an individual's body image and quality of life. It may also be associated with disease progression and lack of control. Lymphoedema predisposes individuals to infection. Skin integrity may be compromised by swelling while more pronounced skin folds and raised protein levels in lymphatic fluid provide ideal conditions for bacterial growth. The incidence of lymphoedema in lymphoma is unknown as most studies have been conducted with women with breast cancer (Rymal 2001).

Skin care to maintain or improve the integrity of the skin and prevent infection, massage, compression and exercise/movement are considered to be the four main components of lymphoedema care. Skin care includes avoiding trauma, moisturising skin and prompt treatment of infection with antibiotics. Use of a high-factor suncream (SPF 15 or above) should be advised (Rymal 2001). Exercise and movement encourage lymph flow and venous return while avoiding overexertion, which increases blood flow too much.

Massage aims to aid lymphatic drainage and two types exist. Simple lymphatic drainage can be taught to patients and carers whereas manual lymphatic drainage requires a trained therapist. Compression utilises elastic compression garments which cover the limb or multi-layered bandaging. Exercise and movement are encouraged while wearing compression garments to encourage lymph flow and venous return (Rymal 2001). Individuals with lymphoedema should be referred to trained lymphoedema practitioners to ensure accurate assessment and appropriate treatment.

Case study 6.2

Isobel, a 63-year-old widow diagnosed with diffuse large B-cell NHL involving clavicular, axillary and retroperitoneal lymph nodes, developed venous obstruction and secondary left deep vein thrombosis due to her lymphoma. She has completed four courses of R-CHOP and is awaiting a CT scan of her chest, abdomen and pelvis before future treatment is planned. If her scan shows a good response, she will receive further treatment up to a maximum of 6–8 courses.

SPECIFIC NURSING ISSUES

In common with individuals with other haematological malignancies individuals with lymphoma are susceptible to a variety of side effects associated with both the disease and its treatment; related nursing issues are discussed in Section 3. A number of psychological effects have been noted for individuals with lymphoma. Isolation, feelings of loss of control and living with uncertainty have been found to be particular issues for individuals with lymphoma and leukaemia (Persson et al 1995). Raised levels of anxiety and depression have also been identified (Devlen et al 1987) and nurses need to be sensitive to individual needs and be ready to provide support (see Chapter 23).

Many lymphomas are potentially curable and individuals may experience prolonged disease-free survival. Younger individuals may want to start or add to their families and infertility may be a problem (see Chapter 20). Further problems may be experienced in relation to work, insurance and financial issues (see Chapter 25).

CONCLUSION

The lymphomas are a diverse group of diseases many of which are potentially curable. For some individuals treatment will be successful and result in long-term disease-free survival. Others will experience a less positive outcome. However, whatever the outcome of treatment individuals with lymphoma and their relatives require both physical and psychological support to enable them to cope with the rigours of treatment, adjust to changed life circumstances and maintain quality of life.

DISCUSSION QUESTIONS

1. Many individuals with lymphoma are elderly. What issues might arise when an elderly person is receiving treatment for lymphoma?

2. What are the educational and informational needs of individuals with lymphoma?

3. What are the rehabilitation needs of individuals who are considered to be cured of their disease?

References

Adami J, Frisch M, Yuen J, Blimelius B, Melby M 1995 Evidence of an association between non-Hodgkin's lymphoma and skin cancer. British Medical Journal 310:1491–1495

Argiris A, Kaklamani V 2004 Hodgkin disease. EMedicine. www.emedicine.com/med/topic1022.htm Accessed 3 April 2005

Baris D, Zahm S H 2000 Epidemiology of lymphomas. Current Opinion in Oncology 12(5):383–394

Bayerdorffer E, Neubauer A, Rudolph B et al and Malt Lymphoma Study Group 1995 Regression of primary gastric lymphoma of mucosa-associated lymphoid tissue type after cure of *Helicobacter pylori* infection. Lancet 345:1591–1594

Bouzourene H, Haefliger T, Delacretaz F et al 1999 The role of *Helicobacter pylori* in primary gastric MALT lymphoma. Histopathology 34:118–123

Cancer Research Campaign 1998 Factsheet 1.1 Incidence – UK. Cancer Research Campaign, London

Cancer Research UK 2004 CancerStats: Mortality – UK. Cancer Research UK, London

Cancer Research UK 2005a CancerStats: Incidence – UK. Cancer Research UK, London

Cancer Research UK 2005b Non-Hodgkin lymphoma – UK. Cancer Research UK, London

Carbone P P, Kaplan H S, Musshof K, Smithers D W, Tubiana M 1971 Report of the Committee on Hodgkin's Disease Staging Classification. Cancer Research 31:1860–1861

Cheson B D 2004 What is new in lymphoma? CA Cancer Journal for Clinicians 54:260–272

Coiffier B 2001 Non-Hodgkin's lymphomas: clinical presentation, treatment and outcome. Roche-Oncology, Basel

Coiffier B, Lepage E, Briere J et al 2002 CHOP chemotherapy plus rituximab compared with CHOP alone in elderly patients with diffuse large-B-cell lymphoma. New England Journal of Medicine 346(4):235–242

Curtis R E, Travis L B, Rowlings P A et al 1999 Risk of lymphoproliferative disorders after bone marrow transplantation: a multi-institutional study. Blood 94:2208–2216

Dal Maso L, Franceschi S 2003 Epidemiology of non-Hodgkin lymphomas and other haemolymphopoietic neoplasms in people with AIDS. Lancet Oncology 4:110–119

DeVita V T J, Canellos G P 1999 The lymphomas. Seminars in Hematology 36(4):84–94

DeVita V T, Hubbard S M 1993 Hodgkin's disease. The New England Journal of Medicine 328(8):560–565.

Devlen J, Maguire P, Phillips P, Crowther D, Chambers H 1987 Psychological problems associated with diagnosis and treatment of lymphomas. British Medical Journal 295:953–957

Diehl V, Thomas R K, Re D 2004 Part II: Hodgkin's lymphoma – diagnosis and treatment. Lancet Oncology 5:19–26

Diehl V, Stein H, Hummel M, Zollinger R, Connors J M 2003 Hodgkin's lymphoma: biology and treatment strategies for primary, refractory and relapsed disease. Hematology 1:225–247

European Organisation for Research and Treatment of Cancer Lymphoma Cooperative Group and GELA 1999 Trial H9 protocol: Prospective controlled trial in clinical stages I–II supradiaphragmatic Hodgkin's disease – evaluation of treatment efficacy, (long-term) toxicity and quality of life in two different prognostic subgroups. EORTC protocol 20982. Cited in: Yung L, Linch D 2003 Hodgkin's lymphoma. Lancet 361:943–951

Evans L S, Hancock B W 2003 Non Hodgkin lymphoma. Lancet 362:139–146

Fisher R I, Dana B W, Le Blanc M et al 2000 Interferon alpha consolidation after intensive chemotherapy does not prolong the progression-free survival of patients with low-grade non-Hodgkin's lymphoma: results of the Southwest Oncology Group randomized phase III study 8809. Journal of Clinical Oncology 18:2010–2016

Flombaum C D 2000 Metabolic emergencies in the cancer patient. Seminars in Oncology 27(3):322–334

Haapoja I S, Blendowski C 1999 Superior vena cava syndrome. Seminars in Oncology Nursing 15(3):183–189

Harris N L, Jaffe E S, Diebold J et al 1999 World Health Organization classification of neoplastic diseases of the hematopoietic and lymphoid tissues: report of the Clinical Advisory Committee Meeting – Airlie House, Virginia, November 1997. Journal of Clinical Oncology 17(12):3835–3849

Harris N L, Jaffe E S, Diebold J et al 2000 Lymphoma classification – from controversy to consensus: the REAL and WHO classification of lymphoid neoplasms. Annals of Oncology 11(Suppl 1):S3–S10

Harris N L, Stein H, Coupland S E et al 2001 New approaches to lymphoma diagnosis. Hematology 1:194–220

Hasenclever D, Diehl V 1998 A prognostic score for advanced Hodgkin's disease. New England Journal of Medicine 339(21):1506–1514

Hoffbrand A V, Pettit J E, Moss P A H 2001 Essential haematology, 4th edn. Blackwell Publishing, Oxford

Hsu J L, Glaser S L 2000 Epstein–Barr virus associated malignancies: epidemiologic patterns and etiologic implications. Critical Reviews in Oncology-Hematology 34:27–53

Jaffe E S, Harris N L, Vardiman J W, Stein H 2001 Pathology and genetics: neoplasms of the hematopoietic and lymphoid tissues. In: Kleihues P, Sobin L (eds) World Health Organization Classification of Tumours. IARC Press, Lyon

Jarrett R F, Armstrong A A, Alexander F A 1996 Epidemiology of EBV and Hodgkin's disease. Annals of Oncology 7(Suppl 4):S5–10

Johnson P W M 1995 The high grade non-Hodgkin's lymphomas. British Journal of Hospital Medicine 53(1/2):14–19

La Vecchia C, Tavani A 2002 Hair dyes and lymphoid neoplasms: an update. European Journal of Cancer Prevention 11:409–412

Leukaemia Research Fund 2003a Hodgkin's lymphoma. www.lrf.org.uk/en/1/dishlyhome.html Accessed 3 April 2005

Leukaemia Research Fund 2003b Non-Hodgkin's lymphoma. http://www.lrf.org.uk/en/1/disnhlhome.html Accessed 3 April 2005

Linch D C, Gosden R G, Tulandi T et al 2000 Hodgkin's lymphoma: choice of therapy and late complications.

Hematology (American Society of Hematology Education Program) 205–221

Lister T A, Crowther D, Sutcliffe S B et al 1989 Report of a committee convened to discuss the evaluation and staging of patients with Hodgkin's disease: Cotswolds meeting. Journal of Clinical Oncology 71(1):1630–1636

Mack T M, Cozen W, Shibata D K et al 1995 Concordance for Hodgkin's disease in identical twins suggesting genetic susceptibility to the young-adult form of the disease. New England Journal of Medicine 332(7):413–418

Mackie M 2001 Hodgkin's disease and non-Hodgkin's lymphoma. In: Scottish Executive Health Department. Cancer scenarios: an aid to planning cancer services in Scotland in the next decade. SEHD, Edinburgh

Manns A, Hisada M, La Grenade L 1999 Human T-lymphotropic virus type I infection. Lancet 353:1951–1958

Marcus R 2003 Current treatment options in aggressive lymphoma. Leukemia & Lymphoma 44(Suppl 4):S15–S27

McCunney R J 1999 Hodgkin's disease, work and the environment: a review. Journal of Occupational Medicine 41:36–46

McLaughlin P 2002 Progress and promise in the treatment of indolent lymphomas. The Oncologist 7:217–225

Meyer R M, Ambinder R F, Stroobants S 2004 Hodgkin's lymphoma: evolving concepts with implications for practice. Hematology (American Society of Hematology Education Program) 184–202.

Milpied N, Deconinck E, Gaillard F et al 2004 Initial treatment of aggressive lymphoma with high-dose chemotherapy and autologous stem-cell support. New England Journal of Medicine 350:1287–1295

Mink S, Armitage J O 2001 High-dose therapy in lymphomas: a review of the current status of allogeneic and autologous stem cell transplantation in Hodgkin's disease and non-Hodgkin's lymphoma. The Oncologist 6:247–256

Mortimer P S 1995 Managing lymphoedema. Clinical and Experimental Dermatology 20:98–106

National Institute For Clinical Excellence 2002 Guidance on the use of rituximab for recurrent or refractory Stage III or IV follicular non-Hodgkin's lymphoma. NICE, London

National Institute For Clinical Excellence 2003 Improving outcomes in haematological cancer: the manual. NICE, London

Opelz G, Henderson R 1993 Incidence of non-Hodgkin lymphoma in kidney and heart transplant recipients. Lancet 342:1514–1516

Patte C, Sakiroglu C, Ansoborlo S et al and Societe Francaise d'Oncologie Pediatrique 2002 Urate-oxidase in the prevention and treatment of metabolic complications in patients with B-cell lymphoma and leukemia, treated in the Societe Francaise d'Oncologie Pediatrique LMB89 protocol. Annals of Oncology 13(5):789–795

Persson L, Hallberg I R, Ohlsson O 1995 Acute leukaemia and malignant lymphoma patients' experiences of disease, treatment and nursing care during the active treatment phase: an exploratory study. European Journal of Cancer Care 4:133–142

Philip T, Guglielmi C, Hagenbeek A et al 1995 Autologous bone marrow transplantation as compared to salvage treatment in relapses of chemotherapy-sensitive non-Hodgkin's lymphoma. New England Journal of Medicine 333:1540–1545

Pileri S A, Ascani A, Leoncini L et al 2002 Hodgkin's lymphoma: the pathologist's viewpoint. Journal of Clinical Pathology 55:162–176

Pui C H, Mahmoud H H, Wiley J M et al 2001 Recombinant urate oxidase for the prophylaxis or treatment of hyperuricemia in patients with leukemia or lymphoma. Journal of Clinical Oncology 19(3):697–704

Quinn M, Babb P, Brock A et al 2001 Cancer trends in England and Wales 1950–1999. TSO, London

Rego M A 1998 Non-Hodgkin's lymphoma risk derived from exposure to organic solvents? A review of epidemiologic studies. Cadernos de Saude Publica 14(Suppl 3):41–66

Ries L A G, Eisner M P, Kosary C L et al 2002 SEER Cancer Statistics Review, 1973–1999. National Cancer Institute, Bethesda, MD

Roggero E, Zucca E, Pinotti G et al 1995 Eradication of *Helicobacter pylori* infection in primary low-grade gastric lymphoma of mucosa-associated lymphoid tissue. Annals of Internal Medicine 122(10):767–769

Rymal C 2001 Lymphedema management in patients with lymphoma. Nursing Clinics of North America 36(4):709–734

Schroeder J C, Olshan A F, Baric R et al 2001 Agricultural risk factors for t(14;18) subtypes of non-Hodgkin's lymphoma. Epidemiology 12:701–709

Shipp M A, Harrington D P, Anderson J R et al 1993 The non-Hodgkin's lymphoma prognostic factors project: a predictive model for aggressive non-Hodgkin's lymphoma. New England Journal of Medicine 329(14):987–994

Simmons E D, Somberg K A 1991 Acute tumor lysis syndrome after intrathecal methotrexate administration. Cancer 67(8):2062–2065

Skinnider B F, Mak T W 2000 The role of cytokines in classical Hodgkin lymphoma. Blood 99(12):4283–4297

Straus S E, Jaffe E S, Puck J M et al 2001 The development of lymphomas in families with autoimmune lymphoproliferative syndrome with germline Fas mutations and defective lymphocyte apoptosis. Blood 98(1):194–200

Sweetenham J 1998 Cancer Research Campaign, Factsheet 27.1 Hodgkin's Disease in Adults – UK. Cancer Research Campaign, London

Swerdlow A J 2003 Epidemiology of Hodgkin's disease and non-Hodgkin's lymphoma. European Journal of Nuclear Medicine and Molecular Imaging 30(Suppl 1):S3–S12

Swerdlow A J, Higgins C D, Hunt B J et al 2000 Risk of lymphoid neoplasia after cardiothoracic transplantation. A cohort study of the relation to Epstein–Barr virus. Transplantation 69(5):897–904

Swerdlow A J, Dos Santos Silva I, Doll R 2001 Cancer incidence and mortality in England and Wales: trends and risk factors. Oxford University Press, Oxford

Thomas R K, Re D, Wolf J, Diehl V 2004 Part 1: Hodgkin's lymphoma – molecular biology of Hodgkin and Reed–Sternberg cells. Lancet Oncology 5:11–18

Vose J, Zhang M, Rowlings P et al 2001 Autologous transplantation for diffuse aggressive non-Hodgkin's lymphoma in patients never achieving remission: a report from the autologous blood and marrow transplant registry. Journal of Clinical Oncology 19:406–413

Vose J M, Chiu B C H, Cheson B D, Dancey J, Wright J 2002 Update on epidemiology and therapeutics for non-Hodgkin's lymphoma. Hematology (American Society of Hematology Education Program) 241–262

Winter J N, Gascoyne R D, Van Besien K 2004 Low-grade lymphoma. Hematology (American Society of Hematology Education Program) 203–220

Yang H, Rosove M H, Figlin R A 1999 Tumor lysis syndrome occurring after the administration of rituximab in lymphoproliferative disorders: high-grade non-Hodgkin's lymphoma and chronic lymphocytic leukemia. American Journal of Hematology 62(4):247–250

Yung L, Linch D 2003 Hodgkin's lymphoma. Lancet 361:943–951

Zhu K, Levine R S, Gu Y et al 1998 Non-Hodgkin's lymphoma and family history of malignant tumours in a case control study (United States). Cancer Causes and Control 9:77–82

Further reading

Persson L, Hallberg I R 2004 Lived experience of survivors of leukemia or malignant lymphoma. Cancer Nursing 27(4):303–313
An original study examining the experience of surviving a haematological cancer.

Rymal C 2001 Lymphedema management in patients with lymphoma. Nursing Clinics of North America 36(4):709–734
An interesting and comprehensive article on an infrequently discussed aspect of practice.

Chapter **7**

Haematological malignancies and children

Deborah Tomlinson

KEY POINTS

- Leukaemia and lymphomas account for approximately 46% of childhood malignancy.
- Acute lymphoblastic leukaemia (ALL) is most common in childhood.
- Treatment protocols can be intense and may occur over extended periods of time, with side effects that are extremely distressing to the child and the family.
- Long-term survival is generally very good.
- Follow-up is essential for detection of relapse and monitoring of late side effects of treatment.

INTRODUCTION

Leukaemia is the most common childhood cancer in 0–14-year-olds, with lymphomas being the third most common (Fig. 7.1). Childhood haematological cancers are treated quite differently from similar diseases in adults and although there remain many similarities in

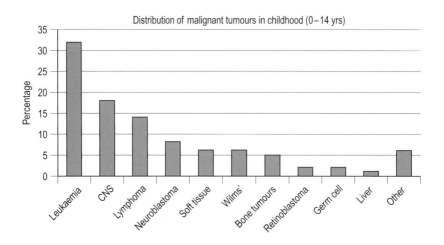

Distribution of malignant tumours in childhood (0–14 yrs)

Figure 7.1
Distribution of malignant
tumours in childhood (0–14
years) (Stiller 2004)

supportive care, there are significant differences in long-term implications. Children have benefited more from improved treatment modalities than adults, particularly in the treatment of acute lymphoblastic leukaemia (Plasschaert et al 2004). With advancing cure rates, the role of the nurse caring for children with malignancy is not only aimed at attempting to reduce and ameliorate symptoms of the disease and treatment but also to prepare children and their families to live with the long-term sequelae of disease and treatment.

LEUKAEMIA IN CHILDHOOD

In childhood the most common leukaemias are:

- acute lymphoblastic leukaemia (ALL) constituting 75–80% of childhood leukaemia
- acute myeloid leukaemia (AML) – 20–25%
- chronic myeloid leukaemia (CML) – <5%.

ACUTE LYMPHOBLASTIC LEUKAEMIA IN CHILDREN

Epidemiology

In childhood ALL affects slightly more males than females (1.2:1); however, a higher preponderance of females are affected in infancy. Peak incidence is between the ages of 2 and 6 years. The highest incidence appears to be in Europe and North America (5 in 100,000 of 0–14-year-olds), with the lowest incidence in Kuwait and Bombay (0.9 in 100,000) (Lilleyman 1997). Generally it has a higher incidence in affluent industrialised nations within white populations.

Aetiological factors

The factors involved in the cause of cancer in children and young people are unclear. Several syndromes have been identified to have hereditary or genetic predisposition to leukaemia including Down's syndrome (trisomy 21); Li-Fraumeni syndrome; neurofibromatosis type 1; Bloom syndrome (Mizutani 1998).

Many risk factors associated with childhood cancer have been investigated with very little evidence of any associations. Clusters of childhood ALL have been reported around nuclear installations. However, recent hypotheses regarding these clusters of ALL have moved away from the thought that background radiation was the cause of these clusters. Kinlen's theory (1995) suggests that population mixing, herd immunity and abnormal response to infection of unusually susceptible children increases the risk of ALL. A possible 'delayed infection' hypothesis or 'hygiene hypothesis' suggests that some infants with a lack of exposure to infection incur an abnormal response following a common infection incurred after mixing with other children in playgroups or schools. Therefore alterations in the pattern of infections in infants may be a contributory factor in the aetiology of ALL.

The few factors that have been found to have an association include the study by Jensen et al (2004) that reports that maternal dietary factors, i.e. consumption of fruits, vegetables and protein sources may play an important role in reducing the risk of ALL; and Naumburg et al (2002) reported that maternal lower genitourinary tract infection in utero increased the risk of childhood leukaemia. This and other studies support the hypothesis that an infectious agent is involved in the aetiology of ALL (Kinlen 1995, Alexander et al 1999, Boutou et al 2002).

REFLECTION POINT

Epidemiological studies are difficult in childhood malignancy. However, public interest and media attention that surround theories of the cause of childhood cancer continues. Why are these studies difficult in this population? Consider the nurse's role in eliciting the parents' thoughts about the cause of their child's disease.

It is known that the transformation or mutation of particular genes leads to the transformation of a normal cell to a malignant cell. The exact number of mutations required is unknown but research indicates that two or more mutations (hits) are involved (Greaves 2004). In childhood ALL:

- the first hit is thought to occur in the womb
- the second hit is then suggested to occur after birth.

This theory has arisen following the observation of high concordance rates of leukaemia in infant monozygotic twins, as well as the study of Guthrie cards (used to collect blood samples from every newborn to screen for phenylketonuria (PKU) and congenital hypothyroidism). The cards collect four spots of blood that allow for testing of other metabolic diseases. It has also been suggested that in childhood ALL the first genetic event may happen in the more mature lymphoid committed

Table 7.1
Signs, symptoms and
attributing causes

Signs and symptoms	Attributing causes
Irritability	Anaemia
Night sweats	Increased metabolic rate
Fatigue	Anaemia
Bone pain may present with limping	Bone marrow impaction
Loss of appetite	General malaise
Pallor and lethargy	Anaemia
Petechiae	Thrombocytopenia
Bruising/unusual bleeding	Thrombocytopenia
Enlarged liver or spleen – protruding abdomen	Increased rate of cell breakdown
Enlarged lymph nodes and fever	Neutropenia and associated infections
Headache, poor school performance, weakness, vomiting, blurred vision, seizures, difficulty maintaining balance	CNS infiltration. (Less than 10% of ALL present with central nervous system involvement)
Coughing, shortness of breath, dysphagia	Thymus involvement; mediastinal mass. (Normally associated with T-cell ALL and occurs in 60–70% of this group)
Testicular swelling	Testicular infiltration
Swelling of head and arms (rare presentation)	Superior vena cava (SVC) obstruction

progenitor cells, compared to the first hit occurring in multipotent stem cells in adult ALL (Plasschaert et al 2004).

Clinical features of ALL

Normally, but not always, symptoms of ALL have a short onset. Symptoms relate to proliferative, immature cells infiltrating the bone marrow and other affected organs (Tomlinson 2004). Reported symptoms may appear like many common childhood illnesses (Table 7.1).

Very rarely, acute leukaemia can present with extremely high blast cell counts causing hyperleucocytosis. This can cause respiratory failure, intracranial bleeding and metabolic abnormalities. The process leading to these complications is known as leucostasis. It was considered that leucostasis was a result of overcrowding blast cells. It is now understood to be the result of adhesive interactions between blast cells and vascular epithelium. Hyperleucocytosis is often treated with leucopheresis to reduce the leucocyte count.

Diagnosis

Diagnostics include:

- full blood count
- blood urea and electrolytes
- chest x-ray
- bone marrow aspiration and trephine
- lumbar puncture.

A lumbar puncture will determine central nervous system (CNS) involvement by examining the cerebrospinal fluid (CSF) for blast cells. A chest x-ray will determine the presence of infection or mediastinal mass. This is particularly significant if a general anaesthetic is being arranged for the bone marrow procedure.

Following diagnosis, prognostic factors (including cell morphology, cytogenetics and immunophenotyping) are used to determine the child's likelihood of relapse or resistance to treatment. This directs the use of protocols, developed through clinical trials, to intensify or reduce the treatment given to ensure adequate cell kill within acceptable levels of toxicity (Tomlinson 2004). Although debate continues about the significance of some prognostic factors, there are several features that have been determined as more favourable prognostic factors. These are known as the Rome/NCI (National Cancer Institute) Criteria (Smith et al 1996):

- WBC $<50,000/m^3$
- female
- 1–9 years of age
- non-T/non-B cell.

All other factors are said to be 'high risk'. The effects of genetic alterations in leukaemia help to explain adverse clinical outcomes. For example, the Philadelphia chromosome produces an active kinase that drives cell proliferation independently of normal requirements for growth factor (see Chapter 4). Apoptosis is also blocked.

Minimal residual disease

Due to the need for more relevant features, minimal residual disease (MRD) has been identified as providing prognostic information (Bruggemann et al 2004, Izraeli & Waldman 2004). MRD (submicroscopic leukaemia) can be detected at specific time points using polymerase chain reaction or flow-cytometry. If there is fast clearance of leukaemic cells, treatment may be able to be reduced. Persistent disease could require treatment modification and intensification.

Treatment

Protocols for childhood ALL generally include the following features:

- induction
- intensification
- CNS-directed therapy
- maintenance.

Treatment normally continues for a period of 2 or 3 years. Infant ALL presents a challenge and infants with the disease are normally treated as a unique subgroup with multiple drugs given at high doses. During induction the drugs used initially will usually induce remission in about 95% of children with ALL.

REFLECTION POINT

Think about how you would explain remission to the family of a young child.

The drugs given usually include oral steroids (prednisolone or dexamethasone), intravenous (iv) vincristine, subcutaneous (sc) L-asparaginase and possibly iv daunorubicin with some protocols. CNS prophylaxis/treatment with intrathecal methotrexate is also started immediately. A uric acid depletory is routinely prescribed (usually allopurinol) as there are associated risks of tumour lysis syndrome (see Chapter 6). Co-trimoxazole (orally if tolerated) is also prescribed as prophylaxis against *Pneumocystis jiroveci* pneumonia (PCP) (previously described as *Pneumocystis carinii* pneumonia). Adverse reactions to co-trimoxazole, including prolonged periods of neutropenia, may indicate the use of alternative options (including aerolised/nebulised pentamidine or oral dapsone).

The intensification block of treatment is usually administered following induction and again about 4 months later. Clinical trials have investigated the introduction of a third block. The drugs used include oral steroids, iv vincristine, iv daunorubicin, iv etoposide, iv cytarabine, oral thioguanine (or mercaptopurine).

CNS-directed therapy is thought essential, as the CNS provides a sanctuary site for leukaemic cells. If this preventative therapy is not given to children with ALL, over 50% would develop CNS disease. Every 12 weeks a lumbar puncture is carried out to administer intrathecal methotrexate. High-dose methotrexate infusions are common in most protocols but the benefits are still under investigation. Cranial radiation may be reserved for children thought to be at high risk of CNS involvement (T cell with high white count at diagnosis) or those with CNS disease at diagnosis.

The maintenance stage mainly consists of oral cytotoxic drugs taken at home. This includes daily oral mercaptopurine and weekly oral methotrexate. Maintenance therapy also includes 4-weekly vincristine, PCP prophylaxis and CNS-directed therapy. High-risk leukaemias may indicate the need for transplantation.

Follow-up

Blood counts will be carried out with decreasing frequency over many years to ensure the detection of relapse. Bone marrow aspiration may also be carried out yearly for the same reason. If relapse occurs, it is usually found in the bone marrow but may also be detected in the CNS or in the testes of boys. The type of treatment offered then depends on the type of relapse; if medullary then reinduction and bone marrow transplant may be offered, whereas for extramedullary relapse chemotherapy and radiotherapy may achieve good success rates if the relapse occurs after the completion of initial treatment. Follow-up also monitors for late side effects of treatment.

ACUTE MYELOID LEUKAEMIA IN CHILDHOOD

Epidemiology

The incidence of AML increases slightly in young people and AML is the most common neonatal leukaemia. Children with Down's syndrome have an increased risk of AML with a 10–15× increased risk over the general childhood population (Hasle et al 2000).

Causes

The various genetic conditions that have a predisposition to AML are generally the same as those of ALL with the addition of myelodysplastic syndrome. Causal environmental risk factors are also the same for ALL and AML.

Signs and symptoms

AML has a similar presentation to ALL, although less specific, with symptoms appearing 1–6 weeks prior to diagnosis and including:

- pallor
- fatigue, weakness
- petechiae
- fever, infection
- sore throat
- lymphadenopathy
- bone pain (less common in AML)
- skin lesions
- gastrointestinal symptoms
- gingival changes or infiltrates
- hepatosplenomegaly is more marked in infants.

The lesions and infiltrates seen in AML are caused by chloromas. Chloromas are localised collections of blast cells. Presentation with bleeding may be due to disseminated intravascular disease (DIC) (see Chapter 16). In a small percentage of children CNS involvement causes similar symptoms as CNS disease involvement in ALL. Presentation may include hyperleucocytosis – 15–20% of children present with leucocyte counts greater than 100×10^9/L. Testicular infiltration is uncommon in AML. Confirmation of diagnosis requires the same procedures applied to the diagnosis of ALL.

Treatment

The best outcomes in the treatment of AML have been achieved by intensive therapy over a brief period of time. This usually includes an induction anthracycline (usually daunorubicin) and cytarabine. Remission is achieved in about 90% of children but the challenge is then to maintain remission. Following first remission, allogeneic stem cell transplant is chosen in 60% of children. If cytogenetics have been found to be favourable, then intensive chemotherapy consolidation may be the chosen option (Sung et al 2003). Transplant should be offered if relapse occurs. CNS treatment is also included.

Patients with Down's syndrome have shown an increased response to therapy allowing for AML protocols to be tailored specifically for this group.

Follow-up

Follow-up that is appropriate and sensitive following treatment for AML is required. AML has an increased incidence of relapse (approximately

45%) and despite improvements the cure rate for children with AML is only 50%.

CHRONIC MYELOID LEUKAEMIA

Chronic myeloid leukaemia (CML) is rarely seen in children and young people, the incidence being less than 1 in 100,000 in patients younger than 20 years of age, with 80% of these cases being over the age of 4 years. The Philadelphia chromosome is normally a 'hallmark' of CML (see Chapter 4). Cytogenetics shows a Philadelphia chromosome in 90% of new patients with CML.

Signs and symptoms

CML has three phases and the signs and symptoms depend on the phase the disease has reached. Table 7.2 highlights the phases and corresponding signs and symptoms.

Treatment

Allogeneic bone marrow transplant is normally the treatment of choice. However, Milot et al (2002) have reported encouraging results with the use of interferon and cytarabine for children with Philadelphia chromosome positive CML.

Follow-up

Remissions are induced but relapse is very common and there are extremely few long-term survivors of CML in children or adolescents.

Juvenile myelomonocytic leukaemia

Juvenile myelomonocytic leukaemia (JMML) is a controversial classification subgroup of CML. This was previously called juvenile chronic myeloid leukaemia. It represents less than 1% of childhood leukaemia. The cells in JMML do not contain the Philadelphia chromosome, although other chromosome abnormalities are present. Allogeneic stem cell transplant is required as soon as possible but prognosis is very poor.

Table 7.2
Phases of chronic myeloid leukaemia

Phase	Time range	Signs and symptoms
Chronic	Lasts about 3 years (can range from few months to 20 months)	Non-specific: fatigue, anorexia, weight loss and excessive sweating. Physical signs: pallor, bruising, low-grade fever, sternal bone pain, splenomegaly
Accelerated	Generally, 3–6 months	Similar to chronic phase with more unexplained fever, lymphadenopathy, bruising and petechiae
Blast crisis	(Resistant to treatment – fatal)	Similar to acute leukaemia

LYMPHOMAS

Lymphomas are malignancies that arise from cells of the immune system (see Chapter 1). They can involve any subpopulation of lymphoid cells and for this reason, although classified as solid tumours, they are often linked with leukaemia. Lymphomas are the most common malignancy in young people. Lymphocytes are primary cells of the immune system. Following differentiation, some circulate in blood but the majority populate the lymph nodes, lymphatic fluid or lymphatic organs, e.g. tonsils. In lymphoma the lymphocytes are malignant cells.

The two main classifications of lymphoma in children and young people are:

- Hodgkin's disease (HD)
- Non-Hodgkin's lymphoma (NHL).

EPIDEMIOLOGY

- HD is more commonly seen in teenagers and young people, with a peak incidence in the teens. It is rare before the age of 5 years.
- In less developed countries, HD is more common in younger children.
- Incidence of NHL rises steadily with increasing age.
- Lymphoma is seen more frequently in immunocompromised patients either inherited (e.g. Wiskott–Aldrich syndrome) or acquired (e.g. HIV).
- In Central Africa, NHL incidence is much higher, causing 50% of childhood malignancies.

HODGKIN'S DISEASE/LYMPHOMA

Hodgkin's disease, first described in 1832 by Dr Thomas Hodgkin, is frequently identified by the presence of Reed–Sternberg cells (Hendershot 2004). These are multinucleated giant cells with an 'owl's eye' appearance (these cells have also been observed in other disorders).

Causes

The cells of origin in this type of lymphoma are, as yet, unknown. There is a suspected association between Epstein–Barr Virus (EBV), which is identified as a co-factor, not a causative agent. There is also an increased incidence of HD among siblings, and multiple family members, possibly indicating a heritable aetiology.

Signs and symptoms

Presentation usually includes:

- Painless lymphadenopathy (60–90% in lower cervical chain).
- Supraclavicular and axillary adenopathy.

- About 30% with mediastinal mass causing respiratory symptoms. Superior vena cava syndrome can also occur due to a mediastinal mass.
- 10–30% with hepatosplenomegaly.
- Systemic symptoms – B symptoms (see Chapter 6) in 30% of patients; including unexplained fever over 38°C for three consecutive days, drenching night sweats, weight loss of 10% or more in the previous 6 months (Chauvenet et al 2000).

Treatment

Treatment for HD is almost always multimodal using chemotherapy and radiation therapy. Surgery is usually only used for tissue biopsy. Most treatment regimens for HD are given on an outpatient basis. Drugs predominantly used in the treatment of HD include: mecloretha-mine, vincristine, prednisone, procarbazine, doxorubicin, methotrexate, bleomycin, vinblastine, etoposide, dacarbazine and cyclophosphamide. Currently treatment is being modified and efforts made to avoid the use of alkylating and other drugs with significant long-term sequelae (see Chapter 9).

Radiation therapy is often used for consolidation following chemo-therapy. Radiation fields for HD include:

- involved field: area of original or residual disease
- mantle field: neck, chest axillae
- inverted-Y field: subdiaphragmatic/pelvis.

Autologous stem cell transplant may be used for refractory or relapsed disease. Follow-up is important, particularly owing to the frequent use of radiation in HD protocols.

NON-HODGKIN'S LYMPHOMA

The three main types of NHL in children and young people are:

- Burkitt's or Burkitt's-like lymphoma (small non-cleaved cell type) is of B-cell origin (40% of NHL)
- lymphoblastic lymphoma is usually of T-cell origin (30% of NHL)
- large cell lymphoma may be of either T- or B-cell origin (30% of NHL).

NHLs are an aggressive form of cancer characterised by rapid cell division and an often high tumour burden at diagnosis (Hendershot 2004). They generally occur twice as often in males as in females.

Signs and symptoms

Due to the rapid doubling time of NHLs, there is often large tumour burden and metastases at diagnosis (see Chapter 9). The timescale between symptom onset and diagnosis is usually short. Clinical features may be life-threatening at diagnosis. Symptoms relate to tumour location and histologic subtype. Pressure from the tumour may cause swelling, pain, respiratory disease or malignant effusions.

The primary presentations are head and neck, abdomen, intrathoracic, mediastinal or hilar adenopathy (Cairo & Perkins 2000). Advanced metastatic disease is present in 70% of children who present with NHL (Cairo & Perkins 2000). Symptoms such as headache, cranial nerve palsies, altered level of consciousness, and other symptoms of menigoencephalitis may be indicative of central nervous system (CNS) disease found most commonly in Burkitt's lymphoma (sporadic type) (Hendershot 2004).

Children with more than 25% of blast cells in their marrow technically have leukaemia. This is mature B-cell leukaemia and is often referred to as Burkitt's leukaemia. Primary presentation of tumour *and* >25% bone marrow involvement is classified as 'Burkitt's leukaemia/lymphoma'. Bone marrow involvement may present with symptoms of infection, fatigue, and bleeding resulting from an underlying pancytopenia. Twenty percent of Burkitt's lymphomas have bone marrow involvement identical to acute lymphoblastic leukaemia (Hendershot 2004).

Early complications can arise with NHL and include respiratory compromise due to mediastinal mass, superior vena cava syndrome or massive pleural effusion, tumour lysis syndrome and renal disease.

Treatment

Initiation of therapy for NHL, although potentially life-saving, may also lead to new complications. Nurses must be prepared to anticipate, diagnose and manage these complications. The primary treatment for NHL is chemotherapy. Multi-agent and intrathecal therapy are used. Treatment protocols depend on type and stage of disease.

Surgery is not used for diagnosis and staging, with the exception of abdominal tumors. Radiation therapy is not generally used in the treatment of these tumours except in emergency situations, including management of airway or CNS disease, resistant disease and palliative treatment for chemotherapy-resistant tumours (Hendershot 2004).

Refractory or recurrent NHL often requires stem cell transplant. Both autologous and allogeneic stem cell transplants have been used, normally dependent on marrow involvement.

CARE OF THE CHILD WITH HAEMATOLOGICAL MALIGNANCY AND THEIR FAMILY

The care of a child with leukaemia or lymphoma is usually planned, in the initial stages, at a regional children's cancer centre (in the UK there are currently 22 centres). Childhood haematological cancers are mainly treated alongside other childhood cancers. In many cases the provision of care is complemented by a system of shared care between the regional centre and a unit in a hospital more local to the child's home. The multidisciplinary team is involved in all cases, providing a range of inpatient, outpatient and community liaison facilities.

The principle of care for a child with haematological cancer follows the model of generalist children's nursing that applies family-centred care. Parents and nurses are in partnership in caring for the child through negotiation and empowerment. This also encourages nurses to explore the effect on the family of the child's illness.

Several of the principles of nursing care of adults with leukaemia and lymphoma may also be applicable. However, there are differing effects of these diseases, differing courses of treatment; age-specific considerations and additional effects on families that are important to consider.

DIAGNOSIS

Childhood cancer is still a rare occurrence and, in context, this means a general practitioner may see only one or two cases throughout a career in medicine (Colliss 1996). This, and the fact that many of the symptoms resemble normal childhood illness, may lead to a delay in diagnosis.

Case study 7.1

Tom, aged 5, had been taken by his parents to the GP with intermittent fevers six times over a period of 4 months. The fever was also, usually, accompanied by flu-type symptoms or sore throats, etc. Initially treated as a viral illness, antipyretics were prescribed. The GP then prescribed antibiotics with little effect on the fevers. The GP then made a referral to a paediatrician at the emergency department of a local hospital. A full blood count was carried out that revealed abnormalities consistent with leukaemia. Tom was referred to a regional cancer centre for further investigations.

REFLECTION POINT Consider the implications of the situation described in case study 7.1. How would Tom's family be feeling about the possible delay in diagnosis?

It is important to acknowledge the distress and difficulties in assimilating information for families at this time and to be available to address their concerns (Harding 2000). To enable confirmation of a diagnosis several investigations that have been described previously need to be carried out. One advantage of transferring the treatment of a child to a specialist centre is the availability of resources that enable the majority of investigations to be carried out in the one hospital. Knowledge about the various tests, preparation and aftercare involved is essential to enable optimum preparation and to be able to answer any queries and concerns of the child and family. Adequate preparation will also assist in the cooperation of the child during the investigation procedures.

On confirmation of a diagnosis the 'bad news' must be given to the family; this is usually carried out in a disclosure interview with the parents by an experienced member of the health-care team. A second health-care professional (often a nurse) is usually present. This enables a second person to be available to answer questions regarding information they have given during the interview. As with anyone, when given a diagnosis of cancer, this fact becomes all-consuming, causing an inability to assimilate any further information. The parents are then faced with the dilemma of how and what to tell the sick child (Harding 2000).

Case study 7.2

The parents of Joan, aged 14, are told that a diagnosis of non-Hodgkin's lymphoma has been confirmed. Following the disclosure interview they stipulate that Joan must not, under any circumstance, be informed of her diagnosis. Joan's aunt recently died of cancer at the age of 30. The parents feel that the diagnosis would be too distressing for her and would affect her ability to cope with the illness. Further meetings and discussions are held with the parents to try to understand their anxieties and to try to enable a solution that would mean that Joan could be told of her diagnosis. A multidisciplinary meeting is called and discussions continued to resolve this dilemma.

REFLECTION POINT

Consider your ethical responsibility to the family and the child in case study 7.2. Think of how you would reply to Joan if she asked you if she had cancer.

The amount and type of information given to the child is dependent on various factors including age, religion and ability. Communication skills are of paramount importance. Knowledge about handling difficult situations and families' coping strategies and functioning may help health-care professionals to develop effective communication strategies (Harding 2000). Confirmation of diagnosis also affects other family members including siblings, grandparents and close friends. Self-awareness, suitable education and support systems must be developed to assist in coping with distressing situations encountered in caring for a child with a haematological cancer.

ADMINISTRATION OF TREATMENT

Chemotherapy

The principles of administration and handling of cytotoxic therapy for children are the same as for adults (see Chapter 9). However, the physical, developmental and psychological/emotional factors in children create various issues that are addressed during their care. The four routes used in children for the administration of chemotherapy are:

- oral
- intravenous
- subcutaneous (usually replaces the intramuscular route, owing to reduced risk of bruising or bleeding)
- intrathecal.

All other routes are not routinely used in paediatrics. Liquid oral preparations of cytotoxic drugs are rarely available due to a small demand and chemical instability (Hooker & Palmer 2000). Suspensions need to be shaken as solid components may settle at the bottom of the bottle. Crushing and breaking tablets destroys the intact protective coating and is not recommended because of the hazardous nature of cytotoxic drugs. However, tablets may be the only available preparation and crushing of tablets may be inevitable. Additional safety precautions are required that include preparation in a draught-free environment; washing and drying of tablet crusher/mortar and pestle and tablet cutters; avoiding the use of spoons to crush tablets. Through encouragement and play activities, and with assistance from nurses and play specialists, small children can be encouraged to swallow tablets (Hooker & Palmer 2000). Oral chemotherapy may be required for long periods of time at home for maintenance therapy and compliance may become an issue (Theurer & Tomlinson 2002).

The main difference in care required for the administration of intravenous preparations in children is in achieving venous access. The majority of protocols for children with haematological cancer would warrant the insertion of a central venous access device, e.g. an implantable port or an external catheter. Treatment for Hodgkin's disease does not usually require central venous access and peripheral access is used. Nursing care includes efforts to reduce the trauma of repeated venepuncture. Topical local anaesthetic cream, e.g. EMLA, is often used but complemented with other coping techniques such as distraction, bubble blowing, use of computer games.

Subcutaneous injections (usually of L-asparaginase in the ALL protocols) are usually administered in the upper leg following the application of local anaesthetic cream. The use of indwelling subcutaneous devices is also common practice. They may be in situ for a week after insertion, again with the use of anaesthetic cream. Preparation through play and/or verbal explanation is imperative (Hooker & Palmer 2000).

Lumbar punctures for the administration of intrathecal chemotherapy can be extremely distressing. Anaesthetic or sedation is frequently used. However, some children are able to accept the lumbar puncture if local anaesthetic cream is applied approximately an hour before the procedure. Local injection of lignocaine may also aid the analgesic effect. It is important to work with the child or family to negotiate an approach that is acceptable (Hooker & Palmer 2000).

Radiation therapy

External beam radiotherapy is often used in the treatment of Hodgkin's disease and, of course, as part of the treatment plan in bone marrow transplant where total body irradiation is required (see Chapter 10). Accuracy of planning is essential; therefore the cooperation of the child will help to optimise the experience. Receiving radiation therapy can be a very frightening ordeal. Good preparation will help to elicit children's cooperation. Parent's anxiety can also impact on the child's anxiety. It may be stressful for everyone that the child is left in the room alone. A play specialist may be particularly valuable in preparing the child and family and can have everyone participate in 'statue' games, etc.

Consider how families could be encouraged to practise at home to encourage the cooperation of a child about to receive external beam radiation.

Immobilisation techniques include:

- head rests, knee rolls
- vacuum bean bags filled with Styrofoam beads
- development of immobilisers/blocks
- plaster of Paris casts
- general anaesthesia.

Children may require a general anaesthetic or sedation due to young age, developmental immaturity or extreme distress. Short-acting drugs such as ketamine may be used. These children will require to be treated early in the day to avoid repeated extended periods of fasting. Hydration and nutrition will need particular attention.

An anaesthetist must be present to monitor the child. This will be with the aid of audiovisual monitoring and electrocardiographic and respiratory monitors for the short period that the child requires to be alone when the radiation treatment is being delivered. Radiotherapy is usually delivered to children in an adult centre and adequate, safe recovery must be assured. If the child requires another procedure such as lumbar puncture, the team will often carry out this procedure under the same anaesthetic.

PHYSICAL SIDE EFFECTS

The principles of supportive care for physical side effects are detailed in Section 3. The nature of children means that there are aspects that require special consideration. Side effects of radiotherapy are dependent on the age of child – younger children are more vulnerable to side effects.

Chemotherapy may erase immunity and periods of prolonged neutropenia are expected. Families require education regarding the care of their child at home if neutropenic. This includes staying out of public places, avoiding public transport, avoiding anyone with an infection and emphasising what steps to take in the event of a fever developing, i.e. contact the nearest centre/unit and bring the child to hospital immediately.

Fungal infections can be life-threatening to immunocompromised children. Oral candidiasis is the most common fungal infection and usually can be prevented by prophylaxis using nystatin suspension, clotrimazole, or systemically by oral fluconazole. Aggressive mouth care (every four hours) decreases the severity of these infections.

Aspergillus can be particularly threatening. Spores can be inhaled and in a person with a normal immune system cause no problems. In the immunocompromised child, life-limiting pneumonias and other organ infections can develop. Treatment initially is with intravenous amphotericin. When the disease is under control, the child may require a prolonged course of oral antifungal agents.

When a foreign body, e.g. central venous access device, is in place, fevers are significant, even when the neutrophil count is normal. Cardiac prophylaxis may be needed if children are at risk for developing subacute bacterial endocarditis.

Contact with chickenpox may be common in children. The earlier varicella zoster immune globulin (VZIG) is given after exposure, the greater the effectiveness. If VZIG is given and the child develops chickenpox, it prevents immunity from developing, in most cases, so future exposures will require a repeat dose of VZIG (Salisbury & Begg 1996). Children who have received varicella virus vaccine have the same risk of shingles as patients who have had actual chickenpox (Salisbury & Begg 1996). Institutional policies vary regarding treatment of shingles and chickenpox.

Hearing loss may be caused by platinum drugs, intravenous frusemide, vancomycin and aminoglycoside antibiotics – they damage the 8th cranial nerve. Radiation damages the lubrication-secreting cells of the ear and cerumen becomes very hard and dry. Hearing can be impaired by the auditory canal becoming packed with cerumen, so it is important to teach avoidance of the use of cotton buds. To conserve all remaining hearing, patients should be encouraged to use earplugs for activities with high-decibel noise levels, and to play music at lower levels than what might be considered 'cool'. After therapy is completed, hearing should be monitored at 6 months, then annually. Preferential seating may be needed within the classroom setting. Hearing aids may also be needed.

Low doses of radiation (600–1000 cGy) will slow bony growth. Doses of only 2000 cGy are high enough to *prevent* bone growth by causing premature closure of the epiphyseal plate. Radiation can affect how enamel is laid down and teeth become more susceptible to disease. Teeth, like bones, can have arrested development from relatively low doses of radiation.

Pain in children is often under-treated due to a variety of issues. Education of all team members, including parents, nurses, doctors and play specialists, is essential to overcome these barriers and implement best standard practices for pain management. Nurses are often the facilitators in this process as they observe, support, and educate the patient and family. A child's pain is a sensory experience with an emotional and cognitive response. Helping children to describe their pain in objective, measurable terms can improve the treatment. It is important to use a tool that is appropriate for the child's developmental age and when possible it should be introduced prior to the painful experience. For example the Wong–Baker Faces Pain Rating Scale (Whaley & Wong 1987) uses faces and a numerical scale for a child to assess pain by pointing at the face or number that best describes how they feel. When obtaining a child's self report it is imperative to be aware of their developmental level. Non-verbal cues are critical to assess in all patients, but they are especially important in infants and very young children,

Nutritional status is important. Children often lose weight due to cancer cachexia, anorexia, mucositis, nausea and vomiting. Active and prophylactic treatment is essential and growth velocity must be maintained. Enteral and parenteral nutrition is often considered. It must also be remembered that children receiving steroids, particularly during induction therapy for ALL, are likely to gain weight.

Hair loss is not life-threatening and temporary in almost all patients but is often the most visible sign of cancer and one of the most devastating for the child and family. Conversely, many parents are concerned when there is no hair loss, and need to be reassured that hair loss is not a 100% occurrence and some children will have minimal to no hair loss, depending on the treatment regimen.

PSYCHOSOCIAL ISSUES

Supportive care regarding some psychosocial needs of the child and family are encompassed in the above sections on administration and physical side effects of treatment. Other aspects that affect children include the long periods of hospitalisation, neutropenia and outpatient visits that can disrupt schooling; education can be delivered by hospital teachers. Visits by liaison nurses are usually made to the school to inform teachers about the needs of the child prior to their return to the school system. It is also important that nurses emphasise to parents that children can go to school during treatment at home assuming that they are not neutropenic.

Support for parents is imperative. This may be derived from family members and friends, as well as members of the multidisciplinary team and support agencies and groups. Helping parents to cope with diagnosis and treatment can be facilitated by encouraging their involvement in the child's care while in hospital and ensuring they are fully informed at all stages. Concurrent life events must also be considered.

Research regarding the impact of the experience on siblings has increased over the last two decades. The attention given to the sick child and separation from one or two parents during periods of hospitalisation disrupts siblings' lives (Slade 2000). Siblings will have their own anxieties about their family as well as their own health, relationships, school, etc. Recognition that the well child remains as much a part of the family as they have always done is essential and siblings need regular, frequent contact with their parents and the sick child.

REFLECTION POINT Consider the types of support that could be offered to well siblings of children with leukaemia or lymphoma.

SURVIVORSHIP

Improved survival rates for children diagnosed with leukaemia and lymphoma have increased the importance surrounding late effects of treatment. Treatment and individual patient-related factors impact on the risk of the occurrence of late effects. Therefore identification of individuals at high-risk, follow-up guidelines and intervention strategies are essential (Robison & Bhatia 2003). In 2003, the Scottish Intercollegiate Guidelines Network developed guidelines for the long-term follow-up of survivors of childhood cancer (SIGN 2003). The delayed consequences may have a greater impact on the lives of these children, as they get older, than the acute side effects they experienced in the past. A multidisciplinary approach is essential to achieving cure while minimising the occurrence of late effects of treatment.

Late effects of treatment can be multiple. The major issues for survivors focus on the risk of developing a secondary malignancy, organ dysfunction (including cardiac, pulmonary, gonadal), growth retardation, decreased fertility, impaired intellectual ability, and reduced quality of life (Robison & Bhatia 2003). Aspects of the effect of some of these issues on adolescents are discussed in Chapter 8.

PALLIATION

Despite improved survival, a percentage of children die from malignant disease. The transition into palliation shifts the emphasis of treatment from cure to symptom control. This transition period may be short and well defined or prolonged and include clinical trials of experimental therapy. It is another particularly distressing time and families that have emphasised a partnership approach that includes respect, negotiation and honesty are more likely to accept the situation than families who feel uninformed or unsupported (Beardsmore & Fitzmaurice 2002). Outreach nurse specialists provide excellent models of practice in paediatric palliative care. They liaise with the multidisciplinary team to help to ensure that essential components in care are delivered.

In the UK, resources are available to enable most children to die at home if that is their choice and the choice of the family. Discussing with the family what will happen and what must be done when their child dies can prevent the family contacting emergency services in a panic (Beardsmore & Fitzmaurice 2002). Bereavement support is often offered to families following the death of a child. The family may be invited to meet with the physician at the treatment centre. This may be beneficial to some families but it is usually an extremely difficult visit to make.

REFLECTION POINT Consider what guidance a family may require if they appear to develop an unnatural dependency on individual members of the health-care team or the treatment centre.

CONCLUSION

Haematological cancers in children are often treated with complex protocols that mean care is often delivered over an extended period of time. There are many transitions that the child and family must face throughout the disease trajectory. Nurses caring for these children and families must interpret and respond appropriately to the need for information and support during the care journey.

Understanding both the nature of treatment and its consequences, physically and psychologically, is essential. Nurses must also provide knowledgeable and effective care during individual treatment pathways. Partnership approaches are imperative to facilitate appropriate care across the multidisciplinary team. Communication skills are also important as children's cancer nurses are ideally placed to develop relationships with the children and families and ensure that the coordination of care includes access to appropriate resources.

The ability to undertake such a role is developed over time and ongoing education makes a significant contribution to personal development. Nurses must respond to new challenges, and ensure that evidence-based practice continues to be integrated into this specialist field.

DISCUSSION QUESTIONS

1. It has been assumed that the child and family will accept treatment offered for their diseases. What are the implications if a 12-year-old boy and his family refuse blood product infusion treatment, due to religious beliefs, for anaemia and thrombocytopenia following early intensification treatment phase for ALL?

2. Parents of an 8-year-old boy with relapsed ALL, who is the youngest of three children, instigate discussion with you about having another baby in the hope that the umbilical cord blood will provide the donation for the planned transplant. What factors should be considered when entering into this discussion?

References

Alexander F E, Boyle P, Carli P M et al 1999 Population density and childhood leukaemia: results of the EUROCLUS Study. European Journal of Cancer 35(3):439–444

Beardsmore S, Fitzmaurice N 2002 Palliative care in paediatric oncology. European Journal of Cancer 38:1900–1907

Boutou O, Guizard A V, Slama R, Pottier D, Spira A 2002 Population mixing and leukaemia in young people around the la Hague nuclear waste reprocessing plant. British Journal of Cancer 87(7):740–745

Bruggeman M, Pott C, Ritgen M, Kneba M 2004 Significance of minimal residual disease in lymphoid malignancies. Acta Haematologica 112(1–2): 111–119

Cairo M S, Perkins S 2000 Non-Hodgkin's lymphoma in children. In: Bast R C, Kufe D W, Pollock R E, Weichselbaum R R, Holland J F, Frei E (eds) Cancer medicine, 5th edn. B C Decker Inc., Hamilton

Chauvenet A, Schwarz C L, Weiner M A 2000 Hodgkin's disease in children and adolescents. In: Bast R C, Kufe D W, Pollock R E, Weichselbaum R R, Holland J F, Frei E (eds) Cancer medicine, 5th edn. B C Decker Inc., Hamilton

Colliss G 1996 Children having oncology treatment. In: McQuaid L, Huband S, Parker E (eds) Childrens' nursing. Churchill Livingstone, Edinburgh, pp 411–429

Greaves M F 2004 Biological models for leukaemia and lymphoma. International Agency for Research on Cancer (IARC) Science Publications 157:351–372

Harding S 2000 The impact of diagnosis. In: Langton H (ed) The child with cancer: family-centred care in practice. Baillière Tindall, Edinburgh, pp 37–78

Hasle H, Clemmensen I H, Mikelsen M 2000 Risks of leukemia and solid tumors in individuals with Down's syndrome. Lancet 355:165–169

Hendershot E 2004 Solid tumors. In: Tomlinson D, Kline N (eds) Pediatric oncology nursing: advanced clinical handbook. Springer-Verlag, Heidelberg, pp 26–82

Hooker L, Palmer S 2000 Administration of chemotherapy. In: Gibson F, Evans M (eds) Paediatric oncology: acute nursing care. Whurr, London, pp 22–58

Izraeli S, Waldman D 2004 Minimal residual disease in childhood acute lymphoblastic leukemia: current status and challenges. Acta Haematologica 112(1–2):34–39

Jensen C D, Block G, Buffler P, Ma X, Selvin S, Month S 2004 Maternal dietary risk factors in childhood acute lymphoblastic leukemia. Cancer Causes Control 15(6):559–570

Kinlen L J 1995 Epidemiological evidence for an infective basis in childhood leukaemia. British Journal of Cancer 71(1):1–5

Lilleyman J S 1997 Paediatric oncology update: acute lymphoblastic leukaemia. European Journal of Cancer 33(1):85–90

Milot F, Brice P, Phillipe N et al 2002 α-interferon in combination with cytarabine in children with Philadelphia chromosome-positive chronic myeloid leukemia. Journal of Pediatric Hematology/Oncology 24(1):18–22

Mizutani S 1998 Recent advances in the study of the hereditary and environmental basis of childhood leukaemia. International Journal of Hematology 68(2):131–143

Naumburg E, Bellocco R, Cnattinigius S, Jonzon A, Ekbom A 2002 Perinatal exposure to infection and risk to childhood leukemia. Medical and Pediatric Oncology 38(6):391–397

Plasschaert S L, Kamps W A, Vellenga E, de Vries E G, de Bont E S 2004 Prognosis in childhood and adult acute lymphoblastic leukaemia: a question of maturation? Cancer Treatment Review 30(1):37–51

Robison L L, Bhatia S 2003 Late-effects among survivors of leukaemia and lymphoma during childhood and adolescence. British Journal of Haematology 122:345–359

Salisbury D M, Begg N J 1996 Immunisation against infectious diseases. HMSO, London

Scottish Intercollegiate Guidelines Network 2003 Long-term follow-up for survivors of childhood cancer. www.sign.ac.uk. Website updated 24 Nov 2004, accessed 28 Nov 2004.

Slade A 2000 Impact of treatment on the family. In: Langton H (ed) The child with cancer: family centred care in practice. Baillière Tindall, Edinburgh, pp 105–140

Smith M, Arthur D, Camitta B et al 1996. Uniform approach to risk classification and treatment assignment for children with acute lymphoblastic leukemia. Journal of Clinical Oncology 14(1):18–24

Stiller C A 2004. Childhood cancer. In: The health of children and young people. HMSO, London. www.statistics.gov.uk/children/downloads/child_cancer.pdf. Website updated March 2004, accessed November 2004.

Sung L, Buckstein R, Doyle J J, Crump M, Detsky A S 2003 Treatment options for patients with acute myeloid leukemia with a matched sibling donor: a decision analysis. Cancer 97(3):592–600.

Theurer M, Tomlinson D 2002 Increasing children's compliance with oral chemotherapy. Cancer Nursing Practice 1(6):19–24

Tomlinson D 2004 Leukemia. In: Tomlinson D, Kline N E (eds) Pediatric oncology nursing: an advanced clinical handbook. Springer-Verlag, Heidelberg, pp 2–24.

Whaley L, Wong D L (eds) 1987 Nursing care of infants and children, 3rd edn. Mosby, St. Louis, pp 1070

Further reading

Langton H 2000 The child with cancer: family centred care in practice. Baillière Tindall, Edinburgh
This book combines the concepts of psychological impact of disease and quality of life issues with the partnership approach to care. Many research studies in the field of psychosocial care in paediatric oncology are used to inform each of the issues addressed.

Chapter **8**

Adolescents with cancer

Deborah Tomlinson

KEY POINTS

- Leukaemia and lymphomas account for approximately 36% of cancers in adolescence (15–24 years of age).
- Lymphoma is the most common type of malignancy in adolescents.
- Particular requirements of the adolescent population group need to be addressed with relation to the additional devastating diagnosis of cancer.
- The needs of parents, siblings and partners also require consideration within the family-centred care model.
- Long-term survival for adolescents with haematological cancer is generally very good.
- Follow-up is essential for detection of relapse and monitoring of late side effects of treatment.
- Continued research into the experience of cancer for the adolescent population needs to be encouraged.

INTRODUCTION

Adolescents with a diagnosis of cancer face not only the challenges presented by adolescence itself but also the immense challenges of the disease (Hanna 1993). Caring for the adolescent in any medical speciality raises different issues compared to any other population group (Royal College of Paediatrics and Child Health 2003). In haematological cancers there has been some progress towards addressing the services that are provided to this age group of patients. However, from the outset the use of the term 'adolescents' can be contentious; it may have implications that can typecast a patient as rebellious and non-compliant (Michelagnoli et al 2003). Fortunately much of the research that takes this group into consideration also includes the young adult, which includes patients up to their late 20s. 'Teenagers and young adults' or the term 'young people' is becoming more commonly used. The thought is that the young adult needs as much tact, privacy, respect from carers and age-appropriate facilities as the teenager (Michelagnoli et al 2003). Throughout this chapter the term 'adolescents' is used synonymously with teenagers and young adults unless a specific age range is cited.

HAEMATOLOGICAL CANCERS IN ADOLESCENTS

Figure 8.1 shows an approximate distribution of malignancies in the 15–24 age group. Lymphomas are the most common cancer in this population. The age range of this subgroup of patients often varies between studies; however, an interesting observation that highlights the need for individualised services for this subgroup is that of Albritton & Bleyer (2003) who reported that the rate of cancer in 15–19-year-olds was nearly twice the rate in 5–15-year-olds.

There are no types of cancer exclusive to adolescents although some, such as bone tumours, have a peak incidence in teenagers. Hodgkin's disease is higher in adolescents than children but increases steadily in incidence throughout the age spectrum (Craft 2003).

Figure 8.1
Distribution of malignant tumours in young people (data taken from Birch et al 2003)

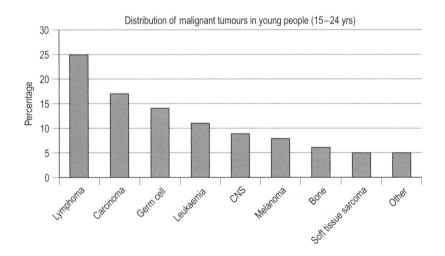

Distribution of malignant tumours in young people (15–24 yrs)

The types of lymphomas or leukaemias seen in adolescents do not change greatly compared with those in children; however Nachman (2003) reports a higher incidence of Philadelphia chromosome positive acute lymphoblastic leukaemia (ALL) and T-cell immunophenotype and lower incidence of extramedullary bulk disease in 16–21-year-olds compared to younger patients. Interestingly, recent reports show that adolescents treated on paediatric protocols for acute lymphoblastic leukaemia and Hodgkin's disease have a better outcome than those managed by adult oncologists (Jeha 2003, Yung et al 2004). However, there remains a shorter overall survival and event-free survival for adolescents with ALL compared to younger children (Irken et al 2002).

The arbitrary referral and differing outcomes for adolescents with haematological cancers has presented challenges in the treatment of this group of patients which require services that will incorporate the needs of this group and consequently improve outcome.

DIAGNOSIS

There is potential within the adolescent group for a delay in diagnosis of cancer (Albritton & Bleyer 2003). Reasons for this may include:

- A sense of invincibility in adolescents and young people that may minimise physical symptoms.
- Denial or embarrassment.
- Low suspicion for a diagnosis of cancer in the adolescent; symptoms may be attributed to school, examination stress, fatigue or excessive physical exertion.
- Parents are not able to see or examine the body of an adolescent as they could a younger child.
- Physicians may be poorly trained in dealing with this population group.

Health education for adolescents should continue to include health awareness and self-examination. Education should also include treatment and cure rates of cancer in children and young people, which would dispel the pessimistic perception that may have arisen through awareness of older individuals with cancer (Albritton & Bleyer 2003). Fortunately, more training programmes for health-care professionals are incorporating sessions specific to the care of adolescents.

COMPLIANCE WITH TREATMENT

Adherence to therapy, particularly oral chemotherapy, has been reported as more problematic in adolescents than in other age groups (Tebbi 1993, Lancaster et al 1997). This may be the oral 6-mercaptopurine or oral methotrexate that is required for the treatment of acute lymphoblastic leukaemia over an extended period of time. Smith et al (1979) measured the compliance of oral prednisolone in adolescents with leukaemia and non-Hodgkin's lymphoma and found that 59% were poorly adherent.

Various social and psychological factors are thought to influence compliance and these include knowledge and understanding, quality of interaction, social support, health beliefs and attitudes, and illness and treatment (Cameron 1996). However, poor rates of compliance can result in the misinterpretation of a drug's effectiveness and can lead to additional tests, dose alterations and hospitalisation (Tebbi 1993). They can lead to both medical and nursing staff feeling powerless, frustrated and becoming emotionally withdrawn from the patient (Nyatanga 1997). Failure to fully comply with oral chemotherapy may in part account for unexplained late relapses (Davies et al 1993, Lilleyman & Lennard 1996).

There has been criticism of the term 'compliance' as there is the potential for the labelling of patients (Playle & Keeley 1998). This could reinforce the view that the professional is dominant, the patient passive and that non-compliance is deviant behaviour (Playle & Keeley 1998). The adolescent should be in a position to understand the treatment regimen in terms of how it will affect his lifestyle and future health, therefore healthcare professionals must refrain from making judgmental responses to non-compliance as this may indeed exacerbate the problem (Cameron 1996, Nyatanga 1997).

To improve patient compliance with chemotherapy it is necessary to have an understanding of the reasons why adolescents do not take prescribed medications. Factors suggested as having an effect on compliance include:

- The process of transition from parental dependency to autonomy in adolescence produces confusion as to who is responsible for medication administration (Tebbi 1993).
- Normal adolescent risk-taking behaviours and disputes with parents about self-care responsibilities may have a negative effect on compliance (Eiser 1996).
- Difficulty in adjusting to the diagnosis and treatment will have an effect on compliance (Fielding & Duff 1999).

Another factor which may contribute to non-compliance in treatment is a lack of knowledge about the condition and the importance of continuing treatment when adolescents perceive themselves as being 'well'. To maximise compliance with chemotherapy treatment, health-care professionals must be aware of the many factors involved and have an in-depth knowledge of the family in their care (Theurer & Tomlinson 2002).

Due to the complexity of non-compliance in adolescents, it is necessary to adopt an individualised approach to promote compliance. The adolescent with cancer is the central focus of care with families and nurses in partnership providing that care. This partnership approach can be effective in promoting compliance with chemotherapy. Partnership may consist of negotiation, sharing, open communication and the transfer of power from the nurse to the adolescent and family (Lee 1999). Difficulties in the model of partnership include that of clarifying and negotiating the partnership roles, alongside issues of power and control within partnerships (Bishop 2000). The degree of collaboration between nurses and the adolescent may depend on a perceived difference of status between health-care professionals and adolescent based on knowledge and attitude. Nurses need to share unbiased and complete information with the adolescent and family in an appropriate and supportive manner; this gives them control and empowerment (McPhee 1995). The emphasis of family care must be on collaboration with the adolescents and their families, recognising their strengths and providing them with assistance to find their own solutions to their own identified needs.

It has been suggested that the issue of non-compliance should be discussed openly from the outset in a non-judgmental manner (Fielding & Duff 1999, Hooker & Palmer 1999). This approach allows parents to discuss any difficulties that they may have or anticipate. In addition, adolescents may appreciate the opportunity to discuss their feelings with health-care professionals regarding long-term oral treatment in private.

Negotiation can also help to minimise later misunderstandings about care and promote the use of choice by both the adolescent and their family. All members of the multidisciplinary team can be involved in negotiation, resulting in a consistent approach to care (Langton 2000). Neill (1996), in a study of parental participation in care, found that the greatest barrier was negotiation. Parents felt that their loss of control along with confusion over their role led to great stress and anxiety and potential conflict. These issues would be of obvious importance to an adolescent who was seeking control of his/her life. The issue of negotiation has been highlighted by Lau et al (1998), who found that the timing of administration of oral chemotherapy was significant in the patient's compliance. This study supports the idea that evening administration of drug therapy is associated with a lower risk of relapse, indicating that it may be easier to remember to administer medication at this more convenient time.

The way children and their families perceive their ability to change or control their lives has a major impact on their willingness or ability to comply with treatment (Cameron 1996). This is particularly relevant to adolescents who have ALL, as the nature of adolescence means that they strive towards autonomy in their personal lives. The continued health of children and adolescents with cancer may be influenced by their self-understanding and self-evaluation (Ishibashi 2001). Therefore the provision of information about the illness and available social support can promote the self-esteem of young people with cancer, which in turn can influence social and emotional health. Ishibashi (2001) believes that it is vital for children and adolescents with cancer to receive information about their illness, as this can reduce uncertainty and negative feelings and assist in their full participation in treatment.

Case study 8.1

Mike, a 15-year-old, was diagnosed with acute lymphoblastic leukaemia. From the point of disclosure of his diagnosis he appeared to be coping with diagnosis and treatment. Generally, he accepted all treatment when in hospital and appeared to understand and cope throughout the first year of diagnosis. He was on maintenance therapy for 3 months when his blood counts, taken at clinic visits, appeared to be higher than expected for someone on oral 6-mercaptopurine and oral methotrexate. Also, he did not require a repeat prescription when it was expected. On questioning Mike and his mother it became unclear when he received his oral medications at home. Now at the age of 16, Mike said that he wanted to have some control of his own treatment and his mother had explained his medications to him. Mike finally admitted to not always remembering to take the medication.

REFLECTION POINT   Consider Mike's situation in case study 8.1. What type of dialogue would you need to have with Mike? What resources/practices could be implemented to assist Mike to continue with his own medication administration?

REFUSAL OF TREATMENT

Refusal of treatment is congruous with complete non-compliance. However, the legal and ethical implications that it raises for health-care professionals are of much greater concern. An adult patient is legally allowed to refuse treatment, despite views of many others who may believe that it is not in the patient's 'best interest' to refuse. An adolescent (or child) under the age of 16 years can legally consent to treatment. Valid consent must follow adequate information, the ability to understand the information, and a formed reasoned decision that is free from coercion (Van Norman & Palmer 2001, Charles-Edwards 2003).

The ability to understand the information is probably the most controversial issue regarding consent in those under the age of 16 years. In the United Kingdom, in 1985, a court case regarding a 15-year-old challenged the adherence to the 16-year-old age limit. The case questioned the decision that a 15-year-old independently requested and received oral contraceptives without the parent's knowledge. The following decision of the House of Lords held that children/adolescents under 16 could consent to receiving medical treatment provided there was sufficient intelligence and understanding of the proposed treatment (*Gillick v West Norfolk and Wisbech Area Health Authority 1985*). Unfortunately, there was no definition of criteria stated for what would become known as '*Gillick Competence*'.

The situation is usually straightforward if the adolescent is willing to consent. However, problems arise when treatment is considered to be in the best interest of the adolescent but he/she refuses. In the under-

16 age group this decision can be overridden by someone who has parental consent. If the parental consent was also refused, the medical professions could then approach the courts to obtain permission to continue with treatment as it could be deemed to be in the best interests of the patient. Therefore, it would appear that those under 16 years of age can consent to treatment but not necessarily refuse (Tomlinson 2004). Consequently, each case must be considered individually.

Most older adolescents have the required capacity to make competent health-care decisions, and health-care professionals must respect this and allow the autonomy of the competent adolescent. Nurses have a role to act as advocates for these adolescents and understanding some of the implications surrounding each individual case can help in assessing and evaluating the situation to achieve the most satisfactory outcome (Tomlinson 2004).

Case study 8.2

Jill, a 16-year-old diagnosed with Hodgkin's disease, has consented to receive treatment. A central venous access device was not considered necessary. Each time Jill receives treatment a peripheral intravenous access device must be inserted. Jill is physically reluctant to undergo this procedure and, consequently, several nurses have to restrain her to enable the device to be inserted. Following insertion Jill is cooperative regarding treatment.

REFLECTION POINT In case study 8.2, Jill is effectively refusing to have an intravenous access device inserted. Consider the ethical implications for health-care staff involved in the insertion procedures. What steps could possibly improve this situation for all concerned?

PSYCHOSOCIAL ISSUES FOR ADOLESCENTS

The psychosocial care of adolescents with cancer can present the greatest challenges when care is compared to that of children. Older adolescents and young adult patients may be living independently with a partner and/or children and they may be employed. Adolescents are beginning to strive for autonomy and independent decision-making – a diagnosis of cancer makes them dependent again and not in control of their lives (Albritton & Bleyer 2003). Several developmental issues become necessary for the adolescent (Albritton & Bleyer 2003):

- Establishing a new self-image (body-image); in relationship to a sexually developed body and autonomous thinking.
- Restructuring future plans.
- Renegotiation of relationships with parents/siblings/partners.
- Forming complicated emotional relationships with individuals.

Health-care professionals must be mindful of the diversity of problems that may seem more intense as an adolescent than at any other time of their life. Adolescents may resist discussing issues with staff – members of the multidisciplinary team must be aware that they may need to be the first to raise issues including career, financial concerns, body image, sexuality and relationships. Making sense of the changes in their lives can be very confusing to the adolescent. Health-care professionals must realise the potential ambiguity and help to develop understanding and positive coping strategies for each patient on an individual basis.

A recent study explored the information needs of adolescents with cancer (13–17 years of age) and the potential role of that information in their cancer experience (Hooker 2004). Some of the important conclusions of the study were:

- Priorities for information included their illness, treatment available and the likelihood of success.
- Individuality between and variation within adolescents regarding information-giving strategies must be expected.
- Teenagers are keen to construct positive attitudes to treatment and value efforts of adults who do the same. They do, however, wish any voiced concerns to be recognised.
- Teenagers may not often ask questions when given the opportunities. When they do ask questions, they deserve optimum attention.

Although there has been an increase in the awareness of the needs of adolescents with cancer, little theoretically based research has been carried out regarding psychosocial needs and the interventions that could be employed to assist them in their coping strategies (Haase 2004). Recent investigators, in the USA, have studied 'resilience' as an important factor that can affect the adolescent's response throughout the disease trajectory, and one that may be influenced by nursing intervention (Nelson et al 2004). A complex model described as the 'Adolescent Resilience Model (ARM)' has been developed and includes the concepts listed below (Haase 2004):

1. Uncertainty in illness
2. Disease- and symptom-related distress
3. Family atmosphere
4. Family support/resources
5. Social integration
6. Health-care resources
7. Defensive coping
8. Courageous coping
9. Derived meaning
10. Resilience
11. Quality of life.

The thought is that the ARM can be used to guide interventions designed to 'target specific protective or risk factors to enhance resilience and quality of life issues' (Haase 2004, p 294). This model would appear to be entirely suitable for this population of patients.

FATIGUE

The symptom of fatigue is recognised as a consequence of both disease and treatment (see Chapter 22). The aetiology of this type of fatigue is complex with many contributing factors (Belmore & Tomlinson 2004):

- Physiological: including anaemia, nutritional status and biochemical changes secondary to disease and treatment. For many adolescent regimens, unlike for adult regimens, dose-limiting parameters do not include fatigue as a side effect (Belmore & Tomlinson 2004).
- Psychological: anxiety and depression potentially lead to fatigue (Langeveld et al 2000). This may become increasingly complex as fatigue may be due to a depressed mood or a person may become depressed if they perceive that they are constantly fatigued (Langeveld et al 2000). Additionally, depression and fatigue may co-occur in cancer patients, as pathology can be the same (Visser & Smets 1998).
- Situational: changes in sleep patterns are common, with stays in hospital; this can contribute to feelings of general lethargy and tiredness.

Research has been instigated in the past few years to investigate how fatigue affects the adolescent during and after treatment for malignancy (Hinds & Hockenberry-Eaton 2001, Edwards et al 2003, Langeveld et al 2003). One study compared overwhelming tiredness in adolescents with cancer (on and off treatment) with that in adolescents who had not had a diagnosis of cancer (Gibson et al 2003). The study compared the themes generated through analysis of interview, diary and focus-group data from groups of adolescents who were on treatment, 2 years off treatment, more than 5 years off treatment, and the group who had not had cancer. Findings showed the presence of overwhelming fatigue in adolescents receiving treatment; variation in fatigue patterns for adolescents 1–2 years out of treatment; with inconsistencies in reports of fatigue from those who were a long time out of therapy (Gibson et al 2003).

Importantly, one of the consistencies reported was the need for adolescents to attempt to lead normal lives and reach their developmental milestones despite having a diagnosis of cancer. Gibson et al (2003) suggest that the symptom of fatigue should be addressed when preparing adolescents from the point of diagnosis, including strategies that have been described as being useful in reducing fatigue. These strategies often mainly consist of planned periods of rest and sleep. The assessment and recording of the experience of fatigue in adolescents and how individuals choose to cope with it should be incorporated into supportive care. Fatigue for adolescents with cancer is a complex concept to understand but patients need support and education to enable them to cope with this symptom. To ensure that these measures are included when planning care, health-care professionals also need to be educated about fatigue.

FERTILITY

Radiotherapy that involves the pelvic area or systemic chemotherapy can cause direct damage to gonadal tissue (the testes and ovaries) resulting in sub-fertility or infertility in both males and females (Tomlinson & McNeill 2004). Adolescents with Hodgkin's lymphoma are also particularly at risk of becoming infertile. In females there may be some loss of oocytes, with or without the occurrence of acute ovarian failure (see Chapter 20). Radiotherapy, even in low doses, involving the uterus in childhood or adolescence is associated with (Tomlinson & McNeill 2004):

- increased incidence of nulliparity
- spontaneous miscarriage
- intrauterine growth retardation with decreased uterine volume and decreased elasticity.

If acute ovarian failure does not occur, there may still be changes that include decreased libido and premature menopause.

Rates of infertility in males appear higher than in females (Albritton & Bleyer 2003). Although fertility preservation options are more feasible and successful for males, there appear to be inconsistencies in the approach to the management of sperm cryopreservation and the corresponding psychosocial support (Shaw et al 2004).

Adolescents and young adult survivors frequently report fertility as a major factor affecting their quality of life (Albritton & Bleyer 2003). Infertility or sub-fertility is frequently documented as a late side effect of treatment. However, many adolescents will not recall sufficient discussions regarding their risk of infertility (Albritton & Bleyer 2003), although the potential for adolescents to repress or deny information concerning sexuality and fertility must be acknowledged. It is therefore important for the health-care professional involved to initiate discussion and provide information regarding the risk of infertility and the option of germ cell preservation prior to the commencement of cytotoxic treatments.

Techniques in preserving fertility continue to be developed. Established options include cryopreservation of spermatozoa and collection of mature oocytes with fertilisation and subsequent cryopreservation of embryos in the female with a partner. Sperm cryopreservation should be discussed with all sexually mature males. Although this may be considered a difficult subject to discuss in the initial stages of the disease, it can be seen as an optimistic view with the adolescent being able to plan for their life after treatment. The collection of a sperm specimen is usually carried out in collaboration with an embryologist from an assisted conception unit (ACU). A consent form must be signed by the adolescent and includes a question about the use of their sperm in the event of their death. It must be pointed out that this is the same form for everyone, not just those about to receive treatment for cancer (Shaw et al 2004). These procedures must be carried out within a few days as it is important that cytotoxic treatment commences. This service and storage is free of charge in the UK; however, other countries such as the USA charge an annual fee for storage.

The knowledge and ability of adolescent males regarding masturbation and ejaculation may be very variable. The embarrassment of the situation or the pain and/or discomfort of the disease may cause inability to produce a specimen. Often parents are included in the discussions or the parent (usually father) may offer to discuss the issue with their teenager. Consideration must also be given to religious and personal views of both masturbation and the soft pornographic materials that are often used in an ACU to assist in the process. It is important that different methods of semen collection be considered, such as transrectal electro-ejaculation or microsurgical aspiration of sperm from the epididymis.

Case study 8.3

Joe, at 15 years of age, was diagnosed with Hodgkin's disease. Joe was informed of treatment and potential acute and late side-effects. The possibility of sperm cryopreservation was discussed with his parents present. Joe and his parents were keen that he should be given this opportunity. The following day a specimen container was brought to Joe's room in the ward and he was told what it was for. He acknowledged this information. Several hours later Joe returned the specimen container to staff. It was noted that it appeared to be urine in the container. After speaking with his parents, a male nurse was able to return to Joe and discuss masturbation with him. The next day Joe was able to go to the ACU, where a room with a couch and some of the reading materials were left. Joe was unable to produce a specimen and treatment had to commence the next day.

REFLECTION POINT   Consider the follow-up counselling that Joe (Case study 8.3) may require. Could anything else have been done to help Joe? Do you think that the ordeal will cause problems for Joe in years to come?

Current and future developments

Experimental strategies are investigating the harvesting and storage of gonadal tissue; cryopreservation of immature spermatogenic cells or oocytes; gonadotrophin suppression and inhibition of follicle apoptosis (Thomson et al 2002). Following cure, stored tissue could possibly be auto-transplanted or matured in vitro until it reached sufficient maturation for fertilisation with assisted reproductive techniques (Brougham et al 2002). Human primordial follicles survive cryopreservation, and ovarian hormonal activity has returned after re-implantation; although as yet no pregnancies have been reported (Thomson et al 2002). These potential developments raise many ethical and legal issues. Adequate regulation of developments is essential (see Chapter 20). These adolescents must be ensured realistic, safe prospects for fertility in the future and patients at risk of sub-fertility must receive appropriate counselling as part of their routine care (Tomlinson & McNeill 2004).

LATE EFFECTS OF TREATMENT

The issues of late side effects of treatment in adolescents are multiple and similar to those of patients treated in childhood. Some aspects of affect on adolescents are particular to this age-range, including fatigue and fertility discussed above. Reports have suggested that, even following completion of treatment, adolescents can have abnormal perceptions of their body and/or their health. Sometimes this is manifested as reckless behaviour or hypochondria (Albritton & Bleyer 2003). Reckless behaviour may be generated through feelings of invincibility, inferiority, insecurity or uncertainty regarding the future. However, this is often a similar view of adolescents who have not had cancer (Hollen & Hobbie 1996). Research investigating these issues has produced conflicting results; including studies around attendance and performance at school and work (Albritton & Bleyer 2003).

Growth

Factors inhibiting growth include cranial irradiation, spinal irradiation, glucocorticoids and chemotherapeutic agents, as well as altered nutrition/inadequate caloric intake. During puberty the sex hormones, along with growth hormone and nutrition, influence growth until epiphyseal fusion is complete and growth is finished. Fortunately the older adolescent will have completed most of their growth dependent on calorific intake and growth hormone.

However, the younger adolescent treated for cancer is less likely to achieve their expected stature unless growth hormone (GH) replacement is given. GH is given as daily subcutaneous injection. GH replacement therapy is normally discontinued once final height has been achieved. However, consideration needs to be given to the continuation of GH replacement beyond this time in order to avoid other adverse consequences associated with GH deficiency including metabolic abnormalities (glucose intolerance); a reduction in bone mineral density; and consequent impaired quality of life (Gleeson et al 2003). Therefore replacement therapy may continue, at a reduced dose, into adulthood (Brougham et al 2002).

Adolescents are often able to self-administer injections of GH at home. However, compliance/adherence and remembering to take it may present issues. Despite GH replacement therapy, expected stature may not be achieved. The adolescent may develop a dependency on the GH and be reluctant to discontinue its use in the hope that some further growth can be achieved. Health-care professionals need to be aware of all the issues surrounding the needs of the adolescent with regard to this aspect of their follow-up care.

PALLIATIVE CARE

Palliative care for adolescents is a relatively new area (George & Hutton 2003). The clinical care of an adolescent receiving palliative care can resemble more of an adult model than that of childhood. However, the adolescent may still be seen as a child within a family and family-centred care remains very important. Also there may be regression of behaviour in some adolescents that can produce difficulties in communication and coping abilities (George & Hutton 2003). They may be able to comprehend the facts and consequences of the incurability of their disease but not be able to cope with the emotional consequences.

Partnerships between the multidisciplinary team and the patient and their family remain vitally important. Truthful discussion and negotiation is essential. However, it must be remembered that honesty can be painful and nurses must be confident in their ability to provide information in a sensitive manner in order to remain supportive to the adolescent and the family (Curnick & Harris 2000). Providing options, such as returning home for the terminal phase, can give an adolescent some control over their lives. Adolescents who choose to stay in hospital may do so for various reasons: it may be difficult for an adolescent to think about having to become dependent on parents again; they may wish to spare their parents the pain of caring for them while they are dying; they may be afraid of death and feel more secure within the hospital. Adolescents may feel that they would like to make a will. It must be recognised that this could be a very difficult issue to raise, particularly with parents, but the patient should be allowed the opportunity to discuss it. Some may go as far as to plan their own funeral. Health-care professionals have a task of allowing adolescents to develop as a 'normal' adolescent but with awareness that the situation is extremely abnormal as they are dying (George & Hutton 2003).

Case study 8.4

Clive was 15 years old when his illness became incurable and palliation commenced. Clive's parents did not want him to know of this decision as they felt that he could not cope emotionally with this prognosis. His parents asked health-care professionals not to mention anything to Clive and made sure someone remained with him in hospital at all times.

Case study 8.5

Sandra, a 16-year-old, in the terminal stages of cancer, was aware that she was dying while at home. However, after realising this she refused to enter into any discussion about dying or death. She carried on with her life as normal until physically unable to do so. This was her choice and her family believed it was the best for Sandra and enabled her, and the family, to cope with the terminal phase of her illness.

TEENAGER CANCER UNITS

The concept of teenage cancer units (TCU) was to provide a specific environment for the adolescent age group patients where appropriate specialist care could be delivered. In the UK, the first TCU was opened in 1990 at the Middlesex Hospital, London. At present there are about 6–8 TCUs in the UK. Some other hospitals have designated adolescent beds or units but not specifically for those with cancer. Although these developments have been viewed optimistically, there is no evidence to demonstrate their benefits and as yet, these units are not part of any coordinated plan for adolescents with cancer. However, despite positive reports, particularly from adolescents treated in them (Geehan 2003), the limitations of TCUs must be acknowledged. The unit must be supported by a skilled multidisciplinary team (Whelan 2003) and this expertise may not be sustainable. The numbers of adolescents requiring admission to a TCU at any one time may be very variable and so staffing numbers may become an issue.

The introduction of the TCU was mainly due to the foundation of the Teenage Cancer Trust (TCT) when inequalities in the UK for adolescents with cancer were realised (Whiteson 2003). The TCT aims to establish a unit in every regional cancer centre in order that every adolescent (between the ages of 13 and 25 years) has access to one of these units. The TCT also organised a conference in 2002 for adolescents themselves. The TCT Multidisciplinary forum meets four times per year and international conferences on 'Cancer and the Adolescent' provide opportunities for the presentation of advances and debate of issues specific to the care of adolescents with cancer (Whiteson 2003). The TCT is also instrumental in the provision of information to schools, regarding health, lifestyles and peers coping with cancer. Further information on the TCT can be obtained from their website, http://www.teencancer.org

CONCLUSION

Adolescents with cancer are becoming more increasingly acknowledged as a group with very specific needs. Communication and the provision of information are vital for this population of patients. Adequate, timely information can assist the adolescent to develop effective coping strategies and help to ensure the best possible psychological outcome (Hooker 2004). Many adolescents with cancer come through the disease and go on to lead something of a normal life. Some may have late effects and unfortunately for some the disease will be incurable (Craft 2003). The particular needs of the adolescent must be considered and they must be supported, to achieve the best possible outcome.

DISCUSSION QUESTIONS

1. The development of Teenage Cancer Units has led to adolescents becoming friendly with others on the unit. Peer support is often encouraged from varying sources. However, this may lead to these adolescents having friends die from their disease. Do you consider it appropriate for peer relationships between patients on these units to be encouraged by way of a 'buddy' system?

2. Adolescent patients are often similar in age to those professionals caring for them. Adolescent patients may develop close relationships with particular health-care professionals in the hospital where the boundaries of a relationship may be questionable. It may be difficult to avoid this situation. What coping strategies could you as a nurse apply to ensure this does not happen?

References

Albritton K, Bleyer W A 2003 The management of cancer in the older adolescent. European Journal of Cancer 39:2584–2599

Belmore J, Tomlinson D 2004 Central nervous system. In: Tomlinson D, Kline N E (eds) Pediatric oncology nursing: advanced clinical handbook. Springer-Verlag, Heidelberg, pp 337–344

Birch J M, Alston R D, Quinn M, Kelsey A M 2003 Incidence of malignant disease by morphological type, in young persons aged 12–24 years in England, 1979–1997. European Journal of Cancer 39:2622–2631

Bishop J 2000 Partnership in care. In: Langton H (ed) The child with cancer: family centred care in practice. Baillière Tindall, Edinburgh, pp 1–20

Brougham M F H, Kelnar C J H, Wallace W H B 2002 The late endocrine effects of childhood cancer. Pediatric Rehabilitation 5(4):191–201

Cameron C 1996 Patient compliance: recognition of factors involved and suggestions for promoting compliance with therapeutic regimens. Journal of Advanced Nursing 24:244–250

Charles-Edwards I 2003 Making health care decisions with children. Cancer Nursing Practice 2(2):29–32

Craft A W 2003 Postscript. European Journal of Cancer 39:2694–2695

Curnick S, Harris A 2000 The dying child. In: Langton H (ed) The child with cancer: family centred care in practice. Baillière Tindall, Edinburgh, pp 355–386

Davies H A, Lennard L, Lilleyman J S 1993 Variable mercaptopurine metabolism in children with leukaemia: a problem of non-compliance? British Medical Journal 306:1239–1240

Edwards J L, Gibson F, Richardson A, Sepion B, Ream E 2003 Fatigue in adolescents with and following a cancer diagnosis: developing the evidence base for practice. European Journal of Cancer 39(18):2671–2680

Eiser C 1996 The impact of treatment: adolescents' views. In: Selby P, Bailey C (eds) Cancer and the adolescent. BMJ Publishing, London, pp 264–275

Fielding D, Duff A 1999 Compliance with treatment protocols: interventions for children with chronic illness. Archives of Disease in Childhood 80:196–200

Geehan S 2003 The benefits and drawbacks of treatment in a specialist teenage unit – a patient's perspective. European Journal of Cancer Nursing 39(18):2681–2683

George R, Hutton S 2003. Palliative care in adolescents. European Journal of Cancer 39(18):2662–2668

Gibson F, Richardson A, Edwards J, Ream E, Sepion B 2003 A descriptive study to explore the impact of cancer and its treatment on adolescents: final report. King's College London, University of London and Institute of Child Health, Great Ormond Street Hospital for Children, London

Gillick v West Norfolk and Wisbeach 3All ER 402 (HL 1985)

Gleeson H K, Stoeter R, Ogilvy-Stuart A L, Gattamaneni H R, Brennan B M, Shalet S M 2003 Improvements in final height over 25 years in growth hormone (GH)-deficient childhood survivors of brain tumors receiving GH replacement. Journal of Clinical Endocrinology and Metabolism 88(8):3682–3689

Haase J E 2004 The adolescent resilience model as a guide to interventions. Journal of Pediatric Oncology Nursing 21(5):289–299

Hanna K M 1993 Health behaviours of adolescents who have been diagnosed with cancer. Issues in Comprehensive Pediatric Nursing 16(4):219–228

Hinds P, Hockenberry-Eaton M 2001 Developing a research program on fatigue in children and adolescents diagnosed with cancer. Journal of Pediatric Oncology Nursing 18(2 Suppl 1):3–12

Hollen P J, Hobbie W L 1996 Decision making and risk behaviors of cancer-surviving adolescents and their peers. Journal of Pediatric Oncology Nursing 13:121–133

Hooker L 2004 Teenagers' information needs. In: Gibson F, Soanes L, Sepion B (eds) Perspectives in paediatric oncology. Whurr, London, pp 158–175

Hooker L, Palmer S 1999 Administration of chemotherapy. In: Gibson F, Evans M (eds) Paediatric oncology acute nursing care. Whurr, London, pp 22–58

Irken G, Oren H, Gulen H et al 2002 Treatment outcome of adolescents with acute lymphoblastic leukemia. Annals of Hematology 81(11):641–645

Ishibashi A 2001 The needs of children and adolescents with cancer for information and social support. Cancer Nursing 24(1):61–67

Jeha S 2003 Who should be treating adolescents and young adults with acute lymphoblastic leukaemia? European Journal of Cancer 39(18):2579–2583

Lancaster D, Lennard L, Lilleyman J S 1997 Profile of non-compliance in lymphoblastic leukaemia. Archives of Disease in Childhood 76:365–366

Langeveld N, Ubbink M, Smets E on behalf of the Dutch Late Effects Study Group 2000 'I don't have any energy': the experience of fatigue in young adult survivors of childhood cancer. European Journal of Oncology Nursing 4(1):20–28

Langeveld N E, Grootenhuis M A, Voute P A, de Haan R J, van den B C 2003 No excess fatigue in young adult survivors of childhood cancer. European Journal of Cancer 39:204–214

Langton H 2000 Negotiating care. In: Langton H (ed) The child with cancer: family centred care in practice. Baillière Tindall, Edinburgh, pp 21–36

Lau R C, Matsui D, Greenberg M, Koren G 1998 Electronic measurement of compliance with mercaptopurine in pediatric patients with acute lymphoblastic leukaemia. Medical and Pediatric Oncology 30(2):85–90

Lee P 1999 Partnership: what does it mean today? Journal of Child Health Care 3(4):28–31

Lilleyman J S, Lennard L 1996 Non-compliance with oral chemotherapy in childhood leukaemia. British Medical Journal 313:1219–1220

McPhee M 1995 The family systems approach and pediatric nursing care. Pediatric Nursing 21(5):417–423

Michelagnoli M P, Pritchard J, Phillips M B 2003. Adolescent oncology – a homeland for the lost tribe. European Journal of Cancer 39:2571–2572

Nachman J B 2003 Adolescents with acute lymphoblastic leukaemia: a new 'age'. Reviews in Clinical and Experimental Hematology 7(3):261–269

Neill S 1996 Parent participation: literature review and methodology. British Journal of Nursing 5(1):34–40

Nelson A E, Haase J, Kupst M J, Clarke-Steffen L, Brace-O'Neill J 2004 Consensus statements: interventions to enhance resilience and quality of life in adolescents with cancer. Journal of Pediatric Oncology Nursing 21(5):305–307

Nyatanga B 1997 Psychosocial theories of patient non-compliance. Professional Nurse 12(5):331–334

Playle J, Keeley P 1998 Non-compliance and professional power. Journal of Advanced Nursing 27:304–311

Royal College of Paediatrics and Child Health 2003 Bridging the gaps: health care for adolescents. RCPCH, London

Shaw N, Wilford H, Sepion B 2004 Semen collection in adolescents with cancer. In: Gibson F, Soanes L, Sepion B (eds) Perspectives in paediatric oncology nursing. Whurr, London, pp 141–157

Smith S D, Rosen D, Trueworthy R C, Lowman J T 1979 A reliable method for evaluating drug compliance in children with cancer. Cancer 43:169–173

Tebbi C K 1993 Treatment compliance in childhood and adolescence. Cancer 71(Suppl 10):3441–3449

Theurer M, Tomlinson D 2002 Increasing children's compliance with oral chemotherapy. Cancer Nursing Practice 1(6):19–24

Thomson A B, Critchley H O D, Kelnar C J H, Wallace W H B 2002 Late reproductive sequelae following treatment of childhood cancer and options for fertility preservation. Best Practice and Research Clinical Endocrinology and Metabolism 16(2):311–334

Tomlinson D 2004 Physical restraint during procedures: issues and implications for practice. Journal of Pediatric Oncology Nursing 21(5):258–263

Tomlinson D, McNeill E 2004 Endocrine system. In: Tomlinson D, Kline N E (eds) Pediatric oncology nursing: advanced clinical handbook. Springer-Verlag, Heidelberg

Van Norman G A, Palmer S K 2001 The ethical boundaries of persuasion: coercion and restraint in clinical anesthesia practice. International Anesthesiology Clinics 39(3):131–143

Visser M R M, Smets E M A 1998 Fatigue, depression and quality of life in cancer patients: how are they related? Supportive Care in Cancer 6:101–108

Whelan J 2003 Where should teenagers with cancer be treated? European Journal of Cancer 39(18):2573–2578

Whiteson M 2003 The Teenage Cancer Trust – advocating a model for teenage cancer services. European Journal of Cancer 39(18):2688–2693

Yung L, Smith P, Hancock B et al 2004 Long term outcome in adolescents with Hodgkin's lymphoma: poor results using regimens designed for adults. Leukaemia and Lymphoma 45(8):1579–1585

Further reading

George R, Hutton S 2003 Palliative care in adolescents. European Journal of Cancer 39(18):2662–2668
This article explores many of the underlying principles of palliative care for adolescents and a model of care that has emerged accordingly.

Morgan S, Hubber D 2004. Setting up an adolescent service. In: Gibson F, Soanes L, Sepion B (eds) Perspectives in paediatric oncology nursing. Whurr, London
This chapter details the background to the development of the Teenage Cancer Trust, processes undertaken in order to set up a teenage cancer unit and some of the psychosocial requirements of adolescents that must be considered when planning services.

SECTION **2**

Treatment

SECTION CONTENTS

Chapter 9

Chemotherapy

Shirley Tervit and Karen Phillips

CHAPTER CONTENTS

KEY POINTS

- Cytotoxic drugs remain the primary therapy for most haematological cancers.
- An understanding of the cell cycle and tumour growth is essential to understand the actions of cytotoxic drugs.
- Safe handling procedures are paramount due to the hazardous nature of the drugs.
- Nursing strategies to minimise toxicity must be in place and are essential to patient care.

INTRODUCTION

Cytotoxic chemotherapy drugs interfere with cell growth and division and are a vital part of disease management in patients with haematological cancers. Chemotherapy is used with curative intent in a variety of diseases and has been shown to improve outcomes and lengthen disease-free survival in a number of others (Preisler et al 1987, Keating et al 1998, Burnett et al 1999).

Nurses are often required to help patients to make sense of their illness and treatment, in order to do this effectively, a basic understanding of cellular biology and the pharmacology of cytotoxic agents used is essential. This chapter focuses on the principles of cytotoxic chemotherapy, including normal and tumour cell kinetics, toxicities, administration issues and implications for nurses.

PRINCIPLES OF CHEMOTHERAPY

Chemotherapeutic agents kill malignant cells but their toxic effects are also seen in normal cells and tissues, particularly those that divide rapidly, e.g. bone marrow, hair follicles, epithelial cells of the gastrointestinal tract and gonads. Normal cells do, however, have a greater capacity for repair and effects are usually reversible (Wujcik 1992). Cyclic chemotherapy remains a common treatment choice in haematological cancers. It aims to destroy malignant cells through delivery of maximum effective drug doses while limiting toxicities by allowing recovery of normal cells between cycles (Perry 2003). Malignant and non-malignant cells have common kinetic properties and an understanding of these is essential in understanding how chemotherapy works.

THE CELL CYCLE

Generally, chemotherapeutic drugs act on the cell cycle within which cellular reproduction occurs (Fig. 9.1). In normal adult tissue cellular division is controlled and is similar to the rate of cell loss, unless there is a physiological need to increase cell numbers, e.g. an increase in white cells (leucocytosis), during infection.

The cell cycle has five phases: G_1, S, G_2, M, G_0. Each describes a period of time for different cellular processes. G refers to gap phases when the cell is preparing for the more active phases of synthesis (S) and mitosis (M) (DeVita 1997).

G1: first growth phase (post–mitotic phase)

The cell prepares for deoxyribonucleic acid (DNA) synthesis by producing ribonucleic acid (RNA), and proteins. Prior to proceeding to the S phase, the cell reaches a restriction point, R. Here, proteins act as a master brake ensuring all necessary events have taken place before the cell can

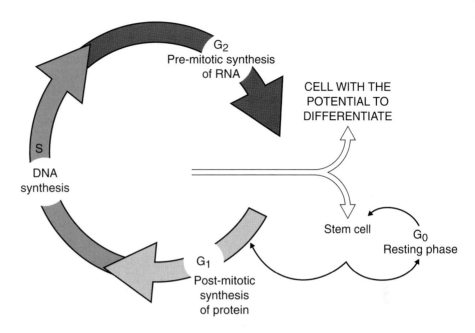

Figure 9.1
The cell cycle (from Maxwell &
Maker 1992, reproduced with
permission)

proceed through the cycle (Sears & Nevins 2002). If irreparable cellular defects are present, the cell will initiate apoptosis (programmed cell death) preventing damaged genetic information being passed to future generations of cells. Once past R, progression through the cell cycle is inevitable. This restriction point is often lacking in malignant cells, perhaps through loss of a major cell cycle control, e.g. the tumour suppressor gene (P^{53}), or other checkpoints allowing them to continue to mitosis with damaged cellular components (Martini 2001).

S (synthesis) phase

During S phase, synthesis of DNA occurs. DNA separates and forms a template to enable genetic information to be copied. The genetic code for the cell is replicated and by the end of S phase the cell has doubled its genetic material to 46 pairs of chromosomes, 23 pairs go to each new daughter cell during mitosis.

G2: second growth phase (pre-mitotic interval)

The cell enlarges and further protein synthesis occurs providing enough protein for two new cells.

Mitosis

This is the physical division of the cellular nucleus. Division of the cytoplasm (cytokinesis) also takes place and these processes result in the creation of two daughter cells (Marieb 2004). Following mitosis, the cell may:

- re-enter G_1 and continue through the cell cycle continually proliferating to replace dying cells

- enter G_0 (resting phase), stop reproduction on reaching normal size (resting, non-proliferating), but retain the capacity for re-entry into the cell cycle if a physiological need occurs
- enter G_0 and differentiate, becoming an end cell (static, terminally differentiated), incapable of further entry into the cell cycle or capable of only a limited number of entries. Cellular apoptosis occurs after the cell has fulfilled its function. Cells in G_0 are not considered to be in the cell cycle and are largely protected from the effects of chemotherapy (Moran 2000).

The time taken to complete the five phases is known as the 'cell cycle time' and varies between tissues and also between normal and malignant cells. The biggest variation is seen in G_1 whilst the other phases remain comparatively constant (Folkman 2001).

TUMOUR CELL KINETICS

Tumour cells can be distinguished from normal cells by their lack of controlled cell division. Their sensitivity to normal controlling factors has been either partially or completely lost (King 2000). Although some tumour cells exhibit a rapid cycling time, the rate is not higher than that seen with normal tissue renewal (Bodnar et al 1998). Malignant cells lack

Table 9.1
Differences between normal and malignant cells (King 2000)

Normal cells	Malignant cells
Restrictive point control: Damage to DNA, high cell density or depletion of essential amino acids, will block the cell in G_1 phase of the cell cycle until repairs are carried out or apoptosis occurs	Loss of restrictive point control (P^{53}). The cell will continue to proliferate despite suboptimal nutrition and damage to DNA
Contact inhibition: Cell growth halts when contact is made with neighbouring cells	Reduced contact inhibition. Cell growth continues and cell will invade without respect for constraints
Anchorage dependence: Normal cells need a surface on which to attach in order to grow, and proliferate	Loss of anchorage dependence. Do not need a surface on which to attach and proliferate
Cells pass through a finite number of doublings then apoptosis occurs	Immortality of transformed cells. Capable of passing through an infinite number of cell doublings if sufficient nutrition and growth factors are available
Cell adhesion molecules mean cells will stay in contact with similar cells within the tissue structure	Reduced adhesiveness. Have increased mobility and will break away from neighbouring cells. Can settle at distant sites (metastasise) with formation of new vascular supply (neoangiogenesis)

sensitivity to the control mechanisms governing normal cell growth and mutations of P^{53} are common (Selivanova et al 1998). Table 9.1 illustrates the differences between normal and malignant cells.

Tumour growth

Tumour growth is affected by doubling time and growth fraction.

Doubling time

This is the time taken for a tumour to double its volume of cells. It is dependent on several factors including:

- histological type
- age of tumour
- whether it is a primary or metastatic growth.

A clinically detectable tumour contains 10^8 cells (1 g) and will have undergone an exponential growth of about 30 doublings. Without treatment the tumour burden would eventually prove fatal (Tannock & Hill 1998). A short doubling time is seen in acute leukaemia and in some forms of non-Hodgkin's lymphoma.

Growth fraction

Growth fraction is the proportion of actively dividing cells within a tumour. In the early stages of tumour growth, cell volume is low yet the ratio of dividing cells (growth fraction) is high. As tumour volume enlarges, hypoxia and lack of perfusion and nutrients occurs resulting in a reduction in growth fraction and a low number of actively dividing cells. This is described as the Gompertzian growth curve (Devita 1991) (Fig. 9.2). During the genesis of a tumour, growth is slow, followed by a period of accelerated growth, which continues into the later stages of growth when the rate slows and a plateau is reached. In some tumours this growth fraction is very high, for example in acute leukaemia, where

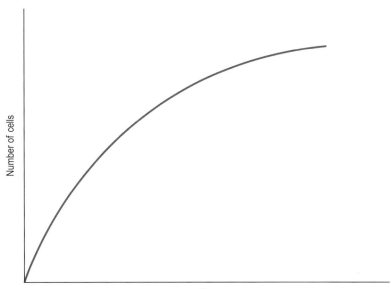

Figure 9.2
Gompertzian growth curve

the bulk of the tumour is composed of actively dividing cells. In other tumours, e.g. the chronic leukaemias, the proportion of cells dividing is low (Kantarjian et al 1998).

In tumours, as in normal tissue, not all cells are actively proliferating at any one time. Tumours are composed of both clonogenic cells (stem cells) and non-clonogenic cells (end cells), some of which may be viable. One of the principles of chemotherapy treatment is to increase the number of non-clonogenic cells. The use of colony stimulating factors (CSFs) is currently being evaluated in clinical trials, as they have shown promise in recruiting viable non-clonogenic cells into the cell cycle. Although controversial, their use may improve cytotoxic cell kill (Estey et al 1994, Burnett et al 2002, Löwenberg 2003).

Cell kill hypothesis

The response of tumour cells to cytotoxic drugs was first recognised in laboratory rat leukaemia cells which reproduced at a constant rate (Skipper 1974). The drugs killed a constant proportion rather than an absolute number of cells each time they were delivered. This is described as log kill. For example, if drug 'A' kills 90% of a tumour containing 10^5 (100,000) cells, one dose of the drug would leave 10^4 (10,000) remaining. A further dose would leave 10^3 (1000) and so on with subsequent doses killing 90% of cells each time the drug is delivered. It would therefore take five doses to reduce the tumour burden to one cell (Tannock & Goldenberg 1998). Host immune-surveillance (or immunity) might then destroy the remaining single cell. There is evidence, however, that one viable tumour cell can reproduce enough times to prove fatal to the host (King 2000). For this reason therapy is often continued even when the disease is not clinically detectable (Pratt et al 1994) and provides the basis for induction (initial therapy), consolidation, intensification and maintenance therapy seen in lymphoma and acute leukaemias (Marcus et al 1989). Consolidation therapy consists of higher doses of the same drugs used in initial (induction) therapy. Intensification uses different drugs to minimise the likelihood of drug resistance. Maintenance therapy consists of treatment with lower doses over a prolonged period of time and is used to treat some lymphomas and acute lymphoblastic leukaemia.

Log kill hypothesis is a theoretical model and makes the assumptions that all cells within the tumour are sensitive to the chemotherapy and that sensitivity does not change (Skipper 1974). The theory has limitations in practice because:

- cells may not be in the correct phase for cell cycle specific drugs to be effective
- perfusion of the tumour varies, which may result in reduced drug delivery
- there may be cancer cells in sanctuary sites which drugs cannot reach (e.g. central nervous system, testis)
- tumour cells may be unresponsive to the drug (primary resistance)
- tumour cells may exhibit initial response but develop resistance (secondary or somatic resistance)

- cell kill may be counterbalanced by cell replication between doses of the drug
- dose-limiting toxicities can delay administration (Kell et al 2003).

Current treatment strategies are guided by cell kill hypothesis and the Gompertzian model of growth (Hussein et al 1998). More recently, targeted therapies have been introduced, some of which have proved to have substantial benefits to patients, especially in terms of reducing toxicity to normal tissue. These agents are discussed in greater depth in Chapter 11.

CLASSIFICATION OF CYTOTOXIC DRUGS

Cytotoxic drugs interfere with the synthesis of DNA, RNA, and proteins or with the proper function of these molecules, leading to cell death. They are classified according to their mode of action and their specificity in the cell cycle although often more than one mechanism is involved. Generally, drugs are divided into two categories: cell cycle phase specific (CCPS) and cell cycle phase non-specific (CCPNS).

Cell cycle phase specific drugs

These drugs act at specific phases within the cell cycle. They are selectively potent if given when a large number of cells are in the appropriate phase of the cell cycle. Unfortunately, there is no guarantee that, when these drugs are delivered, malignant cells will be in that particular phase of the cycle. Table 9.2 shows examples of CCPS drugs.

Cell cycle phase non-specific drugs

CCPNS drugs are effective in all phases of the cell cycle. They have a direct effect on the DNA molecule and are considered more toxic than CCPS drugs (Table 9.3). However, any cells in G_0 phase will be unaffected by the drugs. This has led to the use of continuous infusion of some cytotoxic agents, with subsequent therapeutic benefit. Current therapies combine CCPS and CCPNS drugs in order to achieve maximum cell kill.

COMBINATION CHEMOTHERAPY

Traditionally, intermittent cycles of multiple drugs (combination chemotherapy) have been used for treating haematological cancers. Combining cytotoxic drugs with different modes of action has very important advantages (Grimwade et al 1998):

- they attack tumour cells by different mechanisms
- different drugs may have additive or synergistic effects
- the risk of cumulative adverse effects is reduced as drugs with differing toxicities are used
- it allows normal cells to recover between cycles
- it may bypass potential mechanisms of resistance.

Table 9.2
Cell cycle phase specific
drugs and their actions

Classification	Agents	Mode of action
Antimetabolites	Cytarabine Fludarabine 6-mercaptapurine Methotrexate Thioguanine Hydroxyurea Chlofarabine Cladribine	Structural analogues of metabolites. Mimic naturally produced purines, pyrimidines or folates essential for the formation of nucleic acids. Act by competing with or substituting for other metabolites in such a way that dysfunction and cell death occurs. Active in S phase.
Vinca alkaloids	Vinblastine Vincristine Vinorelbine Vindesine	Derived from the periwinkle plant *Vinca rosea*. Bind rapidly to tubulin in S phase preventing mitotic spindle formation needed during M phase.
Epipodophylotoxins	Etoposide	Extracted from mandrake plant. Inhibits topoisomerase: the enzymes used to break DNA bonds before copying and repair breaks after copying. Halts cell cycle at G_1.
Miscellaneous agents	L-asparaginase	Causes hydrolysis of amino acid asparaginases within the leukaemic cell. Active in G_1.

All drugs used in combination therapy should (Marcus et al 1989):

- be selectively toxic to the tumour in question when used as single agents
- have a differing mode of action from other agents used
- have differing dose-limiting toxicities from other agents used.

Corticosteroids, e.g. prednisolone and dexamethasone, are also used in combination with cytotoxic drugs. Their action is not well understood but it is thought that they render cells more susceptible to chemotherapy (Sheriden 1996). They are thought to work by impeding mitosis and are therefore useful when given in combination with M-phase cytotoxic drugs (Wilkes et al 2003). Prednisolone is widely used in lymphoid malignancies owing to its unique effectiveness against lymphocytes (Wujcik 2000).

PHARMACOLOGY

How a drug behaves once it is in the body is dependent on its pharma-cokinetic properties: how it is absorbed, distributed, metabolised and excreted from the body. All of these factors determine the ability of chemotherapeutic drugs to reach their cellular targets. The route of administration is also important to optimise drug delivery by increasing

Classification	Agents	Mode of action
Alkylating agents	Cyclophosphamide Ifosfamide Carboplatin Chlorambucil Cisplatin Mechlorethamine Melphalan Busulphan	Cross-linking of base pairs and strand breaking. Highly reactive compounds also known as radiomimetic drugs as the effects are similar to radiotherapy.
Nitrosureas	Carmustine Lomustine	Also known as alkylators. Highly lipid-soluble, allowing free passage across membranes achieving effective central nervous system concentrations. Inhibit DNA repair.
Anthracyclines	Doxorubicin Daunorubicin Mitomycin Bleomycin	Antitumour antibiotics isolated from natural substances; various strains of soil fungi. Prevent synthesis of RNA. Intercalate between base pairs similar to alkylators. Cause single- and double-stranded DNA breaks.
Anthracenedione (new class antitumour antibiotic)	Mitoxantrone	Inhibits both DNA and RNA synthesis, intercalating between base pairs and distorting DNA structure.
Platinum agents	Cisplatin Carboplatin	Inorganic heavy metal complexes with similar action to alkylators. Denaturing of DNA.
Miscellaneous	Procarbazine Dacarbazine	Unclear: affects pre-formed DNA and RNA.

the proportion of the drug available for potentially therapeutic effect (bioavailability). Normal function of the liver and kidneys is paramount as these two organs are involved in metabolism and excretion of most cytotoxic agents. Impaired function can lead to increased toxicity or dose reduction, which may lower the therapeutic value of treatment.

Drug resistance

The cellular uptake of a cytotoxic drug is very important and can influence the ability of chemotherapy to induce complete or durable remissions (Perry 1992). Treatment failure and disease recurrence can be a significant problem when treating cancers and the development of drug resistance is the most common explanation for chemotherapy treatment failures. Drug resistance may be temporary, resulting from variations in drug bioavailability, alterations in metabolism or elimination, location of the tumour in sanctuary sites, reduced perfusion of the tumour, host toxicity as well as alteration in cellular kinetics. Resistance, apparent at onset (intrinsic), or evident at relapse after initial response (acquired), poses a much greater problem and is a major barrier to the effectiveness of chemotherapy in curing disease (Gottesman et al 2002, Baird & Kaye 2003).

Substantial research has been undertaken in recent years into the phenomenon known as multidrug resistance (MDR) (Baird & Kaye 2003, Broxterman et al 2003). In MDR, tumour cells are resistant to a variety of organic and functionally unrelated cytotoxic drugs. Figure 9.3 illustrates the mechanisms involved in multidrug resistance, which range from increased degradation of drugs within the cell to decreased drug activation.

The best understood mechanism of MDR is over-expression of P-glycoprotein (P-gp). P-gp uses the energy molecule adenosine triphosphate (ATP) within the cell to actively pump drugs out of the cell (Gottesman et al 2002). As a result of this, cross-resistance has been observed for naturally occurring and semisynthetic drugs such as doxorubicin and etoposide. Multidrug-resistance modulators such as cyclosporin A and PSC 833, a cyclosporin analogue, have been clinically evaluated in an attempt to overcome the phenomenon. Their use, however, has been limited due to organ toxicity (Sonneveld et al 1996).

Dose intensification has been used in recent years as a strategy for overcoming drug resistance, as a definite relationship exists between drug dose and tumour response in sensitive cell populations (Hryniuk & Peter 1987). There is some evidence that increasing the dose of cytarabine both reduces the number of treatment failures due to resistant disease and the subsequent risk of relapse (Mayer et al 1994, Weick et al 1996). Intensification does, however, increase the likelihood of severe toxicity, particularly bone marrow suppression. Haematopoeitic growth factors (HGFs), such as granulocyte-colony stimulating factor (G-CSF) and granulocyte-macrophage colony stimulating factor (GM-CSF), have proved a major advance in supportive care and toxicity reduction. However, their use is limited to non-myeloid malignancies.

Drug interactions

Drug interaction is not uncommon and one drug may alter the action or length of action (half-life) of another. Although substantial therapeutic benefits or toxicities can be seen where a drug enhances the action of another (as in combination therapy), inhibition can lead to a reduced therapeutic effect (Wilkes et al 2003). With the increasingly common use of complementary alternative medicines (CAMs), it is important to be aware that some CAMs may have an adverse effect on patients receiving cytotoxic drugs. For example, echinacea may be harmful in patients receiving treatment for lymphoma (Werneke et al 2004). Another commonly used CAM is St John's wort, it may also interact with some cytotoxic agents causing toxic effects (Izzo & Ernst 2001). It is therefore very

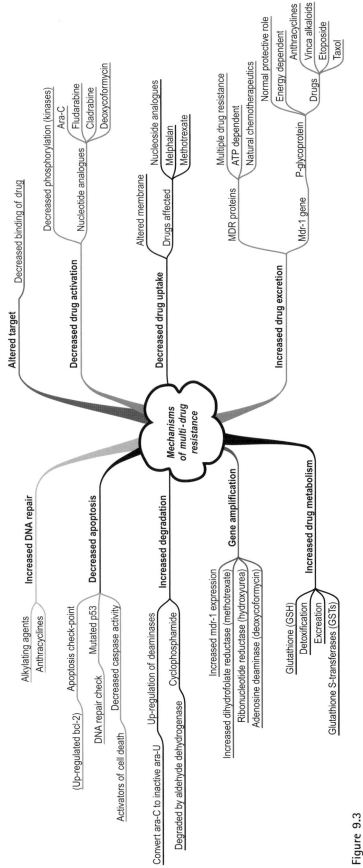

Figure 9.3
Multidrug resistance (reproduced with kind permission of Dr Jonathon Kell)

important to encourage patients to inform health-care professionals of any alternative medications they are taking.

Case study 9.1

John, a 50-year-old married man with two grown-up children, has been diagnosed with AML. Following diagnostic investigations he is entered into the MRC AML-15 trial. He has been randomised to receive fludarabine, cytarabine, G-CSF and mylotarg. This will start within 24 hours.

REFLECTION POINT Consider the key nursing issues relevant at this stage, including the information John requires, his supportive needs, ethical issues and symptom management.

SAFE HANDLING

Antineoplastic drugs are recognised as causing serious health effects including genetic damage, fertility problems, organ toxicity, birth defects and cancer (DesRoche 2003). Safe handling is therefore of paramount importance for all health-care workers who handle cytotoxic drugs and waste. Exposure may occur during drug preparation, transportation, administration and disposal of equipment (Health and Safety Executive 2003). Exposure can occur through inhalation, absorption through skin or mucous membranes, ingestion, or through needle-stick injury (Holmes 1997). There is also the potential for exposure to active drugs in urine, sweat, emesis, faeces and saliva (Royal College of Nursing (RCN) 1998). As a general rule excreta from patients receiving chemotherapy should be treated as hazardous for a minimum of 48 hours (Allwood et al 2001). For extended precautionary periods for handling excreta see Table 9.4.

Work practice guidelines prevent or minimise risks of accidental exposure. The RCN clinical practice guidelines for the administration of cytotoxic chemotherapy (RCN 1998) are the only UK national, evidence-based, multidisciplinary guidelines and currently the best available guidelines for practice. However, nurses also need to familiarise themselves with local policies and procedures. A further useful resource is the Management and Awareness of the Risk of Cytotoxics (MARC) project established in 1999 to update, develop and expand the RCN guidelines (Roberts 2003). Further information can be found at www.marcguidelines.com

Principles of safe handling are summarised in Box 9.1.

Table 9.4
Drugs that require extended precautionary periods when handling excreta (adapted from Allwood et al 2001, reproduced with permission)

Drug	Route	Duration (days) after completion of therapy for which precautions are necessary when handling urine and faeces	
Bleomycin	Injection	3	?
Cisplatin	IV	7	?
Cyclophosphamide	Any	3	5
Dactinomycin	IV	5	7
Daunorubicin	IV	2	7
Doxorubicin	IV	6	7
Epirubicin	IV	7	5
Etoposide	Any	8	7
Melphalan	Oral	9	7
Mercaptopurine	Oral	10	?
Methotrexate	Any	11	7
Mitomycin C	Injection	?	?
Mitoxantrone	IV	12	7
Thiotepa	Injection	13	?
Vinca alkaloids	IV	4	7

? = no information available.

Box 9.1   Principles of safe handling of cytotoxic drugs and waste

All personnel involved in the preparation, transportation, administration and disposal of cytotoxics must receive education regarding the risks of exposure and precautions to minimise risks (RCN 1998). Cytotoxic drugs should be reconstituted in a safety cabinet such as an isolator or laminar flow cabinet by a pharmacist trained in the preparation of these drugs (Aracelli & Hedges 1996, Allwood et al 2001).

Health-care workers involved in the transportation of cytotoxics should receive training regarding exposure hazards and management of spillage. Drugs should be transported using a clearly labelled container indicating cytotoxic contents (RCN 1998).

Only nurses and doctors who have received education and competency training should be involved in the checking, administration and disposal of cytotoxic drugs. Personal protective equipment should be worn at all times when handling cytotoxics. Equipment varies between institutions but should include disposable gloves, plastic apron and eye protection. Eyewash, spillage and extravasation kits should be readily available in areas where chemotherapy is administered. All equipment involved in the preparation and administration of chemotherapy should be treated as hazardous and disposed in clearly labelled, sealed containers (Araceli & Hedges 1996, RCN 1998, Allwood et al 2001).

All staff, patients and carers should be educated in the disposal of excreta. Minimal personal protective equipment of gloves and apron should be worn when handling excreta. In the event of clothing or linen becoming contaminated, items should be doubled-bagged, labelled and disposed of as cytotoxic waste (RCN 1998).

In the case of accidental spillage appropriately trained staff should obtain spillage kit and adorn personal protective equipment which should include latex and neoprene gloves (or similar) >0.45 mm thick, overshoes, gown or plastic apron with armlets, respirator, full face mask and eye protection. Using large absorbent pads the spillage should be worked from the outside area inwards, to avoid spreading the spillage further. All materials should be disposed of as cytotoxic waste and the incident reported as per local policy (RCN 1998).

PRINCIPLES OF ADMINISTRATION

Chemotherapy should only be administered by professionals who have received formal education and can demonstrate competence (RCN 1998). Nurses and doctors need a clear understanding of the purpose of treatment, the drugs used, route of administration and safe administration principles.

ROUTES OF ADMINISTRATION

Intravenous administration

The intravenous route is most frequently used for delivering cytotoxic drugs (Holmes 1997, Dougherty & Bailey 2001). Both peripheral and central venous access devices can be used (see Chapter 12).

Continuous ambulatory infusion

An increasing trend towards continuous ambulatory infusion has dramatically changed cancer treatment (Holmes 1997, Dougherty & Bailey 2001). Drugs such as bleomycin and doxorubicin have relatively short half-lives and are more effective when administered continuously because they are present at constant levels when malignant cells replicate (Dougherty & Bailey 2001). Administering drugs at lower doses over several days avoids peak plasma levels and has been shown to reduce toxicities, e.g. anthracyclines have been shown to be less cardiotoxic when administered continually and are used in this way to treat multiple myeloma (Salmon & Cassidy 1997). Continuous infusions allow patients to go home and receive chemotherapy over a prescribed number of days, e.g. VAD (vincristine and doxorubicin) for myeloma. Careful consideration of potential complications must be discussed with patients and their carers. Complications include the risk of extravasation, precipitation of drugs, spillage and pump malfunction. Patients and carers must be educated in safely troubleshooting any adverse event in order to feel confident about receiving chemotherapy at home.

Oral

The past 20 years have seen an increasing trend towards the use of oral drugs (Skirvin & Lichtman 2002). This trend is likely to continue as, in 2000, an estimated 20–25% of over 300 new antineoplastic agents in development were oral products (Thomas et al 2000). Oral medication is more economical, noninvasive and easier to administer than parenteral administration but no less toxic (Holmes 1997). If adverse side effects such as nausea and vomiting are experienced, patient compliance can be problematic (Dougherty & Bailey 2001, Birner 2003) thereby reducing drug effectiveness. Other factors affecting absorption include: other drugs (e.g. metoclopramide) or physiological conditions that alter normal gut motility (e.g. vomiting, severe diarrhoea) (Birner 2003). Nurses must be aware of these factors and provide education on dose, frequency, safe storage and handling of medication, expected side effects and management of complications to ensure that patients receive an effective drug dose.

Box 9.2   Commonly used oral chemotherapy drugs

- busulfan
- chlorambucil
- cyclophosphamide
- etoposide
- hydroxyurea
- imatinib
- melphalan
- mercaptopurine
- methotrexate
- procarbazine
- thioguanine

Box 9.3   Drugs that can be given subcutaneously and intramuscularly

- bleomycin
- cyclophosphamide
- cytarabine
- L-asparaginase
- methotrexate

Oral cytotoxics have the same potential toxicities as drugs administered by any other route and community nurses need to be aware of this and liaise with hospital staff if excessive side effects inhibit administration or if a patient becomes pyrexial. Safe handling procedures are also required for oral medication. Disposable gloves should be worn and a 'no touch' technique used in dispensing medication (RCN 1998). Commonly used oral cytotoxic drugs are shown in Box 9.2.

Subcutaneous and intramuscular administration

Due to the vesicant and irritant properties of cytotoxic drugs, few agents can be given directly into the tissues (Holmes 1997, Dougherty & Bailey 2001). Drugs that can safely be given subcutaneously and intramuscularly are shown in Box 9.3. When administering these agents the smallest needle that will allow passage of drugs should be used to minimise trauma, using the 'Z-track' technique to avoid leakage (Holmes 1997, Dougherty & Bailey 2001). Sites should be rotated and monitored for any adverse reaction.

Intrathecal and intraventricular administration

Most chemotherapeutic agents are unable to cross the blood–brain barrier (Holmes 1997, Dougherty & Bailey 2001). The central nervous system (CNS) can provide a sanctuary site for tumour cells in certain lymphomas and leukaemia (Allwood et al 2001). Therefore a lumbar puncture is used to administer drugs directly into the cerebrospinal fluid in order to target tumour cells in the CNS. Intrathecal access can be technically difficult, painful for the patient and drugs may reach only the epidural or subdural space (Holmes 1997, Allwood et al 2001, Dougherty & Bailey 2001). Anticancer agents that can be administered intrathecally or intraventricularly are limited to (Allwood et al 2001):

- cytarabine
- hydrocortisone
- methotrexate
- thiotepa.

Unfortunately, there has been an alarming amount of fatal intrathecal drug errors in patients receiving concomitant intravenous therapy (Toft 2001). Consequently the DOH (2001) published guidelines on intrathecal chemotherapy administration. These guidelines state that drugs should be administered in a designated area where intravenous chemotherapy agents are not administered. Drugs should be clearly labelled for intrathecal use, prescribed and stored separately from intravenous medication and administered only by accredited medical staff certified competent in intrathecal administration.

ADVERSE EVENTS

EXTRAVASATION

Extravasation can be defined as the accidental leakage of a drug into the surrounding tissue (How & Brown 1998). Numerous cytotoxic agents are known to cause venous irritation or damage. Box 9.4 and Table 9.5 outline the potential for tissue damage associated with cytotoxic drugs.

Vesicant drugs are considered most problematic when extravasation occurs owing to the drugs' ability to bind to tissue DNA (Skokal 2001). Cells die on contact with these drugs then release active particles back into the tissue; these bind with the next healthy cell. They are capable of continuing their path of destruction for months, causing extensive tissue damage which can lead to surgical debridement, contractures, amputation or mastectomy (depending on the site of infiltration) (Camp-Sorrell 1998) (Plate 9 illustrates damage caused by extravasation of a vesicant).

Early recognition of extravasation is significant in limiting damage. Signs and symptoms are variable, so nurses should observe closely for any signs of extravasation and be able to distinguish these from other conditions producing similar symptoms. Conditions that may result in misdiagnosis are listed in Table 9.6. If there is any doubt about whether extravasation has occurred, the incident should be treated as an extravasation and treated promptly.

Management of cytotoxic extravasation remains ambiguous (How & Brown 1998, Dougherty & Bailey 2001) – nurses administrating cyto-

Box 9.4 Definition of drugs according to their potential to cause serious necrosis when extravasated (adapted from Allwood et al 2001)

Definitions of groups

- Vesicants – capable of causing pain, inflammation and blistering of the local skin, underlying flesh and structures, leading to tissue death and necrosis
- Exfoliants – capable of causing inflammation and shedding of skin, but less likely to cause tissue death
- Irritants – capable of causing inflammation, rarely proceeding to breakdown of tissue
- Inflammatory agents – capable of causing mild to moderate inflammation and flare in local tissues
- Neutral – ostensibly inert or neutral compounds that do not cause inflammation or damage

Table 9.5 Categories of cytotoxic drugs according to their potential to cause serious necrosis when extravasated (from Allwood et al 2001, reproduced with permission)

Vesicants	Exfoliants	Irritants	Inflammatory agents	Neutral
Amsacrine	Aclarubicin	Carboplatin	Etoposide phosphate	Asparaginase
Carmustine	Cisplatin	Etoposide	Fluorouracil	Bleomycin
Dacarbazine	Daunorubicin	Irinotecan	Methotrexate	Cladribine
Dactinomycin	liposomal	Tenoposide	Raltitrexed	Fludarabine
Daunorubicin	Docetaxel			Gemcitabine
Doxorubicin	Doxorubicin			Ifosfamide
Epirubicin	liposomal			Interleukin 2
Idarubicin	Floxuridine			Melphalan
Mitomycin	Mitoxantrone			Pentostatin
Mustine	Oxaliplatin			Thiotepa
Paclitaxel	Topotecan			α-Interferons
Streptozocin				
Treosulfan				
Vinblastine				
Vincristine				
Vindesine				
Vinorelbine				

toxics need to be aware of local policy and procedure. General principles of extravasation management are listed in Table 9.7.

ANAPHYLAXIS, ALLERGIC OR HYPERSENSITIVITY REACTIONS

Nearly all cytotoxic drugs could theoretically produce a hypersensitivity reaction (Allwood et al 2001) and as a general rule, such reactions

Table 9.6
Signs and symptoms of extravasation and factors which can lead to misdiagnosis (Curren et al 1990, Holmes 1997, Allwood et al 2001)

Signs and symptoms of extravasation	Factors which can produce similar symptoms
Swelling	(Always an indication to stop infusion)
Leakage	(Always an indication to stop infusion)
Burning, stinging and pain	pH and osmolarity of cytotoxic drugs can cause venospasm on administration resulting in pain and irritation. Usually differentiated as a 'dull ache' rather than 'burning'.
Erythema	Some agents (doxorubicin, epirubicin, daunorubicin, mitoxantrone) may cause 'flare reaction', which appears as a raised red streak along the vein and can be seen in as many as 17.5% of doxorubicin administrations.
Absence of blood return on aspiration	Not always indicative and may exacerbate an extravasation. Applying negative pressure by aspirating may pull an extravasated cannula back into the vein and provide blood return indicating vein is intact.
Resistance to syringe or lack of free flow of infusion	Giving set may be kinked, venous access device may be positional and require repositioning.

Table 9.7
Management of extravasation (Angel 1995, How & Brown 1998, Allwood et al 2001, Pattison 2002)

Action	Rationale
Stop the infusion	To prevent further infiltration
Mark extravasated area with a pen	If antidote indicated, the area of induration is clearly marked after the cannula has been removed
Attempt to aspirate venous access device	To try and remove any residual drug away from tissues
Remove venous access device (if peripheral)	To allow access to extravasation site
For vesicant drugs administer 100 mg hydrocortisone (2 ml) as six to eight 0.1–0.2 ml subcutaneous injections around the circumference of site	Use of steroids is controversial but is thought to reduce inflammation
For vinca alkaloids administer 1500 units of hyaluronidase in 2 ml of water for injection	As these drugs do not bind to DNA, the aim is to spread and dilute drug to decrease concentration
Apply hydrocortisone 1% cream topically to affected area	To reduce irritation and inflammation
For drugs other than vinca alkaloids – apply ice packs for 24 hours (renewed every 2 hours) to affected area	To localise drug by causing vasoconstriction and decreased absorption and neutralise drug's metabolic effect
If vinca alkaloid extravasation, apply heat packs for 24 hours (renewed every 2 hours) to affected area	To spread and dilute facilitating vasodilation and increasing absorption of drug
Document the area, size and treatment of extravasation in patients' notes, fill out an incidence form and also complete national 'Green Card' reporting scheme	Documentation of adverse event is critical in evaluating healing process. 'Green Card' scheme aims to collate and analyse accurate information on treatments and their effectiveness to devise accurate information and develop predictive index of risks for extravasation, coordinated through St Chad's Unit, City Hospital, Birmingham

occur as a result of over-stimulation of the body's immune system. Drugs more likely to cause reactions (Holmes 1997, Allwood et al 2001) are:

- L-asparaginase
- cisplatin
- daunorubicin
- doxorubicin
- epirubicin
- etoposide
- idarubacin
- melphalan
- rituximab.

The patient receiving cytotoxic chemotherapy should be assessed, observed and supported by professionals who are competent in identifying toxicities and complications (RCN 1998). The patient's allergy history should be discussed prior to administration. For patients with a significant hypersensitivity profile, premedication or test dosing should be considered. Signs and symptoms of hypersensitivity include:

- localised or generalised itching of the skin
- facial or general flushing
- nausea and/or vomiting
- dyspnoea and/or wheezing
- oedema particularly of the face
- light-headedness or headache
- bronchospasm
- respiratory arrest
- cardiac arrest.

Management of hypersensitivity reactions is outlined in Box 9.5. Patients who experience mild hypersensitivity reactions may continue with their treatment provided they have received supportive medication (e.g. hydrocortisone, dexamethasone, antihistamines).

Box 9.5   Management of anaphylactic, hypersensitivity and allergic reactions (adapted from Holmes 1997)

- Stop infusion but maintain intravenous access
- Ensure airway is maintained and administer oxygen if dyspnoeic
- Call for emergency support and medical assistance
- Reassure patient that drug reaction is suspected; provide information of subsequent interventions
- Lie flat and elevate lower limbs
- Obtain baseline observations
- Administer emergency drugs as prescribed, e.g. hydrocortisone, chlorphenamine, adrenaline
- Monitor patient closely until stable
- Document severity of reaction and management

MANAGEMENT OF SIDE EFFECTS

HAEMATOLOGICAL TOXICITIES

Myelosuppression is the most frequent dose-limiting toxicity of chemotherapy and is potentially life-threatening. White blood cells divide every 6–8 hours, and are therefore quickly affected by cytotoxic drugs (Dougherty & Bailey 2001). Loss of white blood cells, particularly neutrophils (neutropenia), occurs rapidly, within 7–14 days, with expected recovery 21–28 days after drug administration (Holmes 1997). The lowest point to which blood cells drop is referred to as the 'nadir'. Some agents (e.g. nitrosoureas) have a delayed nadir (26–63 days) and prolonged recovery (35–89 days) (Skeel 1995). The recovery rate of neutrophils is therefore fundamental in scheduling drugs.

Platelets divide slower than white cells, every 8–10 days, and the onset of thrombocytopenia is more gradual. Red cells divide every 120 days and anaemia occurs later due to cumulative effects of anticancer agents and the disease process (Holmes 1997). Both anaemia and thrombocytopenia are managed with transfusions (see Chapters 12 and 16).

Patients and carers must receive comprehensive education regarding the signs and symptoms of myelosuppression and measures to reduce the risks of infection and bleeding (see Chapters 15 and 16). Temperature should be monitored closely – febrile neutropenia (temp >38°C) must be treated as a medical emergency as systemic sepsis can be rapid when the body has no natural defences.

GASTROINTESTINAL TOXICITIES

Gastrointestinal toxicities are common dose-limiting side effects of chemotherapy. Mucositis is a toxic inflammatory reaction affecting the entire gastrointestinal mucosa, including the oral mucosa (stomatitis) (Wojtaszek 2000). Stomatitis can present as erythema, cracked lips, dysphagia, candidiasis, bleeding and xerostomia, resulting in pain, reduced oral intake and increased risk of oral infection (Wojtaszek 2000, Borbasi et al 2002). Eisen et al (1997) found that 15% of patients undergoing bone marrow transplantation developed systemic fungal infections secondary to stomatitis and one-third of these were fatal. Nursing interventions depend on the extent of stomatitis and are detailed in Chapter 18.

Over the past 20 years clinical and basic research have steadily improved the control of chemotherapy-induced nausea and vomiting (CINV) (Gralla et al 1999). However, CINV has remained the side effect feared most by patients with cancer (Coates et al 1983, Schnell 2003).

Uncontrolled CINV can lead to delays in therapy and dose reductions, both of which can have negative impacts on tumour response rates (Gillespie 2001). It may also result in incalculable distress that can diminish the patient's quality of life (Goodman 1997). Nursing interventions aim to minimise the distress caused to patients and manage any complications of persistent nausea and vomiting (see Chapter 17). Nurses need to be aware of the emetogenic potential of chemotherapy agents and the range of pharmacological options available.

Diarrhoea and constipation can be disturbing side effects of cytotoxic therapy that may result in significant physical and emotional distress for patients (Cope 2001). Furthermore, diarrhoea and constipation may lead to diminished therapy efficacy, treatment delays, dose reductions and, in severe cases, can be life-threatening.

Constipation can be caused by adjuvant therapies (e.g. opiates, anti-emetics) or by the neurotoxic effects of vinca alkaloids causing autonomic nerve dysfunction, resulting in lack of stimulation and peristalsis (Cope 2001).

Nursing interventions for chemotherapy-induced altered bowel habit vary depending on the underlying cause. Overall prompt assessment and appropriate treatment prevents diarrhoea and constipation becoming debilitating for patients, the emphasis being on prevention rather than treatment. Nurses can pre-empt many potential alterations in bowel patterns by developing their knowledge of the gastrointestinal toxicities of chemotherapy agents and providing appropriate patient education.

HAIR LOSS

Hair loss has been cited as the most distressing side effect of chemotherapy and can influence withdrawal from treatment (Love et al 1989, Batchelor 2001). The incidence and severity of chemotherapy-induced alopecia is dependent on several factors including the half-life metabolite of the drug(s), mono or combination therapy, the dose and length of infusion (Batchelor 2001). Onset of hair loss is usually within 7–10 days with marked hair loss within 2–3 weeks (DeSpain 1992, Camp-Sorrel 2000). Body hair divides less frequently than scalp follicles and is therefore less susceptible to damage; however, long-term therapy may result in the loss of pubic, axillary and facial hair (Seipp 1997).

Patients must be reassured that effects on the hair are almost always reversible; regrowth usually appears 4–6 weeks after completion of treatment (Camp-Sorrell 2000). However, approximately 65% of patients experience changes when their hair regrows. Alteration in colour is most common but alterations in texture have also been recorded (Fairlamb 1988). It is important that nurses prepare patients for hair loss. Various strategies can be suggested to help to disguise hair loss, e.g. wigs, scarves, turbans or hats. It is also advisable for patients to consider cutting long hair before treatment to minimise the volume as it starts to fall out, which would hopefully help to minimise their distress (Camp-Sorrel 2000, Batchelor 2001).

FATIGUE

Most patients receiving cytotoxic therapy experience fatigue (Ferrell et al 1996). Nursing management of chemotherapy-related fatigue has traditionally been to recommend frequent rest periods or sleep. However, recent studies reveal that passive strategies compound the fatigue experience and light exercise, hobbies, diversional activities and balancing activity with rest are advocated (Ream & Richardson 1999). For fuller discussion on the psychological impact of fatigue see Chapter 22.

CARDIOTOXICITY

Both acute and chronic cardiotoxicity can result from chemotherapy, and are particularly associated with the anthracycline antibiotics (Holmes 1997, Fristoe 1998, Dougherty & Bailey 2001). Acute toxicity occurs immediately after administration of chemotherapy and is manifested with electrocardiogram abnormalities including tachycardia, and ectopic ventricular and atrial contractions, which are usually transient and resolve without intervention (Holmes 1997, Dougherty & Bailey 2001).

The most critical and dose-limiting cardiotoxicity is cardiomyopathy. Cardiomyopathy induced by anthracyclines usually occurs weeks to months after the last drug dose, but can also occur five or more years later (Fristoe 1998). Associated risks to developing cardiomyopathy include: total cumulative dose >550 mg/m^2, age <15 or >70, pre-existing hypertension or heart disease and previous mediastinal radiotherapy (Van Hoff et al 1982, Camp-Sorrell 1999). Signs and symptoms (Dougherty & Bailey 2001) include:

- tachycardia
- breathlessness
- non-productive cough
- distension of the neck veins
- ankle oedema.

This damage is irreversible – cytotoxic drugs should be discontinued and supportive care commenced.

PULMONARY TOXICITY

The lung is sensitive to the toxic effects of several antineoplastic agents including bleomycin, busulfan, carmustine, chlorambucil, cyclophosphamide, cytarabine, fludarabine, lomustine, melphalan, methotrexate and mitomycin (Holmes 1997, Camp-Sorrell 1999). Researchers have reported the incidence of pulmonary toxicity as high as 40–60% (Ettinger & Turlock 1991). Toxicities can manifest as acute pneumonitis and/or chronic fibrosis (Wickham 1986). The agents most associated with chronic fibrosis are bleomycin and carmustine. Both have cumulative dose ranges where the risk of pulmonary toxicities rises significantly. Awareness of the risk of pulmonary toxicity enables the nurse to be alert for the initial signs and symptoms of dry cough and exertional dyspnoea. Further investigations may then be scheduled to determine the extent of pulmonary damage and an appropriate treatment plan formulated, which usually includes dose reduction or discontinuation.

HEPATOTOXICITY

Hepatotoxicity is an uncommon but serious complication of cytotoxic therapy (Dougherty & Bailey 2001). Liver damage can manifest in elevated liver enzymes, abnormal liver function tests, jaundice or abdominal pain. Drugs known to be hepatotoxic include L-asparaginase, amsacrine, carmustine, cisplatin, chlorambucil, dacarbazine, daunorubicin and methotrexate (Holmes 1997, Dougherty & Bailey 2001). Liver function should always be evaluated prior to cytotoxic therapy and dose reduction or discontinuation considered if abnormalities occur.

NEPHROTOXICITY

Many antineoplastic agents and/or their metabolites are excreted by the kidneys, therefore careful monitoring of renal function before, during and after treatment is fundamental to detection of early renal impairment. Drugs known to be nephrotoxic include cisplatin, methotrexate, mitomycin C, nitrosoureas, ifosfamide and cyclophosphamide (Dougherty & Bailey 2001).

Haemorrhagic cystitis is a major toxicity associated with high-dose cyclophosphamide and ifosfamide. Severity varies from transient cystitis to severe bladder damage resulting in life-threatening haemorrhage (Laffan & Panek 1996). Pre-hydration and adjuvant administration of MESNA (sodium-2-mercapto-ethane-sulphunate) pre-, peri- and post-cytotoxic infusion aims to prevent haemorrhagic cystitis. Similarly, the scheduling of the dose should be carefully considered not to take place overnight as nurses need to ensure patients void >100 ml/h. Strict urinalysis permits early detection of haematuria and additional MESNA can be administered when indicated.

Acute uric acid nephropathy commonly arises in patients with leukaemia or lymphoma who have large, rapidly growing tumors that are very responsive to cytotoxic drugs (Holmes 1997). Massive tumour lysis results in subsequent production of uric acid, which can generally be prevented by prophylactic administration of allopurinol combined with hydration prior to administration of cytotoxic drugs.

NEUROTOXICITY

The exact incidence of neurotoxicity from cytotoxic drugs is unknown (Armstrong et al 1997). Neurotoxicity is usually transient, resolving when treatment is completed, although permanent neurological deficits may result (Holmes 1997). Incidence and severity are affected by the route of administration. For example, methotrexate given intravenously does not cross the blood–brain barrier and therefore minimal neurotoxic effects are seen. However, intrathecal administration can cause meningeal irritation with nausea/vomiting, stiff neck, headache, pyrexia and lethargy (Holmes 1997). Similar side effects can be seen with intrathecal cytarabine.

High-dose ifosfamide has shown to produce neurological toxicity, which manifests as changes in mental status. The patient may gradually deteriorate, progressing from mild confusion to a somnolent state, then becoming comatose, which can be fatal if the drug is not discontinued (Cameron 1993).

Vinca alkaloids are known to cause peripheral neuropathy, which can be dose-limiting. Neuropathy occurs initially in the feet and can progress to ankles and calves; later it presents in the fingers and hands, affecting all aspects of daily living (Smith et al 2002). Nurses must be aware that patients may describe peripheral neuropathy in many ways, such as burning, tingling, pins and needles, or numbness.

GONADAL TOXICITY

Many anticancer agents have a profound and sometimes permanent effect on the ovaries and testes resulting in infertility (McInnes & Schilsky 1996). Chapter 20 provides a fuller discussion on fertility issues.

Secondary malignancies

Secondary malignancies are cancers caused by damage to DNA of normal cells that have been exposed to chemotherapy and radiation therapy. Although secondary malignancies are associated with chemotherapy alone, they are more common following radiation plus chemotherapy (Avery 2001). The most common secondary malignancy is acute myeloid leukaemia following alkylating therapy given for Hodgkin's lymphoma, non-Hodgkin's lymphoma and multiple myeloma (Ronk 2001).

Case study 9.2

John has undergone course 1 and course 2 of his treatment and is due to be randomised for course 3. Treatment has been delayed due to delayed recovery of his bone marrow. He is very tired and frightened to undergo further treatment.

REFLECTION POINT

Consider why bone marrow recovery took so long. What other side effects may John have experienced? What are the nursing issues now in helping him through this next course of chemotherapy?

CONCLUSION

Nursing patients receiving chemotherapy remains challenging. With continual advancements in complex treatments and commitment to effective symptom management the challenge goes on. Gaining theoretical knowledge regarding the drugs' multifaceted effects allows the nurse to predict, prevent, promptly identify and intervene to help patients through their experience.

DISCUSSION QUESTIONS

Choose one chemotherapy regimen commonly used in your area. Relating this directly to a case with which you are familiar explore and discuss the following:

1. What drugs were used? In what phase of the cell cycle do these drugs act and how are they classified?

2. What are the nursing implications of systemic and organic toxicities that may accompany the administration of cytotoxic drugs?

3. What are the informational and educational needs of individuals undergoing treatment and their families?

References

Allwood M, Stanley A, Wright P 2001 The cytotoxics handbook, 4th edn. Radcliffe Medical Press, Oxford

Angel F S 1995 Current controversies in chemotherapy administration. Journal of Intravenous Nursing 8(1):16–23

Araceli A, Hedges L 1996 The challenge of handling chemotherapy in the intensive care unit. Critical Care Nursing 18(4):16–25

Armstrong T, Rust D, Kohtz J 1997 Neurological, pulmonary and cutaneous toxicities of high-dose chemotherapy. Oncology Nursing Forum 24(1):23–33

Avery R 2001 Hodgkin's disease. In: Gates R A, Fink R M (eds) Oncology nursing secrets, 2nd edn. Hanley and Belfus, Philadelphia, pp 153–158

Baird R D, Kaye S B 2003 Drug resistance reversal – are we getting closer? European Journal of Cancer 39(17):2450–2461

Batchelor D 2001 Hair and cancer chemotherapy: consequences and nursing care – a literature study. European Journal of Cancer Care 10:147–163

Birner D 2003 Safe administration of oral chemotherapy. Clinical Journal of Oncology Nursing 7(2):158–162

Bodnar A G, Oulette M, Frolkis M et al 1998 Extension of life span by introduction of telomerase into normal human cells. Science 279:349–352

Borbasi S, Cameron K, Quested B et al 2002 More than just a sore mouth: patients' experience of oral mucositis. Oncology Nursing Forum 29(7):1051–1057

Broxterman H J, Lankelma J, Hoekman K et al 2003 Peripheral blood stem cell transplantation in myeloma using CD34 selected cells. Bone Marrow Transplantation 17(5):723–727

Burnett A K, Goldstone A H, Milligan D W 1999 Daunorubicin versus mitoxantrone as induction for AML in younger adults given intensive chemotherapy: preliminary results of MRC AML 12 Trial. British Journal of Haematology 105(1):67(abs)

Burnett A K, Wheatley K, Goldstone A H, Stevens R F, Hann I M, Rees J K L 2002. The value of allogeneic bone marrow transplant in patients with acute myeloid leukaemia at differing risk of relapse: results of the UK MRC AML 10 Trial. British Journal of Haematology 118(2):385–400

Cameron J 1993 Ifosfamide neurotoxicity: a challenge for nurses; a potential nightmare for patients. Cancer Nursing 16(1):40–46

Camp-Sorrell D 1998 Developing extravasation protocols and monitoring outcomes. Journal of Intravenous Nursing 21:232–239

Camp-Sorrell D 1999 Surviving the cancer, surviving the treatment: acute cardiac and pulmonary toxicity. Oncology Nursing Forum 26(6):983–999

Camp-Sorrell D 2000 Chemotherapy: toxicity management. In: Yarbo C H, Frogge M H, Goodman M, Groenwald S L (eds) Cancer nursing principles and practice, 5th edn. Jones and Bartlett, Boston, pp 470–471

Coates A, Abraham S, Kaye S B et al 1983 On the receiving end: patient perception of the side effects of cancer chemotherapy. European Journal of Cancer and Clinical Oncology 19:203–208

Cope D 2001 Management of chemotherapy-induced diarrhoea and constipation. Nursing Clinics of North America 36(4):695–707

Curren C F, Luce J K, Page J A 1990 Doxorubicin-associated flare reactions. Oncology Nursing Forum 17(3): 387–389

DeSpain J D 1992 Dermatologic toxicity of chemotherapy. Seminars in Oncology 19(5):501–507

Department of Health 2001 National guidance on the safe administration of intrathecal chemotherapy. Department of Health, London

DesRoches P 2003 Cytotoxic drug handlers – monitoring in the occupational health setting. AAOHN Journal 51(3):106–108

DeVita V T 1991 The influence of information on drug resistance on protocol design. Annals of Oncology 2(2):93–106

DeVita V T 1997 Principles of cancer management: chemotherapy. In: DeVita V T, Hellman S, Rosenberg S A (eds) Cancer: principles and practice of oncology, 5th edn. Lippincott, Philadelphia, pp 333–347

Dougherty L, Bailey C 2001 Chemotherapy. In: Corner J, Bailey C (eds) Cancer care in context. Blackwell Science, Oxford, pp 179–221

Eisen D, Essell J, Brown E 1997 Oral cavity complications of bone marrow transplantation. Seminars in Cutaneous Medicine and Surgery 16(4):265–272

Estey E, Thall P, Andreeff M et al 1994 Use of G-CSF before, during and after fludarabine and Ara-C induction chemotherapy of newly diagnosed AML or MDS: comparison with fludarabine + Ara-C without G-CSF. Journal of Clinical Oncology 24:671–678

Ettinger N A, Turlock E P 1991 Pulmonary considerations of organ transplantation. American Review of Respiratory Disorders 144:213–223

Fairlamb D J 1988 Hair changes following cytotoxic drug induced alopecia. Post Graduate Medical Journal 64:757,907

Ferrell B R, Grant M, Dean G E, Funk B, Ly J 1996 'Bone tired': the experience of fatigue and its impact on QOL. Oncology Nursing Forum 23(10):1539–1547

Folkman J 2001 Pharmacology of cancer biotherapeutics: antiangiogenesis agents. In: DeVita V T, Hellman S, Rosenberg S A (eds) Principles and practice of oncology, 6th edn. Lippincott Williams and Wilkins, Philadelphia

Fristoe B 1998 Long-term cardiac and pulmonary complications in cancer care. Nurse Practitioner Forum 9(3):177–184

Gillespie T W 2001 Chemotherapy dose and dose intensity: analyzing data to guide therapeutic decisions. Oncology Nursing Forum 28(2):5–10

Goodman M 1997 Risk factors and antiemetic management of chemotherapy-induced nausea and vomiting. Oncology Nursing Forum 24(7):20–32

Gottesman M M , Fojo T, Bates S E 2002 Multidrug resistance in cancer: role of ATP-dependent transporters. Nature Reviews Cancer 2:48–58

Gralla R J, Osoba D, Kris M G et al 1999 Recommendations for the use of anti-emetics: evidence-based, clinical practice guidelines. Journal of Clinical Oncology 17(9):2971–2994

Grimwade D, Walker H, Oliver F et al 1998 The importance of diagnostic cytogenetics on outcome on AML: analysis of 1,612 patients entered into the MRC AML: 10 Trial. Blood 92:2322–2333

Health and Safety Executive 2003 Safe handling of cytotoxic drugs. Health and Safety Executive, London

Holmes S 1997 Cancer chemotherapy a guide for practice, 2nd edn. Asset Books, Dorking

How C, Brown J 1998 Extravasation of cytotoxic chemotherapy from peripheral veins. European Journal of Oncology Nursing 2(1):51–58

Hryniuk W M, Peter J L 1987 Implications of dose intensity for cancer clinical trials. Seminars in Oncology 14(Suppl 4):1–44

Hussein K K, Dahlberg S, Head E et al 1998 Treatment of acute lymphoblastic leukemia in adults with intensive induction, consolidation and maintenance chemotherapy. Blood 73:57–63

Izzo A A, Ernst E 2001 Interactions between herbal medicines and prescribed drugs: a systematic review. Drugs 61:2163–2175

Kantarjian H M, Giles F J, O'Brien S M et al 1998 Clinical course and therapy of chronic myelogenous leukaemia with interferon-alpha and chemotherapy. Haematology Oncology Clinics of North America 12:31–80

Keating M J, O'Brien S, Kerner S 1998 Long-term follow-up of patients with chronic lymphocytic leukemia (CLL) receiving fludarabine regimens as initial therapy. Blood 92:1165–1171

Kell W J, Burnet A K, Chopra R et al 2003 Simultaneous administration of mylotarg (Gemtuzumab Ozogamicin) with intensive chemotherapy in induction and consolidation in younger patients with acute myeloid leukaemia: a feasibility study. Blood 102:4277–4283

King R J B 2000 Cancer biology, 2nd edn. Pearson Prentice Hall, Harlow

Laffen A, Panek Y 1996 Haemorrhagic cystitis: a nursing issue. Transplant Nursing Journal 5(2):26–28

Love R R, Leventhar H, Easerlig D V, Nerenz D R 1989 Side-effects and emotional distress during cancer chemotherapy. Cancer 63:604–612

Löwenberg B, van Putten W, Theobald M et al 2003 Effect of priming with granulocyte colony-stimulating factor on the outcome of chemotherapy for acute myeloid leukemia. New England Journal of Medicine 349(8):743–752

Marc Guidelines 2003 Management and awareness of the risks of cytotoxics. http://www.marcguidelines.com last updated July 2003. Accessed Dec 2004

Marcus R E, Catovsky D, Johnson S A et al 1989 Adult acute lymphoblastic leukemia: a study of prognostic features and response to treatment over a ten year period. British Journal of Haematology 73:2051–2066

Marieb E N 2004 Human anatomy & physiology, 6th edn. Pearson Benjamin Cummings, San Francisco

Martini F H (ed) 2001 Fundamentals of anatomy & physiology, 5th edn. Prentice Hall, Harlow

Mayer R J, Roger B, Davis C A et al 1994 Intensive postremission chemotherapy in adults with acute myeloid leukemia. New England Journal of Medicine 331:896–903

McInnes S, Schilsky R L 1996 Infertility following cancer chemotherapy. In: Chabner B A, Longo D L (eds) Cancer chemotherapy and biotherapy: principles and practice, 2nd edn. Lippincott-Raven, Philadelphia

Moran P 2000 Cellular effects of cancer chemotherapy administration. Journal of Infusion Nursing 23(1): 44–51

Pattison J 2002 Managing cytotoxic extravasation. Nursing Times 98(44):31–34

Perry M C (ed) 1992 The chemotherapy source book. Williams & Wilkins, Baltimore

Perry M C 2003 Classical chemotherapy: mechanisms, toxicities and the therapeutic window. Cancer Biology & Therapy 2(4 Suppl 1):S2–S4

Pratt W B, Ruddon R W, Ensminger W D et al 1994. The anticancer drugs. Oxford University Press, New York, pp 29–30

Preisler H D, Davis R B, Kirshner J et al 1987 Comparison of three remission induction regimens and two postinduction strategies for the treatment of acute nonlymphocytic leukemia: a cancer and leukemia group B study. Blood 69:1441–1449

Ream E, Richardson A 1999 From theory to practice: designing interventions to reduce fatigue in patients with cancer. Oncology Nursing Forum 26(8): 1295–1305

Roberts R 2003 Reducing the risks. Cancer Nursing Practice 2(4):22–23

Ronk B 2001 Organ toxicities and late effects. In: Gates R A, Fink R M (eds) Oncology nursing secrets, 2nd edn. Hanley and Belfus, Philadelphia, pp 385–390

Royal College of Nursing 1998 Clinical practice guidelines: the administration of cytotoxic chemotherapy. Technical report. RCN, London

Salmon SE, Cassidy J R 1997 Plasma cell neoplasms. In: DeVita V T, Hellman S, Rosenberg S A (eds) Cancer principles and practice of oncology. Lippincott-Raven, Philadelphia, pp 2344–2387

Schnell F M 2003 Chemotherapy-induced nausea and vomiting; the importance of acute anti-emetic control. The Oncologist 8:187–198

Sears R C, Nevins J R 2002 Signaling networks that link cell proliferation and cell fate. Journal of Biological Chemistry 277(14):11617–11620

Seipp C A 1997 Hair loss. In: DeVita V T, Hellman, Rosenberg S A (eds) Cancer: principles and practice of oncology, 5th edn. Lippincott-Raven, Philadelphia, pp 2757–2758

Selivanova G, Kawasaki T, Ryabohenko L et al 1998 Reactivation of mutant p53: a new strategy for cancer therapy. Seminars in Cancer Biology 8:369–378

Sheriden C A 1996 Multiple myeloma. Seminars in Oncology Nursing 12:1–12

Skeel R T 1995 Antineoplastic drugs and biological response modifiers: classification, use and toxicity of clinically useful agents. In: Skell R T, Lachant N A (eds) Handbook of cancer chemotherapy, 4th edn. Little Brown & Co, Boston

Skipper H E 1974 Combination therapy: some concepts and results. Cancer Chemotherapy Reports (part 2) 4(1):137–145

Skirvin J A, Lichtman S M 2002 Pharmacokinetic considerations of oral chemotherapy in elderly patients with cancer. Drugs and Aging 19(1):25–42

Skokal W A 2001 Extravasation. RN 64(9):57–61

Smith E L, Whedon M B, Bookbinder M 2002 Quality improvement of painful peripheral neuropathy. Seminars in Oncology Nursing 18(1):36–43

Sonneveld P, Marie J P, Huesman C 1996 Reversal of multidrug resistance by SDZ PSC 833, with VAD (vincristine, doxorubicin, dexamethasone) in refractory multiple myeloma. A phase 1 study. Leukaemia 10:1741–1750

Tannock I F, Goldenberg G J 1998 Drug resistance and experimental chemotherapy. In: Tannock I F, Hill R P (eds) The basic science of oncology, 3rd edn. McGraw Hill, Maidenhead, Berkshire, pp 392–419

Tannock I F, Hill R P (eds) 1998 The basic science of oncology, 3rd edn. McGraw Hill, Maidenhead

Thomas F W, Cahill A G, Mortenson L E, Schoenfeldt M 2000 Oral chemotherapy, cytostatic and supportive care agents: new opportunities and challenges. Oncology Issues 15:23–25

Toft B 2001 Toft Report: external enquiry into the adverse incident that occurred at Queen's Medical Centre Nottingham 4 March 2001. Department of Health, London

Van Hoff D, Rozencwerg H, Piccart M 1982 The cardiotoxicity of anti-cancer agents. Seminars in Oncology 9(1):23–33

Weick J K, Kopecky K J, Appelbaum F R et al 1996 A randomized investigation of high-dose versus standard dose cytosine arabinoside with daunorubicin in patients with previously untreated acute myeloid leukemia: a Southwest Oncology Group Study. Blood 88(8):2841–2851

Werneke U, Earle J, Seydel C et al 2004 Potential health risks of complementary alternative medicines in cancer patients. British Journal of Cancer 90(2):408–413

Wickham R 1986 Pulmonary toxicity secondary to cancer treatment. Oncology Nursing Forum 13(5):69–76

Wilkes G M, Ingwersen K, Barton-Burke M 2003 Oncology nursing drug handbook. Jones and Bartlett, Boston

Wojtaszek C 2000 Management of chemotherapy-induced stomatitis. Clinical Journal of Oncology Nursing 4(6):263–270

Wujcik D 1992 Current research in side effects of high dose chemotherapy. Seminars in Oncology Nursing 8(2):102–112

Wujcik D 2000 Leukaemia. In: Yarbo C H, Frogge M H, Goodman M, Groenwald S L (eds) Cancer nursing principles and practice, 5th edn. Jones and Bartlett, Boston, pp 1244–1268

Further reading

Barton-Burke M, Wilkes G M, Ingwersen K 2002 Cancer chemotherapy care plans handbook, 3rd edn. Jones and Bartlett, Boston
A compact source book containing commonly used chemotherapeutic agents covering nursing issues relating to toxicity management as well as safety aspects.

Gates R A, Fink R M 2001 Oncology nursing secrets, 2nd edn. Hanley & Belfus, Philadelphia
An easy-to-read text set out in question-and-answer format; appropriate from novice to expert practitioner

Preston F A, Wilfinger C 1997 Memory bank for chemotherapy, 3rd edn. Jones and Bartlett, Boston
Pocket-sized book ideal as a quick reference on individual cytotoxics, indications as well as nursing alerts.

Summerhayes M, Daniels S 2003 Practical chemotherapy – a multidisciplinary guide. Radcliffe, Oxford
An excellent resource laying out commonly used chemotherapy regimens with specific sections for prescribers, pharmacists and nurses.

http://www.marcguidelines.com
MARC guidelines – management and awareness of the risks of cytotoxics. Website established in 1999 to update, develop and expand guidelines developed by the RCN and promote the safe handling of cytotoxic drugs

http://www.extravasation.org.uk
The National Extravasation Information Service aims to be the premier site for information on, the reporting of, and the improved detection, management and hence outcome of extravasation injuries.

Chapter 10

Radiotherapy

Carmen Cule and Joyce Butters

CHAPTER CONTENTS

KEY POINTS

- Radiotherapy is used for radical (curative), adjuvant, prophylactic and palliative treatment in haemato-oncology.
- Radiotherapy can be used alone or in combination with chemotherapy.
- Cells that proliferate rapidly are most sensitive to radiation damage.
- Side-effects depend on the part of the body being treated and the radiation dose given.
- High-quality information and support are vital for individuals receiving radiotherapy.

INTRODUCTION

Radiotherapy is the use of high-energy radiation to destroy cancer cells. In haematological oncology, radiotherapy is used for radical, adjuvant, prophylactic and palliative treatments. Radical radiotherapy treatment aims to cure and is used for non-Hodgkin's lymphoma (NHL) and Hodgkin's lymphoma (HL), either alone or combined with chemotherapy. Further examples of radical treatment include total body irradiation (TBI) given as part of the conditioning treatment prior to bone marrow transplant and treatment for solitary plasmacytoma.

Prophylactic radiotherapy treatment is used in acute lymphoblastic leukaemia (ALL) and B-cell NHL for those at high risk of meningeal relapse (see Chapters 4 & 6). Palliative radiotherapy is used to control symptoms such as pain or swelling in solitary plasmacytoma, myeloma or lymphoma. This chapter explains the use of radiotherapy for haemato-oncological conditions including: the effect of radiation on the cell and what this means in particular treatment situations, the principles of radiotherapy, types of treatment used, how radiotherapy is planned and administered, the side effects of radiotherapy and quality of life issues.

PRINCIPLES OF RADIOTHERAPY

Radiation damages all cells and cannot distinguish between normal and cancer cells. In radiotherapy, x-ray and electron beams are directed at tumour tissue. The beams interact with the constituents of tumour cells (molecules, electrons and nuclei) giving up their energy to them, altering the cells' chemical structure and thus damaging the cells, causing biological changes (Stanton & Stinson 1992). Radiation capable of damaging cellular components in this way is known as ionising radiation. Understanding the principles of radiotherapy requires knowledge of the atomic structure of cells.

ATOMIC STRUCTURE

All living material is composed of atoms. Atoms are structures composed of a few simple particles combined together in different ways (Fig. 10.1). The nucleus of an atom is made up of protons, which are positively charged, and neutrons, which have no charge. The nucleus has negatively charged electrons orbiting around it. The closer the electron is to the nucleus, the stronger the bond between them. For the atom to remain stable, negative and positive charges must balance each other.

IONISING RADIATION

Electrons can escape from the orbit but need extra energy to escape their attraction to the nucleus (Fig. 10.1). The energy caused by radiation

Figure 10.1
Diagrammatic representation
of an atom

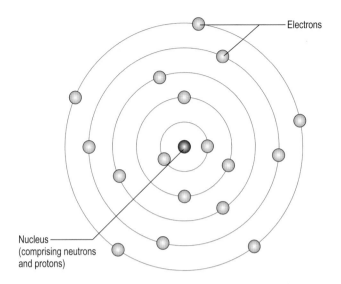

Electrons

Nucleus
(comprising neutrons
and protons)

results in the collision of high-energy photons with atoms, which over-comes the binding energy of the nucleus and allows electrons to escape from their orbit. Electron loss makes the number of positively charged protons and negatively charged electrons unequal, the atom becomes unstable and is known as an ion. The unstable atom breaks down in an attempt to become stable again and ionising radiation is produced during the process. Energy is transferred to electrons when radiation is absorbed by tissues and causes further cellular damage (Adamson 2003).

Various kinds of radiation are emitted from the physical decay of naturally unstable atoms resulting in a more stable state. These are alpha (α), beta (β) and gamma (γ) waves depending on the characteristics of the emission. All these forms of radiation can produce ionisation in tissue but gamma rays are of the greatest use in radiotherapy.

X-rays, a form of electromagnetic radiation, are also used in radiotherapy. The electromagnetic spectrum consists of electric fields. Radio waves are at the lower end of the spectrum with a longer wavelength and lower energy (Fig. 10.2), while x-rays and gamma rays at the top end of the spectrum with a shorter wavelength and higher energy have greater penetration and can cause greater damage to tissues.

Most radiotherapy is delivered as external beam treatment by machines (usually linear accelerators) designed to produce x-rays of sufficient penetrating power (depth dose) to be effective for deep-seated tumours (Souhami & Tobias 1998). The machines can produce clinically useful x-rays of different energies for different depths of tumours. Radiation dose is now measured in grays (Gy).

Biological effects

Radiation damages the cell both directly and indirectly. Direct damage is caused by the chemical bonds of the cell being broken because of the

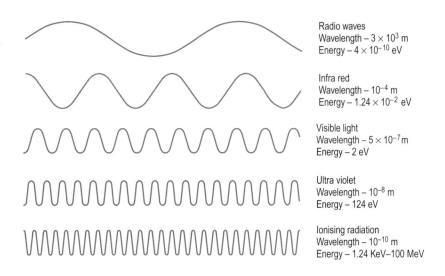

Radio waves
Wavelength – 3×10^3 m
Energy – 4×10^{-10} eV

Infra red
Wavelength – 10^{-4} m
Energy – 1.24×10^{-2} eV

Visible light
Wavelength – 5×10^{-7} m
Energy – 2 eV

Ultra violet
Wavelength – 10^{-8} m
Energy – 124 eV

Ionising radiation
Wavelength – 10^{-10} m
Energy – 1.24 KeV–100 MeV

Figure 10.2
Diagrammatic representation
of the electromagnetic
spectrum

absorption of energy from gamma or x-rays, usually as a result of direct action on cellular DNA. Indirect damage occurs when radiation interacts with the water within a cell and produces other reactive chemicals such as free radicals and oxidising agents, which result in biological damage. This indirect mechanism carries a greater potential for cellular damage because water makes up the bulk of all cells. The most serious effects are because of damage to the chromosomes in the nucleus of the cell (Bomford & Kunkler 2003). Both direct and indirect damage can cause breaks in the single and double strands of cellular DNA and, unless repair is possible, the cell is unable to reproduce. The cell is most likely to be damaged during mitosis and the timing of radiotherapy during the cell cycle is therefore important in inducing cell death (Bomford & Kunkler 2003).

Fractionation

A course of radiotherapy is usually delivered in a number of divided doses (fractions). The number of fractions given varies from one single palliative fraction to daily radical fractions given over several weeks. Improvements in control of some tumours can be achieved by shortening the treatment duration but giving a higher number of small fractions; this is known as hyperfractionation, for example total body irradiation. Two or three fractions may be given with a minimum 6-hour gap between fractions. This allows a larger dose to be given whilst enabling recovery for normal tissues between doses.

Fractionation is important because therapeutic doses of radiation do not usually result in immediate cell death and cells can continue through several cell cycles before death occurs. Response to radiotherapy is affected by cellular:

- oxygenation
- repopulation
- repair
- redistribution.

These factors underpin the rationale for administering radiotherapy in fractions rather than one single dose.

Oxygenation   Hypoxic cells are more radio-resistant than well-oxygenated cells. The degree of oxygenation determines how sensitive a cell is to radiation. Two or three times the radiation dose is needed for tumour death to occur in anoxic cells as opposed to well-oxygenated cells. This is critically important clinically since cells that do not have a good arterial supply will be relatively anoxic and therefore more radio-resistant (Souhami & Tobias 1998).

Repopulation   Repopulation occurs when the stem cells of a tumour regenerate. This can take place during the course of radiotherapy or even between fractions of radiotherapy. Fractionation is planned to prevent repopulation with tumour cells between fractions. Gaps between planned treatments should be avoided to prevent significant repopulation.

Repair   The success of radiotherapy depends on the tumour cell's ability to repair itself (the sensitivity of the cell), compared to the reparative ability of normal cells that are also affected by the radiation. Normal cells have a better and faster capacity for repair than cancer cells. However, all cells will die if exposed to a high enough dose of radiation. The capacity for normal tissue to be able to repair itself more easily than a malignant cell can is the differential between them. The 'therapeutic ratio' is the balance between causing serious damage to normal tissue and curing a cancer. This ratio is the limiting factor to successful cure by radiotherapy.

Redistribution   Radiosensitivity depends on which phase of the cell cycle the cell is in when subjected to radiation (see Chapter 9). The cell is at most risk of damage during the periods when DNA synthesis or cell replication may be disrupted, e.g. in mitosis and G_2 (Holmes 1996, Adamson 2003). Cells that proliferate rapidly are therefore most sensitive to radiation damage. Cells that proliferate slowly take longer to respond to radiotherapy and this helps to explain why radiotherapy side effects can become worse once treatment has been completed. The radiosensitivity of tissues is shown in Table 10.1.

RADICAL RADIOTHERAPY TREATMENTS

LYMPHOMAS

Lymphomas represent the commonest haematological cancer. There are many different types and subtypes, making histological classification

Table 10.1
Radiosensitivity of tissues
(adapted from Souhami &
Tobias 1998)

Highly radiosensitive tissues	Moderately sensitive tissues	Relatively insensitive tissues
Bone marrow	Liver	Bone
Gonads	Kidney	Brain
Gastrointestinal epithelium	Lung	Connective tissue
Lymphoid tissue	Skin	Muscle
Lens of eye	Breast	Spinal cord
	Gut wall	
	Nervous tissue	

Figure 10.3
Mantle technique

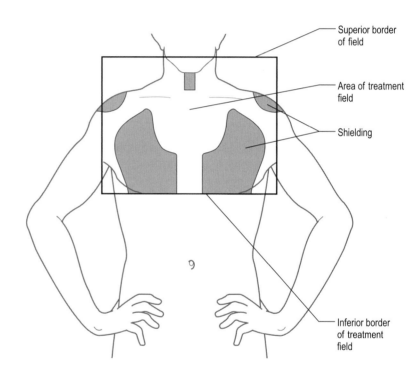

essential for treatment decisions (Sikora & Halnan 1990). Radical radio-therapy results in a high cure rate for stage I and II disease. However, treatment with radiotherapy may be appropriate at different times during the disease (see Chapter 6).

Radiotherapy treatment for HL uses an involved field arrangement to treat affected lymph nodes. If the affected nodes are above the diaphragm, nodes at both sides of the neck, the mediastinum and both axillae are included in the treatment field. This arrangement is called the mantle technique (Fig. 10.3). When the lymph nodes in the para-aortic and iliac regions are involved, the technique is called the Inverted Y (Fig.

Figure 10.4
Inverted-Y technique

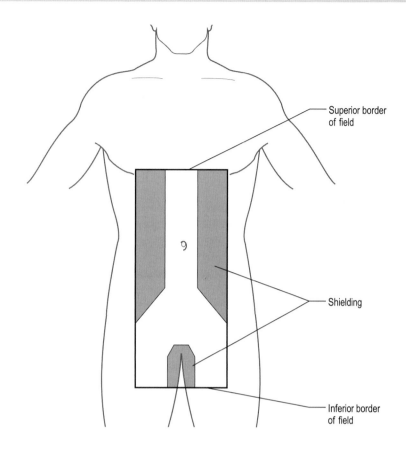

Superior border
of field

Shielding

Inferior border
of field

10.4). Radiotherapy is usually given after a course of chemotherapy, depending on the stage of the disease.

In NHL an involved field arrangement may be used or the specific primary nodal site treated alone, again usually after a course of chemotherapy. This treatment carries a significant long-term risk of future malignancies and infertility, especially for young patients.

Radiotherapy treatment planning

Radiotherapy treatments have to be carefully planned for each patient before treatment begins. Planning takes a considerable length of time and patients are likely to spend more time in the radiotherapy department during planning than for each fraction of radiotherapy. In lymphoma the lymph nodes need to be treated with a high enough dose of radiation to be effective (i.e. kill the tumour cells) but care is required to minimise damage to normal tissue in the treatment field. The mantle technique involves a large treatment area to include all the node areas but also involves the larynx, lungs and the heads of humeri. These areas require to be shielded to avoid damage and are marked in the planning process as well as the areas that require radiation.

A machine called a simulator (a diagnostic x-ray machine that represents the treatment machine) or a CT scanner is used to plan radiotherapy. The patient is positioned carefully on the couch. They must be supine and straight, with their chin extended, this ensures the neck nodes are in the treatment field but avoids treating the mouth. Shoulders should be relaxed and down. Hands are placed on hips with the elbows slightly bent thus enabling axillary nodes to be in the treatment field while avoiding the arms as much as possible. Heels are together with toes apart. It is important that the patient is as comfortable as possible while being in the correct position for treatment. The posterior field is treated under-couch so no movement of the patient is necessary.

For the inverted-Y technique, the patient is positioned supine and straight, a sponge under their head for comfort, their arms relaxed down at their sides, heels together with toes apart. The posterior field is again treated under-couch.

Tiny reference tattoos are marked on the patient's skin to mark the treatment field. Care is taken not to place these in an area that will be shielded. Radio-opaque markers are placed over the tattoos to reference their position and a radiograph taken. For the inverted-Y technique, an intravenous pyelogram (IVP) may also be necessary to ascertain the position of the kidneys. The kidneys will not be able to tolerate the full radical radiation dose and need to be shielded at the tolerance dose (20 Gy). The oncologist draws on the radiograph the areas to be shielded from radiation. Measurements are taken of the distance between the patient's anterior and posterior aspects at the level of the superior edge of the field, the centre of the field and at the inferior edge. An average of these measurements is used to calculate the radiation dose from each field to be prescribed.

The marks drawn on the film are used by the mould room radiographers to make blocks of the exact shape and size to shield areas in the treatment field that are sensitive to radiation, e.g. lungs, larynx and heads of humeri in the mantle technique. The correct position of these blocks is drawn onto perspex plates, which are inserted into the treatment machine and the blocks placed appropriately. A separate plate with blocks is made for the posterior field because the shape will be different due to the divergence of the radiation beam.

When all the planning is complete, the patient returns to the simulator to have x-ray films (anterior and posterior) with the blocks in place. This ensures the treatment is reproducible and exactly as the oncologist prescribed. Any necessary modifications can also be made at this stage.

Radiotherapy treatment –
mantle technique

Patients are positioned exactly as they were in the planning department. The patient is asked to lie still and breathe normally throughout the treatment. The treatment couch is lowered to achieve a distance of 130 cm to the patient's skin, tattoos are lined up with the machine beam centre lights and the patient's position adjusted slightly if necessary. Borders of the treatment field are checked to ensure they are in the correct position.

The plate is inserted into the treatment machine and the shielding blocks placed on the plate in the designated positions. X-ray films are taken to check the position of the blocks on the first treatment. The radiographers leave the treatment room and turn the machine on from outside. Patients are observed during this time using closed circuit television cameras. If any problem occurs, the machine can be immediately switched off so that the radiographers can enter the room. The patient feels nothing when the machine is on. When the first (anterior) field has been treated, the radiographers remove the blocks and the plate. The machine is then moved through 180 degrees and the treatment couch is raised to the correct distance of 130 cm and the posterior plate and blocks are set up. The patient needs to keep as still as possible at this time. This is not usually a problem as treatment is very quick.

Radiation doses prescribed for Hodgkin's lymphoma depend on the stage of disease being treated and whether given in conjunction with chemotherapy. Stage I and II disease require a higher dose than other stages to improve the chance of cure.

TOTAL BODY IRRADIATION (TBI)

High-dose total body irradiation (TBI) is given to some patients with leukaemia and lymphoma prior to bone marrow transplant in conjunction with high-dose chemotherapy (see Chapter 13).

AIM OF TBI

The aim of TBI is to maximise tumour kill while remaining within acceptable levels of damage to normal cells. The potential for lung damage is the greatest dose-limiting factor. The lungs have increased radiation absorption because being full of air they are not dense structures. Other dose-limiting tissues are the kidney, liver, gastrointestinal tract and heart (Dobbs et al 1999).

Benefits of TBI

TBI eliminates tumour cells, by acting on the 'sanctuary sites' (parts of the body which may not be reached by systemic chemotherapy), for example, the meninges, cerebral spinal fluid, ovaries and testes. TBI also kills malignant cells irrespective of their proliferative status. It eradicates all active bone marrow and suppresses the immune system to reduce bone marrow rejection (Sikora & Halnan 1990).

THE BASIC PRINCIPLES OF TBI

Beam energy and delivery

Beam energy of 10 MV photons is required to give a sufficiently even dose distribution.

Dose rates and accuracy

Doses for standard radical radiotherapy treatments are high because a specific small site is targeted but the dose for TBI treatment must be lower as the whole body is included. Single treatments were given when TBI was in its infancy. For many years now, treatment has been hyper-fractionated (twice a day for 4 consecutive days with a 6-hour gap between treatments). Fractionated treatments allow for more accurate control of the dosimetry.

The rate at which the dose is delivered is very important, because of the potential for lung toxicity. In the early days of single treatments the dose rate was critical and was given in the region of 7.5 cGy per minute, which required several hours of treatment time for the patient. Fractionated treatments allow a higher dose rate to be used (in the region of 15 cGy per minute) without affecting lung tolerance. This allows a much shorter beam-on time (10 minutes) for the patient to tolerate.

Homogeneity and lung compensation

To ensure homogeneity and prevent the lungs receiving too high a radiation dose a screen made of two sheets of perspex is placed along-side the patient. In between the perspex sheets, brass sheets are positioned in the head and neck region and the region of the ankles, knees and hips. These compensate for the different separations of the head, neck, shoulders, chest, waist, knees and ankles. Another brass sheet is also positioned to achieve homogeneity and prevent lung tissue receiving too high a radiation dose. These are adjusted for each individual patient and may also be adjusted for each fraction (Fig. 10.5)

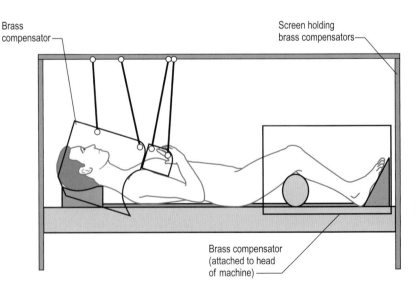

Figure 10.5 An example of Brass compensator set-up

Brass compensator

Screen holding brass compensators

Brass compensator (attached to head of machine)

EXAMPLE OF A RADIOTHERAPY TECHNIQUE FOR TBI

Techniques vary from centre to centre depending on several factors, such as departmental policy, treatment machine availability and a treatment room of sufficient size to allow a field size large enough to encompass the whole body. The requirement is for a treatment distance of 4.5 metres, whereas a standard radiotherapy treatment requires a distance of only 100–130 cm. The following is an example of how one centre in the UK delivers TBI following administration of chemotherapy.

Information/informed consent for TBI

It is very important that patients have a full understanding of what having TBI will mean to them, thus ensuring they are able to give informed consent. One method of achieving this is to arrange a pre-assessment visit to the radiotherapy department prior to the treatment starting. The patient can then meet the radiographer team and visit the treatment room where the process is explained. If the oncology centre is on a different site from the main hospital, a visit can also be made to the ward where the patient will spend the 4 days of treatment. During the visit, all acute and long-term effects can be explained, any questions answered and consent obtained by the consultant oncologist.

Patient position for TBI

Accuracy of beam delivery is vital for any radiotherapy treatment and is equally applicable to TBI. The patient's position is important to ensure that the beam is aligned correctly to administer the planned radiation dose throughout the body. It is therefore essential that the treatment position is reproducible for each fraction. It must be suitable for technical requirements and also comfortable for the patient, enabling them to maintain the position for each fraction.

The patient lies supine, with arms folded across the waist and elbows by their sides (Fig. 10.6). The beam therefore has to pass through the patient's arms before it reaches the lungs, limiting radiation damage to the lungs. The patient's head lies on one square sponge for support and comfort and another sponge is placed as a support under their knees (Fig. 10.7). Treatment is by two beams directed at each side of the patient. The patient spends approximately 45 minutes in the treatment room for each treatment, but beam-on time is only 10 minutes for each side. The remaining time is taken up with setting up and positioning the dosimeters. Set up time becomes faster as treatment proceeds because fewer measurements are required. When the first beam is completed, the patient is turned and the second side treated. Patients are encouraged to bring along their own choice of music to be used as diversion and relaxation therapy. Doses can be measured at the head, neck, shoulders, chest, waist, knees and ankles by attaching small lithium fluoride dosimeters to the patient's skin on each treatment fraction. This allows for any necessary adjustments to be made to the thickness of the brass compensators to deliver the prescribed dose in subsequent fractions. By the final treatment the patient will have received the prescribed dose accurately throughout the body.

Figure 10.6
Diagrammatic representation
of treatment beam and patient
position

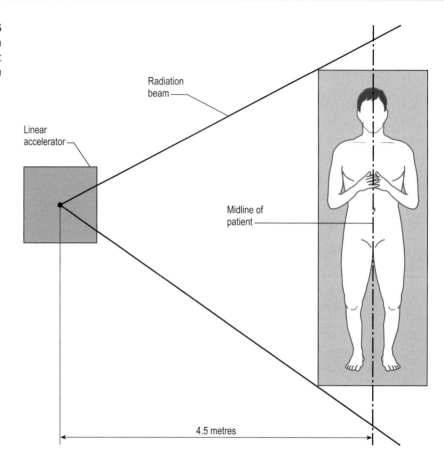

Radiation
beam

Linear
accelerator

Midline of
patient

4.5 metres

Figure 10.7
Patient position for TBI

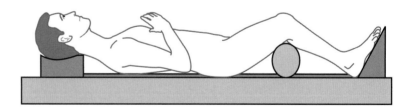

PALLIATIVE RADIOTHERAPY TREATMENT

MYELOMA

Radiotherapy is a valuable palliative treatment in multiple myeloma.
Myeloma cells are sensitive to radiotherapy making it an extremely effective treatment for relieving severe bony pain and improving the strength

of the affected bone, especially where there is a likelihood of spinal cord compression or fracture (Souhami & Tobias 1998). Radiotherapy may also be used once wound healing has occurred following surgical fixation of a pathological fracture.

The number of fractions required depends on the treatment site. For example, average treatment for spinal fields for myeloma is 10 fractions over 2 weeks but this varies depending on the size of the area to be treated. Fractionation takes into account how much of the spinal cord will be in the treatment field. A smaller area would be treated with a shorter fractionation and often one single treatment is safe and effective. This is useful in myeloma as patients frequently require radiotherapy to different sites.

Hemi-body irradiation, to the upper or lower half of the body, is also effective in treating painful bone sites in multiple myeloma.

PROPHYLACTIC RADIOTHERAPY

Acute lymphoblastic leukaemia can recur in the testes; prophylactic radiotherapy can be given to help to prevent this. Prophylactic cranial irradiation has also been used in the past to reduce the risk of CNS relapse. However, long-term consequences can occur and prophylactic treatment is no longer routinely given (see Chapter 4).

EMERGENCY RADIOTHERAPY TREATMENT

Spinal cord compression and superior vena cava obstruction are oncological emergencies and can develop as a result of increasing pressure caused by a growing tumour in either myeloma or lymphoma. Local radiotherapy is the treatment of choice.

SPINAL CORD COMPRESSION

Patients with spinal cord compression may present with symptoms such as weakness in their limbs, back pain and changes in gait, bladder or bowel control (Dobbs et al 1999). Paraesthesia may be present and complete paralysis may occur if the condition goes untreated. A delay in treatment of just hours can lead to permanent disability. Radiotherapy is therefore started as soon as possible after diagnosis is confirmed. Five consecutive radiotherapy treatments (including weekends) are usually given to a dose of 20 Gy at an energy beam of 6 MV (Dobbs et al 1999).

Patients who develop spinal cord compression thought to be due to primary lymphoma need a biopsy to confirm this as treatment by radiotherapy may not be the treatment of choice (Aviles et al 2002).

SUPERIOR VENA CAVA OBSTRUCTION (SVCO)

Superior vena cava obstruction (SVCO) may occur in lymphoma and T-cell acute lymphoblastic leukaemia. If radiotherapy is the treatment of choice (chemotherapy may be an option), dexamethasone is also given to help to reduce oedema. The dexamethasone dose is decreased as response to radiotherapy occurs. A radiation dose of 20 Gy is usually given over five treatments.

MANAGEMENT OF RADIOTHERAPY SIDE EFFECTS

The side effects of radiotherapy, the timing of their occurrence and the severity depend on the part of the body being irradiated, the radiation dose given, rate of cell proliferation and the individual patient. Side effects occur because of damage to normal tissue and may occur during or sometimes after the course of radiotherapy. Any combined chemo-radiation treatment may increase the severity of side effects – it can be difficult to determine the cause of side effects with combination treatments.

Reducing the impact and managing the side effects of radiotherapy is a major part of nursing management. Most patients attend on a daily basis as an outpatient and are encouraged to inform the treatment radiographers of any side effects they may be experiencing so medication and advice can be given. Nursing management of patients undergoing TBI is more intense because side effects are experienced throughout the whole body and more immediately than with more focused treatment. Nursing management of the various side effects is discussed in more detail in Section 3.

SHORT-TERM SIDE EFFECTS

The oral cavity

Xerostomia

The salivary glands are very sensitive to radiation. The amount of saliva produced is reduced and consistency changes, becoming thick and sticky. This leads to a dry mouth and difficulty in swallowing and can be very unpleasant for the patient. Taste changes, oral infections and tooth decay may also occur. Xerostomia may be severe and may start to affect the patient within the first few days of their treatment course (Eisbruch et al 2003). Following TBI, xerostomia may last for months after treatment has finished. It can be alleviated by frequent sips of water, sucking boiled sweets, chewing gum or by the use of medication such as oral pilocarpine (Souhami & Tobias 1998). Some patients find artificial saliva helpful and drinking with meals may help with chewing and swallowing food. Good oral care is also important and is discussed further in Chapter 18. Any necessary dental work should be carried out before radiotherapy starts if the mouth is to be included in the treatment field because of the risk of infection and reduced healing processes.

Mucositis	A sore mouth and throat occurs because mucosal cells have a high rate of proliferation and are therefore very sensitive to radiation. Erythema and soreness of the oral and oesophageal mucosa can lead to severe discomfort when chewing and swallowing. Following TBI a sore mouth and/or throat usually occurs the week following radiotherapy. Pain will require analgesia and is often so severe that diamorphine is required. This can make it difficult for the patient to eat, so food intake must be monitored (see Chapter 19). Alcohol, spicy food, very hot or cold drinks should be avoided. Non-alcohol-based mouthwashes and the use of a soft toothbrush are advised (see Chapter 18).
Parotiditis	Swelling of the parotid gland may occur during the first 24 hours of TBI and usually lasts 1–2 days. Parotid swelling subsides spontaneously and needs no medication.

Gastrointestinal effects

Nausea and vomiting

Nausea and vomiting has a high incidence following TBI (Buchali et al 2000). Anti-emetics, e.g. ondansetron, should be given 30 minutes before TBI to help to prevent nausea and vomiting. For other radiotherapy treatments that may cause nausea or vomiting, anti-emetics are given when necessary. Ongoing assessment of nausea and vomiting should be undertaken with review of the anti-emetic regimen as required. If patients are actively vomiting, fluid intake and output should be closely monitored to avoid dehydration and intravenous fluids administered as needed (for further information on management see Chapter 17).

Diarrhoea

This may occur during the course of radiotherapy to the pelvis and 1–2 weeks after TBI. Abdominal cramps, flatulence and tenesmus may add to patient discomfort. A low-fibre diet and anti-diarrhoeal agents such as loperamide may help. However, there is little evidence to support the efficacy of low-fibre diets (Faithfull 2003a). Uncontrolled diarrhoea can result in dehydration and affect nutritional status. Intake and output of both fluid and food therefore need to be monitored closely. Patients should have good access to washing facilities and emollient creams to prevent anal excoriation and the associated infection risk.

Steatorrhoea and intestinal obstruction

These side effects may occur but are dependent on the amount of damage caused to the mucosal lining.

Bone marrow suppression

Bone marrow is extremely sensitive to radiation, causing anaemia, neutropenia and thrombocytopenia (Souhami & Tobias 1998). A low dose is required if the whole body is irradiated (hence TBI) as bone marrow suppression is a potentially lethal side effect and a dose-limiting factor. Localised treatment can be given to a much higher dose without a major effect on the blood count (see Chapters 13, 15 and 16 for management of bone marrow suppression).

Fatigue

This is a common early and long-term side effect of radiotherapy, unrelated to treatment site. The cause of fatigue is as yet unclear. Following TBI, fatigue can occur by day 4 of treatment. Fatigue can affect global quality of life more than pain, sexual dysfunction and other cancer- or treatment-related symptoms (Stone et al 2000). Increased fatigue, reduced activity, depression and anxiety have also been noted in the family of a patient having radiotherapy treatment. This may be due to the loss of work time and travelling distances imposed on the relatives bringing the patient for their treatment (Jereczek-Fossa et al 2002). Fatigue is discussed further in Chapter 22.

Skin reactions

Skin reactions depend on the radiation dose, the area and situation of skin involved. Radiation skin reactions have four stages:

1. Erythema: the skin becomes pink and warm. It may be tender, slightly itchy and oedematous.
2. Dry desquamation: the skin becomes redder and dry. The epidermis begins to flake and it often feels itchy.
3. Moist desquamation: the skin becomes red and sore with blistering and oozing yellow exudate.
4. Ulceration: deep wounds occur at full skin thickness. Bleeding may occur, wounds are very painful and slow to heal. This stage is rare.

Following TBI skin becomes red, dry and itchy; it peels and colour darkens. At worst, blistering may occur. During the week of TBI, skin will become pink and in the following 10 days the skin becomes more reactive, particularly in the skin folds. Skin reactions (dry, pink and itchy) can be helped with the application of aqueous cream (College of Radiographers 2001). Extra care must be taken to avoid friction in sensitive areas such as the armpit, groin and intra-mammary fold; gentle washing is advised. Advice should be given on exposure to sunlight, the use of high-factor sun creams and protective clothing.

Urinary system

Cystitis and dysuria are common if the bladder is within the treatment area because the mucosa of the bladder is so sensitive to irradiation. Two to three litres of fluid a day will help to reduce the symptoms. Urine specimens should be taken if infection is suspected.

Veno–occlusive liver disease

TBI can contribute to this life-threatening condition. It is diagnosed by biopsy and clinical presentation including the presence of ascites, weight gain, raised serum bilirubin levels and jaundice. Developing veno-occlusive disease after TBI depends on factors such as whether a patient has pre-existing liver disease, their age and diagnosis. For one-third of the patients affected, the condition will be life-threatening (Deeg 1983). Intravenous heparin, weekly liver-function tests and daily weight checks are indicated for this condition.

Alopecia

Alopecia occurs after about 2 weeks but the hair regrows within a few months. Patients receiving TBI or prophylactic cranial irradiation are likely to have already experienced alopecia but it is still important to inform them of this side effect.

Somnolence syndrome (excessive tiredness and lethargy)

Occurs after radiotherapy to the brain. It may occur from 6 to 8 weeks after treatment has finished (Souhami & Tobias 1998).

Case study 10.1

Philip, a 39-year-old man with acute myeloid leukaemia, received chemotherapy and TBI in preparation for a MUD (matched, unrelated donor) transplant. He had few side effects apart from some initial nausea.

He was very positive about his disease and coped by thinking of all the positive issues about his treatment. He found being told of possible negative outcomes (necessary for consent) difficult to cope with and dismissed them, 'I don't need to know that.' He felt that too much emphasis was given to negative information.

Philip had excellent family support but also felt that he needed to help them to cope, by giving them things to do for him while he was in hospital, especially his parents. He also felt that the donor system search should be countrywide from the start. The first donor of choice was local but when this fell through the search widened to the whole country. Philip then had the choice of 12 better matches. 'It was luck I had the best match possible.' This has helped to keep Philip positive.

Philip had good news about the success of his transplant 19 days after the last fraction of radiotherapy. He suffered no short-term effects from his radiotherapy.

LATE SIDE EFFECTS

Late side effects are shown in Table 10.2.

REFLECTION POINT

How would you support a young woman who is being asked to consent to mantle technique radiotherapy when she is told that she has a higher risk of breast cancer in the future?

REFLECTION POINT

How would you support a young man and his wife who are told that his TBI treatment will probably cause infertility?

Long-term follow-up

Long-term follow-up is important to detect early relapse but the development of second cancers (breast and lung), thyroid hypofunction, ischaemic heart disease and malignant melanoma after sunburn are not necessarily detected through long-term follow-up.

Table 10.2
Late side effects of
radiotherapy

Late side effects	Comments
Infertility	Occurs in males with pelvic irradiation treatments and TBI, following quite low doses of radiation. Effective shielding can reduce the dose. In females, a higher radiation dose is necessary to cause permanent cessation of function of the ovaries.
Radiation-induced fibrosis of the lung	Causes a chronic cough, mild orthopnoea and chest discomfort.
Hypothyroidism	May occur during the 5 years following radiotherapy. Individuals will require thyroxine for the rest of their lives.
Radiation-induced heart disease	Usually an asymptomatic pleural effusion but may include constrictive pericarditis, occlusive coronary heart disease and cardiomyopathy.
Cataracts	May develop following TBI as the lens of the eye is very sensitive to the radiation. Radiation-induced cataract can be surgically dealt with without difficulty (Souhami & Tobias 1998).
Interstitial pneumonitis	Can occur 1–6 months after radiotherapy has finished and cause chronic respiratory problems. The patient with pneumonitis may present with a cough and breathlessness. Treatment depends on the severity of the problem (Dobbs et al 1999).
Second primary cancer	Recently a significant increase in the risk of young women developing breast cancer has been found following radiotherapy using the mantle technique (Deniz et al 2003).

QUALITY OF LIFE AND PSYCHOLOGICAL SUPPORT

Cancer and its treatment can create havoc and chaos in a person's life in a way that other, equally serious, diseases do not (Mead 1992). The combination of TBI with high-dose chemotherapy immediately before bone marrow transplant increases the patient's need for psychological support. Many different quality of life questionnaires have been used in clinical trials and have provided great insight into the difficulties faced by cancer patients. However, the perception of quality of life varies for individuals and is therefore very difficult to measure (Faithfull 2003b). Patient's emotions (a mixture of acceptance, anxiety, anger and grief) after a diagnosis of cancer can be directed at health-care staff and this is a challenge for professionals to manage (Souhami & Tobias 1998).

Patients feel that they are being supported, and are more able to overcome panic and restore a sense of control, if they are given accurate, timely and authoritative information (Mead 1992). However, different individuals require different amounts of information and respond to that information in different ways (Jenkins et al 2001). Providing individuals with the amount of information they personally require can help to reduce anxiety, allay panic, increase informed choice and sense of control (Hinds et al 1995). Health-care professionals therefore need to assess problems from the patient's perspective in order to help them to improve their quality of life (Munroe & Potter 1996). Involving patients in discussions and decisions about their care is vital in achieving this.

Anxiety and depression can occur because a patient is worrying about such issues as fatigue, body image, expected side effects and social issues such as not being able to work. Recognition of these conditions early could help the patient to relieve some distress during their treatment (Wells 2003).

Radiotherapy staff welcome and actively encourage questions from patients throughout the course of treatment. Patients are often afraid of their radiotherapy treatment because of misconceptions about what will happen to them such as being burnt or scarred by radiotherapy (Souhami & Tobias 1998). Patients have also been found to rarely ask the clinician important questions (Jenkins et al 2001). An accessible information and support service in radiotherapy departments or a dedicated team member with responsibility for patient information can therefore be invaluable. Both oral explanation and written information should be provided including information about treatment and side effects. It is also important to address any difficulties the patient is experiencing due to side effects from the radiotherapy treatment.

Patients having TBI may also find it more difficult if they have to travel between hospitals to have their radiotherapy at a specialised oncology hospital. They leave the staff they have become familiar with at the main hospital and have to spend 4 days in a different environment with staff they do not know. Explanation and reassurance are vital to help patients to feel safe in this new environment. Nurses and radiotherapy staff at each site must have excellent communication to ensure symptoms are managed and controlled. If a taxi service is used, patients may worry about the risk of infection or experiencing travel sickness. Patients can also feel very bored waiting for their treatment. Providing books and a television may help to pass the time. Encouraging individuals to take something to occupy themselves may also be helpful.

Multidisciplinary teams of oncologists, radiologists, surgeons, pathologists, pharmacists, radiographers, nurses, physiotherapists, occupational therapists, social workers and chaplains working with the patient can be extremely useful in helping all health-care professionals to gain a balanced view of patient needs. Good communication between health-care and other professionals, between staff and patients and across organisational boundaries is vital. Communication between multidisciplinary professionals helps in moving towards the goal of a seamless journey for patients throughout their treatment, thus ensuring continuity of care (Colyer 2003). Good communication between staff and patients helps to reassure the patient that they are being cared for as a person and thus maintain the maximum quality of life possible at this time (Wells & Faithfull 2003).

CONCLUSION

Radiotherapy plays a significant part in the treatment of haemato-oncology disorders. Treatment planning is vital to ensure that treatment is as safe and effective as possible. New technology is enabling extreme accuracy in radiotherapy treatment. This enables the highest dose necessary to be given while minimising side effects. The side effects that a patient may experience depend largely on the treatment site and the dose required. Side effects can be quite difficult for the patient to cope with unless they are observed and managed carefully. Preparing the patient with verbal and written information about radiotherapy and its side effects enhances their ability to cope. Radiotherapy affects the quality of life of a patient and their family. Emotional as well as practical support is necessary to enable the patient to get the best possible results from their treatment. It is the patient's basic human right to feel cared for with dignity and privacy. This together with information-giving must be incorporated into the radiotherapy experience.

DISCUSSION QUESTIONS

1. You overhear a colleague flippantly comparing the patient's experience of TBI with being affected by the Hiroshima bomb. How would you manage your colleague and the effect this may have had on the patient's feelings about radiotherapy?

2. A patient is angry and irritable when speaking to health-care professionals. How would you communicate with this patient to ensure respect for him/her as a person and give high-quality care?

ACKNOWLEDGEMENT

The authors wish to thank Gwenda Innes and Sarah Doherty for their helpful advice and Jim Roach for his help with the illustrations.

References

Adamson D 2003 The radiological basis of radiation side effects. In: Faithfull S, Wells M (eds) Supportive care in radiotherapy. Churchill Livingstone, Edinburgh

Aviles A, Fernandez R, Gonzalez J L et al 2002 Spinal cord compression as a primary manifestation of aggressive lymphomas: long-term analysis of treatments with radiotherapy, chemotherapy or combined therapy. Leukaemia & Lymphoma 43(2): 355–359

Bomford C K, Kunkler I H 2003 Walter and Miller's textbook of radiotherapy: radiation physics, therapy and oncology, 6th edn. Churchill Livingstone, Edinburgh

Buchali A, Feyer P, Groll J et al 2000 Immediate toxicity during fractionated total body irradiation as conditioning for bone marrow transplantation. Radiotherapy and Oncology 54:157–162

College of Radiographers 2001 Summary of intervention for acute radiotherapy skin reactions in cancer patients. The College of Radiographers, London

Colyer H 2003 The context of radiotherapy care. In: Faithfull S, Wells M (eds) Supportive care in radiotherapy. Churchill Livingstone, Edinburgh, pp 1–16

Deeg H J 1983 Acute and delayed toxicities of total body irradiation. International Journal of Radiation Oncology, Biology and Physics 9:1933–1939

Deniz K, O'Mahony S, Ross G, Purushotham A 2003 Breast cancer in women after treatment for Hodgkin's disease. Lancet Oncology 4:207–214

Dobbs J, Barrett A, Ash D 1999 Practical radiotherapy planning, 3rd edn. Edward Arnold, London

Eisbruch A, Rhodus N, Rosenthal D et al 2003 How should we measure and report radiotherapy-induced xerostomia? Seminars in Radiation Oncology 13(3):226–234

Faithfull S 2003a Gastrointestinal effects of radiotherapy. In: Faithfull S, Wells M (eds) Supportive care in radiotherapy. Churchill Livingstone, Edinburgh, pp 247–267

Faithfull S 2003b Assessing the impact of radiotherapy. In: Faithfull S, Wells M (eds) Supportive care in radiotherapy. Churchill Livingstone, Edinburgh, pp 96–117

Hinds C, Streater A, Mood D 1995 Functions and preferred methods of receiving information related to radiotherapy. Cancer Nursing 18(5):374–384

Holmes S 1996 Radiotherapy: a guide for practice. Asset Books, Dorking

Jenkins V, Fallowfield L, Saul J 2001 Information needs of patients with cancer: results from a large study in UK cancer centres. British Journal of Cancer 84(1):48–51

Jereczek-Fossa B A, Marsiglia H R, Orecchia R 2002 Radiotherapy-related fatigue. Critical Reviews in Oncology/Haematology 41:317–325

Mead J M (ed) 1992 Current issues in cancer. BMJ Publishing Group, London

Munroe A J, Potter S 1996 A quantitative approach to the distress caused by symptoms in patients treated with radical radiotherapy. British Journal of Cancer 74:640–647

Sikora K, Halnan K (eds) 1990 Treatment of cancer. Chapman and Hall, London

Souhami R, Tobias J 1998 Cancer and its management, 3rd edn. Blackwell Science, Oxford

Stanton R, Stinson D 1992 An introduction to radiation oncology physics. Medical Physics Publishing, Wisconsin

Stone P, Richardson A, Ream E et al 2000 Cancer-related fatigue: inevitable, unimportant and untreatable? Results of a multi-centre patient survey. Annals of Oncology 11:971–975

Wells M 2003 The treatment trajectory. In: Faithfull S, Wells M (eds) Supportive care in radiotherapy. Churchill Livingstone, Edinburgh, pp 39–59

Wells M, Faithfull S 2003 The future of supportive care in radiotherapy. In: Faithfull S, Wells M (eds) Supportive care in radiotherapy. Churchill Livingstone, Edinburgh, pp 372–382

Further reading

Faithfull S, Wells M 2003 Supportive care in radiotherapy. Churchill Livingstone, Edinburgh

As the title suggests, this book focuses on supportive care of the patient receiving radiotherapy. An excellent text combining the scientific basis of radiotherapy treatment with the patient experience.

Souhami R, Tobias J 1998 Cancer and its management, 3rd edn. Blackwell Science, Oxford

This book gives a thorough introduction to cancer and its problems for all health professionals.

Chapter **11**

Immune modulators and novel therapies

Sylvia Cole and Kathleen Dunne

KEY POINTS

- Immunomodulatory drugs and novel therapies have developed from an increased knowledge of cancer at a molecular level.
- Novel therapies have distinct molecular targets and aim to increase efficacy against malignant cells whilst decreasing toxicity to normal cells.
- Immunotherapy aims to stimulate the body's own immune system to attack tumours.
- Many of these therapies are still at an early stage of development and patients receiving these therapies may be involved in clinical trials.
- Patient and family education is paramount when considering these therapies.
- Nurses must be familiar with the mechanism of action and the management of patients receiving these therapies.

INTRODUCTION

Since the 1950s, haematological cancers have traditionally been treated using cytotoxic chemotherapy. Treatments have been modified over the years in an attempt to increase survival rates and reduce toxicity. The treatment of refractory or relapsed disease remains a challenge, driving the desire to develop novel approaches to disease management. An improved understanding of cancer at a molecular level has resulted in the identification of distinct molecular targets and led to the development of novel therapies with unique mechanisms of action (Cheson et al 2002). These therapies focus on targeting tumour-specific cell surface antigens, stimulation of immune effector cells (cells which become active in response to stimulation) to prevent cancer cell growth, as well as interrupting or blocking proteins associated with specific pathways in the cellular transformation and progression of cancer (Gemill & Idell 2003). They aim to enhance efficacy against malignant cells whilst decreasing toxicity to normal cells. The potential benefits of these agents are being investigated in phase I–phase III clinical trials (Box 11.1), with varying degrees of promise, and offer the hope of remission in relapsed or refractory disease for many patients or, in some cases, complete molecular remission.

This chapter provides a brief synopsis of the action and role of the main immunological and novel therapies currently being investigated in haematological cancers including their development, indications for use, toxicities and implications for nursing care.

Box 11.1   Phases of clinical trials (James & Armitage 2002)
Phase I   Determines the highest dose of a drug that humans can safely tolerate
Phase II   Determines the efficacy and therapeutic dose of the drug
Phase III   Compares the experimental drug or treatment to the standard treatment

GENE THERAPY

It has long been established that cancers result from alterations in the genetic make-up of cells. This knowledge has provided a basis for the development of gene therapy as a treatment for cancer. Gene therapy utilises different approaches (Weiss 1998, Liu 2003):

- a tumour-directed approach delivers therapeutic genetic material into the tumour in an attempt to cause cellular death
- active immunotherapy introduces cytokines or tumour antigens into the tumour with the intent of eliciting an immunological response

where malignant cells will appear 'foreign' to the immune system; this results in stimulation of cytotoxic T cells, which in turn infiltrate and attack the tumour

- adoptive immunotherapy genetically modifies the patient's lymphocytes ex vivo with the intent of enhancing antitumour activity before returning them to the patient.

Gene therapy can be administered either ex vivo or in vivo. The ex-vivo route involves removing the cell of interest from the patient, correcting the genetic defect and returning the corrected genetic material to the patient. The in-vivo route involves the introduction of a corrected gene directly into the target cell and is known as direct gene transfer (Loud et al 2002). Both methods use a vector (a vehicle used to carry the genetic material).

Only a small number of gene therapy studies in haematological cancers are taking place in the United Kingdom, and most of these are currently at the phase I or phase II stage. These studies have investigated the role of immunomodulatory gene therapy in multiple myeloma, lymphoma and leukaemia (Schmidt-Wolf & Schmidt-Wolf 2002). The development of gene therapy is ongoing in an attempt to realise its maximum potential.

TUMOUR VACCINES

Tumour vaccines are used as a therapy to treat rather than prevent disease, as is the aim with classical vaccines. Tumour vaccine preparations contain tumour-associated antigens derived from a particular type of tumour which, when given to patients, initiate an immune response against the antigen it contains. This response may be humoral, cellular or both (Kinzler & Brown 2001) (see Chapter 1). Known as active-specific immunotherapy it aims to override the immunosuppression produced by tumour-derived factors. It can also stimulate specific immunity, resulting in destruction of tumour cells and enhancing the effects of tumour-associated antigens (Rieger 2001).

Response to tumour vaccines has been studied in patients with follicular non-Hodgkin's lymphoma following chemotherapy (vincristine, cyclophosphamide, prednisolone) (Vose 2002). Patients who generated a specific immune response against the idiotype expressed by their lymphoma had significant overall survival in comparison to the patients who did not elicit an immune response. This approach to disease management is now being tested in phase III clinical trials.

CYTOKINES

Cytokines are a family of low molecular weight proteins produced mainly by lymphocytes and phagocytes (Ward 1995). They play a major role in the immune response by controlling cellular growth and differentiation, and regulating immune inflammatory responses (Rieger 2001). Their use as a cancer therapy is to regulate tumour cell growth, initiate a direct cytotoxic effect, stimulate an inflammatory or immune response in the tumour or enhance recovery of normal tissue damaged by cytotoxic agents (Souhami & Tobias 1998). Interferon and interleukin are two cytokines used in the management of haematological cancers.

INTERFERON

There are three types of interferon, alpha, beta and gamma, with alpha predominating in the management of haematological cancers. Interferon alpha has the ability to slow down cell replication by inhibiting protein synthesis and stimulating the activity of natural killer cells, T cells, macrophages and neutrophils (Ward 1995). Its main uses are in the management of hairy cell leukaemia, chronic myeloid leukaemia, low-grade lymphomas and myeloma (Souhami & Tobias 1998).

Case study 11.1

Peter is a 70-year-old gentleman who presented with tiredness and shortness of breath. On admission he was found to be pancytopenic and subsequently received a diagnosis of hairy cell leukaemia. Initially he was treated with interferon alpha three times weekly, which he tolerated very well. However, his response was suboptimal so interferon alpha was discontinued. He is currently receiving deoxycoformycin chemotherapy on a 2-weekly basis.

INTERLEUKIN

Interleukins modulate and regulate immune and inflammatory responses. Approximately 18 variations of interleukins have been identified (Gale & Sorokin 2001). Early studies are in progress to determine the immunological effects of human interleukin-12 following autologous stem cell transplant (Pelloso et al 2004).

HAEMATOPOIETIC GROWTH FACTORS

Haematopoietic growth factors are a family of glycoprotein hormones first discovered in the 1950s and include colony stimulating factors, erythropoietin and thrombopoietin. They act by attaching themselves to receptors on the surface membrane of the target cell, resulting in proliferation, differentiation and maturation of the cell (Wujcik 2001).

Colony stimulating factors

Colony stimulating factors (CSF) are responsible for controlling the formation of neutrophils and monocytes/macrophages. Four main forms of CSF have been identified:

- granulocyte-colony stimulating factor (G-CSF)
- granulocyte-macrophage colony stimulating factor (GM-CSF)
- macrophage colony stimulating factor (M-CSF)
- interleukin (IL)-3.

G-CSF and GM-CSF predominate in clinical practice. G-CSF acts selectively on cells of the granulocyte lineage and is used in the management of chemotherapy-induced neutropenia as well as for the stimulation of peripheral blood progenitor cells (Amgen 2001). GM-CSF has broad activity in the proliferation and differentiation of myeloid lineage progenitor cells, i.e. neutrophils, monocytes, macrophages, eosinophils and dendritic cells (the major antigen-presenting cells) (Buchsel et al 2002).

G-CSF is currently available in a pegylated form (Pegfilgrastim). The prefix 'peg' refers to the polyethylene unit, which has been added to filgrastim resulting in a longer serum half-life of the drug. Pegfilgrastim therefore requires to be given only once per chemotherapy cycle (Phillips 2003). In a phase II study of patients receiving salvage chemotherapy for relapsed or refractory Hodgkin's or non-Hodgkin's lymphoma, the use of pegfilgrastim was compared with filgrastim (administered for 11 days) (Vose et al 2003). Results indicated that a once-only administration of pegfilgrastim was as effective as filgrastim and produced a sustained serum concentration relative to the 11 daily injections of filgrastim.

Erythropoietin

Erythropoietin is a glycoprotein hormone primarily produced by the kidneys in response to a decrease in the level of oxygen in renal tissue, as occurs in anaemia. The kidneys are then stimulated to produce erythropoietin, which in turn stimulates proliferation and differentiation of erythroid cells (Hoffbrand & Pettit 1997).

It has been estimated that anaemia can occur in up to 63% of patients with haematological cancers (Ludwig 2002) resulting in a decrease of the patient's quality of life (QOL) and an increased need for blood transfusion. As human erythropoietin is now available in a recombinant form (rHuEPO, epoietin alfa) studies have been undertaken to ascertain its benefit in the management of anaemia of chronic lymphocytic leukaemia (CLL), multiple myeloma (MM) and low-grade non-Hodgkin's lymphoma (NHL).

Results of a phase III study demonstrated an increase in haemoglobin concentrations, a 50% reduction in the need for blood transfusions after the first 4 weeks of treatment and an improvement in QOL for patients with anaemia of CLL, MM and low-grade NHL (Osterborg et al 2002). Once weekly administration of rHuEPO has now been shown to be as effective as three times weekly administration (Cazzola et al 2003). However, treatment is expensive, requiring a period of 4–8 weeks of therapy before maximum benefit is achieved and effectiveness is only seen in approximately 60% of patients (Samol & Littlewood 2003).

Thrombopoietin

Thrombopoietin is responsible for the regulation of megakaryocyte and platelet development. Thrombopoietin levels usually increase in response to the decline in platelet mass and remain elevated for the duration of thrombocytopenia. Thrombopoietin is now available in a recombinant and a pegylated recombinant form. It is suggested that both preparations can increase the platelet count approximately 5 days after administration with a peak effect 10–12 days later (Kuter & Begley 2002).

Its use is being investigated as an alternative to platelet transfusion or to decrease the frequency of platelet transfusion. However, early clinical trials have not demonstrated significant success, particularly when given in conjunction with myeloablative chemotherapy (Kuter & Begley 2002). Thrombopoietin is also being studied in phase I and phase II clinical trials in the management of cytopenias resulting from aplastic anaemia and myelodysplastic syndrome. Further clinical studies are needed in order to ascertain its maximum potential in the haemato-oncology setting.

SIGNAL TRANSDUCTION INHIBITORS

Part of the process involved in the proliferation and differentiation of cells involves complex signalling pathways, initiated by the use of a growth factor signal, which is transduced through the target cell membrane to the cell nucleus. This in turn begins a series of complex enzymatic activity (Hoffbrand & Pettit 1997). In recent years researchers have been developing therapies which interrupt these signalling pathways with the aim of disrupting proliferation of abnormal cells. One such therapy is imatinib, a tyrosine kinase inhibitor used to block the enzymatic action of the BCR-ABL tyrosine kinase fusion protein, which occurs as a result of the translocation of chromosome 9 and chromosome 22 in chronic myeloid leukaemia (CML) (see Chapter 4). This protein is responsible for driving the transformation and proliferation of leukaemic cells (Goldman & Melo 2003). In clinical trials imatinib has induced complete haematological and major cytogenetic response in a significant number of patients (Kantarjian et al 2002a,b). Its use has now been approved in specified instances for CML (National Institute for Clinical Excellence 2003) (see Chapter 4).

Further studies have been carried out to determine the efficacy of imatinib as a first line therapy in the management of CML. An international phase III study comparing imatinib with interferon and low-dose cytarabine in newly diagnosed patients in the chronic phase of CML found at median follow-up of 19 months a major cytogenetic response of 87.1% in the imatinib group compared with 34.7% in the interferon alpha and cytarabine group (O'Brien et al 2003). Patients receiving imatinib also had clear QOL advantages compared with the other group. Furthermore patients who switched from the interferon alpha group to the imatinib group also experienced a significant improvement in QOL compared with those who remained in the interferon group (Hahn et al 2003).

Although imatinib has revolutionised the management of CML, many questions remain unanswered, particularly regarding the appropriateness of offering an allogeneic stem cell transplant to younger patients who have a matched sibling donor. This may be answered when the long-term data of the experience of using imatinib becomes available (Goldman & Druker 2001).

IMMUNOMODULATORY DRUGS (IMIDS)

One of the ways in which malignant cells can continue to grow is through the development of new blood vessels, a process known as angiogenesis (Callahan & Faragher 1997), provoking the therapeutic use of drugs with antiangiogenic properties in the treatment of cancer. One such drug, thalidomide, has been studied in the management of refractory multiple myeloma and has been shown to overcome classical drug resistance seen with other therapies (Anderson et al 2002). Phase I and phase II studies are now being carried out to determine whether initial administration of thalidomide affects stem cell harvesting or engraftment in newly diagnosed patients, to determine the feasibility and tolerability of thalidomide in addition to standard melphalan and prednisolone in newly diagnosed or relapsed patients and to determine the toxicities associated with its long-term use (UKMF 2004).

As thalidomide has been associated with significant toxicity (including neuropathy and somnolence) other, less toxic immunomodulatory drugs (IMiDs), which are derivatives of thalidomide, are being developed (Tariman 2003). As well as their antiangiogenesis activity, IMiDs stimulate or regulate the function of the immune system by initiating apoptosis, inhibiting growth factors involved in angiogenesis, interfering with cytokine production and stimulating T cells and natural killer cells (Anderson et al 2002).

The use of an IMiD known as CC-5013 (Revimid) is currently being investigated. Early phase I and phase II studies of patients with relapsed or refractory myeloma suggest that it has the ability to overcome drug resistance and cause minimal toxicity (thrombocytopenia and neutropenia), as well as significantly reducing paraprotein levels (Richardson et al 2002). Phase III studies are now underway in the USA to ascertain its efficacy in relapsed or refractory disease.

PROTEASOME INHIBITORS

The proteasome is a large multi-protein particle present in all eukaryotic cells and plays a major role in the protein degradation pathway of the cell. This role is fundamental to the activation or repression of various cellular processes, including cell-cycle progression and apoptosis.

Through this process the proteasome acts as a main link for many cellular regulatory signals and has been acknowledged as a novel target in the treatment of malignant disease (Adams 2002).

PS-341 (Velcade) is an example of a proteasome inhibitor (inhibits 26S proteasome) which has been shown to have antitumour activity in various tumours. Complete blockade, by an inhibitor, of proteolysis initiated by the 26S proteasome results in cellular death (Adams 2002). The results of studies using Velcade in refractory multiple myeloma have demonstrated exciting potential and it is now licensed for the management of MM refractory to other treatment modalities. The PAD trial is now exploring the use of Velcade as a first-line therapy in combination with adriamycin (doxorubicin) and dexamethasone (UKMF 2004).

OTHER AGENTS

ARSENIC TRIOXIDE (TRISENOX)

Arsenic disrupts the cellular transformation process by affecting the biological pathways involved in transformation, resulting in inhibition of proliferation and induction of cellular apoptosis (Norvick & Warrell 2000). The main use of this drug to date has been in the management of relapsed acute promyelocytic leukaemia, where evidence suggests that it causes down-regulation of anti-apoptotic proteins resulting in cellular death (Druker et al 2002). Research is continuing into the use of arsenic trioxide in the management of multiple myeloma, where it has been shown to inhibit proliferation, induce apoptosis and affect tumour growth, as well as inhibiting angiogenesis (Munshi 2001).

TROXACITABINE

This nucleoside analogue has shown antineoplastic activity in some solid tumours. A phase II study of troxacitabine investigated 17 patients in the blast phase of CML. Six patients had failed treatment with imatinib and nine were in the second or later relapse (Giles et al 2002). Results demonstrated that 37% of patients returned to a chronic phase with four patients still in chronic phase after a follow-up of 2–11 months. Research is continuing into this aspect of its use.

HOMOHARRINGTONE

This plant alkaloid, derived from an evergreen tree, is known to have some anti-leukaemic activity. It has been used mainly in the management of acute myeloid leukaemia and more recently in acute promyelocytic leukaemia, myelodysplastic syndrome and the chronic phase of CML (Druker et al 2002). In one study a complete haematological response of 67% and a cytogenetic response rate of 33% were achieved in patients with chronic phase CML who had failed interferon alpha based therapy (O'Brien et al 1995).

REFLECTION POINT

What immunomodulatory drugs and novel therapies are available in your area of practice and what are their implications for your practice?

MONOCLONAL ANTIBODIES

Monoclonal antibodies (MoAbs) are antibodies produced by a single clone of B cells, with the ability to target a specific antigen. On recognition of its specific target the antibody can alter activity of the antigen, stimulate the immune system to destroy the cell and initiate programmed cell death (Gemill & Idell 2003). Effector cells including natural killer cells, killer T cells and macrophages are involved in these processes (Dyer 1999). The targeted cell surface antigen may not be specific to tumour cells alone but may also be expressed on normal cells, which are at a particular stage of differentiation (Souhami & Tobias 1998). Various key characteristics are needed for MoAbs to be effective in destroying their target (Box 11.2).

The use of monoclonal antibodies in the management of cancer developed from the work of Kohler and Milstein's (1975) hybridoma technology (Fig. 11.1), which aimed to produce a cell with the ability to produce mass numbers of a specific antibody to a specific antigen. MoAbs derived from this technology are known as murine MoAbs as they are of mouse origin. These early murine MoAbs were found to have limited therapeutic use as they elicited a human antimurine antibody response in the recipient, resulting in the recipient's immune system directly targeting the treatment itself, thus rendering it ineffective (Capriotti 2001). In attempting to reduce immunogenicity, genetic engineering techniques have been used to develop other types of MoAbs

> **Box 11.2   Key characteristics of target antigens (cited in Schmidt & Wood 2003)**
>
> - The intended antigen target needs to be as specific as possible to lessen toxicity to normal cells
> - A large amount of the target antigen needs to be expressed on the cell surface as the greater the amount of antigen the greater the immune response
> - The targeted antigen must also play a major role in the growth and proliferation of the tumour cell
> - Conjugated MoAbs require a modulating antigen, to internalise the antibody/antigen complex from the cell surface

Figure 11.1
Hybridoma technology (Kohler
& Milstein 1975)

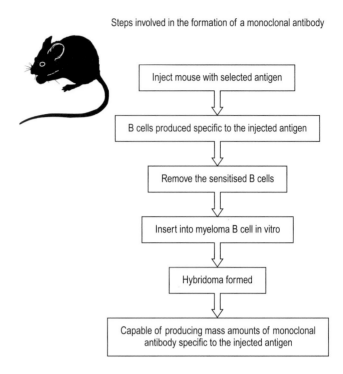

Steps involved in the formation of a monoclonal antibody

Inject mouse with selected antigen

↓

B cells produced specific to the injected antigen

↓

Remove the sensitised B cells

↓

Insert into myeloma B cell in vitro

↓

Hybridoma formed

↓

Capable of producing mass amounts of monoclonal
antibody specific to the injected antigen

ranging from part-mouse/part-human origin, to complete human origin. MoAbs may be used alone to target antigens (unconjugated) or in combination with other agents (conjugated) (Karius & Marriot 1997).

UNCONJUGATED MONOCLONAL ANTIBODIES

Unconjugated forms of MoAbs bind to their targeted cell surface antigens, resulting in initiation of an immune response with the intent of causing cell death by cell lysis (Karius & Marriott 1997). Examples and their indications for use are outlined in Table 11.1.

Case study 11.2

Jane is a 60-year-old female with no relevant past medical history. She presented with abdominal discomfort, loss of appetite and a feeling of fullness. Gastric biopsy confirmed a diffuse large B-cell non-Hodgkin's lymphoma. She received six cycles of RCHOP chemotherapy and is still doing well 8 months later.

Table 11.1
Unconjugated monoclonal antibodies and indications for use

Name	Origin	Target	Indications for use
Rituximab (MabThera)	Chimeric Human/murine MoAb	CD20 antigen found on the surface of normal pre-B2B cells. Expressed on the surface of >90% of B cells in non-Hodgkin's lymphoma.	Has National Institute for Clinical Excellence 2002 approval for: – treatment of patients with Stage III–IV follicular lymphoma who are chemotherapy resistant or in their second or subsequent relapse after chemotherapy. – treatment of patients with CD20 positive diffuse large B-cell non-Hodgkin's lymphoma in combination with chemotherapy. Being investigated in the management of other B-cell conditions (e.g. chronic lymphocytic leukaemia, mantle cell leukaemia, plasmacytoma, Hodgkin's lymphoma), autoimmune disease (e.g. idiopathic thrombocytopenic purpura and autoimmune haemolytic anaemia).
Alemtuzumab (Campath)	Humanised MoAb	CD52 antigen expressed on the surface of B cells, T cells, monocytes, macrophages and natural Killer cells	Licensed for the management of B-cell chronic lymphocytic leukaemia in patients previously treated with alkylating agents who have failed to achieve a complete or partial response or achieved only a short remission (<6 months) following fludarabine therapy.
Epratuzamab	Humanised MoAb	CD22 antigen present on 75% of B lymphocytes	Being investigated in Phase II studies of patients with follicular lymphoma and diffuse large cell lymphomas
Apolizumab	Humanised MoAb	Polymorphic determinant of human leucocyte antigen (HLA-Dr) expressed on normal and malignant B cells	Being investigated in Phase II studies of patients with B-cell relapsed or refractory follicular lymphomas

Compiled from information in Roche Products 2002, Vose et al 2002, Boye et al 2003, Schering Health Care 2004a.
CD – clusters of differentiation.

CONJUGATED MONOCLONAL ANTIBODIES

Conjugated forms of MoAbs combine the basic antibody (which acts as a delivery mechanism providing targeted specificity) with another agent (a conjugate). There are three main forms of conjugate:

- immunotoxin
- chemoimmunoconjugate
- radioimmunoconjugate.

When the antibody reaches its intrinsic target antigen, the conjugated part is released with the intent of initiating cell death (Schmidt & Wood

Table 11.2
Conjugated monoclonal antibodies and indications for use

Name	Origin	Target	Indications for use
Chemoimmunoconjugate: Gemtuzumab (Mylotarg)	Humanised antibody conjugated with the cytotoxic antitumour antibiotic calicheamicin	CD33 antigen expressed on the surface of leukaemic blasts in ≥80% of patients with acute myeloid leukaemia (AML)	Licensed for the treatment of patients with CD33 positive AML in first relapse ≥60 years of age and who are not considered candidates for cytotoxic chemotherapy
Radioimmunoconjugate: Ibritumomab Tiuxetan (Zevalin)	Murine	CD20 antigen found on the surface of normal pre-B and B cells. Expressed on the surface of >90% of B cells in non-Hodgkin's lymphoma	Now licensed in Europe for the treatment of patients with relapsed or refractory low-grade follicular or transformed B-cell non-Hodgkin's lymphoma and patients with Rituximab refractory non-Hodgkin's lymphoma
Iodine-131 Tositumomab (Bexxar)	Murine	CD20 antigen. Iodine-131 labelling allows for targeted delivery of beta radiation to CD20 cells	Chemotherapy refractory low-grade or transformed low-grade B-cell non-Hodgkin's lymphoma. Has not yet received a licence for use in Europe

Compiled from information in Vose et al 2002, Schering Health Care 2004b, Wyeth Pharmaceuticals 2004.

2003). Examples of conjugated MoAbs and indications for use are outlined in Table 11.2.

Immunotoxin

Immunotoxins are formed by attaching MoAbs to highly lethal cellular toxins mainly of plant (e.g. ricin) or bacterial (e.g. *Pseudomonas exotoxin*) origin. Immunotoxins have been used in clinical trials in the management of both solid and haematological tumours. However, they have been associated with marked toxicities, limiting their therapeutic use (Weiner 1999).

Chemoimmunoconjugate

Chemoimmunoconjugates use the antibody as a vehicle by which to deliver conventional cytotoxic drugs to a targeted tumour site.

Radioimmunoconjugate

Radioimmunoconjugates combine the use of a MoAb with the effects of radiation. This is an ideal therapy for the treatment of non-Hodgkin's lymphoma as lymphoma cells have increased sensitivity to radiation (Vose 2002). Radioconjugates induce lethal deoxyribonucleic acid (DNA) damage to the targeted cell but also to nearby cells that do not necessarily express the target antigen (Vose 2002).

TOXICITIES

Toxicities associated with MoAbs vary depending on the type of MoAb. The majority of side effects are mild to moderate infusion-related toxicities and resolve on completion of therapy. Nurses should be familiar with the specific product's characteristic data before administering MoAbs.

Infusion–related side effects

This is the most frequent toxicity seen with the use of MoAbs and has been attributed to the rapid release of cytokines in response to treatment (Boye et al 2003). Signs and symptoms include flu-like symptoms, rigors, chills, pyrexia, nausea, diarrhoea, mucosal congestion, urticaria, bronchospasm and hypotension (Roche Products 2002). These can occur at various stages during the infusion depending on the MoAb being administered.

To reduce the occurrence or intensity of infusion-related side effects the stipulated premedication as per the specific product's characteristic data should be given as per the manufacturer's guidance. Premedication normally consists of an antihistamine and oral paracetamol. MoAbs are administered via intravenous infusion rather than by bolus injection and are commenced at a slow rate or low dose and gradually escalated at varying intervals (Capriotti 2001).

Rituximab

Reactions in 50% of patients most frequently occur 30 minutes to 2 hours after initiation of the first infusion. Reactions are likely to be more severe if the patient has bulky disease or a high number of circulating malignant cells (Roche Products 2002).

Alemtuzumab

Effects normally occur during the first week of therapy effecting approximately 80% of patients (Schering Health Care 2004a). Significant infusion-related toxicity has been associated with this drug during the first 1–2 weeks of administration (Lundin et al 2002).

Gemtuzumab

Infusion-related events most commonly occur after the 2-hour infusion and resolve 2–4 hours later with supportive management. Symptoms include hyperglycaemia, hypoxia, hypertension and dyspnoea (Wyeth Pharmaceuticals 2004). Hypotension can occur several hours following administration (Sievers et al 2001).

Tumour lysis syndrome

Tumour lysis syndrome can occur as a result of rapid tumour breakdown causing renal insufficiency. This is manifested by nausea, vomiting, hyperuricaemia, hyperkalaemia, hyperphosphataemia, hypocalcaemia and acute renal failure (Roche Products 2002). Patients with bulky tumours or a high number of circulating malignant cells are at an increased risk (Roche Products 2002, Schering Health Care 2004a).

Byrd et al (1999) have reported a unique syndrome experienced by patients receiving rituximab who have a high number of tumour cells in the blood. Symptoms included thrombocytopenia, rapid decrement in circulating tumour cell load and mild electrolyte evidence of tumour lysis.

Haematological toxicity

Haematological toxicities vary. With rituximab, thrombocytopenia and neutropenia can occur in up to 10% of patients but is normally mild and transient (Roche Products 2002). Alemtuzumab and gemtuzumab can both cause severe myelosuppression resulting in neutropenia and thrombocytopenia.

Neutropenia

With alemtuzumab neutropenia generally occurs by weeks 5–8 of treatment, increasing the potential for the development of various infections including (Schering Health Care 2004a):

- Herpes simplex
- Pneumonia
- Opportunistic infections:
  - *Pneumocystis carinii* pneumonia
  - Cytomegalovirus
  - Aspergillus pneumonia
  - Herpes zoster
- Rhinocerebral mucomycosis (uncommon).

Infection risk is also increased due to the profound lymphopenia, which can occur particularly with patients who have been heavily pre-treated or who do not receive antibiotic prophylactic therapy (Rai et al 2002). Prophylactic antibiotics against opportunistic infections, e.g. co-trimoxazole, and an oral anti-herpes agent, e.g. famciclovir, is recommended throughout treatment and for approximately 4 months post-treatment with alemtuzumab (Schering Health Care 2004a).

Myelosuppression resulting from gemtuzumab has been attributed to its pharmacological goal as it targets CD33 cells expressed by haematopoietic precursor cells (Sievers et al 2001). The average recovery of absolute neutrophil count to 0.5×10^9 is approximately 40 days after the first dose (Wyeth Pharmaceuticals 2004). The use of prophylactic antibiotics should be considered (Viele 2002).

Thrombocytopenia

Thrombocytopenia associated with alemtuzumab occurs during the first 2 weeks of therapy and normally improves during the remainder of treatment (Schering Health Care 2004a). Thrombocytopenia occurs in most patients receiving gemtuzumab and requires close monitoring of the platelet count. Median time to recovery of platelets to 25×10^9 is approximately 39 days after the first infusion (Wyeth Pharmaceuticals 2004).

Hepatic toxicity

Gemtuzumab has been associated with hepatic toxicity including severe veno-occlusive disease (VOD). In a review of studies, 12% of patients treated with gemtuzumab developed VOD (Giles et al 2001). Patients with underlying hepatic disease or abnormal liver function tests and patients receiving gemtuzumab in combination with other chemotherapy may be at increased risk for developing severe VOD. Gemtuzumab should not be administered if the bilirubin level is greater than 2 mg/dL (Wyeth Pharmaceuticals 2004).

Cardiac toxicity

Cardiovascular events have been reported in patients receiving MoAbs including hypotension, hypertension, myocardial infarction and cardiac arrest. Care should be exercised when treating patients with known cardiac problems (Roche Products 2002, Schering Health Care 2004a).

Toxicities associated with radiolabelled MoAbs

Adverse effects associated with radioimmunotherapy are mainly myelosuppression, primarily resulting in leukopenia and thrombocytopenia (Witzig et al 1999, Vose et al 2000). This tends to occur approximately 5–7 weeks after treatment and takes 2–4 weeks to return to pre-treatment levels (Dillman 2002). It is recommended that monitoring of blood counts should be continued for at least 3 months post-treatment (Clayton 2003). The degree of haematological toxicity is relative to the degree of disease in the bone marrow prior to treatment, hence the recommendation that only patients with less than 25% bone marrow involvement should be considered for treatment (Riley 2003).

Myelodysplastic syndrome has been documented in small numbers of patients treated with Y-90 and I-131 (Kaminski et al 2001, Gordon et al 2004). However, it is unclear whether this is directly related to radioimmunotherapy as these patients were heavily treated with cytotoxic regimes prior to receiving radiolabelled antibodies.

Non-haematological toxicities have been reported in approximately 98% of patients who experienced at least one adverse effect. These included fatigue, nausea, fever, vomiting, infection, hypotension, pruritis and rash (Vose et al 2000, Kaminski et al 2001).

Other toxicities observed include the development of human antimurine antibodies in 8% of patients treated with tositumomab and 2% receiving ibritumomab (tiuxetan) (Kaminski et al 2001, Gordon et al 2004). Hypothyroidism is a also a delayed effect associated with tositumomab, occurring in a small percentage of patients (Kaminski et al 2001).

Fertility issues

Evidence relating to the effects of monoclonal antibodies on pregnancy is scarce. However, it is recommended that patients who are pregnant should not receive MoAbs. Patients receiving MoAbs should avoid pregnancy during treatment and for up to 12 months following completion of therapy (Roche Products 2002, Schering Health Care 2004a, Wyeth Pharmaceuticals 2004).

NURSING MANAGEMENT OF PATIENTS RECEIVING MONOCLONAL ANTIBODIES

The management of side effects encountered with the use of MoAbs varies greatly from that of conventional treatments used in the management of haematological cancers. In order to plan patient care, nurses must have a thorough knowledge of the prescribed treatment and the relevant nursing issues including:

- type of MoAb
- conjugated or unconjugated
- mode of action
- drug's intended target
- indications for use
- precautions
- recommended pre-medication
- contraindications
- possible side effects
- timing of side effects
- prophylactic measures to be taken to prevent side effects
- management of toxicities
- applicable safety regulations for handling and disposal of MoAb.

MoAbs should be administered only in clinical areas where patients can be closely monitored. Cardiopulmonary resuscitation equipment and emergency drugs should be available and easily accessible (Viele 2002).

Patient assessment and pre-treatment issues

Prior to proceeding with treatment the patient should have a thorough physical and psychological assessment carried out. The physical assessment should include the patient's baseline laboratory results, allergy history, medical history, medications, general condition and establish risk factors for infection and tumour lysis (Seeley & DeMeyer 2002, Viele 2002, Riley 2003). Additionally, psychological effects on the patient and family members should also be considered, as the impact of a diagnosis of haematological cancer can never be underestimated.

Emotional support

It is important to remember that many patients who are receiving MoAbs have relapsed disease. As well as coping with the uncertainty that relapsed disease presents, patients are also confronted with the side effects of treatment. Health-care professionals need to take cognisance of these facts and facilitate patients in expressing their fears and anxieties. The importance of using basic counselling skills such as active listening and attending, using open questions, reflecting content and feelings, summarising and checking for understanding (Burnard 1991) cannot be overemphasised in these circumstances.

Observation

Patients must be closely monitored for infusion-related side effects such as chills, fevers, rigors, itch, hypotension, and urticaria. Baseline observations of blood pressure, pulse, temperature, respirations and SAO_2 levels should be recorded, as well as the general condition of the patient. Vital signs should continue to be monitored throughout the infusion. With the use of gemtuzumab, observation of blood pressure and pulse should be continued post-infusion because of the potential for hypotension to occur several hours following completion of therapy (Sievers et al 2001).

Management of side effects

If side effects occur, the infusion should be stopped, an assessment made of the patient's condition and medical assistance requested. Vital signs should be recorded and supportive care administered depending on the type of reaction encountered. In the event of rigors patients should be kept warm until shivering has subsided (Kosits & Callaghan 2000). Supportive measures such as the administration of corticosteroids or antihistamines may be effective for infusion-related side effects (Kosits & Callaghan 2000, Seeley & DeMeyer 2002). When symptoms subside and the patient's condition allows, the infusion may be recommenced according to the manufacturer's instructions. The patient must be closely monitored for further reactions. In the event of severe hypersensitivity or anaphylactic-type reaction, management should be aimed at maintaining renal perfusion and tissue oxygenation (Kosits & Callaghan 2000). Patients at risk of tumour lysis syndrome should be well hydrated and closely monitored. Prophylactic use of allopurinol may be appropriate (Viele 2002, Lynn et al 2003).

It is imperative that patients and carers should be educated about the signs and symptoms associated with cytopenias. In particular patients should be asked to observe for signs of infection, i.e. fever of 38°C or higher, sore throat, cough, oral thrush or dysuria (Viele 2002). The importance of drug schedules and adherence to the use of prophylactic antibiotics should be emphasised. Patients should be advised of signs of a low platelet count, in particular bleeding from the nose, mouth, gums, presence of blood in sputum, urine or stools, bruising or petechial rash (Viele 2002). A contact number should be provided in order that patients can access prompt assistance should they become unwell.

Specific drug considerations

It is important to establish and adhere to any specific recommendations pertaining to the prescribed treatment. Gemtuzumab is light sensitive and must be protected from both direct and indirect light (Viele 2002). Lymphopenia associated with alemtuzumab places patients at increased risk of developing transfusion-related graft-versus-host disease. Therefore blood products should be irradiated until lymphopenia has resolved (Schering Health Care 2004a). Patients receiving therapy on an outpatient basis should avoid driving after treatment owing to the sedative effects of the premedication. Owing to its hypotensive effects patients receiving rituximab may need to omit antihypertensive medication on the day of treatment (Roche Products 2002).

Radiolabelled MoAbs

The administration of radiolabelled antibodies is prescribed in legislation and requires strict adherence to radiological safety regulations and precautions in order to minimise radiation exposure to patients, relatives and medical personnel (Statutory Instrument 2000). These therapies can be administered only by personnel with the appropriate licence and training for handling radionuclides as stipulated by the Administration of Radioactive Substances Advisory Committee (ARSAC 2003). The extent of precautions initiated depends on the type of radiolabelled drug used. Local radiation protection guidelines should be adhered to.

REFLECTION POINT

REFLECTION POINT Identify the educational and psychological needs of patients, and their families, who are receiving novel therapies in your area of practice. What strategies are in place to meet their needs?

Patient and family education

Patient and family education is paramount when administering MoAbs. Education is particularly important when radiolabelled MoAbs are to be given in order to ensure radiation safety measures are adhered to and fears allayed (Clayton 2003). Education should include information about the type of treatment to be given, action, aim of treatment, potential adverse effects, administration schedule, management of adverse effects, signs and symptoms requiring action – including signs and symptoms of infection and bleeding (Viele 2002). The importance of adhering to prophylactic antibiotics must also be stressed. Contraceptive advice and counselling must be provided and appropriate referrals made. Materials such as videos can support education and information leaflets, which are provided by the drug companies (Capriotti 2001).

CLINICAL TRIALS AND THE ROLE OF THE NURSE

As many of the novel therapies discussed are still at an early stage of development, many patients will be involved in clinical trials. The aim of clinical trials is to establish whether a new treatment or new combinations of treatments are better than the current gold standard available (James & Armitage 2002). In order to empower patients to be able to make decisions about treatment and to give informed consent nurses must be familiar with (James & Armitage 2002):

- the aim of the trial
- the possible treatment options within the trial
- side effects of the proposed treatment
- benefits and drawbacks of each treatment option
- administration protocol.

With this knowledge, nurses will be better equipped to provide effective communication to support patients and alleviate fears and anxieties (James & Armitage 2002).

CONCLUSION

Immune modulators and novel therapies are increasingly being used in the treatment and management of patients with haematological conditions. As this approach to disease management is relatively new, there is much room for further research in order to add to the body of knowledge and evidence base of practice. There are many complex physical and psychological issues involved when embarking on treatment therapy with much of the ongoing work at clinical trial level. Nurses therefore need to be fully appraised of ongoing research and developments in this emerging science so that they are fully aware of the effects, side effects and involved management of patients.

ACKNOWLEDGEMENT

The authors are deeply indebted to Dr Jeremy Hamilton, Consultant Haematologist, for his support and advice in the writing of this chapter.

DISCUSSION QUESTIONS

1. How has the introduction and development of novel therapies impacted on the management of haematological cancers?

2. In what ways can immunomodulatory drugs assist the immune system in its attack against cancer?

3. How do the action and side effects of monoclonal antibodies differ from those of conventional cytotoxic chemotherapy?

4. What information and support should be provided for patients entering clinical trials?

References

Adams J 2002 Development of the proteasome inhibitor PS-341. The Oncologist 7(1):9–16

Administration of Radioactive Substances Advisory Committee 2003 www.advisorybodies.doh.gov.uk/arsac Accessed 29 October 2004

Amgen 2001 Neupogen, summary of product characteristics. Amgen Europe, The Netherlands

Anderson K, Shaughnessy J, Biology B et al 2002 Multiple myeloma. American Society of Haematology Education Program Book, Philadelphia, pp 214–240

Boye J, Elter T, Engert A 2003 An overview of the current clinical use of the anti-CD20 monoclonal antibody rituximab. Annals of Oncology 14:520–535

Buchsel P, Forgey A, Grape F et al 2002 Granulocyte macrophage colony-stimulating factor: current practice and novel approaches. Clinical Journal of Oncology Nursing 6(4):198–205

Burnard P 1991 Acquiring minimal counselling skills. Nursing Standard 5(46):37–40

Byrd J, Waselenko J, Maneatis T et al 1999 Rituximab therapy in haematologic malignancy patients with circulating blood tumour cells: association with increased infusion-related side effects and rapid blood tumour clearance. Journal of Clinical Oncology 17(3):791–795

Callahan R, Faragher D 1997 Biology of cancer. In: Gates R, Fink R (eds) Oncology nursing secrets. Hanley and Belfus, Philadelphia, pp 1–5

Capriotti T 2001 Monoclonal antibodies: drugs that combine pharmacology and biotechnology. MedSurg Nursing 10(2):89–95

Cazzola M, Beguin Y, Kloczko J et al 2003 Once-weekly epoietin beta is highly effective in treating anaemic patients with lymphoproliferative malignancy and defective endogenous erythropoietin production. British Journal of Haematology 122:386–393

Cheson B D, Dancey J, Wright J 2002 Novel agents for non-Hodgkin's lymphoma. In: Vose J, Chiu B, Cheson B et al (eds) Update on epidemiology and therapeutics for non-Hodgkin's lymphoma. American Society of Haematology Education Program Book, Philadelphia, pp 241–262

Clayton J 2003 Nursing a patient during and after 90Y-ibritumomab tiuxetan (Zevalin) therapy. Leukaemia & Lymphoma 44(Suppl 4):S49–S53

Dillman R O 2002 Radiolabelled anti-CD20 monoclonal antibodies for the treatment of B-cell lymphoma. Journal of Clinical Oncology 20(16):3545–3557

Druker J, O'Brien S, Cortes J et al 2002 Chronic myelogenous leukemia. American Society of Haematology Education Program Book, Philadelphia, pp 111–135

Dyer M 1999 The role of CAMPATH-1 antibodies in the treatment of lymphoid malignancies. Seminars in Oncology 26(5 Suppl 14):52–57

Gale D, Sorokin P 2001 The interleukins in biotherapy: a comprehensive review, 2nd edn. Jones and Bartlett, Boston, pp 195–244

Gemill R, Idell C 2003 Biological advances for new treatment approaches. Seminars in Oncology Nursing 19(3):162–168

Giles F, Kantarjuan H, Kornblau S et al 2001 Mylotarg (gemtuzumab ozogamicin) therapy is associated with hepatic venoocclusive disease in patients who have not received stem cell transplantation. Cancer 92:406–413

Giles F, Garcia-Manero G, Cortes J et al 2002 Phase II study of troxacitabine, a novel dioxolane nucleoside analogue in patients with refractory leukaemia. Journal of Clinical Oncology 20:656–664

Goldman J, Druker B 2001 Chronic myeloid leukaemia: current treatment options. Blood 98:2039–2042

Goldman J, Melo J 2003 Chronic myeloid leukaemia – advances in biology and new approaches to treatment. New England Journal of Medicine 349(15):1451–1464

Gordon L, Molina A, Witzig T et al 2004 Durable responses after ibritumomab tiuxetan radioimmunotherapy for CD20+ B-cell lymphoma: long term follow-up of a phase I/II study. Blood 103(12):4429–4431

Hahn E, Glendenning A, Sorensa M et al 2003 Quality of life in patients with newly diagnosed chronic phase chronic myeloid leukaemia on imatinib versus interferon alfa plus low dose cytarabine: results from the IRIS study. Journal of Clinical Oncology 21(11):2138–2146

Hoffbrand A, Pettit J 1997 Essential haematology, 3rd edn. Blackwell Science, Oxford

James W, Armitage F 2002 The importance of clinical trials in cancer care. Cancer Nursing Practice 1(9):24–29

Kaminski M, Zelenetz A, Press O et al 2001 Pivotal study of iodine I 131 tositumomab for chemotherapy-refractory low-grade or transformed low-grade B-cell non-Hodgkin's lymphomas. Journal of Clinical Oncology 19(19):3918–3928

Kantarjian H M, Sawyers C, Hochhaus A et al for the International ST1571 CML Study Group 2002a Hematologic and cytogenetic responses to imatinib mesylate in chronic myelogenous leukaemia. New England Journal of Medicine 346:645–652

Kantarjian H M, Talpaz M, O'Brien S et al 2002b Imatinib mesylate for Philadelphia chromosome-positive, chronic-phase myeloid leukemia after failure of interferon alpha: follow up results. Clinical Cancer Research 8:2177–2187

Karius D, Marriott M 1997 Immunologic advances in monoclonal antibody therapy: implications for oncology nursing. Oncology Nursing Forum 24(3):483–494

Kinzler D, Brown C 2001 Cancer vaccines. In: Rieger P (ed) Biotherapy a comprehensive review, 2nd edn. Jones and Bartlett, Boston, pp 357–382

Kohler G, Milstein C 1975 Continuous cultures of fused cells secreting antibody of predefined specificity. Nature 256:495–497

Kosits C, Callaghan M 2000 Rituximab: a new monoclonal antibody therapy for non-Hodgkin's lymphoma. Oncology Nursing Forum 27(1):51–59

Kuter D, Begley C 2002 Recombinant human thrombopoietin: basic biology and evaluation of clinical studies. Blood 100(10):3457–3469

Liu K 2003 Breakthroughs in cancer gene therapy. Seminars in Oncology Nursing 19(3):217–226

Loud J, Peters J, Fraser M et al 2002 Applications of advances in molecular biology and genomics to clinical cancer care. Cancer Nursing 25(2):110–122

Ludwig H 2002 Anaemia of hematologic malignancies: what are the treatment options? Seminars in Oncology 29(3 Suppl 8):45–54

Lundin J, Kumby E, Bjortholm M et al 2002 Phase II trial of subcutaneous anti-CD52 monoclonal antibody alemtuzumab (Campath-H) as a first line treatment for patients with B-cell chronic lymphocytic leukaemia. Blood 100:768–773

Lynn A, Williams M, Sickler J et al 2003 Treatment of chronic lymphocytic leukaemia with alemtuzumab: a review for nurses. Oncology Nursing Forum 30(4):689–696

Munshi N 2001 Arsenic trioxide: an emerging therapy for multiple myeloma. The Oncologist 6(Suppl 2):17–21

National Institute for Clinical Excellence 2002 Guidance on the use of Rituximab for recurrent or refractory Stage III or IV follicular non-Hodgkins lymphoma NICE, London

National Institute for Clinical Excellence 2003 Technology appraisal: leukaemia (chronic myeloid – imatinib) No. 50. www.nice.org

Norvick S, Warrell R Jr 2000 Arsenicals in haematologic cancers. Seminars in Oncology 27:495–501

O'Brien S, Kantarjian H, Keating M et al 1995 Homoharringtonine therapy induces responses in patients with chronic myelogenous leukaemia in late chronic phase. Blood 86:3322–3326

O'Brien S, Guilhot F, Larson R et al 2003 Imatinib compared with interferon and low dose cytarabine for newly diagnosed chronic-phase chronic myeloid leukaemia. New England Journal of Medicine 348(11):994–1004

Osterborg A, Brandberg Y, Molostova V et al 2002 Randomised, double-blind, placebo-controlled trial of recombinant human erythropoietin, epoietin beta in haematological malignancies. Journal of Clinical Oncology 20(10):2486–2494

Pelloso D, Cryan K, Timmons L et al 2004 Immunological consequences of interleukin-12 administration after autologous stem cell transplantation. Clinical Cancer Research 10(6):1935–1942

Phillips M 2003 Pegfilgrastim. Clinical Journal of Oncology Nursing 7(2):238–239

Rai K, Freter C, Mercier M 2002 Alemtuzumab in previously treated chronic lymphocytic leukaemia patients who had also received fludarabine. Journal of Clinical Oncology 20(18):3891–3897

Richardson P, Jagannath S, Schlossman R et al 2002 A multi-centre randomised phase II study to evaluate the efficacy and safety of two CC-5013 dose regimens when used alone or in combination with dexamethasone for the treatment of relapsed or refractory multiple myeloma. Blood 100(11 Abstract 386):104a

Rieger P 2001 Biotherapy an overview. In: Rieger P (ed) Biotherapy a comprehensive overview, 2nd edn. Jones and Bartlett, Boston, pp 3–37

Riley M 2003 Ibritumomab tiuxetan. Clinical Journal of Oncology Nursing 7(1):110–112

Roche Products Limited 2002 MabThera 500 mgs. Roche Products Limited, Hertfordshire

Samol J, Littlewood T 2003 The efficacy of rHuEPO in cancer-related anaemia. British Journal of Haematology 121:3–11

Schering Health Care Limited 2004a MabCampath. Schering Health Care Limited, West Sussex

Schering Health Care Limited 2004b Zevalin. Schering Health Care Limited, West Sussex

Schmidt K, Wood B 2003 Trends in cancer therapy: role of monoclonal antibodies. Seminars in Oncology Nursing 19(3):169–179

Schmidt-Wolf G D, Schmidt-Wolf I G 2002 Immunomodulatory gene therapy for haematological malignancies. British Journal of Haematology 117(1):23–32

Seeley K, DeMeyer E 2002 Nursing care of patients receiving campath. Clinical Journal of Oncology Nursing 6(3):138–143

Sievers E, Larson R, Stadtmauer A et al 2001 Efficacy and safety of gemtuzumab ozogamicin in patients with CD33-positive acute myeloid leukaemia in first relapse. Journal of Clinical Oncology 19(13):3244–3254

Souhami R, Tobias J 1998 Cancer and its management, 3rd edn. Blackwell Science, Oxford

Statutory Instrument 2000 No: 1059 The ionising radiation (medical exposure regulations) 2000. HMSO, London

Tariman J 2003 Understanding novel therapeutic agents for multiple myeloma. Clinical Journal of Oncology Nursing 7(5):521–528

United Kingdom Myeloma Forum UKMF 2004 Clinical trials in multiple myeloma. www.ukmf.org.uk/trials.html Accessed 20 May 2004

Viele C 2002 Gemtuzumab ozogamicin. Clinical Journal of Oncology Nursing 6(5):298–300

Vose J 2002 Immunotherapy for non-Hodgkin's lymphoma In: Vose J, Chiu B, Cheson B et al (eds) Update on epidemiology and therapeutics for non-Hodgkin's lymphoma. American Society of Haematology Education Program Book, Philadelphia, pp 241–262

Vose J, Wahl R, Saleh M et al 2000 Multicentre phase II study of Iodine-131 tositumomab for chemotherapy-relapsed/refractory low grade transformed low grade B-cell non-Hodgkin's lymphomas. Journal of Clinical Oncology 18(6):1316–1323

Vose J, Chiu B, Cheson B et al 2002 Update on epidemiology and therapeutics for non-Hodgkin's lymphoma. American Society of Haematology Education Program Book, Philadelphia

Vose J, Crump M, Lazarus H et al 2003 Randomised, multicenter, open-label study of pegfilgrastim compared with daily filgrastim after chemotherapy for lymphoma. Journal of Clinical Oncology 21(3): 514–519

Ward U 1995 Biological therapy in the treatment of cancer. British Journal of Nursing 4(15):869–891

Weiner L 1999 An overview of monoclonal antibody therapy of cancer. Seminars in Oncology 26(4 Suppl 12):41–50

Weiss R 1998 Some conclusions and prospects. In: Franks L, Teich N (eds) Cellular and molecular biology of cancer, 3rd edn. Oxford University Press, Oxford, pp 415–425

Witzig T, White C, Wiseman G et al 1999 Phase I/II trial of IDEC-Y2B8 radioimmunotherapy for treatment of relapsed or refractory CD20+ B cell non-Hodgkin's lymphoma. Journal of Clinical Oncology 17(12):3793–3803

Wujcik D 2001 Hematopoietic growth factors. In: Rieger P (ed) Biotherapy a comprehensive overview, 2nd edn. Jones and Bartlett, Boston pp 245–282

Wyeth Pharmaceuticals 2004 Mylotarg. Wyeth Pharmaceuticals, Berkshire

Further reading

Bruno B, Rota M, Giaccone L et al 2004 New drugs for the treatment of multiple myeloma. Lancet Oncology 5(7):430–442
Contains a comprehensive review of thalidomide, IMiDs, proteasome inhibitors and arsenic in the management of multiple myeloma.

Frankel A, Neville D, Brigge T et al 2003 Immunotoxin therapy of haematological malignancies. Seminars in Oncology 30(4):545–557
Detailed discussion of the use and action of immunotoxin therapy in relation to haematological malignancies.

Rieger P 2001 The role of oncology nurses in gene therapy. Lancet Oncology 2(4):233–238
Outlines the nurse's role in the administration of gene therapy.

Straus D 2002 Epoietin alfa as a supportive measure in haematologic malignancies. Seminars in Haematology 39(4):25–31
Comprehensive review of the role of epoietin alfa in myelodysplastic syndromes, chronic lymphocytic leukaemia and multiple myeloma.

Stull D 2003 Targeted therapies for the treatment of leukaemia. Seminars in Oncology Nursing 19(2):90–97
Easy-to-read discussion of the role of gemtuzumab, arsenic trioxide, imatinib and alemtuzumab as treatments of leukaemia.

Wienda W, Kipps T 2000 Gene therapy of hematologic malignancies. Seminars in Oncology 27(5):502–511
An interesting analysis of the application of gene therapy in haematological malignancies.

Chapter **12**

Blood component support

Alexandra Gray

KEY POINTS

- Transfusion of the wrong blood is the most common cause of acute transfusion reactions, which can be fatal.
- Safe transfusion practice depends on accurate identification of the patient at every stage of the process.
- The final patient identity check at the bedside is the crucial opportunity to prevent an error.
- The patient should be monitored throughout the transfusion episode for signs and symptoms of a transfusion reaction.

INTRODUCTION

Patients with haematological cancers have a frequent requirement for blood component support, usually related to the effects of treatment. The purpose of this chapter is to facilitate understanding of good practice in relation to blood transfusion and recognition of the importance of providing information in simple and comprehensible language to patients who may require a transfusion. This chapter deals with the transfusion process from donor to recipient, including topics such as technical aspects of blood administration, adverse event reporting and management, blood component therapy and patient information.

SAFE AND APPROPRIATE TRANSFUSION PRACTICE

UK transfusion services have invested enormous resources to provide blood that is amongst the safest in the world. No blood component, however, can be considered to be completely free of risk. It is therefore the responsibility of each practitioner who prescribes and administers blood components to ensure safe and appropriate transfusion practice, i.e. the administration of the correct blood component, which has been stored under optimal conditions, only when there is a clear clinical indication for transfusion. The UK Departments of Health (DOH 1998b, 2002) have issued advice on how to improve the safety of the blood transfusion process. However, despite these initiatives, transfusion errors continue to occur.

The potential risks associated with transfusion have been highlighted by the Serious Hazards of Transfusion (SHOT) Scheme, launched in November 1996. It is a voluntary, anonymised reporting scheme covering both NHS and private hospitals in the UK. In the 6 years since the SHOT reporting scheme commenced, the number of submitted reports has increased by 47% (Stainsby et al 2003). The largest number of serious adverse events reported to SHOT was in the category of 'Incorrect Blood Component Transfused' (IBCT) – 1045 cases, 64% of all reports (Fig. 12.1). The majority of these incidents involved the administration of a unit of blood either intended for another patient or one which was unsuitable, e.g. the patient was in a susceptible group but was not transfused with an irradiated blood component. A total of 193 ABO blood group incompatible transfusions occurred, with 27 deaths, 5 of which were definitely related to the transfusion and 10 probably or possibly related to the transfusion; 69 patients suffered major morbidity, e.g. resulting in admission to intensive care requiring ventilation or experiencing a major haemorrhage from transfusion-induced coagulopathy.

Errors resulting in the transfusion of an incorrect blood component were due to:

- the blood sample being drawn from the wrong patient
- patient details recorded incorrectly on the blood sample label or the blood request form
- the incorrect unit collected from the blood refrigerator
- the formal identity check at the patient's bedside omitted or performed incorrectly at the time of the administration of the blood or blood component (Stainsby et al 2003).

In some instances, more than one error occurred in the course of the transfusion episode. In 481 cases (46%) two or more errors occurred, and

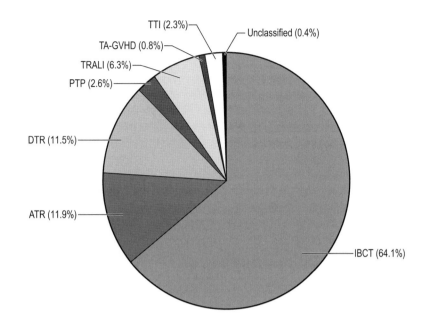

as many as seven errors were reported in three cases. Errors during the collection and/or administration of the unit of blood were common (51% of cases) (Fig. 12.2).

'Wrong blood incidents are without exception avoidable errors'

(Love et al 2002)

Guidelines for best practice in the administration of blood components published by the British Committee for Standards in Haematology (BCSH 1999) should form the basis for local transfusion protocols:

- Request forms should be clearly written and contain full patient details, including identification number, location of patient, details of blood component required, transfusion history, the patient's diagnosis and reason for request.
- Only one patient should be bled at a time to minimise error. Patient details should be verified at blood sampling and the sample should be clearly labelled immediately after the blood has been added to the tube. A pre-labelled tube *must not* be used.
- Poor sampling practices have been identified as a cause of inappropriate requests for blood components (Stainsby et al 2003). Practitioners should avoid taking blood samples from the arm where the infusion is sited because this may result in a diluted sample being sent to the laboratory for analysis or a spurious result being obtained.
- Collection and storage of blood components continues to be a major source of identification error (Stainsby et al 2003). Hospitals should have a policy for collection of blood components and transport to the clinical area. Red blood cells should be stored only in authorised blood refrigerators and should be transported in boxes specifically designed

Figure 12.2
Distribution of errors resulting in the transfusion of an incompatible blood component (reproduced from Stainsby et al 2003, with permission from the Serious Hazards of Transfusion Steering Group)

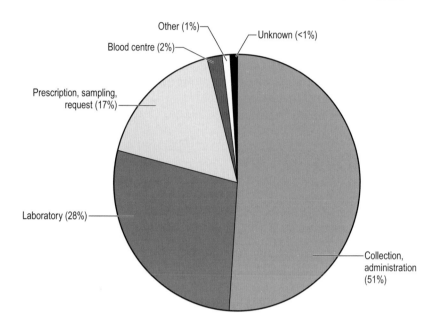

for this purpose. The person collecting the blood component must have documented patient identification details and withdrawals from the refrigerator or hospital transfusion laboratory must be documented.

- Administration of blood components, final patient/component identification checks and the identification of staff responsibilities should be clearly defined by local policies.
- The final patient identity check is crucial in preventing transfusion errors and has been identified as the single most important cause of transfusion error. The patient must be positively identified and their details checked against the patient identification wristband before commencing the transfusion.
- The patient identity checking procedure should be undertaken by at least one person who must be a registered nurse or medical officer.
- Temperature, pulse and blood pressure should be measured and recorded before the start of the transfusion, 15 minutes after the start of each unit and at the end of each transfusion episode. Further observations should be defined in the local transfusion policy for each clinical area.
- No other infusion solution or drug should be added to blood components as they may cause clotting or red cell lysis.
- Infusion pumps should be used only if they have been verified as safe for the administration of blood components and must be used according to the manufacturer's instruction.
- Blood should be warmed using only a device specifically designed for this purpose and must have a visible thermometer and audible alarm (Wilkins 2000).

The 2001/02 SHOT report also recommends that all staff who participate in the transfusion process must receive training in the procedures they undertake and that their competency should be formally assessed and recorded (Stainsby et al 2003). Safety is paramount throughout the entire transfusion process – from donor to recipient. It is useful to understand how blood is collected and tested because these processes affect the final choice and delivery of the product to the clinical area.

DONATION PROCESS

Figure 12.3 illustrates the processing of blood from the donor to the patient. The selection of blood donors is intended to maintain a safe and adequate blood supply. In the UK every blood donation is tested for evidence of hepatitis B (HBV), hepatitis C (HCV), human immunodeficiency virus-1/-2 (HIV-1/-2), human T-cell leukaemia virus-I/II (HTLV-1/-II) and syphilis (McClelland 2001). Since 1998, in order to reduce the unknown risk that variant Creutzfeldt–Jakob disease (vCJD) might be transmissible by blood, a number of initiatives have been implemented by the UK Transfusion Services. These include the manufacture of all plasma products from non-UK plasma (DOH 1998a), the introduction of universal leucodepletion (BCSH 1998), and the importation of clinical fresh frozen plasma for patients born after January 1, 1996 (Standing Advisory Committee on Transfusion Transmitted Infections 2004). The rationale for this decision was that children born after 1996 are considered to have had minimal exposure to the bovine spongiform encephalopathy (BSE) agent because of government measures to prevent BSE entering the food chain. In 2004, the UK transfusion services also deferred all whole blood and apheresis donors who state they have received a blood transfusion in the UK since 1980 (Standing Advisory Committee on Transfusion Transmitted Infections 2004).

Each blood donation is also tested to determine the ABO and RhD (formerly known as Rhesus) blood group.

ABO AND RHD BLOOD GROUPS

A large number of different molecules are present on the surface of the red cells. The molecules (antigens) determine the blood groups. There

Figure 12.3
Preparation of blood
components from donor to
patient (adapted from
McClelland 2001, with
permission from the editor of
the Handbook of Transfusion
Medicine)

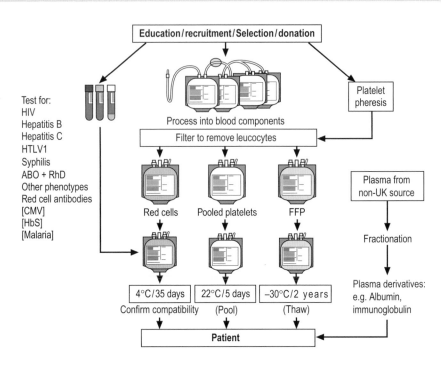

Test for:
HIV
Hepatitis B
Hepatitis C
HTLV1
Syphilis
ABO + RhD
Other phenotypes
Red cell antibodies
[CMV]
[HbS]
[Malaria]

are over 100 different types of antigen but, for the purposes of safe transfusion practice, the most important are the antigens that produce the ABO groups. Also of importance is the RhD antigen, which determines whether someone is 'Rh-positive' (cells carry the D antigen) or 'Rh-negative' (cells lack the D antigen).

Antibodies may develop to each of these antigens if a patient is transfused with blood that is of a different group from their own. Transfused blood will almost never be completely identical with that of the patient unless they have pre-donated their own blood. It is therefore accepted in transfusion practice that there is an approximate 1 in 20 chance that a transfused patient will develop a red cell antibody after transfusion. This does not normally cause any problems, but does need to be taken into account when selecting blood on subsequent occasions.

There are four different ABO blood groups. An individual's ABO group is determined by whether or not their red cells carry the A antigen, the B antigen, both A and B antigens or neither A nor B antigens. In the ABO groups, individuals produce antibodies (immunoglobulins) against the antigens that are not present on their own red cells. Thus, group O individuals have, in their plasma, antibodies to both group A and group B. Group AB individuals have neither of these antibodies, as shown in Figure 12.4.

The transfusion of only a few mL of the wrong (incompatible) ABO group can trigger a massive immune response, leading to shock and disseminated intravascular coagulation (see Chapter 16). Patients may die from circulatory collapse, severe bleeding or renal failure within

Figure 12.4
ABO Blood Group Serology
(reproduced from the Better
Blood Transfusion Continuing
Education Safe Transfusion
Practice module, with
permission from the Scottish
National Blood Transfusion
Service)

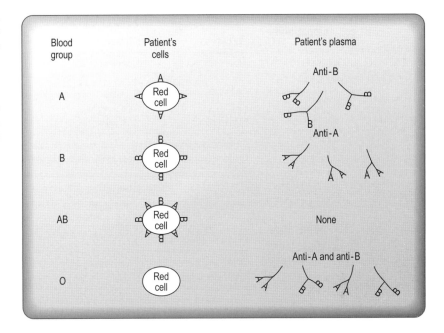

hours of receiving a small volume of blood. Table 12.1 shows the blood group of the component that is compatible with the blood group of the recipient.

It is generally the case that an RhD negative patient is given RhD negative blood when being transfused. RhD positive blood can stimulate the production of anti-D if transfused to an RhD negative recipient. This will normally not cause any acute problem as the antibody will usually appear several days after the transfusion and will not lead to rapid red cell destruction. It is particularly important, however, to use RhD negative red cells when transfusing RhD negative females of childbearing potential. The transfusion of RhD positive blood to an RhD negative female child or woman might sensitise her to produce anti-D. Anti-D might cross the placenta in any subsequent pregnancy and destroy fetal red cells, thereby causing haemolytic disease of the newborn. Table 12.2 shows the blood group of the component that is RhD compatible with the blood group of the recipient.

COMPATIBILITY TESTING

When blood is required for a patient, the hospital transfusion laboratory must carry out a number of tests to select the most appropriate units. The patient's blood sample is first tested to determine the ABO group and the Rh group. In addition, the patient's plasma or serum is mixed with a range of red cells to determine whether or not the patient has antibodies

Table 12.1
Red cell compatibility

Patient blood group	Antigens on cell surface	Antibodies in plasma	Compatible red cells
O	None	Anti-A, anti-B	O
A	A	Anti-B	A, O
B	B	Anti-A	B, O
AB	A, B	None	AB, A, B, O
Unknown	Unknown	Unknown	O

Reproduced from the Better Blood Transfusion Continuing Education Safe Transfusion Practice module, with permission from the Scottish National Blood Transfusion Service.

Table 12.2
RhD compatibility

Patient Rh group	Compatible red cells
RhD positive	RhD positive or RhD negative
RhD negative	RhD negative

Reproduced from the Better Blood Transfusion Continuing Education Safe Transfusion Practice module, with permission from the Scottish National Blood Transfusion Service.

to red cells as a result of a previous transfusion or pregnancy. This combination of tests is known as a 'group and screen' or 'type and screen' and is the most important part of the compatibility testing procedure. It takes the laboratory about 30–40 minutes to perform these tests following receipt of the blood sample.

Once the ABO and Rh group is known and the antibody screen has been shown to be negative (as it is in 99% of cases), blood can be selected for the patient very quickly. If a patient is found to have atypical red cell antibodies, however, finding 'compatible' blood can be very difficult and time-consuming as blood must be selected that lacks the antigen to which the patient has developed an antibody. In some instances, for example, perhaps only 1 in 1000 units will be suitable. The multiple transfusions received by individuals with haemato-oncological disorders predispose them to development of red cell antibodies.

BLOOD COMPONENT SUPPORT

Patients undergoing intensive therapy for haematological cancer have a frequent requirement for blood transfusion due to the myelosuppressive/myeloablative effects of their treatment (Murphy & Pamphilon 2001). Although there is no 'universal trigger' for red cell transfusion (BCSH 2001), it is recommended that the level of haemoglobin, which is used to trigger transfusion in patients receiving intensive treatment, be in the range of 8–10 g/dL (Murphy & Pamphilon 2001).

RED BLOOD CELLS

All available red cell components in the UK are prepared from whole blood donations from voluntary, non-remunerated UK donors. During the manufacturing process, the white cells are removed by passing the blood through a filter (a process called leucodepletion). This reduces the total white cell count in a unit of red cells to less than 5×10^6. The majority of red blood cells issued in the UK are in optimal additive solution, i.e. the plasma is removed from whole blood and replaced with SAGM solution (saline, adenine, glucose and mannitol). SAGM helps to maintain red cell function and viability and reduces the haematocrit to produce flow characteristics similar to those of whole blood. A suspension of red cells in optimal additive solution has an approximate total volume of 300 mL with a haematocrit of 0.55–0.65%.

Red cells have a shelf life of up to 35 days and must be stored in a validated blood refrigerator within a temperature range of $4 \pm 2°C$. Storage temperatures below 2°C cause red cell breakdown, resulting in haemolysis; above 4°C increases the potential for bacterial growth or metabolic activity of the red cells, leading to deterioration of function. It is vital to keep red cells in the refrigerator at all times other than when they are actually being checked or transfused. All blood components should be transfused within 4 hours of removal from the blood fridge or hospital transfusion laboratory.

The transfusion rate for blood components is dependent on the condition of the patient. Red blood cell transfusion rates can vary from 10 minutes in patients with acute blood loss to 4 hours in elderly patients with circulatory overload.

Special requirements

Individuals with haematological cancers are susceptible to transfusion-related complications because of their immunocompromised status and their need for continuing transfusion support. It is the responsibility of the prescribing doctor to identify these requirements and clearly state them on the blood request form. In the 2001/02 SHOT report, 60 patients were put at risk due to a failure to request appropriate components (Stainsby et al 2003). When treating haematology or immuno-deficient patients, it is important to be aware of local protocols for requesting cytomegalovirus (CMV) negative and/or irradiated blood components.

CMV negative components

CMV negative components are produced from donations that have been specifically screened for cytomegalovirus by serological techniques and have been found to be negative. CMV may cause significant morbidity and mortality in immunocompromised patients, mainly due to pneumonia (Murphy & Pamphilon 2001). CMV negative components are currently indicated for transfusion in the following groups of CMV seronegative patients:

- all allogeneic and autologous stem cell transplants
- all potential recipients of allogeneic stem cell transplants (Murphy & Pamphilon 2001).

Irradiated components

Irradiation is used to destroy any T lymphocytes remaining in the blood donation, since these may cause graft-versus-host disease in immuno-compromised patients. Irradiated blood is currently indicated for transfusion in the following groups of haematology patients:

- All autologous bone marrow or peripheral blood stem progenitor cell transplants – during and 7 days before the harvest of haemopoietic cells, and then from the initiation of conditioning therapy until 3 months post-transplant (6 months if total body irradiation is used).
- All allogeneic bone marrow or peripheral blood progenitor cell transplants – from the time of initiation of conditioning therapy and continuing while the patient remains on graft-versus-host disease (GvHD) prophylaxis (usually 6 months).
- Patients with Hodgkin's disease.
- Patients treated with the purine analogue drugs, e.g. fludarabine, deoxycoformycin or cladribine, for 6 months from the last treatment.
- All HLA-matched platelet transfusions (Murphy & Pamphilon 2001).

BCSH guidelines (1996a,b) are also available on the use of irradiated blood components.

PLATELETS

The development of platelet concentrates has had an unquestionable affect on the treatment of patients with haematological cancers in reducing the potential for life-threatening haemorrhage (Freireich 2000). Platelet transfusions are indicated for the treatment and prevention of haemorrhage in patients with thrombocytopenia or an inherited or acquired functional defect (BCSH 2003).

Platelets can be obtained from whole blood donations or by apheresis. All platelets for transfusion are leucodepleted. A single adult dose of platelets should contain $> 240 \times 10^9$ platelets.

Platelets from whole blood donations (pooled platelets)

If anticoagulated blood is left to stand for long enough, the cellular components settle into discrete layers according to their density. The combined layers of white cells and platelets are referred to as the 'buffy coat'. Buffy coats from four or five whole blood donations are pooled together with plasma from one donor to form one platelet pool (a standard adult dose). The pool is centrifuged again and filtered to separate the white cells from the platelets.

Apheresis platelets

'Apheresis' means to 'selectively remove'. The apheresis machines currently in routine use in the UK use centrifugation to separate platelets from anticoagulated whole blood drawn from volunteer donors. Platelet-rich plasma is collected, while the remaining blood constituents are returned to the donor. By apheresis, it is possible to collect the equivalent of five donations' worth of platelets from a single donor during a procedure, which takes approximately 1 hour. Apheresis units have the advantage of reducing the number of donors to which the recipient is exposed during transfusion (i.e. one donor instead of four or five if pooled platelets are used). This reduces the risk of transfusion-transmitted infections and the immune complications of transfusion.

Platelets are stored at a monitored temperature of $22 \pm 2°C$ and are gently agitated throughout the storage period to encourage gas transfer through the semi-permeable storage bag. They should never be refrigerated. Platelets currently have a shelf life of 5 days, which means they expire just before midnight on the fifth day after collection from the donor, the day of collection being day 0. This short shelf life is a challenge to providing adequate supplies of platelets.

Platelets are the component at most risk of bacterial contamination. Between 1997 and 2002 out of 21 bacterial cases reported to SHOT, 17 cases involved platelet units (Stainsby et al 2003).

Indications for platelet transfusion

The normal range for the platelet count in peripheral blood at all ages is $150–400 \times 10^9/L$. A platelet count below this level (thrombocytopenia) is not, in itself, justification for the administration of a platelet transfusion. In deciding whether or not platelet transfusion is warranted for a given level of thrombocytopenia, the following criteria should also be considered:

- the underlying cause of the thrombocytopenia
- any other clinical factors that may predispose to bleeding.

The British Society for Haematology has published national guidelines (2003) on the use of platelet transfusions. Most of the platelet transfusions that are currently administered are given to prevent bleeding in patients with bone marrow failure following treatment with chemotherapy or radiotherapy which has resulted in significant thrombocytopenia. Although there may be no current bleeding, the risk of serious haemorrhage into, for example, the gut or brain, is perceived to be so high that platelet transfusion is warranted.

There has been extensive debate over the level of thrombocytopenia that justifies prophylactic platelet transfusion. Spontaneous bleeding is minimal until the platelet count is less than $5 \times 10^9/L$. Currently $10 \times 10^9/L$ is widely accepted as the limit below which prophylactic platelet transfusion is justified in an otherwise stable patient (BCSH 2003). This approach should, of course, be modified in the presence of other complicating factors such as fever, sepsis or in patients at increased risk of bleeding (see Chapter 16).

Therapeutic platelet transfusions are indicated when patients present with active bleeding due to bone marrow failure or the effects of treatment (BCSH 2003). The recommended infusion time for a platelet transfusion is over a 30-minute period.

Platelet refractoriness

Platelet refractoriness is defined as a failure to achieve the expected platelet increment after two consecutive transfusions. The main causes of platelet refractoriness can be divided into two categories: immune and non-immune. The main immune cause is human leucocyte antigen (HLA) alloimmunisation; other causes include ABO incompatibility and platelet autoantibodies. Since the introduction of leucodepletion in 1999, the incidence of platelet refractoriness has declined (BCSH 2003). Non-immune platelet refractoriness is associated with clinical features such as infection and its concomitant treatments (e.g. antibiotics or antifungal drugs), disseminated intravascular coagulation (DIC) and splenomegaly (BCSH 2003).

GRANULOCYTES

Severe neutropenia in patients with haematological malignancies can limit the treatment/recovery phase following stem cell transplants. The use of granulocyte-colony stimulating factor (G-CSF)-mobilised granulocytes collected by apheresis has renewed interest in this blood component. The use of high-dose granulocyte transfusions can be indicated in patients who are at increased risk of life-threatening bacterial and fungal infections (Murphy & Pamphilon 2001). Granulocytes should be administered within 6 hours of collection.

REFLECTION POINT

Think about the patient observations you undertake before, during and on completion of a unit of red cells. Do you omit any of these observations when administering a unit of platelets or FFP? Do you have a protocol for observing the transfused patient in your clinical area?

THE TECHNICAL ASPECTS OF ADMINISTERING BLOOD COMPONENTS

Blood transfusion can be given successfully through a needle as small as 23 gauge; however, the gauge selection should be dependent on the size of the vein and the desired speed at which the blood is to be transfused. Many haematology patients have venous access established by the use of short-term or indwelling central lines (see Chapter 14). These are generally suitable for the transfusion of blood components. When a multi-lumen catheter is used, the lumen specified for blood components should be used for transfusion. When a very rapid transfusion is to be administered through a central catheter terminating in or near the right atrium, the blood should be warmed. However, this is unnecessary for routine transfusion.

All blood components must be transfused through a blood administration set with an integral mesh filter (170–200 μm pore size) (BCSH 1999). The filter removes macroaggregates, composed of white cells, platelets and coagulum, which can obstruct the cannula. Platelets can be administered through a normal blood or a platelet administration set. Platelets should not be transfused through an administration set that has previously been used for red cells or other blood components as this may cause aggregation and retention of platelets in the line. For patients requiring ongoing transfusion, the infusion line should be changed at least every 12 hours. The administration set should be changed following completion of the prescribed transfusion.

No pharmaceutical agent or solution other than 0.9% saline should be infused through a lumen that is used for the transfusion of blood components as the pH, osmolarity or chemical composition of the drug solution may damage the red cells, platelets or coagulation factors. Blood components must not be given through an infusion set that has been primed with dextrose as this solution may cause haemolysis. Similarly, Ringers Lactate Solution should not be used to flush administration sets as this may lead to clotting of the transfused component in the infusion tubing.

Due to the risk of bacterial proliferation or loss of function, once a blood component has been removed from the hospital transfusion laboratory or blood fridge it must be transfused within 4 hours of spiking the pack.

Case study

Joe, a 66-year-old patient with chronic lymphocytic anaemia, was receiving fludarabine. He was attending the outpatient clinic and reported feeling breathless and fatigued. Joe has been prescribed two units of red cells, as his Hb was 7.6 g/dL. The first unit has arrived in the day bed area and as you are performing the pre-administration checking procedure you note that the laboratory has not provided irradiated red cells.

■ What action should you take?
■ Why is it important that Joe receives irradiated blood components?
■ What can be done to prevent this from happening in the future?

COMPLICATIONS OF TRANSFUSION

ACUTE TRANSFUSION REACTIONS

Acute transfusion reactions occur within the first 24 hours of the transfusion. The most common type of reaction is the development of fever (without haemolysis) affecting 1–2% of red cell recipients and more commonly seen in plasma component recipients. Fluid overload, where the transfusion is administered too rapidly or when an excessive volume is given, is also a frequent acute complication of transfusion. The presenting signs and symptoms and the immediate management of acute transfusion reactions are summarised in Table 12.3.

Table 12.3
Acute transfusion reactions

Reaction	Signs	Symptoms	Management
Febrile non-haemolytic transfusion reaction	Fever >1°C Flushing Tachycardia Rigors	Shivering Headache	Slow or stop the transfusion Administer antipyretic, e.g. paracetamol 1 g orally Recommence transfusion at slower rate Keep the patient warm Continue to monitor the patient
Mild allergic reaction	Urticaria Angioedema	Pruritis (itch) Wheeze (chest tightness)	*Stop* the transfusion and treat according to the severity of the reaction: administer antihistamine, e.g. chlorphenamine 10 mg iv, and/or inhaled steroid
Severe allergic reaction anaphylaxis	Urticaria Hypotension Bronchospasm Laryngeal oedema Vomiting	Pruritis (itch) Dyspnoea Chest pain Abdominal pain Nausea	*Stop* the transfusion Give high-concentration oxygen Administer antihistamine, e.g., chlorphenamine Hydrocortisone Adrenaline Salbutamol by nebuliser
Acute haemolytic reaction	Rigors Fever Chills Restlessness Hypotension Tachycardia Haemoglobinuria Unexpected bleeding (DIC)	Pain at infusion site Anxiety Chest/loin/back pain Respiratory distress Dyspnoea Nausea and vomiting	*Stop* the transfusion Replace the administration set and keep the iv line open with normal saline to maintain systolic blood pressure Notify the doctor immediately Commence appropriate resuscitation treatment: Maintain airway and give high flow O_2 Check urine for signs of haemoglobinuria Inform hospital transfusion laboratory/contact haematologist Send blood unit + giving set + new blood samples and blood cultures for investigation Reassess patient and treat appropriately Seek expert advice if patient's condition continues to deteriorate

Table 12.3
Acute transfusion reactions – Cont'd

Reaction	Signs	Symptoms	Management
Bacterial contamination/ septic shock	Rigors Fever Restlessness Hypotension Tachycardia Haemoglobinuria Unexpected bleeding (DIC)	Anxiety Chest/loin/back pain Respiratory distress Dyspnoea	*Stop* the transfusion Replace the administration set and keep the iv line open with normal saline Notify the doctor immediately Commence appropriate resuscitation treatment as required, e.g. inotropic agents/ diuretics to maintain urine output Give broad-spectrum antibiotics until blood culture results are available NB: Retain all packs for investigation
Transfusion-related acute lung injury	Fever Severe hypoxia Severe bilateral pulmonary oedema Diffuse bilateral shadowing of the lungs	Acute respiratory distress	Administer high concentration oxygen Give inotropes and mechanical ventilation support as required
Fluid overload	Acute dyspnoea Tachypnoea Non-productive cough Raised JVP Basal lung crackles Hypertension Tachycardia	Respiratory distress	*Stop* the transfusion Give high concentration of oxygen Administer a diuretic, e.g. frusemide 20–40 mg by slow iv injection

Remember – If an acute reaction occurs:
Check the patient and component compatibility – if there is any discrepancy *stop* the transfusion and contact your hospital transfusion laboratory immediately.
A mild reaction may be the beginnings of a severe reaction – *do not ignore it.*
Document all adverse events in patient case notes.

Serious or life-threatening acute reactions are extremely rare and include:

- acute intravascular haemolysis
- septic shock
- anaphylaxis
- transfusion-related acute lung injury (TRALI).

Many acute transfusion reactions have very similar initial presentations and rapid, appropriate management can have a major impact on the outcome.

Acute intravascular haemolytic transfusion reaction

Intravascular haemolytic transfusion reactions are caused by incompatible red cells reacting with the patient's anti-A or anti-B antibodies. If an ABO incompatible blood component is transfused to the patient, the red cells are destroyed in the circulation. This can lead to disseminated intravascular coagulation (DIC) and renal failure. Even a few millilitres of incompatible blood can cause an acute transfusion reaction within minutes of the transfusion commencing. If an acute intravascular haemolytic reaction is suspected, the transfusion should be stopped immediately, a new administration set with normal saline should be used and a member of the medical staff notified immediately (Table 12.3).

Septic transfusion reaction

Septic transfusion reactions are more commonly seen during platelet transfusions, but can also occur with red cell transfusions. As large amounts of endotoxin may be present in the blood bag, the reaction can be overwhelming, with hypotension, hypoxia and circulatory failure. The patient may not be pyrexial initially. Inspection of the bag may reveal clumps of platelets or discoloration/haemolysis in a red cell pack. Initial management is the same as for intravascular haemolytic transfusion reactions. If a septic transfusion reaction is suspected, the transfusion must be stopped immediately and the appropriate treatment commenced (Table 12.3).

Severe allergic or anaphylactic type reactions

Severe allergic or anaphylactic type reactions are rare but can be life-threatening. Complications usually occur early in the transfusion. These types of reaction are most commonly seen with the administration of plasma-containing components, e.g. platelets and fresh frozen plasma. Again initial management is the same as for intravascular haemolytic transfusion reactions – stop the transfusion immediately and commence the appropriate treatment (Table 12.3).

Transfusion–related acute lung injury

Transfusion-related acute lung injury (TRALI) is frequently an under-diagnosed acute transfusion reaction; many cases are missed or mis-diagnosed as adult respiratory distress syndrome (ARDS). The SHOT scheme has shown that TRALI is the second most common cause of transfusion-related death, second only to ABO incompatible transfusions (Stainsby et al 2003). The cause of TRALI is often found to be donor antibodies that react strongly against the patient's white cells. Antibodies in the donor unit bind to the patient's white cells, which then lodge in the lung and stimulate a local immune reaction. The signs, symptoms and management of TRALI are summarised in Table 12.3.

DELAYED TRANSFUSION REACTIONS

Delayed transfusion reactions can occur days, months or even years following transfusion and essentially fall into two categories, non-infectious reactions and transfusion-transmitted infections.

Non-infectious reactions

Non-infectious delayed transfusion reactions can be categorised as:

- delayed haemolytic reaction
- alloimmunisation
- post-transfusion purpura
- transfusion associated graft-versus-host disease
- iron overload in patients receiving repeated transfusions.

Non-infectious delayed reactions are generally less serious, although occasionally they can be life-threatening. The signs, symptoms and management of delayed transfusion reactions are summarised in Table 12.4.

Transfusion-transmitted infections

The recognised infections that can be transmitted by blood transfusion are:

- HIV (1 & 2)
- Hepatitis A

Table 12.4
Delayed transfusion reactions

Reaction	Signs	Symptoms	Management
Delayed haemolytic transfusion reaction (DHTR)	Fever Fall in haemoglobin concentration Jaundice Haemoglobinuria Rarely hypotension/ renal failure		Majority of DHTRs require no treatment as the red cell destruction process occurs gradually Expert medical advice should be sought for the treatment of hypotension/renal failure
Post-transfusion purpura (PTP)	Purpura/severe thrombocytopenia usually occurring 5–10 days following transfusion	Bleeding from mucous membranes, gastrointestinal and urinary tracts	High-dose intravenous immunoglobulin (iv IgG) – 2 g/kg given over 2–5 days)
Transfusion-associated graft-versus-host disease (TA-GvHD)	Fever Erythematous skin rash	Diarrhoea Jaundice	There is no effective treatment for TA-GvHD NB: it is imperative that patients at risk of developing TA-GvHD should receive irradiated blood components to prevent donor lymphocyte proliferation
Haemosiderosis/iron overload in frequently transfused patients	Skin pigmentation Cirrhosis of the liver Heart failure/ arrhythmias		Iron chelation therapy when the serum ferritin level >1000 µ/L and the total-iron binding capacity >10.8 Subcutaneous infusion of desferrioxamine: 30–50 mg/kg body weight/day using a syringe driver pump over 8–12 hours at least 5 times a week

- Hepatitis B
- Hepatitis C
- CMV
- Chagas disease
- Malaria
- Syphilis
- HTLV-I & II.

Effective laboratory and donor selection tests have been developed and introduced to detect and exclude blood donations that could transmit these infections to a recipient (McClelland 2001). As a result, the incidence of these infections is very low. In the UK in 2001, the risk that a unit of blood might transmit one of the viruses for which every donation is tested was estimated as less than 1 in 4 million for HIV, around 1 in 100,000 for hepatitis B and less than 1 in 400,000 for hepatitis C (anti-HCV tested). For components tested for both anti-HCV and HCV RNA the risk was less than 1 in a million (McClelland 2001). Bacterial infection remains the largest infection-related risk reported in the UK, over a 7-year period 26 of the 40 confirmed cases reported to SHOT involved bacterial-contaminated units (Stainsby et al 2003).

Transfusion services have taken steps to reduce the number of possible infections. These include the diversion of the first few ml of the donation (likely to contain any organisms entering the collection needle from the venepuncture site), improvements in cleansing techniques of donors' arms, and the introduction of bacterial culture of platelets before issue from the hospital transfusion laboratory. Practitioners should ensure that when administering any blood component a visual inspection of the unit for any irregular appearances is undertaken to prevent this avoidable complication of transfusion.

The risk of acquiring vCJD from a blood transfusion remains uncertain. In late 2003, the first possible transmission of variant Creutzfeldt–Jakob Disease (vCJD) by blood transfusion was described (Llewellyn et al 2004). A second possible transmission was reported in 2004 (Peden et al 2004).

Having a blood transfusion can never be totally without risk; however, correctly used blood products can save lives and improve quality of life for patients undergoing life-threatening treatments. The UK Departments of Health have promoted the appropriate use of blood and alternatives throughout the NHS by publishing advice for clinical staff involved in the transfusion process (DOH 1998b, 2002, SEHD 1999). Local protocols (based on national guidelines wherever possible) should guide practice. Where guidelines are unavailable practice should be based on best available evidence.

CONSENT FOR TRANSFUSION

At present, there is no legal requirement in the UK to gain specific consent from a patient for the transfusion of blood components. It is, however, usually sought as part of general consent (DOH 2001). Consent to transfusion may be given implicitly, orally or in writing and must be bestowed voluntarily and not under any form of duress or undue influence. For the consent process to be valid, the patient must be competent and have received sufficient information to make an informed decision, i.e. about the benefits, risks and expected outcomes of the transfusion. Patient information leaflets are useful aids to promoting discussion with a patient who may, or is about to, undergo transfusion therapy for the treatment of a haematological cancer. They should never be used, however, as a substitute for providing specific guidance or advice on transfusion therapy to the patient. Transfusion leaflets are available from the UK blood transfusion services.

CONCLUSION

The Nursing and Midwifery Council has stated that administering medicines, which include blood components, is 'not a mechanistic task'. Rather, the process requires reflection and exercise of professional judgement in order to minimise risk to the patient (NMC 2002). Nurses can demonstrate their skill and competency when involved in the blood transfusion process by ensuring compliance to protocols and guidelines in areas such as patient identification and record-keeping. If patients with haematological cancers are to continue to benefit from transfusion support, we must ensure that we provide safe and effective treatment during each and every transfusion episode.

DISCUSSION QUESTIONS

1. A patient who has been newly diagnosed with acute leukaemia is about to commence her conditioning treatment before haemopoietic stem cell transplant. She confides in you that she is concerned about the risks associated with blood transfusion and would like more information before she proceeds with her treatment. What can you do to ensure that the patient receives the appropriate information and support?

2. In your clinical area are there initiatives that could be undertaken to improve the safety for individuals receiving blood component therapy?

References

British Committee for Standards in Haematology 1996a Guidelines on gamma irradiation of blood components for the prevention of transfusion-associated graft-versus-host disease. Transfusion Medicine 6:261–271

British Committee for Standards in Haematology 1996b Guidelines on pre-transfusion compatibility procedures in blood transfusion laboratories. Transfusion Medicine 6:273–283

British Committee for Standards in Haematology 1998 Guidelines on the clinical use of leucocyte-depleted blood components. Transfusion Medicine 8:59–71

British Committee for Standards in Haematology 1999 Guidelines for the administration of blood and blood components and the management of transfused patients. Transfusion Medicine 9: 227–238

British Committee for Standards in Haematology 2001 Guidelines for the clinical use of red cell transfusions. British Journal of Haematology 113:24–31

British Committee for Standards in Haematology 2003 Guidelines for platelet transfusions. British Journal of Haematology 122:10–23

Department of Health 1998a Press release: Committee on Safety of Medicines – Review of Blood Products. DOH, London

Department of Health 1998b Better Blood Transfusion, HSC 1998/224. DOH, London

Department of Health 2001 Good practice in consent implementation guideline: consent to examination or treatment. Health Services Circular 2001/023. DOH, London

Department of Health 2002 Better Blood Transfusion – Appropriate Use of Blood. HSC 2002/009 (England); WHC 2002/137 (Wales); HSS(MD) 6/03 (Northern Ireland); NHSHDL 2003/19 (Scotland)

Freireich E J 2000 Supportive care for patients with blood disorders. British Journal of Haematology 111:68–77

Llewellyn C A, Hewitt P E, Knight R S G et al 2004 Possible transmission of variant Creutzfeldt–Jakob disease by blood transfusion. Lancet 363:417–421

Love E M, Jones H, Williamson A et al 2002 Serious hazards of transfusion annual report 2000/2001. SHOT, London

McClelland D B L (ed) 2001 Handbook of transfusion medicine, 3rd edn. HMSO, London

Murphy M F, Pamphilon D H 2001 Practical transfusion medicine. Blackwell Science, Oxford

Nursing & Midwifery Council 2002 Guidelines for administration of medicines. NMC, London

Peden A H, Head M W, Ritchie D L et al 2004 Preclinical vCJD after blood transfusion in a PRNP codon 129 heterozygous patient. Lancet 364:527–529

Scottish Executive Health Department 1999 NHSMEL Better Blood Transfusion. SEHD, Edinburgh

Stainsby D, Jones H, Knowles S et al 2003 Serious hazards of transfusion annual report 2001–2002. SHOT, London

Standing Advisory Committee on Transfusion Transmitted Infections 2004 Creutzfeldt–Jakob Disease: United Kingdom Blood Transfusion Services Position Statement. vCJD Working Party

Wilkins P 2000 Blood component support. In: Grundy M (ed) Nursing in haematological oncology. Baillière Tindall, Edinburgh, pp 156–170

Further reading

British Committee for Standards in Haematology (BCSH) Guidelines http://www.bcshguidelines.com
An excellent resource which allows you to download all the current UK transfusion guidelines.

McClelland D B L (ed) 2001 Handbook of transfusion medicine, 3rd edn. HMSO, London. http://www.transfusionguidelines.org
A comprehensive online resource covering all aspects of transfusion medicine.

Murphy M F, Pamphilon D H 2001 Practical transfusion medicine. Blackwell Science, Oxford
An in-depth book, useful for those wanting a greater understanding of transfusion medicine.

Royal College of Nursing 2004 RCN guidance on improving transfusion practice: right blood, right patient, right time. RCN, London. http://rcn.org.uk

An essential practical guide to the transfusion process for nurses involved in administering blood component therapy.

Scottish National Blood Transfusion Service. Better Blood Transfusion Continuing Education Programme: Safe Transfusion Practice. http://www.learnbloodtransfusion.org.uk
An online continuing education programme which has been designed to assist practitioners involved in the transfusion process in providing consistently high standards of care.

Serious Hazards of Transfusion Reporting Scheme http://www.shot-org.uk
Provides access to the most up-to-date haemovigilance data from the UK reporting scheme.

Chapter 13

Blood and marrow transplantation

Carol Richardson and Joanne Atkinson

KEY POINTS

- Blood and marrow transplantation is a complex undertaking that requires expert care and an up-to-date knowledge base.
- The aim of haemopoietic transplantation is the elimination of the underlying disease in the recipient, together with the full restoration of haemopoietic and immune function.
- Care continues for years post-transplant and long-term follow-up is essential.

INTRODUCTION

Blood and marrow transplantation is an evolutionary sphere of clinical practice. Bone marrow (BM) and peripheral blood stem cell (PBSC) transplantation have emerged as important treatments for many people with both malignant and non-malignant conditions who would otherwise have died of their disease. In the last two decades transplantation has developed from an experimental therapy to a treatment of choice for some diseases. Dramatic knowledge development and scientific breakthroughs have increased survival and improved quality of life for the transplant patient.

A transplant is the infusion of haemopoietic stem cells, the source of which may be bone marrow, peripheral blood or umbilical cord blood. Before receiving stem cells, patients are given a preparatory regime, known as conditioning. This is comprised of high-dose chemotherapy and/or total body irradiation (radiotherapy). Conditioning regimens destroy all myeloid and lymphoid blood cells, causing immunosuppression and destroying all protection against infection. Following infusion the transplanted stem cells repopulate the bone marrow (engraftment) allowing recovery from myelosuppression (Whedon & Wujcik 1997). The concept of transplanting cells appears simple; however, life-threatening side effects and toxicities make caring for transplant patients extremely complex. It requires a highly specialised team of health-care professionals, specialised technology, a strong scientific interface and an appropriate environment. Transplant nurses play a major role in the success of transplantation.

DISEASES REQUIRING TRANSPLANTATION

Haemopoietic stem cell transplant is the sole chance of cure for a number of haematological conditions and can also be considered the best possible treatment option for a number of other diseases as it may prolong disease-free survival. The indications for transplantation are constantly being evaluated through randomised controlled studies (RCTs) particularly in relation to haematological cancers. Transplants may be either allogeneic (from a donor) or autologous (patients own cells). Different types of transplant are suitable for different diseases and these are illustrated in Tables 13.1 and 13.2.

Table 13.1
Diseases for which allogeneic transplant is used (adapted from Duncombe 1997)

Sole chance of cure	Improved disease–free survival over conventional treatment
Primary immunodeficiency syndromes	Acute myeloid leukaemia (AML) (first or second remission)
Aplastic anaemia	Acute lymphoblastic leukaemia (ALL) (first or second remission adults only)
Thalassaemia	Myelodysplasia
Sickle cell disease	Multiple myeloma
Inborn errors of metabolism	
Chronic myeloid leukaemia (CML)	

Table 13.2
Diseases for which
autologous transplant is used
(adapted from Duncombe
1997)

Proven benefit in RCT	Probable benefit	Possible benefit
Non-Hodgkin's lymphoma	Relapsed Hodgkin's lymphoma	Chronic myeloid leukaemia
Acute myeloid leukaemia	Acute lymphoblastic leukaemia	Disseminated breast cancer
Multiple myeloma	Relapsed testicular cancer	Disseminated lung cancer Other solid tumours Severe autoimmune disease

PATIENT SELECTION

As haemopoietic stem cell transplantation has evolved, the procedure has become more refined and outcomes have improved. An individual's eligibility for transplant is assessed by several factors including:

- age
- response of disease to treatment
- stage of disease
- disease-free stem cell source.

Over time newer treatment modalities have become available, changing the parameters for patient selection. However, consideration must be given to organ function, performance status and overall disease status, as well as the psychosocial status of the individual (Wingard 1994). These are essential considerations as transplantation includes aggressive therapy and the individual needs to be in the best possible health to withstand this treatment (Outhwaite 2000).

TYPES OF TRANSPLANT

Transplants are categorised according to the type of donor (Balsdon & Craig 2003).

AUTOLOGOUS TRANSPLANTS

Autologous transplantation uses the patient's own cells, in other words the donor and the recipient are the same person. Stem cells are harvested when the patient is in clinical remission and either used at the time of harvest or cryopreserved to be used at a later date. Autologous transplantation is a very different procedure from allogeneic transplant, largely due to decreased toxicity and fewer side effects (Outhwaite 2000). For this reason autologous transplant can be used for the older person and individuals who are less able to withstand more aggressive treatments, e.g. those with co-morbidity. There are concerns about the greater risk of relapse with autologous transplants because of the potential for malignant cells to remain in the marrow and reproduce. However, for most patients the improvement in quality of life far outweighs the risk.

Autologous transplant can also be used when dose escalation of chemotherapy is required to prevent catastrophic side effects from prolonged pancytopenia. This has application in the solid tumour setting. Although transplantation with the patient's own haemopoietic stem cells will not cause the same toxic side effects as a donor transplant, the difficulty of the procedure must not be underestimated. Expert care and support are required for the transplant to be successful.

Numerous studies have been undertaken in order to minimise relapse and select certain types of cells for transplant, in the hope that restoration of marrow function could be expedited and disease-free survival improved. The results of such trials have so far been disappointing. However, the advent of new therapeutics and novel approaches with monoclonal antibodies continue to be reviewed.

ALLOGENEIC TRANSPLANTS

A human leucocyte antigen (HLA) matched donor is required for an allogeneic transplant. Allogeneic transplantation is a more complex procedure than autologous transplantation. It results in greater toxicity from the conditioning regimens and marrow aplasia, as well as from other complications related to the transplant process such as graft-versus-host disease (GvHD), veno-occlusive disease of the liver and interstitial pneumonitis. However, toxicity is balanced against the advantages of this procedure – receiving disease-free cells and the immunological graft-versus-leukaemia (GvL) effect that can reduce the risk of disease relapse (Balsdon & Craig 2003).

GvL or graft-versus-tumour (GvT) effects are believed to be the main reason that haemopoietic stem cell transplantation leads to long-term disease-free survival. These effects occur when the donor's immune cells, principally T lymphocytes and natural killer (NK) cells, recognise and kill any remaining tumour cells in the recipient's haematopoietic and lymphoid system. As GvL is part of the donor's immune response against the recipient, it is associated with the occurrence of GvHD. Patients who suffer GvHD are, on average, more likely to benefit from GvL effects than patients who do not develop GvHD. Although GvHD can be prevented with strong prophylaxis, such as donor T-cell depletion, this may increase the risk of relapse owing to a lack of GvL. In general, it is desirable to achieve a mild to moderate level of GvHD after transplantation to foster some degree of GvL. However, not every patient who suffers GvHD will have an effective GvL response and unfortunately some will still relapse. The effect of GvL also varies from one disease to another, with CML stimulating the best GvL response and ALL probably the weakest.

Tissue typing

Tissue typing is the process of matching donor and recipient tissue. Potential donors are tested for HLA compatibility and are HLA-typed by at least two blood tests that can detect human leucocyte antigen (expressed on the cell's surface). The first blood test is used to detect the unique combination of antigens which determines the tissue type. The second blood test, such as the mixed lymphocyte/culture (MLC) test, is used to assess whether or not the patient and donor's bone marrow interact adversely.

Scientific developments have led to more precise HLA typing through the examination of DNA. DNA has enabled HLA matching to be detected at a molecular level ensuring greater precision in the HLA typing process. The HLA complex is located on chromosome 6 and consists of HLA A, B, C, DR, DQ and DP antigens or loci. For transplant purposes antigens are split into two classes. Class 1 antigens are found on the surface of most human cells and are easily detected on leucocytes, they include antigens or loci A, B and C. Class 2 antigens are widely distributed and are especially evident on B lymphocytes; they include DR, DP and DQ loci or antigens. The search for compatibility involves comparing HLA A, B and DR antigens. These antigens are the most important to consider in relation to the patient's predisposition to develop GvHD. From each of these three loci, two antigens should be matched ideally (Whedon & Wujcik 1997).

The ideal donor is identical to the recipient, although ABO blood group mismatch may be considered. However, if donor and recipient are ABO mismatched, great caution needs to be exercised during the recovery phase when the patient requires repeated blood product support. Planning and discussion are required pre-transplant in the case of ABO mismatch in order to deplete red cells in the donated marrow and minimise major incompatibility and transfusion hazard. Donors are routinely screened in the same way as the recipients for infections and viruses. Within many transplant centres blood is taken to analyse polymorphic markers in donor DNA. Results of these tests are used to determine the numbers of donor cells and recipient cells in the blood and marrow of the recipient post-transplant and are known as chimerism studies. The term originates from the name of a mythic beast, the Chimera (part lion, goat and snake), and is used to describe a situation where there is effectively a mixture of two individuals present after transplantation.

Full medical history is also required and special attention should be given to psychological morbidity to ensure donors are able to cope with the process of blood or marrow cell donation, the potential for an adverse outcome for the recipient, and the impact donation may have on the recipient.

Distinctions are made between different types of allogeneic transplant.

Sibling allogeneic transplant

The ideal donor and the patient's greatest chance of a full HLA match is with a sibling. An average recipient in western countries has about a 1 in 4 chance of having a sibling who is fully HLA matched (Duncombe 1997).

Syngeneic transplants

Transplants between identical twins are termed syngeneic. This type of transplant is rare. Stem cells are collected from a genetically identical twin. Although this type of transplant uses a donor, in effect it may be comparable to an autologous transplant. There is said to be very little GvL effect and hence a greater risk of relapse (Balsdon & Craig 2003).

Volunteer unrelated transplant

Whilst a compatible sibling offers the best chance of an HLA-matched donor, the majority of patients will require a search for a volunteer donor from a donor panel (Duncombe 1997). Volunteer bone marrow donor registries have been established internationally and healthy volunteers act as HLA-matched donors for patients requiring transplant. National and international donor registries keep details of blood donors/bone marrow donors, including their HLA type, and use computerised systems to find the donor with the best match for the potential transplant recipient.

The two main donor registries in the United Kingdom are the Anthony Nolan Bone Marrow Transplant Trust and the British Bone Marrow and Platelet Donor Panel. The chance of obtaining a match from a bone marrow registry is dependent on how frequently a person's HLA profile appears in the donor population (Campbell 1997). Although the size of bone marrow registries is increasing, the heterogeneity of the HLA complex means there is still a shortage of appropriately matched donors for all potential recipients. Recipients from ethnic minorities have even less probability of achieving an HLA match through this route as they are seriously under-represented on the marrow registries (Outhwaite 2000).

CORD BLOOD TRANSPLANTS

Cord blood transplantation remains a specialised procedure more relevant for some areas of transplantation than others, e.g. in the paediatric setting. Cord blood banks were established to increase the number of different HLA-type donations available (Balsdon & Craig 2003). However, the number of stem cells present may only be sufficient to transplant a child. Further research may advance this area of practice, although it is an established treatment in both paediatric and adult settings (Rocha et al 2004, Barker et al 2005).

THE TRANSPLANT PROCESS

PRE-TRANSPLANT PHASE

The risks of transplant are considered with the patient in this phase. The type of transplant procedure performed should be the least toxic for the patient to achieve potential cure or long-term remission from their disease (Balsdon & Craig 2003). Prior to transplant patients must undergo physical as well as psychological assessments to determine their eligibility for the procedure (Whedon & Wujcik 1997) – the pre-transplant work up. A multidisciplinary team delivers effective transplant care and ideally at this stage the patient should be introduced to all members of this team. The main issues to be considered with the patient will include:

- consent for transplant
- risks and benefits of transplant – this is closely linked to the consent process
- fertility issues – sperm banking and egg cryopreservation should be discussed
- dental appointment – remedial treatment may be required to minimise the infection risk during transplant
- pre-transplant appointments – for example if radiotherapy is to be included in the conditioning regimen, then referral to a specialist oncology centre is required to discuss planning and short- and long-term side effects
- long line insertion
- pre-transplant investigations
  - full blood count
  - blood group
  - kidney function tests
  - liver function tests
  - biochemistry
  - virology specimens
  - samples for specialist analysis, e.g. bcr-abl oncogene in CML (see Chapter 4)
  - ethylene diaminetetracetic acid (EDTA)
  - lung function tests
  - electrocardiogram (ECG)/echocardiogram
  - chest x-ray
  - swabs and samples for infection screening.

The specialist nurse plays a key role in the coordination and delivery of pre-transplant care. The role includes the planning and organisation of investigations and procedures, searches for potential donors from the donor registries and siblings, harvesting of bone marrow and, most especially, assessment of the recipient. Careful assessment can highlight issues that may be problematic in the recovery phase and enable the transplant team to carefully plan possible interventions and support for patients and their families. The role of the bone marrow transplant specialist is firmly rooted in the multidisciplinary team to ensure quality and continuity.

Psychological assessment is essential to fully prepare the patient for this intensive procedure. Individuals may require input from other members of the multidisciplinary team, for example social workers and clinical psychologists. The needs of carers should also be considered at this time. Written information regarding the transplant work-up and the transplant process should be given to the patient and their carers. It is essential that everyone is made aware of the implications of having a dysfunctional bone marrow. This is an extremely stressful and anxious time for both patients and their families and it is imperative that nurses allow sufficient time for everyone to ask questions and express their concerns and fears.

HARVESTING PROCEDURES

Harvesting refers to the procedures used to obtain haemopoietic stem cells for transplantation.

Sources of stem cells

Stem cells may be obtained from bone marrow, peripheral blood or the umbilical cord. Traditionally the bone marrow was used as the primary source of stem cells for transplantation. However, more recently alternative sources of stem cells have been used and, due to scientific and technological advances, the use of peripheral blood stem cells (PBSCs) has superseded bone marrow in many transplant centres. PBSCs are now used in both allogeneic and autologous settings, with the advantage of more rapid engraftment (Soutar & King 1995).

Harvesting bone marrow

Bone marrow harvest requires a general anaesthetic whether the procedure is undertaken for donors or recipients. Standard preoperative care is essential and a full patient profile is required, which includes chest x-ray and ECG, full haematological blood screen, biochemistry, blood group, and safe and autologous blood donations for use if blood transfusion is required. Full viral screen is essential to establish previous viral infections and highlight the need for surveillance of viral reactivation post-transplant. This must include human immunodeficiency virus (HIV), hepatitis screen, cytomegalovirus (CMV), herpes simplex virus (HSV), and varicella zoster virus (VZV).

The patient is taken to theatre and laid prone. Bone marrow biopsy needles are inserted into the posterior iliac crests and repeated aspirations performed. Once a sufficient number of cells have been gathered, the marrow is either frozen and stored or given fresh to the recipient. The usual volume of bone marrow removed is 800–1000 mL in order to acquire 100–300 million cells per kilogram of the recipient's body weight (Outhwaite 2000). Despite the volume of marrow retrieved at harvest it is quickly regenerated and has little effect on the donor's haemodynamic status, although occasionally a top-up blood transfusion is required. Usually an autologous blood donation is used. Donating marrow can be a painful procedure and there is obviously a small anaesthetic risk. Both donors and recipients are given time to discuss these issues during the pre-transplant work up.

Mobilisation and harvesting cells from peripheral blood

Fewer stem cells are normally found in the bloodstream than in the bone marrow. Mobilisation of progenitor cells is therefore required in order to expand the number available for harvest. Chemotherapy causes an increase in the number of circulating progenitor cells in the peripheral blood, and stem cells can therefore be collected from the peripheral blood following chemotherapy. However, the true revolution in the mobilisation and collection of peripheral blood stem cells followed the development of specific haemopoietic growth factors such as granulocyte-colony stimulating factor (G-CSF) and granulocyte-monocyte colony stimulating factor (GM-CSF), which elevate the number of progenitor cells in the peripheral blood. In some patients both chemotherapy and growth factors are utilised to stimulate progenitor cell proliferation. For donors chemotherapy cannot be used and G-CSF alone is administered.

Collection or harvest of stem cells is performed using an apheresis machine. Good venous access is required, which may require long line insertion if access is poor. Regular observations are undertaken and although side effects are minimal, transient hypocalcaemia may occur. Bone pain and flu-like symptoms as a result of G-CSF therapy may also occur. Blood counts are monitored closely during the pre-harvest period in order to determine the increase in circulating white cells and establish the optimum time for harvest. Most specialist centres now use cluster of differentiation 34 (CD34) analysis (the most established surrogate stem cell marker) to decide when apheresis starts. Ideally peripheral blood CD34 counts should exceed $20/\mu L$ before harvesting commences. Post-harvest, cells may be used immediately or cryopreserved for use at a later date.

Harvesting peripheral blood stem cells is a far less invasive procedure than harvesting bone marrow. Engraftment is also faster with the use of peripheral blood stem cells. One of the explanations for more rapid engraftment is that a higher number of more mature progenitor cells are present in peripheral stem cell grafts than in marrow grafts (Gisselbrecht et al 1994). Whilst it can be argued that faster engraftment results in less supportive therapy and reduced risk of infectious complications, studies have failed to show a marked reduction in the number of febrile episodes or verified infections (Larsson et al 1998).

Although collecting stem cells from peripheral blood offers donors a far less invasive procedure than marrow harvest, the use of growth factors requires careful discussion and should be backed up with written information. Risks to a healthy donor such as bone pain and flu-like illnesses are significantly less than previously thought. Consent is of paramount importance and the British Bone Marrow Registry has produced an information resource on the use of G-CSF for healthy donors.

CONDITIONING TREATMENTS

Following physical and psychological assessment and harvesting of haemopoietic stem cells preparatory conditioning therapy is administered. Conditioning refers to the chemotherapy and/or radiotherapy given prior to stem cell infusion and is intended to (Apperley et al 1998):

- eradicate residual disease
- promote immunosuppression in order to prevent rejection although this increases the risk of infection
- create bone marrow space.

Conditioning regimens vary according to the disease and medical condition of the patient. High-dose chemotherapy may be given alone or in conjunction with total body irradiation (TBI), this is dependent on the disease process and status, and careful patient selection. In allogeneic transplantation immunosuppressive therapy is also commenced to reduce the potential for GvHD (Balsdon & Craig 2003). Figures 13.1, 13.2 and 13.3 illustrate conditioning protocols for allogeneic and autologous transplant.

The ideal preparatory regimen is capable of eradicating any remaining malignant cells and it is a fine balancing act achieving sufficient immunosuppressive effect and tolerable morbidity without mortality (Forman & Bloome 1994). This is especially important as chemotherapy and radiotherapy doses used in conditioning regimens are much higher than those normally used; consequently the side effects and toxicities are much greater. Combination conditioning further exacerbates toxicities.

However, recent developments have allowed adjustments to be made to conditioning regimens to reduce overall toxicity in allogeneic or unrelated donor settings; this is called non-myeloablative, reduced intensity or mini-transplantation (Balsdon & Craig 2003). These transplants rely on the immune component (GvL effect) to destroy disease rather than high doses of chemo/radiotherapy, allowing transplant to be used in a wider range of patients. However, long-term effects on disease have not been established and relapse remains a significant risk.

THE TRANSPLANT

The transplant takes place within 24–48 hours of completing conditioning treatment. Stem cells are infused through a blood product administration set via a central venous catheter. The day of the transplant is generally considered as Day 0. The cells migrate to the bone marrow space by a poorly understood mechanism; however normal haemopoiesis does not commence at this point (Soutar & King 1995).

THE PROCESS

Patients may receive fresh or cryopreserved cells. Cells are cryopreserved using dimethylsulfoxide (DMSO), which can induce nausea, vomiting, chills and fever (Balsdon & Craig 2003). If the cells have been cryopreserved, they are thawed in a water bath at approximately 37°C and need to be infused quickly to prevent cell death. The patient must be closely monitored and informed that side effects similar to those experienced during blood component administration may occur. The preservative

Figure 13.1
Allogeneic transplant protocol:
Busulphan 16 mg/kg;
Cyclophosphamide 120 mg/kg

RECIPIENT

Name		Number		Dr	
dd.mm.yy	cm	kg	kg ideal	m² ideal	

Indication:					

HLA	A	B	Cw	DR	DQ	DP
CMV:			GROUP:			

DONOR

Name		Number	
dd.mm.yy/yrs	parity:	relationship:	

HLA:	Stem cells:
CMV:	GROUP:

PROCEDURE

Admission:	Long line:
Transplant:	
Blood products:	
Drug allergy:	
Other requirements:	

Day	Mo 200		
−8	T		Phenytoin 1 g
−7	W		Busulphan 4 mg/kg Start Phenytoin 300 mg daily
−6	Th		Busulphan 4 mg/kg
−5	F		Busulphan 4 mg/kg
−4	S		Busulphan 4 mg/kg
−3	S		MESNA 25 mg/kg; Cyclophosphamide 60 mg/kg/1 h MESNA 95 mg/kg/22 h
−2	M		MESNA 25 mg/kg; Cyclophosphamide 60 mg/kg/1 h MESNA 95 mg/kg/22 h
−1	T		Ciclosporin 5 mg/kg daily
0	W		STEM CELL INFUSION
1	Th		Reduce Ciclosporin to 3 mg/kg daily MTX 15 mg/m²
2	F		FOLINIC ACID Stop Phenytoin 300 mg daily
3	S		MTX 10 mg/m²
4	S		FOLINIC ACID
5	M		Check Ciclosporin TARGET 300 mg/ml
6	T		MTX 10 mg/m²
7	W		FOLINIC ACID

Figure 13.2
Allogeneic transplant protocol:
Fludarabine 150 mg/m²;
Melphalan 140 mg/m²;
CAMPATH 100 mg

RECIPIENT

Name		Number		Dr	
dd.mm.yy	cm	kg	kg ideal	m² ideal	

Disease: diagnosed: stage at transplant:

HLA						
A*	B*	Cw*	DRB1*	DQB1*	DPB1*	
CMV:				GROUP:		

DONOR

Name		Number	
dd.mm.yy/yrs	parity:	relationship:	
HLA:		Stem cells:	
CMV:		GROUP:	

PROCEDURE

Admission:	Long line:
Transplant:	
Blood products:	
Drug allergy:	
Other requirements:	

Day	Mo 200		
−7	W		Fludarabine 30 mg/m²
			Methylprednisolone 2 mg/kg; CAMPATH 20 mg
−6	Th		Fludarabine 30 mg/m²; CAMPATH 20 mg
−5	F		Fludarabine 30 mg/m²; CAMPATH 20 mg
−4	S		Fludarabine 30 mg/m²; CAMPATH 20 mg
−3	S		Fludarabine 30 mg/m²; CAMPATH 20 mg
−2	M		Melphalan 140 mg/m²
−1	T		Start Ciclosporin 5 mg/kg daily
0	W		STEM CELL INFUSION
1	Th		Reduce Ciclosporin to 3 mg/kg
2	F		Check Ciclosporin level TARGET 200 mg/mL

Figure 13.3
Autologous transplant
protocol: PBSC + Melphalan
only

PATIENT

Name		Number		Dr	
dd.mm.yy	cm	kg	kg ideal	m² ideal ()	

Indication: Myeloma diagnosed
CXR:
ECG:
GFR: ml/min/1.7 m²

PBSC

Stored on:
CD34/kg:
Reinfusion:

PROCEDURE

Admission:
Long line:
Transplant:
Drug allergy:
Other requirements:

Day	Feb 2004		
−2	M	23	Melphalan 200 mg/m²
−1	T	24	
0	Th	25	STEM CELL INFUSION (afternoon)

used may cause unpleasant side effects. Patients report a strange taste and a sweet unpleasant smell exudes from the patient's breath and sweat. The smell diffuses around the patient and is present in the atmosphere in the area for around 24–48 hours. Apart from the unpleasant taste and smell all other side effects can be minimised by prophylactic steroids and antihistamines.

For many patients the psychological impact of reaching the day of transplant is overwhelming. They are aware of the implications of not having a functioning bone marrow and are also cognisant of the difficult recovery process ahead. There is often a sense of anticlimax and anticipation. It is essential that health-care professionals caring for patients and their families at this stage of transplant are supportive, knowledgeable and understanding. Most importantly the psychological impact of transplantation should be acknowledged.

SUPPORTIVE CARE DURING ENGRAFTMENT

The 2–4 weeks immediately following transplant when patients are pancytopenic due to the conditioning therapy are critical. Engraftment is said to have occurred when the transplanted cells have migrated to the bone marrow and normal haemopoiesis has returned. This is patient and transplant dependent and can take 10–21 days. Expert nursing knowledge and skills are required at this time to assess, detect, prevent and manage what are often difficult complications impeding patient recovery. Complications are largely dependent on the type of transplant, age and general condition of the patient and the conditioning regimen. Some of the side effects of transplantation experienced as a result of high-dose therapy are discussed in Chapters 9 and 10. However, it is important to consider specific acute and chronic complications that occur post-transplant.

ACUTE COMPLICATIONS POST-TRANSPLANT

Infection

Post-allogeneic and post-autologous transplant patients are inevitably at risk from bacterial, viral and fungal infections. When assessing patients it is important to consider a number of variables including (Wujcik et al 1994):

- previous history of viral infection
- type of transplant
- damaged oral or gastrointestinal mucosa
- degree of neutropenia
- use of central venous catheters
- conditioning regimen.

In the allogeneic setting patients have an added risk from immunosuppressive therapy. Prevention of infection is a key priority and includes prophylactic antibacterial and antiviral therapy administered according to local and national protocols. Protective isolation is standard following transplant, although there is conflicting information on the value of isolation and hepa-filtration for patients undergoing transplantation (National Institute for Clinical Excellence (NICE) 2003). However, there are no robust randomised studies addressing these issues. Although bone marrow registry data analysis of large numbers of patients nursed in isolation suggest that hepa-filtration and laminar airflow are beneficial, other randomised studies have found that similar outcomes (in terms of infection rates) can be achieved using standard room isolation (NICE 2003); further research is required (Parker 1999). This lack of robust evidence means that different units may adopt different policies and apply these for varying periods of time (Kelly 2000).

The psychological impact of isolation needs to be carefully assessed. Patients may feel very vulnerable and out of control. They are removed from their familiar surroundings and also have limited contact with the outside world (Baker et al 1999). Acknowledging these difficulties can help patients to feel more supported and able to discuss their fears and anxieties with the transplant team.

Bacterial infections

Bacterial infections are the most common infections post-transplant. Key issues in managing bacterial infection are vigilance, early detection and prompt treatment (see Chapter 15). In the transplant setting management of bacterial infection often results in the use of a combination of antibiotics (according to local guidelines). Most antibiotic regimens are designed to cover Gram-negative and Gram-positive organisms. Empiric treatment is usually initiated when patients become febrile. Close liaison with the microbiologist is essential.

Viral infections

The most common viral infections following transplantation are reactivation of cytomegalovirus (CMV) and herpes simplex virus (HSV). Management of HSV begins with prophylaxis. Acyclovir is a common antiviral agent administered to prevent the reactivation of the HSV and to treat other herpes infections. It is usually commenced 7 days prior to transplant, although this may vary according to local guidelines. CMV reactivation is more common in the allogeneic setting. Blood surveillance should be commenced on or around Day +14 post-transplant to obtain baseline levels and for the detection of reactivation which occurs from around day +21 as engraftment occurs. Early detection and treatment with ganciclovir is essential. Other common viral infections include respiratory syncytial virus (RSV), parainfluenza viruses and adenovirus. The management of viral infections has been transformed in the last decade due to better surveillance and increased treatment options.

Fungal infections

During the acute phase post-transplant the risk of developing a fungal infection is directly related to the duration and severity of neutropenia (Whedon & Wujcik 1997). Environmental factors such as nearby construction and renovation work can contribute to the development of fungal infections such as aspergillus and candida species. Prophylaxis with antifungal agents is administered as per local protocols.

Anaemia and thrombocytopenia

Thrombocytopenia can be problematic post-transplant and may be prolonged in some patients. Platelet transfusions minimise the risk of bleeding complications. Guidelines and local policies related to platelet counts are in place in order to safeguard the patient. Platelet counts should ideally be kept over $10 \times 10^9/L$ with regular platelet transfusions as required (Whedon & Wujcik 1997). Whilst clear parameters are useful, in some cases excessive platelet consumption may require very regular platelet transfusions, e.g. in the case of infection or haemorrhage (see Chapter 16). Prophylactic platelet transfusions are given prior to invasive procedures.

Anaemia can also be problematic post-transplant. Ideally the patient's haemoglobin should be maintained over 10g/L (Whedon & Wujcik 1997). However, the transplant team should pay heed to the number of blood transfusions given to the patient as previous transfusions may have elevated the patient's ferritin levels. Excessive ferritin can lead to liver impairment post-transplant and patients may require venesection. Sensitive thought needs to be employed in order to balance patient comfort during transplant with post-transplant complications. When dealing with anaemia and thrombocytopenia, the key issue is careful assessment and monitoring for the clinical manifestations that arise as a result of these problems.

Pulmonary complications

Pulmonary complications are a major cause of morbidity, affecting 40–60% of patients (Height & Shields 1995), and are the most common cause of death in the early post-transplant period. Complications include infection, fluid overload, cardiac failure, bleeding and non-infectious events (Balsdon & Craig 2003). Patients may develop pulmonary problems as a result of bacterial infection; *Pneumocystis carinii* pneumonia (PCP) is a common opportunistic infection that can affect patients in the transplant setting.

One of the major pulmonary complications is interstitial pneumonitis, a general term that refers to an inflammatory process involving the intra-alveolar lining of the lung, occuring most frequently between 30 and 100 days post-transplant. Many complex interacting factors contribute to its development including:

- immunosuppression
- existing lung damage
- conditioning treatment
- viruses – most commonly CMV.

Broncheoalveolar lavage remains the gold standard for diagnosing pneumonitis following transplant. The condition can be very difficult to treat and management is complex. If a specific pathogen or process is identified, tailored drug therapy can be instituted. The rapidity with which a specific diagnosis is made and effective therapy commenced is the most important variable in successful therapy (Quabeck 1994).

Gastrointestinal complications

Gastrointestinal complications can be both difficult to manage and difficult for the patient to tolerate. Many patients experience nausea and vomiting due to conditioning therapy and the drugs given as supportive therapy. Assessment and management of these symptoms with anti-emetic prophylaxis is very important (see Chapter 17).

Mucositis is a predictable consequence of conditioning therapy. Incidence rates vary – McGuire et al (1993) report 86% of patients undergoing allogeneic and autologous transplant develop mucositis. Conditioning regimens, particularly regimens containing busulphan, melphalan, etoposide and total body irradiation, predispose the patient to developing severe mucositis. Both conditioning and the transplant produce serious direct and indirect alterations in the oral mucosa owing to immunosuppression and acute GvHD. This may result in infection, bleeding and pain, and may significantly reduce the intake of food and fluids. Mucosal lesions typically present as burning and erythema progressing to diffuse, extensive painful oral ulcerations (Woo et al 1993). It can be difficult to distinguish between mucositis and acute graft-versus-host disease (GvHD).

The impact of mucositis on patients is huge, interfering with social interaction and causing psychological distress (Gaston-Johansson et al 1992). Patients undergoing transplant have stated that acute oral pain, mucositis and inability to eat are major sources of distress (Larson et al 1993). Pain needs careful assessment; management with intravenous opiates is indicated for effective pain relief. Pre-transplant dental referral, good oral hygiene, patient education and careful assessment cannot prevent the problem but may minimise the risk of superimposed infections.

Diarrhoea can occur as a direct result of effects of conditioning therapy on the gastrointestinal mucosa or from bacterial/viral infection. Diarrhoea in the immediate post-transplant period can be one of the most distressing side effects for the patient. Careful monitoring of fluid and electrolyte balance and assessment with regular screening is required. Again a distinction needs to be made between diarrhoea and acute GvHD of the gastrointestinal tract.

Hepatic complications

Abnormalities in liver function tests (LFTs) are common after transplantation, often as a result of infection or sepsis (Balsdon & Craig 2003). However, LFTs are carefully monitored to detect the onset of GvHD or veno-occlusive (VOD) disease of the liver. VOD of the liver can occur 1–3 weeks following allogeneic transplant. Patients with a previous history of liver disease are most susceptible, as are those who have received conditioning agents such as busulphan. Some transplant centres offer prophylactic defibrotide for the high-risk patient; however, this is not standard treatment and is dependent on the transplant centre.

Hepatic VOD is a serious complication that results from damage to the endothelium of the small intra-hepatic venules, with obstruction and hepatocyte destruction. It is a result of high-dose chemotherapy and/or total body irradiation, drug-induced toxicities associated with support medications, GvHD and infection (Whedon & Wujcik 1997). Symptoms include jaundice, tender hepatomegaly, abdominal distension from ascites and weight gain, which is dependent on the degree of VOD. Treatment of VOD is difficult and depends upon good fluid and electrolyte balance, which is managed by accurate fluid restriction and use of diuretics. Anti-thrombotic agents such as tissue plasminogen activator (tPA), defibrotide (Richardson et al 1998) and anticoagulants (Bearman et al 1997) may also be given. However, despite treatment, mortality is around 60% (Balsdon & Craig 2003).

Graft–versus–host disease in allografts

GvHD is caused by immunologically competent lymphocytes infused with the donor stem cells recognising the host tissue (recipient) as foreign and mounting an immune response. This inflammatory reaction is targeted at one or all of the following systems:

- the skin
- the liver
- the gastrointestinal tract.

GvHD can be classified as acute (less than 100 days after transplant) and chronic, which largely occurs after the first 3 months. Acute GvHD is not necessarily a precursor to the development of chronic GvHD; however, the majority of patients who develop the acute form will develop chronic GvHD.

Acute GvHD

Acute GvHD is graded according to severity, grade 1 being mild and grade 3–4 severe, often life-threatening.

- Skin – Usually an erythematous, maculopapular, pruritic rash appears, often on the hands and soles of the feet or behind the ears. The rash can spread to the face, trunk and extremities and in its most severe form can have the appearance of second-degree burns. A skin biopsy will confirm diagnosis and show lymphocyte infiltration and epithelial damage.
- Liver – involvement is manifested by an increase in serum bilirubin and enzymes. In its worst form fulminant liver failure may develop associated with a grave diagnosis. Liver biopsy is difficult to perform in patients with GvHD owing to problems with blood clotting and low platelet counts.
- Gastrointestinal tract – loss of epithelial tissue results in secretory diarrhoea, which may well be excessive (Table 13.3). Strict monitoring of fluid loss is required as this can lead to electrolyte imbalance. Chemotherapy-induced mucositis can often confound the diagnosis. Denudation of the GI tract may create a portal of entry for enteric organisms, which can lead to infection. GvHD can also be isolated to the upper GI tract with symptoms of anorexia, dyspepsia, nausea and vomiting. Biopsies are performed to confirm diagnosis and show similar findings to those of skin biopsy. Table 13.3 illustrates the classification of GvHD.

Prophylaxis One of the most important concepts of transplantation medicine is the prevention of GvHD through the use of immunosup-

Grade	Skin	Liver	GI tract	Quality of life change
1	1–2	0	0	None
2	1–3	1	1	Mild
3	2–3	2–3	2–3	Marked
4	2–4	2–4	2–4	Extreme

Key:
Skin – Determined by the extent of the rash on the body surface. 1 = <25%, 2 = 25–50%, 3 = generalised erythroedema, 4 = desquamation and bullae.
Liver – Determined by bilirubin concentration. 1 = 2.0–2.9 mg/dL, 2 = 3.0–5.9 mg/dL, 3 = 6.0–14.9 mg/dL, 4 = >15.0 mg/dL.
GI tract – Determined by daily volume of diarrhoea. 1 = 500–1000 mL, 2 = 1000–2000 mL, 3 = 1500–2000 mL, 4 = >2000 mL.

pressants. Ciclosporin is a potent immunosuppressant drug and the dose can be manipulated to increase or decrease immunosuppressant activity. When used in conjunction with methotrexate, the severity of GvHD and associated morbidity are reduced (Weaver et al 1994). However, the greater the T-cell depletion as a result of immunosuppression the higher the incidence of relapse. There is a fine balance between preventing GvHD and reducing the incidence of relapse as GvHD accounts for a significant morbidity and mortality rate in allogeneic transplantation. Ciclosporin is commenced prior to infusion of stem cells according to local policy, and regular monitoring of blood parameters is undertaken.

Treatment   The mainstay of treatment for GvHD is the use of high-dose corticosteroids in conjunction with ciclosporin therapy. Pulsed doses of corticosteroids are used to minimise side effects such as infection, high blood glucose, weight gain and Cushingoid appearance. If response is poor, other immunosuppressants such as tacrolimus may be used.

Chronic GvHD   Chronic GvHD normally develops around 3 months post-transplant; however, there have been reports of it occurring up to 2 years later (Whedon & Wujcik 1997). Chronic GvHD presents rather like autoimmune diseases such as scleroderma as it causes fibrosis and atrophy of one or more organs. The fibrotic and inflammatory changes that occur in chronic GvHD are marked and of prolonged duration. Although acute GvHD is often an antecedent of chronic GvHD, it may occur de novo. Chronic GvHD is a cause of significant morbidity and mortality for the transplant patient (Balsdon & Craig 2003) and has a serious effect on quality of life. Symptomatic management is very important to keep individuals as well as possible and promote a better quality of life. Table 13.4 illustrates the complexities and clinical manifestations of chronic GvHD. (Chronic GvHD of the mouth is shown in Plates 12 & 13; Plate 14 shows chronic GvHD of the skin.)

Table 13.4
Clinical manifestations of
chronic GvHD

Organ	Clinical features
Skin	Sclerodermatous skin, thinning and tightening, functional impact, red rash (lichenoid changes)
Hair	Thinning or alopecia, change in hair texture
Mouth	Dry, sensitive to heat and extremes of taste, white plaques on the inside of the cheeks and tongue (lichen planus), painful ulceration, mucosal scleroderma
Gastrointestinal system	Strictures, abnormal gut motility, weight loss
Liver	Cholestasis, abnormal liver function tests
Respiratory system	Bronchiolitis obliterans, chronic respiratory infections, sinusitis
Musculoskeletal system	Fasciitis, pain, osteoporosis
Eyes	Dry, risk of corneal abrasion and infection
Immune system	Profound immunosuppression, risk of sepsis, e.g. pneumococcal, pneumocystis and fungal infections
Haemopoietic system	Cytopenias, eosinophilia

LATE COMPLICATIONS OF TRANSPLANT

Graft rejection

Graft rejection can be defined as the inability of the recipient to accept the graft and is not to be confused with relapse. Rejection is uncommon but can occur up to 4 months following transplant, causing graft destruction by the immunologically competent cells of the host. Treatment consists of the administration of back-up autologous cells to 'rescue' the patient.

Relapse

Scientific advances enable potential relapse to be identified earlier. Molecular and chimerism studies have facilitated understanding of the pattern of relapse. Chimerism testing helps determine the state of engraftment and immune reconstitution, and detects early relapse. Most commonly chimerism results are expressed in terms of 'percentage donor' (the percentage of donor cells to recipient cells). Several misnomers abound: a patient is said to be a 'complete' or 'full' donor chimera when blood or bone marrow are 100% donor-derived and a 'partial' or 'incomplete' chimera when there are still recipient cells present.

Patients who have developed GvHD are more likely to be 100% donor than those who have not, because GvHD allows donor immunity to become fully established and eradicate any residual recipient cells from the blood or bone marrow. Partial donor chimerism may result from graft rejection, incomplete donor immune reconstitution, relapse or a combination of these.

Generally speaking, it is desirable to achieve nearly 100% donor chimerism as this ensures complete engraftment, full donor immune reconstitution and freedom from relapse. Partial donor chimerism after transplantation for malignant disease may herald relapse, either directly because tumour cells are starting to reappear in the blood or indirectly because donor immune reconstitution is not complete and relapse ensues due to inadequate GvL. Partial donor chimerism is more common after reduced intensity transplantation than myeloablative transplantation. Regular monitoring is important, as partial donor chimerism can be rectified by giving further donor lymphocyte infusions (DLI) before a relapse occurs. Donor lymphocytes produce an immune response against the recipient's cells. When DLI is given for partial chimerism, it is not uncommon to see a rise in donor chimerism at the same time as GvHD appears. As a fairly recent advance, longitudinal data related to survival following DLI are sparse; however, numerous studies are ongoing. Preliminary findings are favourable, particularly for specific diseases (e.g. CML).

Chronic infection

Late infectious complications are a multi-facetted phenomenon and can be a major cause of mortality due to functional hyposplenism or continued immunosuppression, particularly for those with chronic GvHD. The combined immunodeficiency affecting B and T cells may take months or even years to recover. The most common types of late infections include encapsulated organisms such as pneumococcal infections and viral infections. All patients need to be vaccinated 6–12 months following transplant depending on local protocols. Vaccination against tetanus, diphtheria, polio (inactivated), pneumococci, influenza and *Haemophilus influenzae* type B (HIB) needs to be undertaken as immunity to these organisms is lost through transplant.

Endocrine problems

The majority of allogeneic transplant patients will be rendered infertile. Both alkylating agents and total body irradiation result in gonadal failure; the role of combination therapy remains unclear (Balsdon & Craig 2003). In women the risk of premature menopause increases with age. Adequate hormone replacement post-transplant will help to reduce menopausal symptoms and minimise the risk of osteoporosis (see Chapter 20). Endocrine status and thyroid function should be checked post-transplant at regular intervals. Hypothyroidism can occur as an early or late complication and is treated with thyroid replacement therapy.

Secondary malignancies

This is a recognised consequence of transplantation. Secondary myelodysplastic syndromes and acute leukaemias have a cumulative incidence of 4% at 5 years with an onset of between 3 and 8 years post-transplant. Solid organ tumours also occur but develop later than haematological malignancies (Deeg & Socie 1998). Although the incidence of secondary malignancies is low, survivorship is increasing and careful follow-up must be continued for many years to detect their onset.

Case study 13.1

Peter, a 41-year-old car salesman, married with two sons aged 15 and 17, presented with a history of recurrent chest infections that had been treated with limited success by his GP. After several courses of antibiotics he developed bruising; a full blood count was taken and he was immediately referred to the haematologist at the local district general hospital. A diagnosis of Philadelphia positive acute lymphoblastic leukaemia was made and all chemotherapy was given at his local hospital. A transplant was considered as the best treatment option because of the high risk of relapse. Peter's two brothers were tested to determine their suitability as sibling donors with the youngest proving to be an HLA match. Peter was referred to the regional haematology unit for transplantation; he met with the transplant team to discuss the pros and cons of the procedure and the consequences of the transplant. Following tissue typing at the district general hospital his donor met with the transplant team with and without his brother to discuss the procedure and they were both offered support and advice. Peter was very well when he was admitted for transplant, he had a positive outlook and a supportive family. His family required a lot of psychosocial support at this time as both sons were undertaking public examinations and his wife was obviously distressed.

The transplant process itself was fairly straightforward; Peter was very anxious throughout and dependent on the ward team. The main complications at this time were acute graft-versus-host disease, treated with steroids and ciclosporin, and repeated chest infections that required numerous antibiotics and antifungal agents. Three weeks after transplant Peter was discharged and followed-up in a dedicated post-transplant clinic every other day. One of Peter's main issues was his inability to cope with his change of role and the lack of control he felt over his situation; he became profoundly depressed, compounded by the fact that he had been given total body irradiation as part of his conditioning therapy, which in itself can cause neurocognitive dysfunction (Balsdon & Craig 2003).

Immunosuppressive therapy was slowly reduced at which time chronic GvHD became problematic. His skin was severely affected, especially the lower limbs and, as control of GvHD was difficult, a number of agents were used. At this time Peter also developed erectile dysfunction and GvHD of the eyes. Over a period of 6 months Peter started to develop shortness of breath, oedema and fatigue; he was referred for an echocardiogram and to a cardiologist. Pericardial thickening was diagnosed causing a degree of heart failure, drug therapy was administered and the pericardium removed. Peter has had to live with chronic illness, fatigue and a degree of organ failure, all of which impact upon his quality of life; he has, however, been given the support required to return to work and is able to cope with his life. When Peter is asked whether he ever wished that he had not had his transplant, he says no for without it he would have died from his disease.

POST-TRANSPLANT FOLLOW-UP

As stem cell transplantation has advanced, increasing numbers of patients are surviving disease-free for longer periods of time. Quality of life for individuals experiencing cure through this procedure is therefore extremely important and the question of whether individuals can return to 'normal life' following transplantation has been raised (Gruber et al 2003). Wettergren et al (1997) report that generally impaired social relationships and financial problems have a huge impact on individuals' rehabilitation and perception of their quality of life.

After intensive inpatient care, patients are followed-up in a clearly identified outpatient setting. Advances in techniques and developments in therapeutics have led to early discharge and appropriate knowledge and skills are required to support these patients. Many patients require intensive physical, social and psychological support whilst at home and this can be an extremely stressful period for the patient and their family. The greatest challenge for many patients is re-integration into society and achieving an acceptable quality of life (Baker et al 1999); a number of issues negatively impact upon this process.

Psychological issues

The post-transplant period can be fraught with difficulties; many patients appear to have psychological morbidity. It is important to make the distinction between a pathological reaction that will be problematic in terms of the individual's psychological recovery and normal emotional reactions to a life-threatening disease and treatments that are followed by many uncertainties. Experience shows that the main consideration for the post-transplant patient is living with the fear of rejection and relapse (Baker et al 1999). Regular monitoring of blood and bone marrow refreshes this fear for some patients. Health-care professionals caring for the patient and their family need to be cognisant of this issue and considerate of their needs. Education, information and support help this process, minimising the fear of living with a disease.

Body image

Upon discharge patients often contemplate the way they looked prior to transplant, which impacts upon their confidence and perception of their body image. Their body reality has often changed as a result of treatment and weight loss, and often perceptions change as a result of this. It is important that an open and honest dialogue is maintained throughout the recovery period so the patient feels comfortable enough to discuss concerns related to the way they appear and their relationships. Body image is discussed further in Chapter 23.

Sexuality

Body image has a direct impact on the patient's sexuality; feeling unattractive potentiates sexual difficulties. Post-transplant individuals will be predominantly infertile and females are plunged into a menopausal state (see Chapter 20). Baker et al (1999) state that 37% of patients experience sexual dissatisfaction and dysfunction one year post-transplant. These problems may persist, with some commentators reporting 25% of patients still suffering difficulties several years post-transplant (Wingard et al 1992). The main areas of sexual dysfunction are problems with orgasm, negative body image and reduced sexual satisfaction (Molassiotis et al 1996). However, from a physiological perspective pain due to vaginal dryness and/or stenosis and persistent vaginal candida can cause dyspareunia in females. For males a poor libido, erectile and ejaculatory dysfunction can lead to sexual difficulties.

Whatever the problem, the transplant team need to firstly promote the kind of relationship in which patients feel comfortable to share such intimate information. Individuals should be considered in the context of their relationship. Good assessment and management will enable the transplant team to establish whether the cause of sexual difficulties is physical, psychological or a mixture of both. Support and appropriate referral are essential.

Employment

Returning to a normal role in society is a challenge post-transplant. Wettergren et al (1997) consider this issue, identifying impaired social relationships and financial problems as key difficulties. Many patients resume their previous employment; this is a key determinant in re-establishing their social roles. In the transplant population, return to employment appears high with 75% of patients having resumed their professional role one year post-transplant (Duell et al 1997). However, for some patients the contrary applies and job discrimination is common for the cancer survivor (see Chapter 25).

Family-focussed care

Having a family member who has undergone a bone marrow transplant exerts a massive burden on the family unit. For many this involves care being delivered in a centre which may well be many miles from home, which exacerbates separation anxiety. It is often difficult to support patients as a result of the significant disruption a transplant causes to the family unit. There are numerous changing roles within the family unit which have to be adjusted to in order to maintain equilibrium, for example grandparents often adopt a parental role. For children, changes in behaviour may well reflect their ability or inability to cope with what is happening to their parent. Close liaison between parents, the extended family, social workers and school will help to facilitate adjustment. The challenge for the patient following transplant is to re-establish their sense of identity within the family unit. Family issues are discussed further in Chapter 24.

REFLECTION POINT

In blood and bone marrow transplantation specialist knowledge and skills are needed to support the patient through the intensive care they require. The nature of the procedure and immediate recovery make it easy for nurses to consider patient care from a physical perspective. As survival continues to improve and technology develops, nurses have a responsibility to support the patient and their carers living with the effects of their transplant and enable them to cope with the consequences. Consider the psychosocial implications of transplantation in the context of your professional practice and review the supportive strategies in place for this group of patients.

FUTURE DIRECTIONS

With improved survival following bone marrow transplantation, the incidence of late complications has increased. Chronic GvHD, late infections, secondary malignancies and multi-organ toxicities exert a huge health burden on the patient. Service development in BMT needs to account for such issues. One development helping to address these issues is the implementation of late complication clinics. Such clinics should have a strong nurse-led focus; however, both human and financial resources are finite and health-care professionals need to be able to clearly articulate their priorities and promote a culture that will develop practitioners with the necessary knowledge and skills.

A strong multidisciplinary team to ensure the delivery of quality care and expertise is essential. Nurses must seize this opportunity to extend their skills and knowledge to enhance patient care. There are many examples of nurse-led initiatives, research and practice development. Nurses have expanded their roles to perform apheresis, bone marrow aspiration, nurse prescribing and the insertion of central venous access, and no doubt will continue to do so. However transplant nurses develop their roles in the future they must be combined with the knowledge and expertise to continue with what is arguably their central role, supporting patients and their carers.

CONCLUSION

Bone marrow transplantation care is a challenging area of clinical practice. Care delivery should be in specialist centres equipped to deal with the plethora of difficulties that arise from this procedure (NICE 2003). A holistic approach to care integrating psychological, physical and social strands should be used. Consistency across the multidisciplinary team is important, with the cornerstone being good communication. Patients must be helped to live with the problems they have as a result of their transplant whilst appreciating that as a result of treatment they are free from a malignancy that might otherwise have been incurable.

DISCUSSION QUESTIONS

1. What are the physical and psychological implications of protective isolation?

2. Should all types of blood and marrow transplants be undertaken in specialist centres? Consider this issue from both a policy and a clinical perspective.

3. The management of late complications following transplant should integrate all clinical services. How can this be best facilitated and coordinated in practice?

4. What support is offered to donors, especially in the light of current clinical developments such as donor lymphocyte infusions?

5. What are the ethical challenges highlighted in this sphere of practice?

References

Apperley J, Girinsky T, Friedrich W et al 1998 Conditioning regimens. In: The EBMT handbook: blood and marrow transplantation. European School of Haematology, Paris

Baker F, Zabora J, Polland A et al 1999 Reintegration after bone marrow transplant. Cancer Practice 7(4):190–197

Balsdon H, Craig J I O 2003 Bone marrow and peripheral stem cell transplantation. In: Booth S, Bruera E (eds) Palliative care consultations in haemato-oncology. Oxford University Press, Oxford

Barker J, Weisdorf D, DeFor T et al 2005 Transplantation of two partially HLA matched umbilical cord blood units to enhance engraftment in adults with haematological malignancy. Blood 105(3):1343–1347

Bearman S L, Lee J, Baron A E et al 1997 Treatment of hepatic veno-occlusive disease with recombinant human tissue plasminogen activator and heparin in forty-two transplant patients. Blood 89:1501–1506

Campbell K 1997 Types of bone marrow and stem cell transplant. Nursing Times 93(7):44–46

Deeg H J, Socie G 1998 Malignancies after haemopoietic stem cell transplantation, many questions some answers. Blood 9:1833–1844

Duell T, Van Lint M, Ljungman D et al 1997 Health and functional status of long term survivors of bone marrow transplantation. Annals of Internal Medicine 126:184–192

Duncombe A 1997 ABC of clinical haematology bone marrow and stem cell transplantation. British Medical Journal 314:1179–1191

Forman S J, Bloome K G 1994 Bone marrow transplantation. Blackwell Science, Boston

Gaston-Johansson F, Franco T, Zimmerman L 1992 Pain and psychological distress in patients receiving preparative chemotherapy and bone marrow transplantation. Oncology Nursing Forum 20:81–88

Gisselbrecht C, Prentice H G, Bacigalupo A 1994 Placebo controlled phase three trial of lenograstim in bone marrow transplantation. The Lancet 343:698–700

Gruber U, Fegg M, Buchmann M et al 2003 The long term psychosocial effects of haematopoetic stem cell transplantation. European Journal of Cancer Care 12:249–256

Height S, Shields M 1995 Problems following bone marrow transplantation. In: Treleaven J, Wienik P (eds) Colour atlas and text of bone marrow transplantation. Mosby-Wolfe, London

Kelly D 2000 Death, dying and emotional labour: problematic dimensions of the BMT nursing role. Journal of Advanced Nursing 34(4):952–960

Larson P J, Viele C S, Coleman S et al 1993 Comparison of perceived symptoms of patients undergoing bone marrow transplantation and the nurses caring for them. Oncology Nursing Forum 20:81–88

Larsson K, Bjorkstrand B, Ljungmen P 1998 Faster engraftment but no reduction in infectious complications after a PBSC transplantation compared to autologous bone marrow transplantation. Supportive Care in Cancer 6:378–383

McGuire D B, Altomonte V, Peterson D E et al 1993 Patterns of mucositis and pain in patients receiving preparative chemotherapy and bone marrow transplantation. Oncology Nursing Forum 20:1493–1502

Molassiotis A, Van der Akker O, Milligan D et al 1996 Psychological adaptation and symptom distress in bone marrow recipients. Psycho-Oncology 5:9–22

National Institute for Clinical Excellence 2003 Guidance on cancer services. Improving outcomes in haematological cancer. The manual. NICE, London

Outhwaite H 2000 Blood and marrow transplantation. In: Grundy M (ed) Nursing in haematological oncology. Baillière Tindall, Edinburgh

Parker L J 1999 Current recommendations for isolation practices in nursing. British Journal of Nursing 8(13):881–887

Quabeck K 1994 The lung as a critical organ in transplantation. Bone Marrow Transplantation 14:519–528

Richardson P G, Elias A D, Krishnan A 1998 Treatment of severe VOD with defibrotide: compassionate use results in response without severe toxicity in a high-risk population. Blood 92(3):737–744

Rocha V, Labopin M, Sanz G et al 2004 Transplants of umbilical-cord blood or bone marrow from unrelated donors in adults with acute leukaemia. New England Journal of Medicine 351:2276–2285

Soutar R L, King D J 1995 Fortnightly review: bone marrow transplant. British Medical Journal 310:31–36

Weaver C H, Clift R A, Deeg H J et al 1994 Effect of graft versus host disease prophylaxis on relapse in patients transplanted for acute myeloid leukaemia. Bone Marrow Transplantation 14:885–893

Wettergren L, Langius A, Bjorkholm M et al 1997 Physical and psychosocial functioning in patients undergoing autologous bone marrow transplant. A prospective study. Bone Marrow Transplantation 20:497–502

Whedon M B, Wujcik D 1997 Blood and marrow stem cell transplantation: principles, practice and nursing insights. Jones and Bartlett, London

Wingard J R 1994 Functional ability and quality of life of patients after allogeneic transplantation. Bone Marrow Transplantation 14(Suppl):S29–33

Wingard J, Curbow B, Baker F et al 1992 Sexual satisfaction in survivors of bone marrow transplantation. Bone Marrow Transplantation 9:185–190

Woo S B, Sonis S T, Monopoli M M et al 1993 A longitudinal study of oral ulcerative mucositis in bone marrow recipients. Cancer 72:1612–1617

Wujcik D, Ballard B, Camp-Sorrell D 1994 Selected complications of allogeneic bone marrow transplantation. Seminars in Oncology Nursing 10(1):28–41

Further reading

Baker F, Zabora J, Polland A et al 1999 Reintegration after bone marrow transplant. Cancer Practice 7(4):190–197
An interesting research paper that highlights many of the issues patients feel are priorities post transplant. Discussion is from a physical, psychological and social perspective. Clinical considerations are included.

Booth S, Bruera E 2003 Palliative care consultations in haemato-oncology. Oxford University Press, Oxford
An excellent text that should be an indicative resource for all haematology nurses. Palliative care should be an integral part of care in specialist haematology; this resource offers an overview of symptom management.

Duncombe A 1997 ABC of clinical haematology bone marrow and stem cell transplantation. British Medical Journal 314:1179–1191
Factual and concise, a good overview of marrow and stem cell transplantation.

Gruber U, Fegg M, Buchmann M et al 2003 The long term psychosocial effects of haematopoetic stem cell transplantation. European Journal of Cancer Care 12:249–256
A useful paper that considers an important component of transplantation care that may well become of secondary importance to the physical perspective.

Whedon M B, Wujcik D 1997 Blood and marrow stem cell transplantation: principles, practice and nursing insights. Jones and Bartlett, London
A detailed and interesting text, considers issues that are important for the health-care professional working in transplantation – offers an alternative perspective.

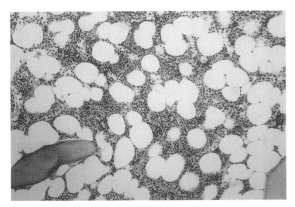

Plate 1 Normal bone marrow showing normal mixed haematopoiesis (courtesy of Dr David Swirsky, with permission of Dr Iderjeet Dokal, Hammersmith Hospital, London)

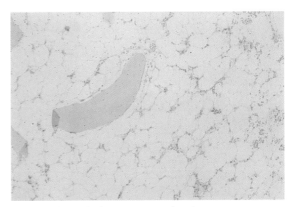

Plate 2 Aplastic bone marrow showing gross hypocellularity with replacement by fat cells (courtesy of Dr David Swirsky, with permission of Dr Inderjeet Dokal, Hammersmith Hospital, London)

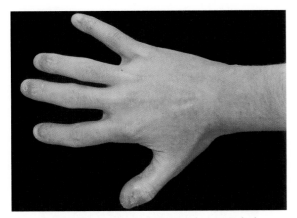

Plate 3 Nail dystrophy in dyskeratosis congenital (courtesy of Dr David Swirsky, with permission of Dr Inderjeet Dokal, Hammersmith Hospital, London)

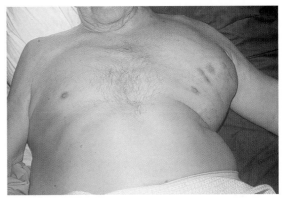

Plate 4 Gross axillary lymphadenopathy in lymphoma (courtesy of Dr Dominic Culligan, Aberdeen Royal Infirmary)

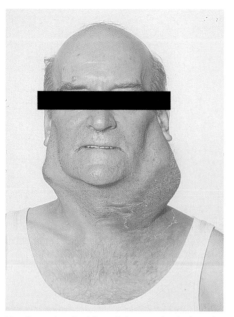

Plate 5 Gross cervical lymphdenopathy in lymphoma (courtesy of Dr Dominic Culligan, Aberdeen Royal Infirmary)

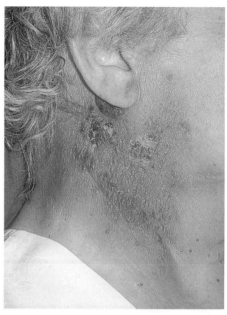

Plate 6 Neutropenic sepsis cellulitis of the neck in acute leukaemia (courtesy of Dr Dominic Culligan, Aberdeen Royal Infirmary)

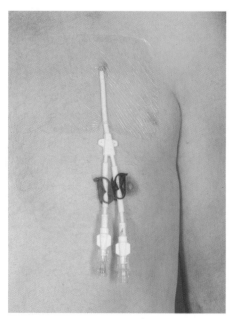

Plate 7 Hickman-type catheter (courtesy of Dr Rachel Green and Mr Douglas Watson, Glasgow Royal Infirmary)

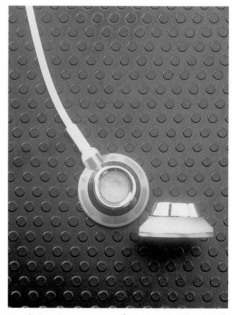

Plate 8 Subcutaneous port (courtesy of Bard Ltd)

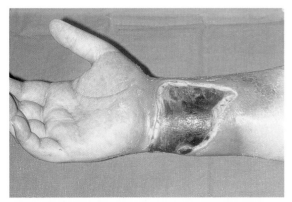

Plate 9 Extravasation of vesicant cytotoxic drug (courtesy of Dr Andrew Hutcheon, Aberdeen Royal Infirmary)

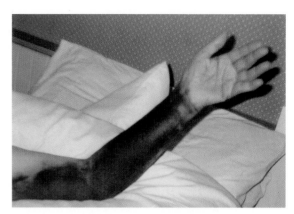

Plate 10 Bruising in thrombocytopenia

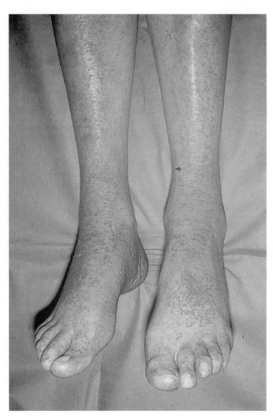

Plate 11 Throbocytopenic purpura (courtesy of Grampian University Hospitals Trust; now NHS Grampian)

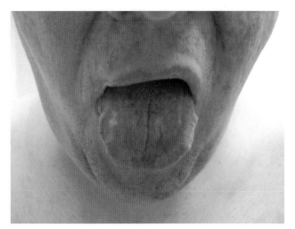

Plate 12 GvHD of the mouth

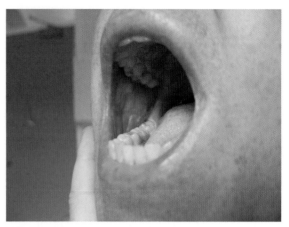

Plate 13 GvHD of the mouth

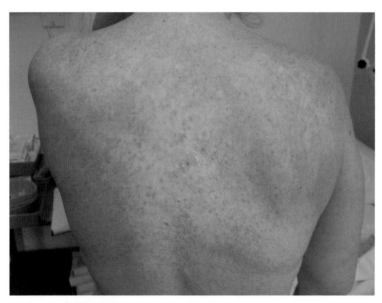

Plate 14 GvHD of the skin

SECTION 3

Nursing issues

SECTION CONTENTS

Chapter **14**

Vascular access

Janice Gabriel

INTRODUCTION

Safe, simple and reliable venous access is the objective in meeting the needs of any patient requiring intravenous therapy. The majority of patients admitted to hospital at the beginning of the 21st century will become a recipient of a vascular access device; haemato-oncology patients are no exception (Petersen 2002). Haemato-oncology patients will require innumerable venepunctures in order to obtain blood samples and for the delivery of treatment. The injury to patients' veins, from both venepunctures and treatment, present challenges for health-care professionals caring for this group of patients (Schelper 2003). Advancements in technology have resulted in the availability of an increased range of vascular access devices (VADs) to meet both clinical requirements and lifestyles of individual patients. Nurses therefore have a responsibility to ensure that patients benefit from the most appropriate VADs from the earliest opportunity, thus also ensuring appropriate use of health-care resources (Lamb 1999, Gabriel 2000, Kayley 2003).

In recent years, the role of the nurse in infusion therapy has developed rapidly, especially within the specialities of oncology and haematology (Gabriel 1996a). Nurses are responsible for coordinating and administering complex treatment regimens and placing a variety of VADs, ranging from peripheral cannulae to skin tunnelled catheters, while ensuring the uneventful longevity of these devices by careful management. With the majority of haemato-oncology patients receiving complex and protracted treatments, it is vital that each individual receives the most appropriate care and management in relation to infusion therapy (Lamb 1999, RCN 2003, Schelper 2003). This chapter discusses the potential trauma to a vessel caused by venepuncture, the range of VADs currently available, and the prevention and management of their potential complications.

THE CIRCULATORY SYSTEM

BLOOD VESSEL STRUCTURE

With the exception of capillaries, all blood vessels are constructed in three layers, i.e. tunica intima (internal layer), tunica media (middle layer) and tunica adventitia (outer layer) (Fig. 14.1).

Figure 14.1
Blood vessel structure

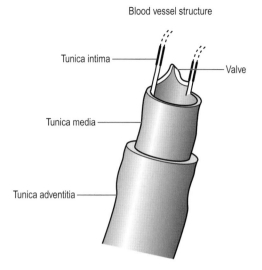

Blood vessel structure

Tunica intima ———— Valve

Tunica media ————

Tunica adventitia ————

Tunica intima

This internal layer of the vessel is composed of endothelium cells laid longitudinally. There is also subendothelial connective tissue throughout the vessel. The endothelial cells can be easily damaged (Hadaway 1995, Weinstein 1997).

Tunica media

The tunica media is constructed from smooth muscle fibres and elastic tissue. Arteries have less elastic tissue than veins, making them more rigid. Muscle fibres enable these vessels to expand and constrict, which can result in spasm as a consequence of temperature change or irritation from infusates or the VAD (Weinstein 1997).

Tunica adventitia

The tunica adventitia supports the vessels and is composed of collagen and nerve fibres. The amount of fibrous tissue varies, with arteries having thicker layers than veins (Scales 1999).

ARTERIAL SYSTEM

Blood is circulated throughout the body from the heart. The ascending aorta, which is the largest blood vessel, with a diameter of 2.5 cm, leaves the left side of the heart, divides and continues to subdivide to supply blood throughout the body (Scales 1999). Routine administration of drugs via the arterial system is contraindicated because it can lead to arterial spasm and limb ischaemia. However, there are occasions when it is indicated, e.g. angiography and treatment of pulmonary embolism with antithrombolitic agents (Scales 1999).

CAPILLARIES

Capillaries are fine vessels composed of a single layer of endothelial cells. These vessels supply each cell with blood and nutrients while facilitating the exchange of gas and collection of waste products from cell metabolism through selective permeability (Scales 1999).

VEINS

Veins collect the blood from the capillaries and return it to the heart, where it is re-oxygenated and starts its journey around the body again. As the veins progress closer to the heart, their diameter increases. Valves play an important role in maintaining the flow of blood through the venous system and back to the heart. A valve is a fold of the tunica intima supported by connective tissue. A fully functioning valve will prevent reflux of blood into a lower part of the vein (Fig. 14.2).

Movement of a limb will cause the muscles to contract and relax. Muscle contraction causes pressure on the adjacent vein, resulting in displacement of the blood within the vessel. The valves prevent blood refluxing into the vein when the muscle is relaxed. In an immobile patient blood flow through the vessels of the lower limbs can become impaired. As the blood flow through the veins of the lower limbs and arms is slower than through those of the larger, central veins, these vessels should not be considered for any patient requiring the administration of vesicant and irritating infusates (Gabriel 1999, Scales 1999).

With increasing age tissue atrophies and skin becomes increasingly transparent. This process does not leave blood vessels unaffected. Ageing causes veins to become more scarred and fragile. Combine this with an elderly patient requiring venous access for chronic leukaemia and obtaining peripheral venous access can become very challenging (Schelper 2003).

PATIENT ASSESSMENT

Before any vascular access device is considered it is vital to undertake a full assessment of the individual patient, their diagnosis, clinical requirements and, if appropriate, their lifestyle. Lifestyle away from the hospital environment will greatly influence the uneventful longevity of the VAD selected, especially if the patient is requiring intermittent or continuous parenteral therapy over a prolonged period of time (Dougherty 1999, Gabriel, 2003). Patient assessment should include:

- diagnosis
- type of intended therapy
- length of proposed therapy
- where the treatment will take place, e.g. hospital, outpatient, homecare or self-administered

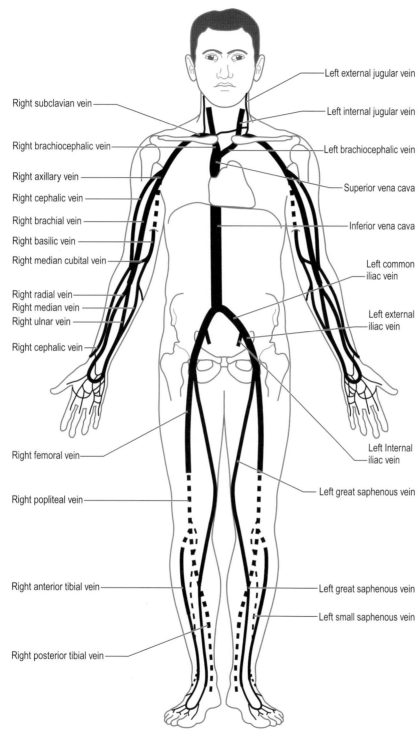

Figure 14.2
Venous system (adapted from Dougherty 1999 with permission)

- condition of veins and limb if appropriate
- age of the patient
- previous problems with venepunctures/VADs
- relevant medical history
- for recipients of a central venous access device (CVAD) any contraindications for the device or site selected
- patient preference
- need for an anaesthetic agent/sedation.

TYPE OF INTENDED THERAPY

It is important to consider the potential effects of the solution and/or drugs to be infused on the patients' veins. Will the patient require the administration of large volumes or highly viscous infusions, e.g. blood products, total parenteral nutrition (TPN)? Is the intended treatment vesicant or irritant to the blood vessel, e.g. a vesicant cytotoxic agent? Is the treatment likely to continue for a number of weeks? As the answer to the majority, if not all, of these questions is likely to be 'yes' for a haemato-oncology patient, then a CVAD, as opposed to a peripheral cannula, should be considered from the outset (Dougherty 1999, Gabriel 1999).

LOCATION OF TREATMENT

It is important to consider where treatment is to take place. If it is hospital-based, it is reasonable to assume that there will be ready access to suitably skilled staff who can manage the patient's device for them and if necessary re-site it. However, if treatment is to take place in the community, or indeed if the patient will be administering their own treatment, the level of support they can access needs to be considered. Although a patient may live close to a hospital, they may have transport problems, or the hospital may be unable to support the requirements of this individual, especially 'out of hours'. Not all patients have access to a specialist iv nurse in the community (Kayley 2003).

CONDITION OF THE PATIENT'S VEINS AND LIMBS

Existing or past injury to a limb may exclude it from being used to establish venous access, e.g. if the patient has experienced a cerebrovascular accident, thrombosis or has an existing fracture resulting in immobilisation of the limb. Routine cannulation should also be avoided in patients with lymphoedematous arms and those who have arteriofistulae or grafts. If a cannula is being used, it is advisable to site the first device in the most distal vein and work upwards as the VAD is re-sited (Dougherty 1999).

PREVIOUS PROBLEMS WITH VENEPUNCTURES/VADS

Patients are ideally placed to be able to advise health professionals of previous problems they may have experienced with venepunctures or cannulation. For example, a patient will know if he/she always has a problem with the left arm when taking blood. It is therefore sensible to ask about problems, where possible, before attempting the venepuncture. If patients have experienced a problem with a CVAD, it is important to take the time to identify exactly what the problem was, so hopefully a repeat scenario can be avoided. Haemato-oncology patients will have a tremendous amount of experience of previous venepunctures.

RELEVANT MEDICAL HISTORY

Patients with certain medical conditions, e.g. mucin-secreting adenocarcinomas, promyelocytic leukaemia, myeloproliferative disorders, are at increased risk of thrombosis if they have a CVAD (Camp-Sorrell 1992). If such a device is required, careful selection of the particular CVAD and its construction material, together with considering the use of prophylactic antithrombolitic therapy, may greatly diminish their risk of experiencing a thrombosis.

Some patients may be at increased risk of bleeding from placement of a VAD, especially a CVAD. If a patient is receiving anticoagulant therapy, or is potentially thrombocytopenic, a blood count and clotting screen should be undertaken before placing a CVAD. A decision to temporarily suspend their anticoagulant therapy should be discussed with the clinician in charge of their care. For patients who are thrombocytopenic it may be appropriate to place a CVAD under the cover of a platelet infusion, but this needs to be discussed with their clinician (Richardson & Bruso 1993).

CVADs can be placed in immunocompromised patients, but the routine placement of such devices in patients who are experiencing neutropenic sepsis should be avoided, where possible, until negative blood cultures are obtained.

SITE SELECTION FOR RECIPIENTS OF A CVAD

The common veins used for placing a CVAD, i.e. tunnelled and non-tunnelled catheters and chest-placed ports, are the internal and external jugular and subclavian veins (see Fig. 14.2). The cephalic, basilic and median cubital veins can be used for peripherally-inserted central catheters (PICCs) and peripherally-placed injection ports (Gabriel 1999). However, the following veins can also be used (Gormon & Buzby 1995):

- saphenous
- inferior epigastric

- gonadal
- lumbar
- intrathoracic
- femoral.

When selecting the vein it is essential to ensure that the passage of the CVAD is not impeded in any way. For example, if the patient has experienced/is experiencing any of the following:

- enlarged axillary/supraclavicular nodes
- surgery/radiotherapy to axilla
- tumour mass
- previous history of thrombosis
- fractured clavicle
- cardiac pacemaker in situ.

If the patient has experienced any of the above, placement of the CVAD should be attempted on the opposite side where possible. If it is not possible, problems may be encountered in advancing the catheter along the vein (Gabriel 1996b).

PATIENT PREFERENCE

In the non-emergency setting, the individual should be consulted regarding their preference for the site of the VAD. Indeed, if more than one type of device will meet the requirements of the individual, they should be invited to participate in the decision about which device they would prefer. Patients have reported that certain locations are more uncomfortable than others for the site of a peripheral cannula (Gabriel 2000). If another site is equally accessible, but more acceptable to the patient, this should be the site of choice. The health professional siting the cannula walks away from the patient once the procedure is completed. The patient will 'live' with the device for the entire time it remains in situ. If a patient has a needle phobia, an injection port should not be considered when a tunnelled catheter or PICC may meet their needs (Dougherty 1999, Gabriel 2000).

NEED FOR AN ANAESTHETIC AGENT/SEDATION

Dougherty (1999) discusses how venepuncture and cannulation have become routine procedures for health professionals to perform. However, for the patient, who is far less familiar with the procedure, it can become a potential fearful experience. When cannulation is a planned procedure, little additional effort or expense is incurred if a topical anaesthetic is used. Local anaesthetic cream or intra-dermal injection should be offered prior to cannulation. Topical anaesthetic cream is now used routinely in the placement of PICCs, with the majority of non-tunnelled, skin-tunnelled lines and injection ports placed using subcutaneous lidocaine (Gabriel 1999). It is now rare for a skin-tunnelled catheter or injection port to be placed as an isolated procedure under general anaesthetic, the exception being children (Bravery 1999).

How are patients in your area of practice prepared for insertion of a CVAD? Could any of the points raised in this chapter help you to enhance the care currently provided?

VASCULAR ACCESS DEVICES

PERIPHERAL CANNULAE

Peripheral cannulae are available in a variety of gauge sizes and lengths, but should not exceed 3.5 cm in length (RCN 2003). Some have stabilisation wings and some injection ports.

MIDLINE CATHETERS

Midline catheters are inserted into a vein in the antecubital area. Sometimes these devices are referred to as peripherally-inserted catheters (PICs). The catheter is advanced along the vein in the upper arm, but does not extend further than the axillary vein due to its overall length, 7.5–20 cm (RCN 2003). Midline catheters are suitable for patients who have difficult venous access in the lower part of the arm and/or require parenteral therapy for up to several weeks, but do not require the placement of a CVAD to meet their clinical needs, e.g. do not require the administration of vesicant agents.

CENTRAL VENOUS ACCESS DEVICES

A central venous access device is a catheter whose tip terminates in the superior vena cava (Goodwin & Carlson 1993, Vesley 2003). Four main groups of CVADs exist:

- non-tunnelled catheters
- skin-tunnelled catheters
- injection ports
- peripherally-inserted central catheters (PICCs).

Non-tunnelled catheters

Non-tunnelled catheters are usually used for short-term access to the central venous system. Access can be achieved from a number of approaches including the internal and external jugular, femoral and subclavian veins (Scales 1999).

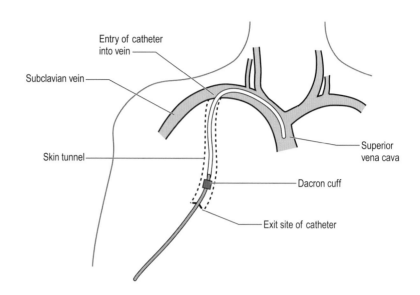

Figure 14.3
Skin-tunnelled catheter

Entry of catheter into vein

Subclavian vein

Skin tunnel

Superior vena cava

Dacron cuff

Exit site of catheter

Tunnelled catheters

These catheters are tunnelled under the patient's skin, usually on the chest wall, and usually access the central venous system via the external/internal jugular or subclavian veins (Fig. 14.3) (a Hickman-type catheter is shown in Plate 7). The design of the catheter incorporates a 'Dacron' cuff on the portion of the catheter sited in the skin tunnel (Broviac et al 1973).

Injection ports

These devices consist of a subcutaneous injection port attached to a venous catheter. The port can be placed peripherally, e.g. under the skin on the arm, or centrally, e.g. under the skin on the chest (Plate 8). The catheter is then tunnelled under the skin until the desired venous access point is reached (Soo et al 1985). Access to the port is achieved by a specifically designed 'Huber' needle to minimise the risk of 'coring', which can result in leakage when the needle is withdrawn from the port through the patient's skin (Haindl 1989). Ports are available with one or two lumens.

Peripherally-inserted central catheters

Peripherally-inserted central catheters (PICCs) are a group of single, dual and more recently developed triple lumen CVADs. Venous access is achieved by cannulating a peripheral vein in the arm, then gradually advancing the catheter until it reaches the superior vena cava (Gabriel 1999).

After placement and before they are used for the first time all CVADs should have verification of their tip location recorded in the patient's notes (RCN 2003). If the device was not placed using image guidance, a chest x-ray should be performed, again with the result clearly documented in the patient's notes (Hadaway 1989, RCN 2003).

> **Box 14.1   Example of lumen sizes**
>
> | Gauge | French |
> |-------|--------|
> | • 16 ga | • 5.0 Fr |
> | • 18 ga | • 4.0 Fr |
> | • 20 ga | • 3.0 Fr |
> | • 23 ga | • 2.0 Fr |

GAUGE SIZE

VADs are produced in standardised gauge sizes. The gauge size will refer to the external diameter of the VAD and be expressed as either 'French' (Fr) or 'gauge' (ga) size, e.g. 5.0 Fr or 16 ga. With multi-lumen CVADs it is the overall diameter of the device that is stated, e.g. 5 Fr (16 ga). Examples of gauge sizes are shown in Box 14.1.

When assessing a patient for a VAD, whether peripheral or central, it is important to consider the gauge size. If a patient has small veins, a large gauge VAD has the potential to irritate the wall of the blood vessel and subsequently give rise to the development of phlebitis.

VAD CONSTRUCTION MATERIAL

All VADs should be radio-opaque. Peripheral cannulae can be polyvinylchloride, teflon or polyurethane. CVADs are commonly polyurethane or silicone rubber (Dougherty 1999, Gabriel 1999). The ideal material is one that causes minimal irritation to the vessel wall, as this will greatly reduce the incidence of phlebitis and subsequent risk of thrombosis to the patient (Strumpfer 1991). Devices constructed from silicone rubber are much softer, resulting in less trauma to the wall of the blood vessel. Rigid materials, such as polyurethane, have an inability to recover from kinking and bending, and are more prone to breakage than silicone rubber.

However, polyurethane can achieve higher flow rates, as the lumen walls of devices constructed from this material are thinner compared to VADs constructed from silicone rubber. This results in a larger internal diameter, meaning that the flow rate of a 4.0 Fr CVAD constructed from polyurethane will be higher than the same size device constructed from silicone rubber (Gabriel 1999). Assessment of the patient's requirements will indicate the most appropriate material for the device selected.

VALVED VADS

Midline and CVADs are available as 'open-ended' or 'valved'. An open-ended device will require clamping when the injection hub is removed, or if the catheter is damaged, to minimise the risk of an air embolism by the introduction of air into the venous circulation via the VAD. An open-ended catheter is also associated with a higher incidence of intraluminal occlusion as a consequence of reflux of blood into its lumen(s). Valved catheters have a valve situated at either the distal or proximal end of the catheter. In the absence of a negative or positive pressure the valve remains closed, therefore when the injection hub is removed, or there is trauma leading to damage of the catheter, the potential for air entry into the patient's circulation via the VAD is greatly diminished, as is the risk of catheter occlusion as a consequence of blood reflux (Mayo & Pearson 1995, Gabriel 1999)

PLACEMENT OF VADS

Once the patient has been assessed, appropriate device selected and site chosen, preparation for the procedure should be undertaken. This not only entails adequate explanation to, and consent from, the patient, but ensuring insertion complications are minimised. Once the device has been placed, the date and time of the procedure should be recorded in the patient's notes, together with who undertook the procedure, where the device was placed (site location) and dressing used. Details of the device should also be recorded including type of device, manufacturer, size and batch number. If a CVAD was placed, a record of who verified the tip location should also be recorded (RCN 2003).

MINIMISING POTENTIAL FOR INSERTION COMPLICATIONS

HAEMATOMA

A haematoma can develop during the insertion procedure as a direct consequence of damage to the patient's vein. It can be caused by:

- perforation of the posterior wall of the vein
- over-advancement of the needle/introducer during cannulation
- tourniquet left in situ for too long
- failure to release tourniquet before removing needle/introducer
- fragile veins
- low platelet count
- anticoagulant therapy
- incorrect choice of VAD
- inadequate pressure on venepuncture site.

ARTERIAL PUNCTURE

Arterial puncture can occur if an artery is cannulated or punctured during the insertion procedure. It is clearly identifiable by the bright red pulsation/spurting of blood. The patient should be reassured and firm pressure applied over the puncture site for at least 5 minutes (Dougherty 1999). If the subclavian artery has been punctured, a chest x-ray should be performed to eliminate a mediastinal haematoma (Richardson & Bruso 1993).

NERVE DAMAGE

Damage to a nerve can occur when the introducer/cannula either touches or severs the nerve during the procedure. Nerve damage is char-acterised as severe, sharp pain radiating down all or part of the affected limb. If this does occur, it should not be ignored, as there is potential for long-term damage resulting in pain and/or loss of movement (Roth 2003a). The patient should be reassured, the introducer/cannula removed and medical assistance sought (Dougherty 2003, Roth 2003a).

AIR EMBOLUS

Potentially an air embolus can occur if air enters the venous circulation during the insertion of a VAD. When inserting a peripheral cannula, midline catheter, PICC or peripherally placed port, the limb involved should be kept below the level of the patient's heart. When placing a non-tunnelled, tunnelled catheter or chest-positioned port, the patient should be placed in the Trendelenburg position or supine (Richardson & Bruso 1993).

PNEUMOTHORAX

A pneumothorax can occur if air enters the space between the pleural lining and the lung. This is most likely to happen with CVADs placed directly into the subclavian vein, where there is a 5% risk of a pneu-mothorax occurring. This is a consequence of the lung being punctured by the introducer during insertion (Richardson & Bruso 1993).

HAEMOTHORAX

Haemothorax can result during placement of non-tunnelled, tunnelled catheters and chest-placed ports. It is a result of puncturing the subcla-vian vein or artery during the insertion procedure, with blood draining into the pleural cavity (Richardson & Bruso 1993, Medical Devices Alert 2003).

CATHETER MALPOSITION

Due to the length of the catheters involved, CVADs have the potential to be malpositioned during the insertion procedure. Recent guidance advocating the use of Doppler and imaging should ensure that all CVADs are indeed centrally placed, i.e. their tips terminate in the lower third of the superior vena cava (SVC) (Hadaway 1989, RCN 2003, Vesley 2003).

If a CVAD is not adequately secured at its insertion site, there is the potential for it to migrate, i.e. it could travel beyond the desired termination point and into the heart, or it could migrate externally leaving the tip resting against the tunica intima of a smaller vessel. The external part of the catheter should be regularly assessed and if there is any cause for concern that migration may have occurred, a chest x-ray should be requested to check the position of the tip (Gabriel 2001, RCN 2003).

PINCH-OFF SYNDROME

Pinch-off syndrome can occur with tunnelled, non-tunnelled and chest-placed ports. It is a result of compression of the catheter between the clavicle and first rib. If left unnoticed, there is a risk of the catheter being broken as a result of the compression between these two structures (Fig. 14.4) (Hinke et al 1990).

ATRIAL FIBRILLATION

Atrial fibrillation can result if the catheter extends beyond the SVC and into the heart.

Figure 14.4
Pinch-off syndrome

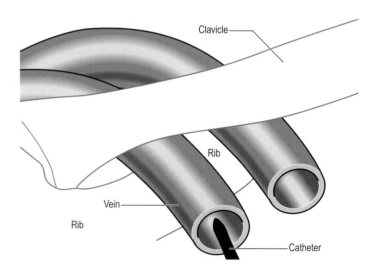

PHLEBITIS

Phlebitis is a result of irritation to the tunica intima and can be caused by the drugs/infusates being administered (chemical phlebitis), irritation by the device (mechanical phlebitis) and by infection (infective phlebitis) (Richardson & Bruso 1993).

Chemical phlebitis

Chemical phlebitis is rarely seen with a correctly positioned CVAD. It is a condition more likely to be experienced in recipients of a peripheral cannula and to a lesser extent in recipients of a midline device. The more acidic or alkaline the therapy being administered the greater the risk of chemical phlebitis. Chemical phlebitis can be prevented by careful assessment of the patient and ensuring the most appropriate device is chosen for the proposed therapy (Richardson & Bruso 1993, Gabriel 1999).

Mechanical phlebitis

Mechanical phlebitis is usually noticeable within the first 7 days following VAD placement. It is a consequence of placing too large a device within the vessel and is more likely to be seen in recipients of peripheral cannulae, midline devices and PICCs. It is also more common in females owing to the smaller size of their veins compared with men (Goodwin & Carlson 1993, Richardson & Bruso 1993). Mechanical phlebitis can be prevented by assessing the patient's veins and carefully selecting the correct size of VAD for the chosen vein, i.e. allowing a sufficient flow of blood around the VAD once it is sited in the vein. Ensuring the VAD is well secured to the patient's skin will also minimise the potential for movement of the device within the vein (Gabriel 2001). If a patient is suspected of having mechanical phlebitis, the application of warm heat for 20 minutes three times a day usually resolves the problem (Richardson & Bruso 1993).

Infective phlebitis

If phlebitis presents several days after insertion, and both mechanical and chemical phlebitis have been excluded, it is probably a result of infection. If infective phlebitis is suspected, local hospital policy should be followed for the management of the patient (RCN 2003).

THROMBOSIS

The development of a thrombosis linked to parenteral therapy is believed to be multifactorial (Ryder 1995). Many patients with haematological cancers will be at increased risk, and the choice of device, construction material, site of insertion and insertion technique can all influence the process. The process of introducing a VAD into a vessel causes trauma to the tunica intima, resulting in the collection of platelets around the damaged areas of the vessel wall – the larger the area of damage, the greater the collection of platelets. This can give rise to the development of thrombi, which may increase in size and eventually break away and flow through the venous system, or remain in situ and occlude the lumen of the vessel (Camp-Sorrell 1992, Ryder 1995).

CVADs inserted percutaneously are associated with a lower incidence of thrombosis than those placed by a surgical cut-down procedure. As PICCs are placed by cannulation of a peripheral vein, the incidence of thrombosis associated with their placement is significantly lower than for other types of CVADs (Gabriel 1999).

The clinical features of thrombosis may not become apparent until the condition is quite advanced. Confirmation of the diagnosis should be undertaken and treatment initiated. It is possible to treat the patient's condition without the removal of the CVAD, but this will depend upon the severity of the symptoms and the patient's general condition (Wickham et al 1992). Treatment can involve removal of the thrombosis by a suitably experienced surgeon/radiologist or the administration of antithrombolytic agents such as tissue-type plasminogen activator (TPA) or urokinase through the affected CVAD. Once the thrombosis has resolved, successful resumption of treatment through the affected CVAD has been reported (Brothers et al 1988).

PREVENTION OF INFECTION

SKIN CLEANSING

Venepuncture and cannulation are the most commonly performed invasive procedures in the UK. To minimise the risk of infection to both the patient and health-care professional, hand washing should be performed before and after clinical procedures. In addition, well-fitting gloves should be used for all infusion-related procedures (RCN 2003).

However sterile the equipment used, the VAD placed has the potential to become infected if inadequate attention is paid to cleaning the patient's skin (Maki et al 1991, Elliott 1993). Contamination of the VAD by bacteria from the patient's skin could result in opportunistic infection to the patient, especially a haemato-oncology patient who may well be immunocompromised. The resulting infection may not be confined to the insertion site, and can develop into a systemic infection, further compromising the patient's health, greatly inconveniencing them and requiring additional health-care resources (Elliott 1993).

Maki and colleagues (1991) published the results of a randomised trial of skin-cleansing agents. They concluded that aqueous chlorhexidine used for cutaneous disinfection prior to placement of an iv device, and for post-insertion site care, significantly reduced the incidence of device-related infection. At the 2002 National Association of Vascular Access Network's (NAVAN) conference in San Diego, Maki reiterated the importance of effective skin cleansing prior to placement of a VAD, advocating the use of aqueous chlorhexidine in a strength of 0.5–2% (Maki 2002).

Administration sets should be changed every 72 hours, or when it is suspected that the integrity of the equipment may have been compromised, or there is suspected contamination (RCN 2003). If the giving set has/is being used for the administration of blood, it will require more frequent changing (RCN 2003) (see Chapter 12).

ACCESSING THE VAD

As long ago as 1985 Linares and colleagues demonstrated that the commonest cause of device-related septicaemia was contamination of the injection hub. Effective decontamination can be achieved by using a pre-saturated alcohol wipe or a chlorhexidine-based solution to clean the hub, and allowing it to adequately dry (drying time is approximately 30 seconds), before accessing the device using an aseptic technique (Gabriel 1999).

There has been much debate over the use of 'ported' cannulae. In the USA they are used far less than in the UK. This is because it is difficult to adequately clean the ports before use, together with the potential for the cap not being changed as frequently as recommended or indeed being absent, resulting in the system being left open for potential contamination (Dougherty 1999).

STABILISATION OF THE VAD

Any vascular access device that is not secured at its point of entry has the potential to migrate. This will not only result in loss of the device but also contribute to the potential for infection (Gabriel 2001). The 'pistoning' effect of an inappropriately secured VAD moving in and out of the vein, and with each movement rubbing against the patient's skin, has the potential to introduce infection. Peripheral cannulae can be adequately secured against the patient's skin with a suitable occlusive dressing, which allows easy observation of the device at its insertion site without the necessity to interfere with the integrity of the dressing. However, midline devices, PICCs and non-tunnelled catheters require additional securement for the entire time they remain in situ. Prior to the development of self-adhesive anchoring devices these VADs were routinely secured with sutures (Fig. 14.5). Sutures were not only uncomfortable for the patient, but also had the potential to significantly increase infection risk and contribute to the risk of needlestick injuries among health-care professionals. Crnich & Maki (2002) demonstrated the effectiveness of self-adhesive anchoring devices in not only minimising VAD migration, but also significantly decreasing the incidence of infection (Gabriel 2001). Sterile, self-adhesive anchoring devices offer a safer alternative to securement of CVADs, especially PICCs, when compared to sutures (Crnich & Maki 2002, RCN 2003).

Once the skin tunnel of a tunnelled CVAD has healed, additional securement is not routinely required. The exception to this would be if the patient is mobile and receiving infusions, potentially placing additional stress on the catheter or injection port.

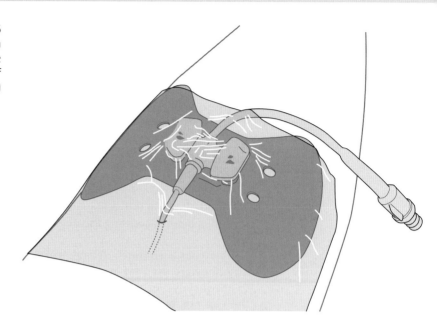

Figure 14.5
Securement of a VAD with
self-adhesive anchoring device
(reproduced with permission of
Venetec International)

DRESSINGS

When the wound overlying the injection well on a subcutaneously implanted port and the skin tunnel for a tunnelled catheter have healed, neither of these devices requires dressings, except when an injection port is in use. However, all other types of VADs require a dressing for the entire period the device remains in situ, as the puncture wound through the skin directly overlays the access point to the patient's vein.

Peripheral cannulae should be covered with a transparent, semipermeable membrane (TSM) dressing. The rationale for the transparency is to ensure easy observation of the VAD and insertion site, without having to compromise the integrity of the dressing. The dressing should be changed if integrity is compromised or moisture or blood is observed, and according to individual organisation's policies. Reasons for dressing changes should be documented in the patient's notes (Dougherty 2003, RCN 2003).

Midline catheters, PICCs and non-tunnelled catheters should also be dressed with a TSM dressing. As there is usually some slight oozing of blood in the first few hours following insertion, it is often necessary to change the initial dressing the day following insertion to minimise the risk of infection. Providing the integrity of the dressing is not compromised and there is no further discharge or accumulation of moisture, Maki et al (1991) recommend a dressing change interval of every 7 days (Gabriel 2001, RCN 2003). For patients who are sensitive to the material used in a TSM dressing, sterile gauze and tape can be used, but these will require more frequent changing to minimise the potential for infection, especially if the integrity of the dressing becomes compromised (RCN 2003).

MAINTAINING PATENCY

INTRALUMINAL OCCLUSION

Occlusion of a VAD can be either intraluminal or extraluminal. Intraluminal occlusion is more commonly associated with the reflux of blood into the lumen of the VAD, leading to a clot (Wickham et al 1992). Occlusion resulting from clotted blood is usually observed as experiencing increasing difficulty when infusing drugs/fluids. This is a result of the blood clot gradually increasing in size until the whole of the lumen is blocked. Intraluminal occlusion from drug/infusate precipitation is usually more sudden in onset.

EXTRALUMINAL OCCLUSION

Extraluminal occlusion can result from a number of factors that lead to external pressure on the VAD. In a CVAD this pressure can result from (Tschirhart & Rao 1988):

- enlarged lymph nodes
- tumour mass
- securing sutures/dressing over the device
- thrombosis
- patient/equipment pressing on the external part of the catheter
- a cardiac pacemaker
- fractured clavicle.

If any problem is experienced in infusing or aspirating from a VAD, assessment of any possible causes of pressure overlying the route of the catheter should be undertaken.

PERSISTENT WITHDRAWAL OCCLUSION

An ability to infuse into a VAD, especially a centrally placed one, combined with the inability to aspirate could be a result of a phenomenon known as 'persistent withdrawal occlusion' (PWO). PWO can be a consequence of an inappropriately placed VAD, for example the tip of the device resting against the wall of the blood vessel. When negative pressure is applied to the VAD, the vessel wall is sucked across the tip of the VAD, preventing aspiration (Gabriel 1997). A more common cause of PWO in CVADs is the formation of a fibrin sheath. Infusion is possible as the positive pressure pushes the fibrin away from the tip of the VAD. However, when aspirating, a negative pressure is applied and the fibrin

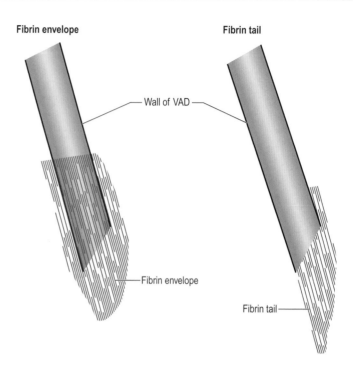

Figure 14.6
Example of fibrin sheaths

is pulled back to cover the tip of the VAD, preventing aspiration (Fig. 14.6) (Gabriel 1997).

Wickham et al (1992) have observed that the development of a fibrin sheath will occur in the majority of CVADs with dwell times in excess of 7 days, yet the majority of these sheaths cause no problems for the patient. A fibrin sheath is a result of the adherence of platelets and fibrin to the outer wall of the VAD. Over a period of time the fibrin extends and can completely envelop the VAD. If this does occur, there is a risk of extravasation of drugs or infusates delivered through the VAD as the drugs/infusates backtrack along the outer wall of the VAD within the envelope of the sheath until an exit point is found. Before attempting to administer any drug or infusion, the patency of the VAD should be established. Failure to do this could result in the patient experiencing extravasation and subsequent litigation (Lawson 2003, Roth 2003a).

EXTRAVASATION

Extravasation is the infiltration of tissue by vesicant drugs or infusates. The incidence of extravasation with a peripheral cannula ranges between 23% and 28%, with an incidence of less than 5% with CVADs (Lawson 2003, Roth 2003b). The commonest causes of extravasation include (Roth 2003b):

- device dislodgement, especially with peripheral cannulae
- inadequate securement of the VAD
- presence of a recent puncture site, e.g. cannulation attempts and/or venepunctures distal to a peripheral cannula
- siting of a peripheral cannula over an area of flexion
- fibrin sheaths
- failure to correctly access an injection port.

FLUSHING SOLUTIONS

Discussion continues about flushing frequencies and most appropriate flush solutions to maintain the patency of VADs. Recent work undertaken by the Royal College of Nursing (RCN) Infusion Therapy (IV) Forum has resulted in the publication of standards to guide nurses involved in infusion therapy (RCN 2003). Standard 6.2 looks specifically at maintaining patency and suggests that, unless otherwise indicated by the CVAD manufacturer, these devices should be flushed with at least twice the prime volume of the catheter, using a concentration of heparin equal to 10 iu in 1 mL of 0.9% sodium chloride. Again, in the absence of specific guidance from a device manufacturer, or if previous occlusion problems have been encountered, 'routine' flushing to maintain patency should take place on a weekly basis. The standard stresses the importance of ensuring the patency of a CVAD before drug/infusate administration by flushing with 0.9% sodium chloride. The device should also be flushed with 0.9% sodium chloride between/after the administration of incompatible drugs/solutions (RCN 2003).

FLUSHING TECHNIQUE

The correct flushing technique has been shown to minimise the incidence of intraluminal occlusion resulting from reflux of blood. When a VAD is flushed, positive pressure is exerted to depress the plunger of the syringe. If the plunger is fully depressed, negative pressure is created when it is removed, causing reflux of blood into the lumen of the VAD. Refluxed blood may develop into a clot with the potential to obstruct the lumen of the VAD (Goodwin & Carlson 1993). In using a positive pressure flush technique, the syringe is removed directly from a valved VAD, or with an open-ended VAD the catheter is clamped, as the practitioner continues to exert pressure on the plunger of the syringe, thus minimising the risk of reflux of blood. In practice this is quite a difficult technique to master and the introduction of positive pressure flush devices has been demonstrated to greatly decrease intraluminal occlusion and infections resulting from the reflux of blood (Gabriel 1997). These flush devices can be used as substitutes for traditional injection hubs to VADs. They function by retaining some of the flush solution when the flushing procedure is commenced. When the syringe is removed, the retained flush solution is then delivered, under positive pressure, into the VAD (Gabriel 1997).

INTRALUMINAL OCCLUSION

Intraluminal occlusion resulting from clotted blood can be managed in CVADs by the instillation of either urokinase 5000 iu or TPA 2 mg left in situ for 10–60 minutes before being aspirated. If difficulty is experienced in instilling the drug, a 10- or 20-mL syringe can be used to deliver the agent. On no account should a syringe smaller than 10 mL be used, as these have the potential to generate too high a pressure, which may result in rupture of the CVAD (Reed 1991). A gentle push/pause technique may help to instil the drug. If this technique fails, a three-way tap may be attached to the end of the CVAD. Two 10 mL syringes are then attached, one containing the urokinase/TPA and the other empty. A gentle rocking action between the syringes, together with manipulation of the three-way tap, will ensure delivery of the drug into the occluded lumen (Gabriel 1997).

DAMAGED VADS

Care should be taken to maintain the integrity of a CVAD by ensuring that it is adequately stabilised and no sharp objects, such as scissors or toothed clamps, come into contact with it.

If a patient breaks the external part of a tunnelled or non-tunnelled catheter, he/she should be immediately laid flat to minimise the risk of an air embolism and the catheter clamped or knotted. If the external part of a PICC is broken, the patient's arm should be kept below the level of their heart and the catheter knotted or clamped. Individual manufacturers of CVADs will be able to provide information relating to repair of their own devices (RCN 2003). Generally speaking it is easier to repair the external part of a CVAD. Whenever a repair takes place it should be documented in the patient's notes and if there is the possibility that the tip of the device has been dislodged, a chest x-ray should be performed to re-confirm its position (Gabriel 1999).

Case study 14.1

John, a 37-year-old married teacher with no children, was diagnosed with acute myeloid leukaemia 3 months ago. He is now in remission and has been identified as having a tissue match with his younger brother. John had a single-lumen skin-tunnelled catheter placed at the time of his diagnosis, which is still in situ. It has been arranged for John to be admitted to a regional teaching hospital, approximately 30 miles from his home, to be prepared for an allogeneic bone marrow transplant. As he will be receiving cytotoxic chemotherapy, blood products, antibiotics and total parenteral nutrition, it is decided to replace his existing single-lumen skin-tunnelled catheter with a triple-lumen device prior to commencement of his treatment. As John has a previous history of a left fractured clavicle, following a football accident in his teens, the replacement skin-tunnelled catheter will follow the same route as the present device.

Case study 14.2

Mary, a 54-year-old solicitor, lives with her husband and two teenage daughters. She has been diagnosed as having non-Hodgkin's lymphoma, for which she has been advised to have CHOP chemotherapy. Although this cytotoxic chemotherapy regimen contains two vesicant agents, i.e. vincristine and doxorubicin, it has been agreed to administer Mary's treatment via a peripheral cannula. The rationale for this is that Mary has good peripheral venous access and will be receiving her treatment on a three-weekly basis. Discussions with Mary identified that she was reluctant to consider a CVAD owing to limitations it would impose on her life in between hospital visits, i.e. the regular flushing of the catheter, the dressing required for a PICC or the visual reminder from a skin-tunnelled catheter. Mary was informed of the potential risks of phlebitis and extravasation from receiving these agents through a peripheral cannula, but weighed these against the possible risks of infection and thrombosis from a CVAD. Mary will reconsider a CVAD should she encounter venous access problems later in her treatment. This conversation was duly recorded in Mary's notes.

CONCLUSION

Parenteral therapy is one of the most commonly undertaken treatments. However, it is an invasive treatment and has the potential to lead to complications, especially in the haemato-oncology patient population. Knowledge regarding the patient's condition, intended treatment, previous medical history and any problems with vascular access devices, together with the types of vascular access devices available, will greatly reduce the potential for complications related to the parenteral therapy. The person placing the VAD should possess the knowledge and skills to assess the patient and place the most suitable device in an appropriate vessel. However, once the device is placed, knowledgeable and skilled management will diminish the potential for complications arising from the procedure and resulting parenteral therapy. Nurses caring for haemato-oncology patients are ideally placed to offer continuity of care to their patients. In so doing, they can often detect the earliest clinical features suggestive of a complication related to the vascular access device or the prescribed treatment. Early intervention can minimise the discomfort for the patient and ultimately ensure the longevity of the device.

DISCUSSION QUESTIONS

1. In your area of practice, what assessment criteria are used to determine the most appropriate VAD for individual patients?

2. What education/information and assessment is required to enable patients to care for their own VAD?

DISCUSSION QUESTIONS – CONT'D

3. How can a multidisciplinary-team approach to care of VADs be implemented and sustained?

4. How can you ensure that guidelines/protocols for care of VADs are based on the most up-to-date evidence?

References

Bravery K 1999 Paediatric intravenous therapy in practice. In: Dougherty L, Lamb J (eds) Intravenous therapy in nursing practice, Churchill Livingstone, Edinburgh, pp 401–445

Brothers T E, Von Moll L K, Arbor A et al 1988 Experiences with subcutaneous infusion ports in three hundred patients. Surgery, Gynaecology & Obstetrics 6(4):295–301

Broviac J, Cole J J, Scribner B H 1973 A silicone rubber atrial catheter for prolonged parenteral alimentation. Surgery, Gynaecology & Obstetrics 136(4):602–606

Camp-Sorrell D 1992 Implantable ports: everything you always wanted to know. Journal of Intravenous Nursing 15(5): 262–272

Crnich C J, Maki D G 2002 The promise of novel technology for the prevention of intravascular device-related bloodstream infection. II. Long-term devices. Healthcare Epidemiology CID 2002(15 May):34

Dougherty L 1999 Obtaining peripheral venous access. In: Dougherty L, Lamb J (eds) Intravenous therapy in nursing practice. Churchill Livingstone, Edinburgh, pp 223–259

Dougherty L 2003 The expert witness: working within the legal system of the United Kingdom. Journal of Vascular Access Devices 8(2):29–35

Elliott T S J 1993 Line associated bacteraemias. Communicable Diseases Report 3(7):R91–96

Gabriel J 1996a Peripherally inserted central catheters: expanding UK nurses' practice. British Journal of Nursing 5(2):71–74

Gabriel J 1996b Care and management of peripherally inserted central catheters. British Journal of Nursing 5(2):71–74

Gabriel J 1997 Fibrin sheaths in vascular access devices. Nursing Times 93(10):56–57

Gabriel J 1999 PICCs: how Doppler ultrasound can extend their use. Nursing Times 95(6):52–53

Gabriel J 2000 Patients' impressions of PICCs. Journal of Vascular Access Devices Winter:26–29

Gabriel J 2001 PICC securement: minimising potential complications. Nursing Standard 11(15): 42–44

Gabriel J 2003 Improved levels of patient care in the UK as nurses gain experience with PICCs. Journal of Vascular Access Devices Summer:18–20

Goodwin M, Carlson I 1993 The peripherally inserted central catheter: a retrospective look at 3 years of insertions. Journal of Intravenous Nursing 12(2): 92–103

Gormon C, Buzby G 1995 Difficult access problems. Surgical Oncology Clinics of North America 4(3):453–473

Hadaway L 1989 An overview of vascular access devices inserted via the antecubital area. Journal of Intravenous Nursing 13(5):297–306

Hadaway L 1995 Anatomy and physiology related to intravenous therapy. In: Terry J, Baranowski L, Lonsway R A, Hedrick C (eds) Intravenous therapy; clinical principles and practices. W B Saunders, Philadelphia, pp 81–110

Haindl H 1989 Technical complications of port-catheter systems. Regional Cancer Treatment 2:238–242

Hinke D H, Zandt-Stastny M D, Goodman L R, Quebbeman E J, Kyzwda E A, Andris D A 1990 Pinch-off syndrome: a complication of implantable subclavian venous access devices. Radiology 177: 353–356

Kayley J 2003 An overview of community intravenous therapy in the United Kingdom. Journal of Vascular Access Devices Summer:22–26

Lamb J 1999 Legal and professional aspects of intravenous therapy. In: Dougherty, L. Lamb, J (eds) Intravenous therapy in nursing practice, Churchill Livingstone, Edinburgh, pp 3–19

Lawson T 2003 A legal perspective on CVC-related extravasation. Journal of Vascular Access Devices Spring:25–27

Linares J, Sitges-Serra A, Garu J 1985 Pathogenesis of catheter sepsis: a prospective study with quantitative and semi-quantitative cultures of catheter hub and segments. Journal of Clinical Microbiology 21(3):357–360

Maki D G 2002 The promise of novel technology for prevention of intravascular device-related bloodstream infection. National Association of Vascular Access Networks (NAVAN) Conference, San Diego, CA, September 2002

Maki D G, Ringer M, Alvarado C J 1991 Prospective randomised trial of povidone-iodine, alcohol, and chlorhexidine for prevention of infection with central venous and arterial catheters. Lancet 338:339–343

Mayo D, Pearson D 1995 Chemotherapy extravasation: a consequence of fibrin sheath formation around venous access devices. Oncology Nursing Forum. 22(4):675–680

Medical Devices ALERT 2003 MDA/2003/020

Peterson B 2002 Stepping into the future: who will care for healthcare? National Association of Vascular Access Networks (NAVAN) Conference, San Diego, CA, September 2002

Reed W 1991 Intravenous access devices for supportive care of patients with cancer. Current Opinion in Oncology 3: 634–642

Richardson D, Bruso P 1993 Vascular access devices – management of common complications. Journal of Intravenous Nursing 16(1):44–49

Roth D 2003a Legally speaking. Journal of Vascular Access Devices Summer:57–58

Roth D 2003b Extravasation injuries of peripheral veins: a basis for litigation? Journal of Vascular Access Devices Spring:13–19

Royal College of Nursing 2003 RCN IV therapy forum: standards for infusion therapy. RCN, London

Ryder M A 1995 Peripheral access options. Surgical Clinics of North America 4(3):395–427

Scales K 1999 Anatomy and physiology. In: Dougherty L, Lamb J (eds) Intravenous therapy in nursing practice. Churchill Livingstone, Edinburgh, pp 21–43

Schelper R 2003 The aging venous system. Journal of the Association of Vascular Access 8(3):8–10

Soo K C, Davidson T I, Selby P, Westbury G 1985 Long-term venous access using a subcutaneous implantable drug delivery system. Annals of the Royal College of Surgeons of England. 67:263–265

Strumpfer A 1991 Lower incidence of peripheral catheter complications by the use of elastomeric hydrogel catheters in home intravenous therapy patients. Journal of Intravenous Nursing 14(4):261–267

Tschirhart J, Rao M 1988 Mechanism and management of persistent withdrawal occlusion. The American Surgeon 54:326–328

Vesley T 2003 X-ray interpretation: theory to practice. Presentation at 17th National Association of Vascular Access Networks (NAVAN) Conference Atlanta, GA, September 2003

Weinstein S M 1997 Anatomy and physiology applied to intravascular therapy. In: Weinstein S M (ed) Plumer's principles and practice of intravenous therapy, 6th edn. JB Lippincott, Philadelphia, pp 47–49

Wickham R, Purl S, Welker D 1992 Long-term central venous access catheters: issues for care. Seminars in Oncology Nursing 2(8):133–147

Further reading

Dougherty L, Lamb J (eds) 1999 Intravenous therapy in nursing practice. Churchill Livingstone, Edinburgh

Standards of infusion therapy 2003 Royal College of Nursing, London

The contributors to both the book and the standards have expertise and experience in placing and caring for individuals with a variety of VADs. Many of them have published papers relating to their specific areas of practice.

Chapter **15**

Prevention of infection

Sarah Hart

KEY POINTS

- Prevention of infection is a major challenge in the management of patients with haematological cancers.
- Infection risk is directly related to the severity and duration of neutropenia.
- The widespread use of antimicrobial agents for immunocompromised patients has led to an increase in antimicrobial resistance, which constitutes a major threat to public health (National Audit Office 2001).
- Collaborative multi-centre research is required to establish the most effective protective isolation practices.
- Adherence to evidence-based infection control policies and procedures is crucial.

KEY POINTS – CONT'D

- Research and effective quality assurance systems are required to improve infection control practice.
- The basic principles of infection control can be assisted by simple procedures such as handwashing and by ensuring that the patient's physical environment is free of microbial contamination (Pellowe et al 2004).

INTRODUCTION

The treatment of patients with haematological cancers has dramatically improved (Appelbaum 2004). Unfortunately, infectious complications related to the treatment for these diseases continue to have significant risk of mortality and morbidity (Auner et al 2002, Tabata et al 2005). This chapter is intended to be a practical guide to the nursing management of haemato-oncology patients. Wherever possible the information is based on scientific studies, whilst other information is obtained from guidance from evidence-based reviews undertaken by recognised experts or institutions. The references, which include textbooks, provide the reader with the opportunity to extend their knowledge.

RISK OF INFECTION

Infection is a major concern in the management of haemato-oncology patients, as its occurrence can be frequent and potentially life-threatening (Benoit et al 2003). Young (1994) discusses seven studies which show infection as the primary cause of death for patients with haematological cancers. More recently a review of 1011 patients with acute leukaemia treated between 1984 and 2002 also found that infection was the most common cause of death (Rubnitz et al 2004).

A further retrospective study of 114 autologous stem cell transplantation patients found that fever requiring antimicrobial therapy occurred during 80% of all treatment cycles, with 60% of these fevers being diagnosed as 'of unknown origin' (Auner et al 2002). Bowden & Mayers (1994) point out that the more aggressive treatment regimens are associated with a higher incidence of, and mortality from, infection, although it is not always clear whether the increase in infection is related to the underlying illness or its therapy. However, a study to determine whether patients with diverse haematological cancers had differing susceptibility to infectious complications during high-dose chemotherapy found no difference, suggesting all haemato-oncology patients are equally susceptible to infection (Auner et al 2002). Prevention of infection has increased in importance since treatments such as haemopoietic stem cell transplantation (HSCT) have led to steadily improving rates of long-term, disease-free survival for haemato-oncology patients

(Appelbaum 2004). (Plate 6 illustrates an infective episode in acute leukaemia.)

There are four major challenges to be considered in the prevention or reduction of the occurrence of infection:

- Use of increasingly toxic treatments including aggressive antineoplastic chemotherapy, radiotherapy and procedures such as HSCT, causing profound immunosuppression (Meunier 1995).
- The increase in antibiotic-resistant organisms means clinicians can no longer rely on limitless supplies of antibiotics when infections do occur (Communicable Disease Surveillance Centre 2000); infections caused by antibiotic-resistant micro-organisms significantly increase the risk of death (Turnidge 2003).
- Impaired immune response means the usual signs and symptoms of infection are reduced (Schimpff 1995).
- Global travel increases the risk of exposure to new infectious diseases – one example being severe acute respiratory syndrome (SARS) (Lashley 2004).

These challenges substantially increase the difficulty in preventing, treating and detecting infection in individuals. Factors which increase the infection risk for those with haematological disease include:

- *Immunocompromise* due to underlying disease, notably those affecting the bone marrow, but also diseases such as HIV, chronic alcoholism and diabetes mellitus.
- *Immunosuppression* as a consequence of radiotherapy, chemotherapy or steroid therapy causes neutropenia, cellular and humoral immune dysfunction.
- *Presence of colonising organisms* in those who are immunosuppressed. Colonising organisms of otherwise low pathogenicity can cause endogenous infection (Glauser & Calandra 2000).
- *Age* – extremes of age increase susceptibility to infection, as well as affecting recovery from treatment (Tabata et al 2005).
- *Loss of skin and mucous membrane integrity* provides entry for micro-organisms.
- *Antibiotic therapy* – the administration of broad-spectrum antibacterial agents produces a shift in microbial flora, which disrupts their natural ability to prevent colonisation with hospital-acquired pathogens (National Audit Office 2001). In the presence of antibiotics, resistant micro-organisms have a selective advantage (Hart 1998) and the risk of fungal infections is increased (Glauser & Calandra 2000).
- *Poor nutrition* reduces the production of white blood cells required for immunity. Food supplements enhance the immune system (Jiang et al 2004).
- *Multiple invasive procedures* breach the body's natural barriers to infection providing entry for micro-organisms. These include the skin and mucous membranes with intravenous catheters, urinary catheters and biopsy needles.

SOURCES OF MICRO-ORGANISMS

Infection can be grouped into two categories, exogenous, which refers to organisms originating outside or away from the patient's body, and endogenous, attributed to organisms already present in or on the patient's body (Tammelin et al 2003, Rohde et al 2004). The detrimental effects of both can be limited by scrupulous cleanliness of the patient and environment.

About 9% of patients develop a healthcare-associated infection (HCAI) following admission to hospital. This costs the UK National Health Service as much as one billion pounds a year and as many as 5000 patients die from HCAI (National Audit Office 2001). As the incidence and severity of infection are inversely proportional to the degree of immunosuppression (Schimpff 1995), it can be expected that haemato-oncology patients will have an even higher incidence of infection. Adoption and adherence to good infection control principles is therefore vital in reducing the incidence of HCAI (Hospital Infection Working Group 1995).

Schimpff (1995) reviewed infections in a group of cancer patients and found nearly all infections originated from endogenous organisms colonising the patient at or near the site of infection; one-third of these organisms were initially exogenous and had been acquired subsequent to hospital admission. For example, *Pseudomonas aeruginosa* can usually be found colonising the rectum prior to bacteraemia originating from a perianal cellulitis. Similarly the oral cavity harbours many varieties of bacteria which do not cause problems in an immunocompetent person (Safdar & Armstrong 2002). Unfortunately the mucositis which frequently accompanies cytotoxic therapy increases the pathogenicity of these organisms, which can lead to local and systemic infection (Bagg et al 2003, Scully et al 2004).

INFECTING ORGANISMS

Immunosuppressed patients can become infected with any pathogenic micro-organism capable of causing infection in healthy persons and are particularly susceptible to opportunistic micro-organisms which do not normally cause infections in healthy persons (Calandra 2000). Susceptibility to these organisms means that infections are likely to occur in immunosuppressed individuals despite efforts to avoid infection. Measures taken to prevent infection are therefore aimed at minimising the risk from micro-organisms. All micro-organisms are important if they have the ability to be transmitted in the environment, cause infection and produce clinical infection. These may be bacterial, viral, protozoal, helminthic or fungal. Some organisms cannot survive for long outside the body; an example of this is meningococcal meningitis which can be carried harmlessly in the back of the throat of one person but when inhaled by a susceptible host causes significant infection. Other

Table 15.1
Organisms and their vectors

Vector	Organism
Food – Undercooked chicken, eggs – Raw fruit and vegetables	*Salmonella, Listeria, Bacillus* *Pseudomonas, Campylobacter*
Tap water	*Cryptosporidium, Pseudomonas,* *Legionella*

Stagnant water (unsterile humidification
    water, flower water, water-retaining
    toys, etc.)
	Pseudomonas

Soil	*Aspergillus, Clostridium*
Plants and flowers	*Aspergillus, Pseudomonas*
Contaminated intravenous fluids	*Pseudomonas*
Showers, hand basins, baths, toilets	*Pseudomonas, Clostridium difficile,* vancomycin-resistant Enterococci
Bedding	*Staphylococcus aureus* (including MRSA), vancomycin-resistant Enterococci
Air	*Aspergillus*

Furniture, floors, beds	*Staphylococcus aureus* (including MRSA),
	    Staphylococcus epidermidis,
	    vancomycin-resistant Enterococci,
	    Clostridium difficile

Contaminated dressing packs,
    stethoscopes, pens
	Staphylococcus aureus (including MRSA),
	    Staphylococcus epidermidis,
	    vancomycin-resistant Enterococci,
	    Clostridium difficile

organisms such as *Pseudomonas aeruginosa* have the ability to contaminate and survive in the environment prior to reaching a susceptible host (Buttery et al 1998). While others such as methicillin-resistant *Staphylococcus aureus* (MRSA) have the capability of surviving and multiplying within the environment (Dietze et al 2001). Examples of organisms and their vector are shown in Table 15.1.

In the past, bacterial infections have been relatively easily treated with intravenous antibiotics. However, the emergence of antibiotic-resistant organisms has further increased the risk of serious infection by changing the balance of survival in favour of the resistant organism. Coliforms including Klebsiella and Enterobacter are especially important as they have the ability to acquire resistance to many antimicrobial agents. They can be found in the environment and cause opportunistic infections and outbreaks of cross-infection. Recent reports of MRSA acquiring vancomycin resistance (Franchi et al 1999) emphasise the importance of compliance with effective infection control policies.

REFLECTION POINT Suzanne, a 40-year-old diabetic with acute myeloid leukaemia has been admitted for allogeneic HSCT. She has a skin-tunnelled venous catheter in situ, the exit site of which is growing MRSA. Identify the factors which make Suzanne especially susceptible to infection (see end of chapter for suggestions).

Fungal infections tend to have a high mortality rate. Commonly identified pathogens include the Candida group and Aspergillus (Marr et al 2002, Safdar & Armstrong 2002). In one study following allogeneic HSCT, invasive fungal infections accounted for 39% of the non-relapse mortality rate (Fukuda et al 2003).

PRINCIPLES OF INFECTION CONTROL

PROTECTIVE ISOLATION

The risk of infection for haemato-oncology patients is directly related to the severity and duration of immunosuppression. Neutropenia is a predictable result of cancer therapy and the exact level of neutrophils is a useful index of infection risk. The risk of infection rises as the neutrophil count falls, there being a major increase with a rapidly falling count or when the count approaches zero (Kibbler 2003).

Protective isolation procedures have traditionally been used to reduce infection risk for the neutropenic patient. The need for protective isolation has long been debated. Poe et al's (1994) survey of 91 bone marrow transplant programmes in the USA found that all units used some type of protective environment, although practices varied considerably. A later review of Australian and North American paediatric oncology units indicated that protective isolation which includes positive pressure single rooms, low microbial diet and strict handwashing is only required for patients receiving allogeneic transplants (Dadd et al 2003).

Protective isolation practices range from the use of purpose-built units with air filtration systems and plastic isolators to single rooms on a general ward or shared rooms within a controlled environment on a general ward (Dougherty & Lister 2004). Protective measures taken within these environments also vary. In complete protective environments a strict aseptic approach may be taken, with staff wearing sterile clothing and patients undergoing gut decontamination and receiving a sterile diet. At the other end of the range practices may be limited to common-sense measures such as handwashing and avoiding people with obvious infections. In between are a variety of practices including wearing gloves, gowns and masks, and use of a modified or low bacterial diet. Research data demonstrating the effectiveness of protective isolation practices is currently inconclusive (Mank & van der Lelie 2003, Larson & Nirenberg 2004).

Early studies suggest that (expensive to build, maintain and staff) protective isolation units have been seen to reduce infection (Buckner et al

1978). Yet protective isolation only appears to affect long-term survival by reducing graft-versus-host disease (Storb et al 1983). According to Dunleavey (1996), the lack of evidence supporting the effectiveness of protective isolation practices has resulted in many units abandoning these practices. However, there is some evidence to suggest that positive pressure air filtration systems may be effective in reducing the incidence of bacterial and fungal infections especially Aspergillus (Hahn et al 2002). The Center for Disease Control (CDC) (2003) suggests that infection control risk assessments should be conducted to establish the needs of the patient population.

The risk of infection when using single rooms and shared rooms on general wards depends on the general condition of the ward environment and the infectious status of other patients. However, if protective isolation is to be effective, it needs to be instituted on admission, before the patient has the opportunity to become colonised with potentially pathogenic organisms from the hospital environment such as MRSA and vancomycin-resistant Enterococci (VRE) (Duckro et al 2005, Ott et al 2005).

There is a lack of data comparing cross-infection rates in single rooms to those in shared rooms. However, a small study investigating transmission rates of urinary tract infection indicated cross-infection is reduced if catheterised patients are nursed in single rooms (Fryklund et al 1997). The Department of Health's (2004a) Health Building Notes (HBN) 4 consultative document related to inpatient accommodation states that there are many benefits of a single room including: protecting immunosuppressed patients at risk of acquiring an infection from others, and reducing the risk to others from a patient who is admitted with or subsequently develops an infection. Furthermore, NHS Estates (2002) advise that infection control must be included on all stages of the design of new buildings or the renovation of existing buildings and suggest that there is an increasing need for en-suite single rooms with appropriate air conditioning because of the increases in antibiotic-resistant bacteria and immunosuppressed inpatients.

New hospitals have more single rooms for isolation that ever before. Eight of 12 hospitals applying for planning approval in 2004 have 50% single rooms. The four without this provision were asked to review their plans (DoH 2004a), reflecting how the control of infection is being incorporated into the design of hospitals.

In conjunction with protective isolation, microbial suppression of alimentary tract organisms with oral non-absorbable antibiotics has been evaluated as a means of preventing infection (Storring et al 1977). Inconsistent results have been obtained from randomised trials and Wade (1994) outlines the disadvantages of these regimens, including patient poor compliance, nausea and cost. However, their use may reduce infection rates during periods of profound and persistent neutropenia, significant mucosal disruption or recurrent perirectal infections.

A study of infection rates comparing hospitalised patients in single rooms and patients who spent some time at home, where food restrictions and antibiotic prophylaxis continued, found that mortality data compared favourably (Russell et al 1992). This evidence, combined with the incidence of HCAI, supports the need for further investigation into the benefits of early discharge.

Collaborative multi-centre research is required to establish the most effective protective isolation practices, so that national guidelines can be developed. Psychological distress caused by protective isolation also needs to be addressed (Belec 1992) (see Chapter 23) and highlights the importance of attention to all aspects of patient care.

BARRIER NURSING

Whilst handwashing is the simplest and most important measure to prevent healthcare-acquired infection, the isolation of infected patients is key in controlling the transmission of infection (Bowden 2000). Carriers of infection and infected patients must be identified early. The potential for cross-infection should be evaluated and barrier nursing commenced when necessary. For example, patients colonised with MRSA will need barrier nursing whilst patients who are compliant with good handwashing and have *Clostridium difficile* in their stool will not (Sanderson & Richardson 1997). Viral infections such as shingles or chickenpox (herpes zoster) and cytomegalovirus may be easily transmitted between individuals with haematological cancers – patients with these conditions will require strict barrier nursing (Dougherty & Lister 2004). As with those in protective isolation, individuals being barrier nursed because of an infection will need support as they can feel stigmatised and lonely (Knowles 1993). Improved communication between the patient and hospital staff can improve the isolation experience (Ward 2000).

Protective clothing

The choice of protective clothing is decided by expected contact with infected or immunocompromised patients or to comply with universal blood and body fluid precautions. Generally, if protective clothing is worn correctly for universal blood and body fluid precautions, additional protective clothing is not required. Plastic aprons provide a cheap impermeable barrier to micro-organisms and should be worn during close contact with infected, immunosuppressed patients or when blood and body fluids are present; they must be changed between patients. Gloves do not replace handwashing and clean boxed gloves should be worn to protect the wearer from blood and body fluid contamination. Sterile gloves are only required during certain aseptic techniques. Caps and overshoes are not required. Masks and eye protection are rarely required, except to protect the wearer during universal precautions or administering toxic drugs (National Institute for Clinical Excellence (NICE) 2003).

STRATEGY FOR THE PREVENTION OF INFECTION

Attention to the following points will reduce the risk of infection for haemato-oncology patients.

HANDWASHING

Handwashing is the single most important procedure for preventing infection. Hands must be washed before and after patient contact. Rings and wristwatches must be removed and sleeves rolled up. Plain liquid soap is suitable for general tasks and removes transient organisms. Bactericidal detergent will remove both transient and resident organisms and should be used prior to aseptic techniques and providing care for immunocompromised patients. Bactericidal alcoholic handrub is a quick, effective means of cleansing hands (NICE 2003) and can be used when hands are clean and during aseptic techniques. Alcoholic handrub must be at each patient's bed (National Patient Safety Agency (NPSA) 2004).

REFLECTION POINT Review the handwashing techniques of yourself and your colleagues. Compare current practice with the above guidelines.

FIT, HEALTHY STAFF AND VISITORS

Staff caring for those who are immunosuppressed should be free from infection. Visitors should be advised of the potential for cross-infection and the importance of informing ward staff if they are unwell or have been in contact with a contagious disease.

REGULAR OBSERVATIONS

Vital signs must be regularly monitored for signs of infection, and the condition of the mouth and skin observed on at least a daily basis. The body's normal reaction to infection is for tissue macrophages to be attracted to the area in an attempt to remove the organisms inducing an inflammatory response. Phagocytes (neutrophils and macrophages) are attracted to the site of inflammation by the process of chemotaxis, destroying the organism by phagocytosis (Modjtahedi & Clarke 2004). In neutropenic patients this inflammatory response to infection is reduced and the normal signs of inflammation will be reduced or absent. Therefore every sign of infection must be treated as significant. Frequently the only sign of infection is a pyrexia and there may be no obvious indication of the site of infection. In the presence of pyrexia a full infection screen should be undertaken in an attempt to identify the infecting organism. Microbiological samples should be collected, including bacteriological and viral cultures of blood, urine and sputum specimens, nasal and throat swabs, and swabs from any suspicious lesions. A chest x-ray may also be performed. Septicaemic shock can develop rapidly in an immunosuppressed individual and may result in death. It is therefore imperative that broad-spectrum intravenous antibiotics are commenced immediately when signs of infection are detected.

PATIENT HYGIENE

Daily showers or baths and regular hairwashes should be encouraged to remove micro-organisms and improve patient comfort. Individuals must be provided with clean towels and disposable wash clothes. Baths must be cleaned carefully after each patient. The Essence of Care (DoH 2001), which includes personal and oral hygiene, provides a tool to help to identify best practice and to develop action plans to improve care.

MOUTH CARE

Mouth care will help to keep mouth and lips clean, moist and intact, and will reduce pain and infection. Regular assessment of the mouth and oral care is essential (Scully et al 2004, Wohlschaegar 2004) (see Chapter 18).

MAINTENANCE OF BODY'S NATURAL DEFENCES

Care should be taken to minimise the potential for infection at venous access sites (see Chapter 14). Care should also be taken to maintain skin integrity, with attention to pressure areas if the individual has reduced mobility. Keeping fingernails and toenails clean and short will also help to prevent individuals accidentally injuring themselves. Avoidance of constipation will reduce the possibility of damage to the rectal mucosa. If constipation does occur, use of suppositories and enemas should be avoided, again to prevent damage to the rectal mucosa.

ENVIRONMENTAL CLEANLINESS

The patient environment and equipment shared by more than one patient can become contaminated with potentially pathogenic micro-organisms. One study found that shared hospital equipment as diverse as bed tables, bed linen and blood pressure cuffs can become contaminated with MRSA, and can act as a reservoir of infection for future patients on whom the equipment is used (Boyce et al 1997). The use of carpets and soft furnishings in patient areas should also be avoided (NHS Estates 2002, CDC 2003). A clean hospital environment provides the right setting for good infection control (DoH 2004b). Over 3000 matrons have been appointed since 1999 whose responsibilities include improving cleaning standards (NHS Estates 2004).

Thorough daily cleaning using hot soapy water will remove most organisms; disinfectants are not generally required (Ayliffe et al 2000). Microbial contamination can be removed by thorough cleaning with soap and water or destroyed by sterilisation or disinfection (Ayliffe et al 2000). Equipment that is only used on intact skin can be cleaned with detergent and water. Generally, equipment which penetrates skin, mucous membranes or sterile cavities should be sterile disposable or sterilised by autoclaving. Equipment which has contact with mucous membranes should preferably be sterilised by autoclaving but may be thoroughly cleaned and disinfected. Care must be taken to comply with the Control of Substances Hazardous to Health Regulations (COSHH 2002) when using disinfectants. On discharge the room and furniture should be cleared and terminally cleaned. Use of a bleach solution is required when the patient is colonised with VRE (Kearns et al 1995). Communal ward kitchen equipment and working surfaces are reservoirs for infection and must be meticulously cleaned and maintained (Ayliffe et al 2000).

Restrict plants and flowers

Fresh and dried flowers and potted plants should be restricted in the rooms of immunosuppressed individuals as they are a reservoir for potential pathogens (CDC 2003).

Aseptic techniques

Aseptic techniques must be adopted during all tasks that bypass the body's natural defence mechanisms and when handling equipment such as intravenous catheters (see Chapter 14). Aseptic techniques help to prevent contamination of wounds and other susceptible sites (Dougherty & Lister 2004).

Clean food

Raw fruit and vegetables and undercooked fish, eggs and meat are a potential infection risk (Pattison 1993). Food restrictions vary between units and may be dependent on the treatment being administered. Greater restrictions may be placed on those undergoing HSCT. However, in general raw fruit and vegetables and foods known to carry bacteria, such as soft cheeses, should be avoided. Other foods should be well cooked for those who are immunosuppressed (see Chapter 19).

Drinking water and ice

The 1989 United Kingdom Water act requires that drinking water is tested at every stage of its treatment. Tap water is also chlorinated to ensure that any remaining bacteria are killed. Unfortunately drinking water and ice may be contaminated through incorrect handling by staff, patients or visitors and environmental factors such as dirty ice machines and contaminated taps (Wilson et al 1997). For especially immunosuppressed patients such as HSCT patients, drinking water and ice should be provided from boiled or filtered water (NHS Estates 2002). Bottled drinking water has become very popular; this water is not governed by the strict legislation of tap water and in the past has been found to be contaminated (Walker 1992). Therefore, filtered tap water remains the water of choice.

Disinfecting bedpan washer

Mechanically clean and disinfect bedpans and urinals. All shared equipment must be heat treated between uses.

Reliable hospital laundry

Used linen must be thermally disinfected to remove micro-organisms by a laundry which complies with the Department of Health's (1995) Regulations. Clean linen should be transported and stored in a safe, clean manner.

PATIENT EDUCATION

Patient education is important so that individuals are aware of the actions they can take to minimise the infection risk, recognise signs of infection and be aware of the need to report these signs promptly. Patients should be informed that their risk of infection will be minimised if signs of infection are detected early and treated promptly. Information should be provided of the likely signs of infection that may occur, both as an inpatient and whilst they are at home, and whom they should inform of these problems. Symptoms for which advice should be sought include increased respiratory, heart and pulse rate, pyrexia, productive cough, rash, skin lesions, infected wound, frequency of micturition, bleeding, and gastrointestinal disturbances such as mucositis or diarrhoea (Bowden 2000).

Education increases patient satisfaction and enhances compliance with prevention of infection practices (Richards 1998). Additionally it empowers individuals to participate in their care while improving quality of care (Kreps 2003).

VISITOR AND FAMILY CARER EDUCATION

Carers who are present when health-care professionals are providing information to patients experience a decrease in anxiety and greater satisfaction, and the patient experiences fewer problems post-discharge (Driscoll 2000). Educated visitors are more likely to comply themselves and encourage the patient to comply with infection control procedures. Research studies have indicated that the majority of family carers wish to be further involved in decision-making and care (Walker & Dewar 2001). Similarly, preparation of patients prior to, during and after transplantation can help to alleviate anxieties throughout care (Buchsel et al 1996).

DISCHARGE PLANNING

Immune recovery after treatment such as HSCT will be delayed long after the patient has been discharged from hospital (Vossen & Handgretinger 2001). Discharge planning of immunocompromised patients involves the medical and nursing team from the hospital and the community, as well as the significant family or friends who will be providing help and support in the community (Dougherty & Lister 2004). Once at home patients need to be alert to signs and symptoms of infection so that they know to contact their doctor or the hospital immediately if problems occur. The risk of acquiring an infection in the community can be reduced by taking precautions when shopping, storing and preparing food, and avoiding foods known to contain bacteria. Whilst discharged patients can mix with other people, they must avoid persons with colds, influenza and other infections. For these reasons it is sensible to avoid crowded pubs, theatres, shops or restaurants. Health-care professionals should advise outpatients when they can mix more freely with people again, as this will depend on the underlying disease and treatment programmes.

Animals are generally restricted from the clinical setting. Whilst contact with animals by terminally ill immunocompromised patients should continue, for patients currently receiving or recovering from immunosuppressive therapy caution must continue following discharge and contact should be restricted to known, well cared for, fit pets. Contact with animal faeces, saliva and urine should be avoided (CDC 2003). Nurses have a key role in preparing patients for life after a haematological cancer and discharge planning should begin at the time of admission (Fernsler & Fanuele 1998).

Case study 15.1

Joe is an 18-year-old diagnosed with acute lymphoblastic leukaemia 12 months ago. During this time he has been treated with intensive chemotherapy and spent prolonged periods of time in the isolation area of the haematology unit. Joe is currently receiving treatment as an outpatient in the day case unit.

Eight days after his latest chemotherapy treatment Joe arrived on the unit unexpectedly one morning as he had developed a pyrexia. His temperature was found to be 38.9°C with a pulse of 110 and blood pressure of 110/70. A full blood count showed a haemoglobin of 9.8 g/L, white cell count of 0.7×10^9/L, an absolute neutrophil count of 0.04×10^9/L and a platelet count of 179×10^9/L.

Joe was admitted to an isolation room to protect him from further infection and screening was begun to establish the origin and causative agent of his infection. Blood was taken peripherally and from both lumens of Joe's Hickman line for culture. Swabs were taken from the central line exit site for microscopy, culture and sensitivity. A throat swab and specimens of urine, faeces and sputum were also obtained for analysis.

Joe was examined by the doctor and a chest x-ray performed. He was commenced on intravenous antibiotics as per hospital protocol for patients with a neutropenic septic episode. Joe's temperature and pulse were initially monitored 2-hourly until he became more stable and his general condition was closely observed for signs of deterioration. Fluid intake and urine output were monitored to ensure adequate hydration and oxygen saturation levels were measured.

Blood counts were taken daily to check Joe's white count and renal and liver function. The source and causative organism for Joe's infection were never isolated. He became apyrexial after 24 hours but continued to be closely observed throughout his admission. Remaining apyrexial he completed 5 days of intravenous antibiotics and was discharged home.

MEANS OF IMPROVING INFECTION CONTROL PRACTICE

RESEARCH

Research allows the development of the scientific knowledge base for nursing practice by seeking ways to improve and standardise practice. The demands placed on nurses working in the rapidly changing field of oncology mean that clinical research to identify new and effective strategies to prevent infection is essential.

STANDARDS

Standards can be used as the basis for measuring quality of care provided to patients and underpin effective infection control programmes (Infection Control Standards Working Party 1993, Luthert & Robinson 1993).

AUDIT

Audit is a systematic critical and continuing analysis of quality of care and use of resources to identify where improvements can be made (Millward et al 1993). Most aspects of infection control such as mouth care, care of central lines, compliance to handwashing can be audited. The Infection Control Nurses Association (ICNA), working in partnership with the Department of Health, has produced an audit tool which provides a reliable, agreed, repeatable infection control audit which can be used in all areas of the hospital (ICNA 2004).

POLICES AND PROCEDURES

Approved policies and procedures which are regularly reviewed and updated to take account of new research and high-dose chemotherapy regimens should be available for all infection control issues (Dougherty & Lister 2004). Compliance with infection control policies and procedures is variable. Moore (1997) stresses that reducing infection requires ongoing education of staff in view of the high turnover of nursing and medical staff. Houang & Hurley (1997) suggest that education programmes based on psychological principles improve motivation and compliance; Teare & Peacock (1996) found that the introduction of an infection control link nurse system raised the profile of infection control by disseminating knowledge and changing behaviour and attitudes. Adoption of one or both of these strategies may help adherence to infection control policies.

CONCLUSION

This chapter has reviewed strategies which will help to reduce the incidence of infection. Whilst controversy surrounds the nursing management of the haemato-oncology patient, nurses need to be familiar with the principles and rationale for good infection control practices.

DISCUSSION QUESTIONS

1. Why are haemato-oncology patients especially susceptible to infection?

2. What elements of nursing care are most useful in preventing infection in immunocompromised patients?

3. Which clinical features indicate that protective isolation is required?

4. Which common infections seen on your ward require barrier nursing?

5. What are the strengths and weaknesses of protective isolation in your place of work?

6. How might infection control practices be improved in your place of work?

7. How can communication with the infection control team be strengthened?

SUGGESTIONS FOR FIRST REFLECTION POINT

Factors which increase patient's risk of infection:

- diabetic
- disease of bone marrow
- previous treatment with chemotherapy and antibiotics
- allogeneic HSCT, necessitating the use of immunosuppressive drugs to prevent graft-vs-host disease
- already colonised with a potentially pathogenic organism.

References

Appelbaum F R 2004 Bone marrow transplantation for leukaemia current status and strategy for improvement. Annals of the Academy of Medicine Singapore 33(5 Suppl):S4–S6

Auner H W, Sill H, Mulabecirovic A et al 2002 Infectious complications after autologous hematopoietic stem cell transplantation: comparison of patients with acute myeloid leukaemia, malignant lymphoma, and multiple myeloma. Annals of Hematology 81(7):374–377

Ayliffe G A J, Fraise A P, Geddes A M, Mitchell K 2000 Control of hospital infection: a practical handbook, 4th edn. Chapman & Hall, London

Bagg J, Sweeney M P, Lewis M A et al 2003 High prevalence of non-albicans yeasts and detection of anti-fungal resistance in the oral flora of patients with advanced cancer. Palliative Medicine 17(6):477–481

Belec R H 1992 Quality of life: perceptions of long term survivors of bone marrow transplantation. Oncology Nursing Forum 19(1):31–37

Benoit D D, Vandewoude K H, Decruyenaere J M et al 2003 Outcome and early prognostic indicators in patients with a hematologic malignancy admitted to the intensive care unit for life-threatening complication. Critical Care Medicine 31(1):104–112

Bowden R A 2000 Infections in blood and bone marrow transplant patients: allogeneic and autologous transplantation. In: Glauser M P, Pizzo P A (eds) Management of infections in immunocompromised patients. WB Saunders, London, pp 189–218

Bowden R A, Mayers J D 1994 Infection complicating bone marrow transplantation In: Rubins R H, Young L S (eds) Clinical approach to infection in the compromised host, 3rd edn. Plenum, New York, pp 601–628

Boyce J M, Potter-Bynoe G, Chenevert C, King T 1997 Environmental contamination due to methicillin-resistant *Staphylococcus aureus*: possible infection control implications. Infection Control & Hospital Epidemiology 18(9):622–627

Buchsel P C, Leum E W, Randolph S R 1996 Delayed complications of bone marrow transplantation: an update. Oncology Nursing Forum 23(8):1267–1291

Buckner C D, Clift R A, Sanders J E 1978 Protective environment for marrow transplant recipients. A prospective study. Annals of Internal Medicine 89:893–901

Buttery J P, Alabaster S J, Heine R G et al 1998 Multiresistant *Pseudomonas aeruginosa* outbreak in a pediatric oncology ward related to bath toys. Pediatric Infectious Diseases 17(6):509–513

Calandra T 2000 Components of the natural host defence systems against infection. In: Glauser M P, Pizzo P A (eds) Management of infections in immunocompromised patients. WB Saunders, London, pp 3–6

Center for Disease Control (CDC) 2003 Guidelines for environmental infection control in healthcare facilities. Morbidity Mortality Weekly Report 52(RR10)1–42

Communicable Disease Surveillance Centre 2000 Antimicrobial resistance in 2000 England and Wales. Public Health Laboratory Service, London

Control of Substances Hazardous to Health Regulations (COSHH) 2002 HMSO, London

Dadd G, McMinn P, Monterosso L 2003 Protective isolation in hemopoietic stem cell transplants: a review of the literature and single institution experience. Journal of Pediatric Oncology Nursing 20(6):293–300

Department of Health 1995 Hospital laundry arrangements for used and infected linen. HSG(95)18. HMSO, London

Department of Health 2001 The essence of care. Patient focussed benchmarking for health care practitioners. HMSO, London

Department of Health 2004a HBN 4 Inpatients accommodation. Supplement 1: Isolation facilities in acute settings. HMSO, London

Department of Health 2004b Towards cleaner hospitals and lower rates of infection. A summary of action. HMSO, London

Dietze B, Rath A, Wendt C et al 2001 Survival of MRSA on sterile goods packaging. Journal of Hospital Infection 49(4):255–261

Dougherty L, Lister S 2004 The Royal Marsden Hospital manual of clinical nursing procedures, 6th edn. Blackwell, Oxford

Driscoll A 2000 Managing post discharge care at home; an analysis of patients' and their carers' perception of information received during their stay in hospital. Journal of Advanced Nursing 31(5):1165–1173

Duckro A N, Blom D W, Lyle E A et al 2005 Transfer of vancomycin-resistant enterococci via health care workers' hands. Archives of Internal Medicine 165(3):302–307

Dunleavey R 1996 Isolation in BMT: a protection or a privation? British Journal of Nursing 5(11):663–668

Fernsler J, Fanuele J S 1998 Lymphomas: long term sequelae and survivorship issues. Seminars in Oncology Nursing 14(4):321–328

Franchi D, Climo M W, Wong A H et al 1999 Seeking vancomycin resistant *Staphylococcus aureus* among patients with vancomycin resistant enterococci. Clinical Infectious Diseases 29(6):1566–1568

Fryklund B, Haeggman S, Burman LG 1997 Transmission of urinary bacterial strains between patients with indwelling catheters: nursing in the same room and in separate rooms compared. Journal of Hospital Infection 36:147–153

Fukuda T, Boeckh M, Carter R A et al 2003 Risks and outcomes of invasive fungal infection in recipients of allogeneic hematopoietic stem cell transplant after nonmyeloablative conditioning. Blood 102(3):827–833

Glauser M P, Calandra T 2000 Infections in patients with hematologic malignancies. In: Glauser M P, Pizzo P A (eds) Management of infections in immunocompromised patients. WB Saunders, London, pp 141–188

Hahn T, Cummings K M, Michalek A M et al 2002 Efficacy of high-efficiency particulate air filtration in preventing aspergillosis in immunocompromised patients with haematological malignancies. Infection Control & Hospital Epidemiology 23(9):525–531

Hart C A 1998 Antibiotic resistance: an increasing problem? British Medical Journal 316:1255–1256

Hospital Infection Working Group 1995 Hospital infection control. Department of Health, London

Houang E T S, Hurley R 1997 Anonymous questionnaire survey on the knowledge and practices of hospital staff in infection control. Journal of Hospital Infection 35:301–306

Infection Control Nurses Association working in partnership with the Department of Health 2004 Audit tools for monitoring infection control standards. Fitwise, Edinburgh

Infection Control Standards Working Party 1993 Standards in infection control in hospitals. Department of Health, London

Jiang X H, Li N, Zhu W M et al 2004 Effect of post operative immune-enhancing enteral nutrition on the immune system, inflammatory responses, and clinical outcome. Clinical Medical Journal 117(6):835–839

Kearns A M, Freeman R, Lightfoot N F 1995 Nosocomial enterococci resistance to heat and sodium hypochlorite. Journal of Hospital Infection 30:193–199

Kibbler C 2003 Infections associated with neutropenia and transplantation. In: Finch R G, Greenwood D, Norrby S R, Whitley R J (eds) Antibiotic and chemotherapy anti-infective agents and their use in therapy, 8th edn. Churchill Livingstone, Edinburgh, pp 545–561

Knowles H E 1993 The experience of infectious patients in isolation. Nursing Times 89(30):53–56

Kreps G J 2003 The impact of communication on cancer risk, incidence morbidity, mortality and quality of life. Health Communication 15(2):161–169

Larson E, Nirenberg A 2004 Evidence-based nursing practice to prevent infection in hospitalized neutropenic patients with cancer. Oncology Nursing Forum 31(4):717–725

Lashley F R 2004 Emerging infectious diseases: vulnerability, contributing factors and approaches. Expert Review of Anti-Infective Therapy 2(2):299–316

Luthert J M, Robinson L 1993 The Royal Marsden Hospital manual of standards of care. Blackwell Science, Oxford

Mank A, van der Lelie H 2003 Is there still a indication for nursing patients with prolonged neutropenia in protective isolation? European Journal of Oncology Nursing 7(1):17–23.

Marr K A, Carter R A, Boeckh M, Martin P, Corey L 2002 Invasive aspergillosis in allogeneic stem cell transplant recipient changes in epidemiology and risk factors. Blood 100(13):4358–4366

Meunier F 1995 Infections in patients with acute leukaemia and lymphoma. In: Mandel G L, Dolin R (eds) Principles and practices of infectious diseases, 4th edn. Churchill Livingstone, Edinburgh

Millward S, Barnett J, Thomlinson D 1993 A clinical infection control audit programme. Journal of Infection Control 24:219–232

Modjtahedi H, Clarke A 2004 The immune system. In: Gabriel J (ed) The biology of cancer. Whurr, London, pp 96–109

Moore A 1997 Hospital bugbear. The Health Service Journal 107(5577 Suppl 1):1–4

National Audit Office 2001 The challenge of hospital acquired infection. HMSO, London

National Health Service (NHS) Estates 2002 Infection control in the built environment. HMSO, London

National Health Service (NHS) Estates 2004 A matron's charter: an action plan for cleaner hospitals. HMSO, London

National Institute for Clinical Excellence (NICE) 2003 Infection control: prevention of healthcare-associated infection in primary and community care. NICE, London

National Patient Safety Agency (NPSA) 2004 Clean your hands campaign. NHS Direct, London

Ott M, Shen J, Sherwood S 2005 Evidence-based practice for control of methicillin-resistant Staphylococcus aureus. AORN Journal 81(2):361–364

Pattison A J 1993 Review of current practice in clean diets in the UK. Journal of Human Nutrition and Dietetics 6:3–11

Pellowe C M, Pratt R J, Loveday H P et al 2004 The EPIC project. Updating the evidence-base for national evidence-based guidelines for preventing healthcare-associated infections in NHS hospitals in England: a report with recommendations. British Journal of Infection Control 5(6):10–16

Poe S S, Larson E, McGuire D, Krumm S 1994 A national survey of infection prevention practices on bone marrow transplant units. Oncology Nursing Forum 21(10):1687–1694

Richards T 1998 Partnership with patients British Medical Journal 316:85–86

Rohde H, Kalitzky M, Kroger N et al 2004 Detection of virulence-associated genes not useful for discriminating between invasive and commensal Staphylococcus epidermidis from a bone marrow transplant unit. Journal of Clinical Microbiology 42(12):5614–5619

Rubnitz J E, Lensing S, Zhou Y et al 2004 Death during induction therapy and first remission of acute leukaemia in childhood: the St Jude experience. Cancer 10(7):1677–1684

Russell J A, Poon M C, Jones A R et al 1992 Allogeneic bone marrow transplantation without protective isolation in adults with malignant disease. Lancet 339:38–40

Safdar A, Armstrong D 2002 Prospective evaluation of Candida species colonization in hospitalized cancer patients: impact on short-term survival in recipients of marrow transplantation and patients with haematological malignancies. Bone Marrow Transplantation 30(12):931–935

Sanderson P, Richardson D 1997 Do patients with clostridium need to be isolated. Journal of Infection Control 36(2):157–158

Schimpff S C 1995 Infections in the cancer patient. In: Mandell G L, Bennett J E, Dolin R (eds) Principles and practices of infectious diseases. Churchill Livingstone, Edinburgh, pp 2666–2686

Scully C, Epstein J, Sonis S 2004 Oral mucositis: a challenging complication of radiotherapy, chemotherapy and radio-chemotherapy. Part 2 diagnosis and management of mucositis. Head and Neck 26(1):77–84

Storb R, Prentice R L, Buckner C D 1983 Graft-versus-host disease and survival in patients with aplastic anemia treated by marrow graft from HLA-identical siblings. New England Journal of Medicine 308:302–307

Storring R A, Jameson B, McElwain T J, Wiltshaw E 1977 Oral non-absorbed antibiotics prevent infection in acute non-lymphoblastic leukaemia. Lancet 2:837–840

Tabata M, Kai S, Satake A et al 2005 Relationships between hematological recovery and overall survival in older adults undergoing allogeneic bone marrow transplantation. Internal Medicine 44(1):35–40

Tammelin A, Klotz F, Hambraeus A, Stahle E et al 2003. Nasal and hand carriage of Staphylococcus aureus in staff at the department of thoracic and cardiovascular surgery: endogenous or exogenous source. Infection Control & Hospital Epidemiology 24(9):686–689

Teare E L, Peacock A 1996 The development of an infection control link-nurse programme in a district general hospital. Journal of Infection Control 34: 267–278

Turnidge J 2003 Impact of antibiotic resistance on the treatment of sepsis. Scandinavian Journal of Infectious Disease 35(9):677–682

Vossen J M, Handgretinger R 2001 Immune recovery and immunotherapy after stem cell transplantation in children. Bone Marrow Transplantation 28(Suppl 1):S14–S15

Wade J C 1994 Epidemiology and prevention of infection in the compromised host. In: Rubins R H, Young L S (eds) Clinical approach to infection in the compromised host, 3rd edn. Plenum, New York, pp 5–31

Walker A 1992 Drinking water, doubts about quality. British Medical Journal 304:175–178

Walker E, Dewar B J 2001 How do we facilitate carers' involvement in decision making. Journal of Advanced Nursing 34(3):329–337

Ward D 2000 Infection control: reducing the psychological effects of isolation. British Journal of Nursing 9(3):162–170

Wilson I G, Hogg G M, Barr J G 1997 Microbiological quality of ice in hospital and community. Journal of Hospital Infection 36:171–180

Wohlschaeger A 2004 Prevention and treatment of mucositis: a guide for nurses. Journal of Pediatric Oncology Nursing 21(5):281–287

Young L S 1994 Management of infections in leukemia and lymphoma. In: Rubins R H, Young L S (eds) Clinical approach to infection in the compromised host, 3rd edn. Plenum, New York, pp 551–575

Further reading

Ayliffe G A J, Lowbury E J L, Geddes A M, Williams J D (eds) 2000 Control of hospital infection: a practical handbook, 4th edn. Chapman and Hall, London
This handbook provides practical guidance and information on effective ways of controlling infection, and is an interesting and useful guide for all health-care professionals.

Barrett J, Treleaven J (eds) 1998 The clinical practice of stem cell transplantation, vols 1 and 2. Isis Medical Media, Oxford
This book provides information related to research, nursing and medical care of this rapidly expanding and changing treatment. A useful resource to health-care workers in the field of bone marrow transplantation.

British Committee for Standards in Haematology Clinical Task Force 1995 Guidelines on the provision of facilities for the care of adult patients with haematological malignancies (including leukaemia and lymphoma and severe bone marrow failure). Clinical and Laboratory Haematology 17:3–10
This useful report defines four levels of care for the management of adult patients with haematological

malignancies and marrow failure, outlining the extra specialist expertise, staffing and resources required to provide this care.

Gabriel J 2004 The biology of cancer. Whurr, London
This book presents a comprehensive account of the biology of cancer and provides a thorough knowledge base for nurses caring for patients with cancer.

Glauser M P, Pizzo P A 2000 Management of infections in immunocompromised patients. WB Saunders, London
This book provides the general principles of the immune response, guide to diagnostic procedures, plus the practical management of infection, which is divided into specific conditions.

Wilson J 2001 Infection control in clinical practice. Baillière Tindall, Edinburgh
This book provides practical, relevant, readable, research-based information on the prevention and control of infection and includes chapters on microbiology and immunology. This sound scientific information provides a basis for the formulation of standards of care in infection control.

Chapter 16

Haemorrhagic problems

Jan Green and Shelley Dolan

KEY POINTS

- Bleeding may be a consequence of disease or treatment.
- Thrombocytopenia is the commonest cause of bleeding in haemato-oncology.
- Bleeding episodes are potentially life-threatening.
- Bleeding episodes can be extremely frightening for patients and their relatives.
- Prompt recognition and management of bleeding episodes is essential.

INTRODUCTION

Nursing patients with haematological cancer is multifaceted due to the unpredictability of the disease, its treatment and outcomes. Patients also have complex needs ranging from the emotional to the practical. It is in this context that haematology nurses need to recognise the haemorrhagic or bleeding problems that can arise either as a side effect of treatment or disease progression, or as a separate issue altogether, such as the patient with Hodgkin's disease (HD) who develops idiopathic thrombocytopenia purpura (ITP).

Nurses need the knowledge and competence to prevent and manage bleeding episodes if they occur, whilst also being patient educators and compassionate supporters. The patient and the family also need to be aware of the potentially life-threatening consequences of bleeding and the need to prevent bleeding. This chapter considers the various causes of bleeding, patient education in the prevention and management of bleeding, and associated nursing management.

CAUSES OF BLEEDING

Bleeding can be attributed to:

1. Low platelet count (thrombocytopenia) caused by:
   - disease progression and infiltration of the bone marrow subsequently depressing platelet production
   - treatment
   - idiopathic thrombocytopenic purpura (ITP)
   - grossly enlarged spleen
2. Disseminated intravascular coagulation (DIC)
3. Thrombotic thrombocytopenic purpura (TTP)
4. Blood vessel erosion such as tumour infiltration or chemotherapy causing damage
5. Platelet dysfunctions such as in myeloma.

THROMBOCYTOPENIA

Thrombocytopenia refers to any condition in which there is a deficiency of platelets. Platelets have an integral function in blood clotting and a reduction in their number results in either slower blood clotting or an inability to clot depending on the severity of thrombocytopenia (see Chapter 1). Thrombocytopenia is the commonest cause of bleeding in patients with haematological cancers (Cohen 2002).

Disease–related infiltration of the bone marrow

This is the commonest cause of thrombocytopenia in haematological cancers. Leukaemia, lymphoma, aplastic anaemia and myelodysplastic syndromes inhibit bone marrow function and consequently platelet production (Liesner & Machin 1998). This phenomenon also occurs when solid tumours invade bone marrow space, consequently suppressing normal bone marrow function.

Treatment

Several treatments for haematological cancers result in thrombocytopenia. Cytotoxic drugs have an adverse effect on bone marrow function with varying degrees of severity (see Chapter 9). Some drugs such as carmustine have a delayed rather than immediate effect on platelet counts. Patients may have severe effects prompting a bleeding episode some time after treatment, when it would appear that their platelet count should be settling. Nurses need to be aware of the side effects of the drugs they are giving so they can advise patients appropriately.

Radiotherapy also has an adverse effect on bone marrow function. Platelet recovery is slow after treatment, especially if treatment has been focussed on areas with high bone marrow content (see Chapter 10).

For patients who have undergone bone marrow transplantation (BMT) or more commonly peripheral stem cell transplantation (PSCT) the platelet cell line is the last to recover. Recovery of the platelet count varies from patient to patient and can sometimes take several months.

Idiopathic thrombocytopenic purpura

Idiopathic thrombocytopenic purpura (ITP) is caused by platelet sensitisation to autoantibodies resulting in their premature death and removal from the circulation (Hoffbrand et al 2001). It can be an acute or chronic condition, is usually idiopathic but is sometimes associated with chronic lymphatic leukaemia (CLL) and Hodgkin's disease (Hoffbrand et al 2001). Treatment is related to platelet count:

- If the patient is asymptomatic, not actively bleeding and has a platelet count above 50,000/mm^3, no treatment is required. However, if there is active bleeding, high-dose corticosteroids are required. Early dose reduction is advised due to the well-known multiple side effects of steroids. Corticosteroids suppress platelet sensitisation to autoantibodies, thus preventing their death (BNF 2002).
- Intravenous immunoglobulin (IVIG) can also be used to induce a quick short-term rise in the platelet count. The mode of action is unclear (Cohen et al 2001) but consideration must be given to longer-term treatment.
- Splenectomy is recommended for those patients who do not respond to steroids or IVIG. All splenic tissue must be removed so as to prevent regrowth and subsequent relapse (Hoffbrand et al 2001).
- Immunosuppressive drugs such as cyclophosphamide, cyclosporin, vincristine and azathioprine can be used alone or in combination and are usually given only to those patients who do not respond to steroids and splenectomy (Hoffbrand et al 2001).
- Platelet transfusion is not indicated in the long-term management of ITP as transfused platelets are destroyed in the same way as the patient's own platelets exposing individuals to a blood component inappropriately. However, platelets must be administered in acute life-threatening situations before longer-term treatment can be established (Hoffbrand et al 2001).

Enlarged spleen

A grossly enlarged spleen is not always associated with bleeding. Yet the full blood count may indicate thrombocytopenia due to the pooling and increased platelet destruction in the enlarged spleen reducing circulating cell numbers. Platelets have a normal lifespan and the remaining circulating platelets usually have normal function (Hoffbrand et al 2001). This condition mainly affects patients with chronic myeloproliferative and lymphoproliferative disorders, e.g. chronic myeloid leukaemia (CML).

DISSEMINATED INTRAVASCULAR COAGULATION

Disseminated intravascular coagulation (DIC) is an extremely complex systemic thrombo-haemorrhagic disorder which can develop very quickly and swiftly progress into a life-threatening situation (Furlong 2001). DIC has a mortality rate of 50% (Tan 2002). DIC has many causes but within haemato-oncology is most frequently associated with acute promyelocytic leukaemia (APL) and septicaemia. However, in recent years the introduction of all-trans-retinoic acid as a treatment for APL has dramatically reduced the incidence of DIC (Levi & ten Cate 1999). DIC is thought to be caused by the release of procoagulant material, in the form of cytokines, and tissue factors into the circulation (Furlong 2001, Hoffbrand et al 2001).

In DIC the coagulation cascade becomes severely disrupted, as the balance between plasmin and thrombin production becomes uncontrolled. The complex biofeedback between these two enzymes controls the bleeding/clotting balance. Fibrin deposits in the small blood vessels stimulate the development of blood clots in blood vessels and organs which can lead to hypoperfusion, localised ischaemia, pulmonary embolism, cerebrovascular accident and ultimately organ damage and failure (Furlong 2001). Clot formation results in depletion of platelets, fibrinogen and other clotting factors, leading to thombocytopenia and excessive bleeding from multiple sites, which can be very difficult to control (Liesner & Machin 1998, Moake 2003). Bleeding can be very distressing for patients and their relatives and a great deal of support and sensitivity is required.

Diagnosis is made clinically with confirmation by laboratory results. A combination of tests of haemostasis is used to confirm DIC as no single test is diagnostic. Expected values include (Tan 2002):

- low platelet count
- prolonged prothrombin time
- prolonged activated partial thromboplastin time
- prolonged thrombin time
- decreased antithrombin III
- decreased fibrinogen
- increased fibrin degradation products, e.g. D-Dimer test (highly responsive test for DIC).

Treatment is aimed at correcting the underlying cause of DIC and consists of transfusions of platelets, fresh frozen plasma, cryoprecipitate and red cells as required. Protein C concentrates have recently shown some promise in DIC caused by sepsis (Toh & Dennis 2003).

THROMBOTIC THROMBOCYTOPENIC PURPURA

Thrombotic thrombocytopenic purpura (TTP) is usually associated with drug usage such as cytotoxic chemotherapy, e.g. cyclophosphamide, or continued use of antibiotics (Hoffbrand et al 2001). Platelets clump together due to the development of an inhibitory antibody, which may be stimulated by infection. Tiny clots form in the small blood vessels, causing damage and weakness to their walls resulting in rupture and subsequent bleeding. Treatment includes:

- plasma exchange
- steroids
- red cell transfusion to correct anaemia
- oral folic acid
- platelet transfusions (in life-threatening bleeds only).

BLOOD VESSEL EROSION

Tumour infiltration or infective processes can cause blood vessel erosion resulting in cataclysmic haemorrhage, especially if a major vessel is involved. This may be fatal if no immediate action is taken (Dolan 2000).

PLATELET DYSFUNCTION

Whilst there are many causes of platelet dysfunction, in haematological cancers platelet function is most commonly adversely affected by abnormal immunoglobulins produced by conditions such as myeloma (see Chapter 5). Some drugs, food supplements and alternative therapies can also affect platelet function including:

- aspirin (most common) decreases platelet aggregation and inhibits thrombus formation (BNF 2002)
- non-steroidal anti-inflammatory drugs (NSAIDs), e.g. ibuprofen or diclofenac, can cause gastrointestinal mucosal damage and precipitate ulceration and bleeding (BNF 2002)
- beta-lactam antibiotics such as penicillins and cephalosporins are known to cause thrombocytopenia, especially if the patient is septic and has renal impairment (BNF 2002).
- fish oils
- alcohol (Liesner & Machin 1998)
- heparin (Hoffbrand et al 2001)
- St John's wort, an alternative therapy used to treat mild depression, can interfere with the efficacy of some chemotherapy drugs and is thought to affect platelet function.

It is therefore important to ascertain whether the patient is taking any medication which could inhibit platelet function prior to commencing cytotoxic chemotherapy.

Case study 16.1

Dave, aged 34, was diagnosed with high-grade non-Hodgkin's lymphoma and treated successfully with cyclophosphamide, doxorubicin (Adriamycin), vincristine (Oncovin) and prednisolone (CHOP chemotherapy) as an outpatient. He made an excellent recovery with complete remission (CR) by all disease markers. However, 6 months post-treatment at routine follow-up, his platelets showed a marked fall to 25,000/mm³. His blood count was rechecked to ensure there were no errors in the reading or that platelets were not clumping together (clumping platelets often give a misleading incorrect low reading). However, no error was detected.

A bone marrow aspiration was performed and a diagnosis of idiopathic thrombocytopenic purpura (ITP) was made. Dave had no symptoms of bruising or bleeding so no treatment was indicated for his ITP at that time.

Dave was followed-up in the general haematology clinic to ensure his platelet count remained stable and any trends or changes noted. He was given written information relating to ITP and has contact details should he need urgent consultation or treatment.

SPONTANEOUS BLEEDING

Spontaneous major bleeding can occur when the platelet count falls below 20,000/mm³. The lower the count the worse the bleeding is likely to be. However, bleeding also depends on platelet function. If platelet function is good, then bleeding will be less, although each patient's physiological response to a low platelet count will be vastly different (Chen & Graber 2003). Patients with counts below 100,000/mm³ can experience a prolonged bleeding time but are unlikely to experience abnormal spontaneous bleeding, whilst those with a platelet count between 50,000/mm³ and 20,000/mm³ may report 'bruising easily'.

The release of bacterial endotoxins in the acutely septic patient increases platelet consumption, causing a rapid drop in the count (Dolan 2000). A rapidly dropping platelet count is more likely to cause severe spontaneous bleeding episodes than a more slowly falling count (Chen & Graber 2003). Patients who are septic and receiving beta-lactam antibiotics are susceptible to rapidly falling platelet counts and require close monitoring because of the increased risk of spontaneous bleeding.

PREVENTION OF SPONTANEOUS BLEEDING

Preventative strategies, which may help to reduce the potential for spontaneous bleeding, include:

- prophylactic platelet infusions if levels fall below a predetermined threshold, usually 10,000/mm³ (British Committee for Standards in Haematology 2003)

- platelet transfusion before any invasive procedure where the count is below 50,000/mm^3.

Recognising spontaneous bleeding

Nurses need to monitor the patient and act promptly on any signs of bleeding. Patients and their carers also need to be educated in prevention and recognition of the signs and symptoms associated with bleeding. Educating patients to recognise the early symptoms of a bleed and knowing what to do about it is vital, especially with the growing number of patients receiving toxic treatment as outpatients. It is important that patients and carers are aware of the potentially life-threatening consequences of bleeding and the necessity of immediately reporting problems to the medical and nursing team to ensure they receive urgent treatment. A balance needs to be struck between giving the patient and their carers enough information to make them aware of the potential dangers of bleeding and overemphasising the issue so that the individual is afraid of living a normal life.

Patients may be afraid of the unknown – giving them precise verbal information followed by accurate and easily understood written information should be the aim of all involved in health care. Giving the patient written information is important (Department of Health (DoH) 2000). However, nurses should ensure that they explain the information to patients and ensure that there is understanding of potential problems and who to contact if bleeding is either suspected or occurs. It has been suggested that just giving patients literature is insufficient, as many people never read leaflets and subsequently state they have never been informed (DoH 2003). Whitman-Obert (1996) notes that information given to patients and their carers is not always retained or understood, so it is essential that nurses are aware of the need to repeat information to enhance memory and understanding. It can also be useful to underline pertinent points within an information leaflet to highlight what patients have been told.

It would appear that patients often do not recognise the life-threatening nature of bleeding problems and often delay seeking urgent medical attention, sometimes with fatal consequences. This is because they are afraid of bothering medical and nursing staff with what they believe is an inconsequential problem. There is some evidence to support this, with Faithfull (1995) observing that patients do not report symptoms they perceive to be trivial or for which they feel there is nothing that can be done to help. Helping individuals to recognise the significance of bleeding problems is therefore a challenge for nurses. Cooley et al (1995) suggest that nurses need to develop innovative means of educating patients to their level of understanding and educational ability so they fully understand the implications of the information given to them.

MINOR BLEEDING EVENTS

These are most likely to occur when the platelet count has fallen, below 20,000/mm^3 or more often below 10,000/mm^3. Minor vascular assaults can occur in the mucosa of the mouth (especially the gums around the tooth margins) and nose. The aim of nursing care is to facilitate patient understanding of the causes of bleeding, thereby helping to prevent these events, recognising and managing problems if they occur, and seeking prompt aid. Both patients and nurses need to be vigilant for signs and symptoms of bleeding including:

- unpleasant taste (of blood) in the mouth
- slight oozing of blood around the gum margins
- excess of blood observed when blowing the nose
- blood blisters.

CONTROL OF SMALL BLEEDS

Small bleeds can usually be well managed by the use of:

- firm pressure applied to the bleeding point
- using ice pressure packs or sucking ice chips
- topical vasoconstrictive preparations such as adrenaline
- topical preparations, e.g. tranexamic acid and sucralfate, to the lips
- oral drugs, e.g. tranexamic acid
- platelet transfusion or, more rarely, fresh frozen plasma.

Careful observation of the patient is important, including measurement of vital signs: blood pressure, pulse and temperature. Daily physical examination is an integral part of nursing care and should include observation of the following for any signs of bleeding:

- skin integrity and signs of purpura or bruising (Plates 10 & 11)
- mouth and gums
- perianal region
- urine and faeces.

Patients should be advised to observe for signs of bleeding. Individuals should be educated to prevent assaults on the oral mucosa, by maintaining careful oral hygiene (see Chapter 18). It is also important for patients to be aware that should mucosal integrity be compromised by infection, prompt diagnosis and treatment should be sought so that the risk of bleeding is minimised (Groenwald et al 1997).

Epistaxis can be caused by excessive nose blowing or manipulation and these activities should be discouraged. Whilst generally not serious, these events can nevertheless be very frightening for the patient and their carers and could be the precursor to a major bleed. What starts as a minor bleed may develop quickly into something more substantial and the nasal cavity may require packing with topical vasoconstrictive agents to control bleeding.

Every care must be taken to avoid compromising skin integrity, especially if the patient is bed-bound as this group of patients is at high risk of developing pressure sores, which may bleed or become infected. Careful monitoring of patient risk using well-established assessment tools such as the Waterlow scale (Waterlow 1985) will indicate patient susceptibility to pressure sores and may prevent their development. This is easy to do for the inpatient but outpatients too can be inactive and need to be aware of the problems encountered by the development of pressure sores. Advice should be given to patients and their carers on prevention.

Men should be advised against wet shaving as this may precipitate a bleeding event, which is sometimes extraordinarily difficult to stop even though blood loss itself may be minimal. Topical clotting preparations such as tranexamic acid and vasoconstrictive agents such as adrenaline, as well as ice, are useful in stopping bleeding.

Menstrual bleeding can be a problem for many female patients during their treatment and can become severe. Menstruating women are commenced on progesterone preparations prior to treatment, to suppress menses.

Invasive procedures

Invasive procedures such as intramuscular injections should be avoided as they may cause painful bleeding that may be difficult to stop – necrosis and permanent damage may result. Many drugs, such as low molecular weight heparin and granulocyte-colony stimulating factor (G-CSF) are, however, given by subcutaneous injection and great care must be exercised in administration to ensure vascular integrity. Pressure applied to the site for 5 minutes after the injection will help to prevent any bleeding.

Consideration should be given to the exit site when removing intravenous devices – the application of continuous pressure to the site for at least 5 minutes will prevent excessive bleeding.

Use of enemas and suppositories should be avoided where possible as damage to the rectal mucosa may occur, causing a break in skin integrity and subsequent bleeding. Where possible, drugs should be given intravenously or orally.

REFLECTION POINT

Does your ward or department produce written information highlighting the safety issues surrounding bleeding problems following treatment? Consider a patient whom you have cared for and how you managed to convey to them the potentially life-threatening consequences of bleeding. Reflect on the difficulties patients may experience in understanding the implications of this. How do you ensure that you provide sufficient information to meet patient needs without increasing fears about their well-being? What resources are available to you to help you to get your point across?

MAJOR HAEMORRHAGE

Massive haemorrhage can be devastating and potentially fatal, especially if prompt action and treatment are not initiated. Common sites of major haemorrhage are:

- bladder (haemorrhagic cystitis)
- upper gastrointestinal tract
- lower gastrointestinal tract
- central nervous system.

BLADDER – HAEMORRHAGIC CYSTITIS

Haemorrhagic cystitis (HC) is defined as bladder inflammation with macroscopic haematuria. It is generally the result of a chemical or other traumatic insult to the bladder (chemotherapy, radiation therapy) (Medical Dictionary Online 2002/3). Following bone marrow transplantation patients are especially vulnerable and HC is a major cause of morbidity and occasional mortality. Patients need intensive support and treatment. Those with mild HC have a better outcome than those with severe HC (Leung et al 2001).

Patients receiving cyclophosphamide as a conditioning therapy prior to blood and marrow transplant are particularly susceptible and up to 40% of patients will develop HC (Amersham Health 2003). HC occurs as a result of the effects of the waste product of cyclophosphamide (a metabolite called acrolein), which causes ulceration and vasculitis of the bladder mucosa. Spasmodic intermittent pain is the accompanying feature of HC, which worsens if a blood clot is passed. Intraluminal filling defects due to blood clots are known to cause pain (Amersham Health 2003). Other causative factors include:

- radiation – which is a relatively rare problem but does require treatment due to its progressive nature (Crew et al 2001)
- acute and chronic graft-versus-host disease (GvHD) (Leung et al 2002)
- adenovirus – which may be reactivated in the immunocompromised patient, especially following bone marrow transplantation (Leung et al 2001)
- BK virus – can also be reactivated in the immunocompromised, especially bone marrow transplant recipients (Crew et al 2001, Leung et al 2002)
- other chemotherapeutic conditioning treatments such as busulphan.

Prevention and treatment strategies for HC include the maintenance of forced hydration and the infusion of Mesna during treatment with cyclophosphamide. Mesna combines with the metabolite acrolein, preventing its toxic effect of erosion on the bladder mucosa (BNF 2002).

Bleeding can be severe, on occasion leading to impaired renal function, and can be fatal if not treated (Leung et al 2002). Investigations include a full blood count, clotting profile, and monitoring of urea and electrolytes to assess renal function. Urine output should be observed and bladder irrigation should be commenced at the first sign of urinary retention or if blood clots are passed. Pain associated with HC should be managed with analgesia. Blood component transfusion may also be required.

UPPER GASTROINTESTINAL TRACT

Massive haemorrhage from the upper gastrointestinal (GI) tract is caused by:

- pre-existing ulceration
- stress-induced ulceration of the endothelium
- endothelial damage from either radiotherapy or chemotherapy leading to tissue ulceration and bleeding
- viral, fungal and bacterial infections causing ulceration and tissue frailty leading to breakdown and bleeding
- acute GvHD.

Acute GvHD can, in severe cases, cause ulceration to the endothelium in the upper GI tract leading to nausea and sickness followed by melaena (Franklin 2001). Onset can be insidious, resulting in massive haemorrhage that may require organ support in critical care and can be fatal. The mainstay of treatment is prevention with immunosuppressive drugs such as cyclosporin, methotrexate and steroids (Franklin 2001). Recent research has also shown monoclonal antibodies such as rituximab and alemuzumab and the purine analogue pentostatin to be useful in the prevention and treatment of GvHD.

LOWER GASTROINTESTINAL TRACT

Massive haemorrhage of the lower GI tract is caused by:

- Severe infection. Individuals with haematological cancer receive many courses of antibiotics and ultimately drug resistance may develop. Infection can therefore become overwhelming, requiring stronger and more toxic antibiotics. The gut becomes increasingly inflamed and ulcerated, leading to bleeding. As this cycle continues, the risk of haemorrhage becomes greater and more difficult to manage.
- Pseudomembranous colitis. The naturally occurring gut bacterium *Clostridium difficile* grows out of control during persistent and continual antibiotic treatment. *Clostridium difficile* produces a toxin, which causes the gut lining to become inflamed and ulcerated leading to bleeding (Muir 2002).
- Ischaemic ulceration. Steroids and NSAIDs are often included in treatment or supportive therapy for the patient with haematological cancers. However, these drugs can cause gastric irritation, ulceration and consequently bleeding. Prophylactic treatment is therefore very important as prevention is always better than cure. The use of proton pump inhibitors or an H_2-receptor antagonist such as ranitidine, given at twice the usual dose to reduce gastric pH levels, is recommended to prevent this potentially fatal side effect (BNF 2002). Prophylactic treatment should be prescribed routinely for all patients who are taking steroids.

Clinical signs of a GI bleed

There are no obvious early presenting symptoms of an impending haemorrhage of the upper or lower GI tract, making diagnosis very difficult. However, if the patient becomes shocked and displays the following clinical signs, a diagnosis of an acute GI bleed should be suspected, investigated and excluded:

- loss of blood pressure
- tachycardia
- sweating
- pallor
- melaena (upper GI bleed)
- fresh blood loss (lower GI bleed)
- occasionally haematemesis.

Investigations of GI tract bleeding include:

- full blood count
- clotting profile
- plain abdominal x-ray
- CT scan of the abdomen
- endoscopic examination.

Endoscopic examination is an invasive procedure and carries the risk of causing trauma and inducing bleeding. Use of endoscopy needs careful evaluation for the severely neutropenic patient as there is an added risk of introducing further infection. Gastroscopy is easier to perform in the presence of haemorrhage than colonoscopy.

Treatment options include:

- Blood component support.
- Management of any clotting deficiencies.
- Direct endoscopic treatment if a bleeding point is identified with diathermy or bleeding point necrosis with adrenaline. Intravenous protamine sulphate may reduce severe bleeding but should be administered only when intensive monitoring is available owing to severe cardiovascular side effects (Dolan 2000).
- Laparotomy may be appropriate in rare circumstances when there is no other option and the patient's life is at risk. This should be performed only with input from haematologists and anaesthetists who can provide expert support and advice regarding management of thrombocytopenia and clotting dysfunction, as well as care of an immunocompromised patient. Close monitoring in a high-dependency area is required.
- Recombinant Factor VIIa has recently shown promise in the treatment of massive overwhelming haemorrhage. Its use in this area is still new, undergoing evaluation and tightly controlled by protocol.

CENTRAL NERVOUS SYSTEM

Massive CNS bleeds are fortuitously rare, as their consequences can be devastating. A CNS bleed can be due to:

- infection
- disease
- drug toxicity.

There are, however, certain preventative strategies that may help to reduce the potential for a cerebral bleed, including prophylactic platelet transfusion before any invasive procedure when the platelet count is below 50,000/mm^3. Cerebral irritation may be caused by drugs such as cyclophosphamide, with the sequelae of seizures and possible cerebral trauma leading to bleeding; prophylactic anticonvulsants should be administered. Nurses need to be alert to possibility of a CNS bleed and it is important that changes in each patient's consciousness levels are carefully monitored.

If a CNS bleed is suspected, urgent investigations should be initiated including:

- CT scan of the brain
- full blood count to determine platelet count
- clotting screen.

Treatment is dependent upon bone marrow function and clotting profile. If the patient is thrombocytopenic, platelets are transfused and consciousness level is closely monitored. Any changes should be reported instantly. In the worst case scenario, where consciousness deteriorates, surgery may be indicated to relieve an acute rise in intra-cranial pressure (ICP).

CONCLUSION

Individuals with haematological cancers make many demands on haematology nurses. Nurses need to be experienced and knowledgeable with the skills and expertise to both care for and educate patients and their carers, thereby helping them to gain confidence in preventing, recognising and managing bleeding problems.

DISCUSSION QUESTIONS

1. What advice should you give a patient who is taking NSAIDs for arthritis and has just started on cyclophosphamide as part of the treatment?

2. What would you do if you saw a patient with a gradually falling platelet count over 2 or 3 days who was starting to slur speech?

3. A patient receiving chemotherapy treatment at home calls to say he has a rash over the feet. What action would you take?

4. Jim is recovering from a bone marrow transplant. He likes to shave every day and is feeling 'dirty and unkempt'. How would you support Jim and what advice would you give him?

References

Amersham Health 2003 Cystitis, chemotherapy-related. The encyclopaedia of medical imaging Volume IV:2. http://www.amershamhealth.com/medcyclopaedia/medical/volume%20iv%202/cystitis%20chemotherapy%20related.asp Accessed 23 Nov 2003

British Committee for Standards in Haematology, Blood Transfusion Task Force 2003 Guidelines for the use of platelet transfusions. British Journal of Haematology 122:10–23

BNF 2002 British National Formulary 44. British Medical Association and Royal Pharmaceutical Society of Great Britain, London

Chen K, Graber M A 2003 Hematologic, electrolyte and metabolic disorders: bleeding disorders. University of Iowa family practice handbook, 4th edn. http://www.vh.org/adult/provider/familymedicine/FPHandbook/Chapter06/01-6.html Accessed 6 Nov 2003

Cohen E E W 2002 Medline Plus Medical Encyclopaedia: thrombocytopenia. http://www.nlm.nih.gov/medlineplus/ency/article/000586.htm. Accessed 30 Oct 2003

Cohen H, Kernoff P B A, Colvin B B T 2001 Plasma, plasma products and indications for their use. In: Contreras M (ed) ABC of transfusion, 3rd edn. BMJ Books, London, pp 40–44

Cooley M E, Moriarty H, Berger M S, Selm-Orr D, Coyle B, Short T 1995 Patient literacy and the readability of written cancer educational materials. Oncology Nursing Forum 22(9):1345–1351

Crew J, Jephcott C, Reynard J 2001 Radiation-induced haemorrhagic cystitis. European Urology 40:111–123

Department of Health 2000 The NHS plan: a plan for investment, a plan for reform. http://www.dh.gov.uk/PublicationsAndStatistics/Publications/PublicationsPolicyAndGuidance/PublicationsPolicyAndGuidanceArticle/fs/en?CONTENT_ID = 4002960&chk = 07GL5R Accessed 16 Aug 2004

Department of Health 2003 Toolkit for producing patient information. HMSO, London

Dolan S 2000 Haemorrhagic problems In: Grundy M (ed) Nursing in haematological oncology. Baillière Tindall, Edinburgh, pp 201–210

Faithfull S 1995 'Just grin and bear it and hope that it will go away': coping with urinary symptoms from pelvic radiotherapy. European Journal of Cancer Care 4:158–165

Franklin I 2001 Cytokines, stem cells and immunotherapy. In: Murphy M, Pamphilon D (eds) Practical transfusion medicine. Blackwell Science, Oxford, pp 287–307

Furlong M 2001 Disseminated intravascular coagulation. http://www.emedicine.com/EMERG/topic150.htm Accessed 30 Nov 2003

Groenwald S L, Frogge M L, Goodman M, Yarbro C H 1997 Cancer nursing: principles and practice, 4th edn. Jones and Bartlett, Boston, p 202

Hoffbrand A V, Pettit J E, Moss P A H 2001 Essential haematology, 4th edn. Blackwell Science, Oxford

Leung A Y, Mak R, Lie A K et al 2002 Clinicopathological features and risk factors of clinically overt haemorrhagic cystitis complicating bone marrow transplantation. Bone Marrow Transplantation 29(6):509–513

Leung A, Suen C, Lie A, Liang R, Yuen K, Kwong Y 2001 Quantification of polyoma BK virus in hemorrhagic cystitis complicating bone marrow transplantation. Blood 98(6):1971–1978

Levi M, ten Cate H 1999 Current concepts: disseminated intravascular coagulation. New England Journal of Medicine 341(8):586–592

Liesner R J, Machin S J 1998 Platelet disorders. In: Provan D, Henson A (eds) ABC of clinical haematology. BMJ Publishing, London, pp 29–31

Medical Dictionary Online 2002–3 http://www.books.md/H/dic/haemorrhagiccystitis.php Accessed 23 Nov 2003

Moake J L 2003 The Merck manual of medical information – second home edition 1995–2003. http://www.merck.com/mmhe/sec14/ch173/ch173d.html Accessed 30 Nov 2003

Muir A 2002 Pseudomembranous colitis. Yahoo Health Encyclopaedia http://health.yahoo.com/health/encyclopedia/000259/1.html Accessed 27 Nov 2003

Tan S J 2002 Recognition and treatment of oncological emergencies. Journal of Infusion Nursing 25(3):182–188

Toh C H, Dennis M 2003. Disseminated intravascular coagulation: old disease, new hope. British Medical Journal 327:974–977

Waterlow J 1985 Pressure sores: a risk assessment card. Nursing Times 81(48):49,51,55

Whitman-Obert H 1996. Patient information handouts: taking care of yourself – a self-help guide for patients with cancer. Oncology Nursing Forum 23(9):1443–1446

Further reading

The following further reading is recommended to extend understanding of the physiology of haemorrhagic problems, the use of blood and blood components, and the clinical expertise required from the haematology nurse in providing psychological support for patients.

Contreras M (ed) 2001 ABC of transfusion, 3rd edn. BMJ Books, London

Green D, Ludlam C 2004 Fast facts – bleeding disorders. Health Press, Oxford

Hoffbrand A V, Pettit J E, Moss P A H 2001 Essential haematology, 4th edn. Blackwell Science, Oxford

Kearney N, Richardson A, Di Giulio P (eds) 2001 Cancer nursing practice: a textbook for the specialist nurse. Churchill Livingstone, Edinburgh

Further information on TTP can be found at http://www.netdoctor.co.uk/diseases/facts/ttp.htm

Chapter **17**

Nausea and vomiting

Jan Hawthorn

KEY POINTS
- Nausea and vomiting are the most distressing side effects of chemotherapy and radiotherapy.
- Therapeutic agents and non-pharmacological supportive techniques are available to prevent or treat nausea and vomiting.
- Nursing interventions aim to minimise the distress caused to patients by these unpleasant side effects.

INTRODUCTION

For patients, nausea and vomiting are arguably the most distressing aspect of cancer treatment (Coates et al 1983, Giffin et al 1996, Passik et al 2001) to the extent that 25–50% of patients may delay or even refuse potentially curative treatment (Ritter et al 1998). Nausea and vomiting may cause a variety of debilitating medical problems such as dehydration or poor nutrition, as well as leading to low morale, depression, poor compliance, less satisfaction with treatment, and a lower quality of life (Martin et al 2003). Patients with haematological cancers are often given aggressive and highly emetogenic chemotherapy regimens, and those undergoing bone marrow transplantation (BMT) will receive toxic chemotherapy and/or total body irradiation on consecutive days. For these patients, poor anti-emetic control adds to the burden of such treatment and can make the whole experience even more distressing. It is important, therefore, that nurses take an active role in prevention of these untoward side effects in vulnerable patients. This chapter briefly outlines what we know about the process of nausea and vomiting and discusses appropriate treatments (both pharmacological and supportive) for chemotherapy- and radiotherapy-induced vomiting. Nursing interventions that minimise the risk of vomiting occurring and help to ameliorate symptoms are also discussed.

WHY DOES CHEMOTHERAPY OR RADIOTHERAPY CAUSE NAUSEA AND VOMITING?

Biologically, vomiting is essentially a protective mechanism designed to remove ingested poisons. Although chemotherapy is given for therapeutic purposes, it is still essentially a 'poison', which will be identified as such by the body and hence the vomiting response will be activated. Similarly, radiotherapy will be perceived as a damaging or 'poisonous' experience and it is possible that radiation damage releases unusually high concentrations of cellular contents into the circulation, which also activate the emetic reflex (Andrews & Davis 1993).

Vomiting is orchestrated by the 'vomiting centre' in the brainstem. This region (which is a centre in a functional rather than anatomical sense) comprises the area postrema (AP) and the associated chemo-receptor trigger zone (CTZ), the nucleus tractus solitarius (NTS) and the dorsal motor nucleus of the vagus (DMV), also known as the dorsal vagal complex (Hawthorn 1995). The AP, near the floor of the fourth ventricle, is outside the blood–brain barrier and so can detect noxious substances in the blood and pass messages to the CTZ. The vagus, the main nerve taking information from the gut, passes information to the NTS. Information from the ear and from higher cortical parts of the brain (e.g. those involved with emotion, conditioning, fear) also passes to the vomiting centre. So the vomiting centre receives both chemical and neural inputs from various parts of the body. The DMV then coordinates the output of the centre and orchestrates the process of vomiting. Despite the name the CTZ is thought to be less involved than the gut in chemotherapy-induced vomiting (Andrews & Davis 1993).

Some neurotransmitters are released by chemotherapeutic agents and radiotherapy – these include serotonin (or 5-hydroxytryptamine, 5-HT), which is released in the gut and detected by vagal afferents, and substance P, which is released in the NTS (Stahl 2003) and stimulates neurokinin 1 (NK1) receptors. Thus stimulation of the gut and of the AP will release substance P. Preventing the action of these two neuro-transmitters has formed the basis for the development of the latest anti-emetics.

THE PROCESS OF NAUSEA AND VOMITING

Nausea is the prodromal feeling that vomiting is about to occur. Feelings of nausea are due to changes in the gut, especially the stomach, which stops its rhythmic squeezing movements and becomes static (a very large or fatty meal can also cause gastric stasis and feelings of nausea). The nauseated individual usually appears pale, cold and clammy, may be sweating, and have tachycardia – all signs of activation of the sympathetic nervous system. They will also be producing a lot of saliva from parasympathetic activation. The nauseated individual tends to focus on their own lack of wellbeing and becomes disinterested in external surroundings.

Nausea is followed by retching (rhythmic movements of the respiratory and abdominal muscles), the pyloric sphincter closes (to prevent the gastric contents moving into the duodenum), the cardiac sphincter opens, and forceful contraction of the respiratory muscles causes the active expulsion of the stomach contents through the mouth. The epiglottis moves to prevent stomach contents entering the airways. In everyday circumstances vomiting brings immediate relief of the nausea, but for those receiving chemotherapy this is often not the case and nausea may persist unabated, in spite of actively vomiting, for several hours; such nausea is often more distressing to the individual than vomiting itself.

TYPES OF EMESIS

Nausea and vomiting associated with chemotherapy can be classified as acute, delayed or anticipatory. Acute nausea and vomiting occur within 24 hours of chemotherapy, while delayed nausea and vomiting are usually defined as commencing more than 24 hours after chemotherapy, although there has been a suggestion that delayed symptoms may occur as soon as 16 hours post-chemotherapy (Mantovani et al 1998). Additionally the terms 'breakthrough vomiting' or 'refractory vomiting' may be used for vomiting that occurs despite anti-emetic cover. Delayed emesis can impact as much, if not more than, acute emesis on patients' morale and quality of life and remains a major challenge as it does not respond so well to the majority of anti-emetics as acute symptoms. It is, however, still important to achieve good control of acute emesis, since patients who are well controlled during the first 24 hours develop less delayed symptoms and are likely to experience better control of emesis in subsequent cycles of therapy.

Anticipatory vomiting can develop in some patients, especially where the nausea and vomiting after treatment has been severe. If this occurs, certain aspects of the treatment or surroundings become 'cues' that can make the patient feel nauseous or actually vomit. Common cues are the treatment nurse or sight or smell of the hospital. Anticipatory symptoms can develop after only one pulse of chemotherapy, although it is more common after 3–4 pulses.

This phenomenon can remain with the patient for many years after treatment has ceased and anticipatory symptoms, being psychological in origin, respond poorly to anti-emetics. It is important, therefore, to prevent emetic symptoms as much as possible from the outset and to identify especially vulnerable patients who may need more potent anti-emetics. If anti-emetic control is efficient, anticipatory symptoms do not have the opportunity to become established.

RISK OF VOMITING AFTER TREATMENT

Not every patient will be sick after cancer treatment; it depends on a variety of patient- and treatment-related factors. For chemotherapy, which is generally more emetic than radiotherapy, the most influential factor on the risk of vomiting is the drug(s) used. Table 17.1 lists the common chemotherapeutic drugs in relation to their emetic potential. This table is only a guide – the dose and route of administration of drugs can alter their emetogenicity and the combination of several chemotherapeutic agents can enhance overall emetic potential. It must also be remembered that the characteristics of the vomiting, such as the frequency, intensity, duration and latency to feeling nausea or vomiting, after administration of the drug is often not accurately known.

For radiotherapy, the dose per fraction, field size and region of the body being irradiated are important. The higher the dose rate or greater the field size the more emesis is experienced. Total body or hemibody irradiation and radiation to the abdomen is the most emetogenic; radiotherapy to the skin or limbs rarely causes vomiting. Emesis induced by radiation is an acute event occurring 30 minutes to 4 hours after treatment.

PATIENT FACTORS

Individuals also vary in responses to therapy; factors predicting a greater emetic response include:

- gender – women are more prone to vomiting (Zook & Yasko 1983, Roila et al 1988)
- age – patients <6 or >50 years are more susceptible to chemotherapy (Roila et al 1988, 1989)
- young patients are less susceptible to radiotherapy (Priestman 1988)
- anxiety – exacerbates post-treatment symptoms (Andrykowski & Gregg 1992)
- course of treatment – emesis is more easily controlled following the first dose of chemotherapy or radiotherapy (Gralla et al 1981, Roila et al 1989)
- alcohol intake – there is a lower incidence in people consuming >10 units of alcohol/week (Schnell 2003)
- experiences of vomiting in pregnancy

Table 17.1
Emetic potential of cytotoxic
drugs used in haemato-
oncology

Frequency of emesis	Agent
<10%	Vincristine
	Bleomycin
	Fludarabine
	2-Chlorodeoxyadenosine
	6-Thioguanine (po)
	Chlorambucil (po)
	Cyclophosphamide (po)
	Busulphan
	Capecitabine
	Bevacizumab
10–30%	Methotrexate $<250\,mg/m^2$
	Mitomycin
	Vinblastine
	Vinorbeline
	Bleomycin
	Etoposide
	Mercaptopurine
	Melphalan
	Hydroxyurea
	Paclitaxel
	Docetaxel
	Bortezomib
	Cetuximab
	Trastuzumab
	Gemcitabine
	Imatinib
30–60%	Methotrexate $250–1000\,mg/m^2$
	Cyclophosphamide $\leq750\,mg/m^2$
	Doxorubicin $20–60\,mg/m^2$
	Mitoxantrone
	Daunorubicin
	Idarubicin
	Ifosfamide
60–90%	Dacarbazine
	Cyclophosphamide >750 $\leq1500\,mg/m^2$
	Doxorubicin $60\,mg/m^2$
	Procarbazine (po)
	Amsacrine
	Methotrexate $>1000\,mg/m^2$
	Carmustine $\leq250\,mg/m^2$
	Cytarabine $>1\,g/m^2$
>90%	Cyclophosphamide $>1500\,mg/m^2$
	Carmustine $>250\,mg/m^2$
	Streptozotocin
	Mechlorethamine
	Cisplatin

Adapted from Lindley et al 1989, Merrifield & Chaffee 1989, Hesketh et al 1995, Allwood et al 1997, MASCC 2004.

- treatment setting – anti-emetic control is less efficient in outpatient chemotherapy settings than in hospital (Roila et al 1989).

There is also evidence of an interaction between these factors. In one study patients having no risk factors showed considerably less nausea and vomiting (20%) that those having four risk factors (76%) (Osoba et al 1997).

REFLECTION POINT   What factors would alert you to check that appropriate anti-emetics have been prescribed for an individual due to commence chemotherapy? Would you look for the same characteristics in someone due to commence radiotherapy?

TREATMENT OF NAUSEA AND VOMITING

PHARMACOLOGICAL

There are several anti-emetic drugs available to control nausea and vomiting induced by chemotherapy or radiotherapy (Table 17.2). Since the introduction of the four 5HT3 receptor antagonists, ondansetron, granisetron, tropisetron and dolasetron (the 'setrons') in the 1990s (dolasetron is not available in the UK), many studies have been conducted into their efficacy and they are now regarded as the treatment of choice or 'gold standard' for moderately and highly emetogenic chemotherapy (Italian Group for Antiemetic Research 1992, Cunningham et al 1996, Schnell 2003).

A fifth 5HT3 receptor antagonist, palonosetron, which has a long half-life (about 40 hours) is under development (Stacher 2002). In comparison with ondansetron and dolasetron it has shown some superiority in complete protection from acute and delayed emesis (Aapro et al 2003), but these findings require further confirmation.

Some of the studies discussed here relate to cisplatin-induced vomiting, and although this drug is not routinely used in haemato-oncology these data are still important since cisplatin is the most emetogenic drug known and as such can be used as a yard stick by which to measure anti-emetic potential. Moreover, patient risk factors can influence emetogenicity of drugs so that patients with a large number of risk factors may require anti-emetic treatment typically prescribed for a highly emetogenic regimen even when the chemotherapy regimen is considered moderately emetogenic (Doherty 1999). So high-risk patients receiving drugs such as daunorubicin and cyclophosphamide may require potent anti-emetic cover.

As single agents, the 5HT3 antagonists can achieve complete control of cisplatin-induced vomiting in 40–60% of cases (Del Favero et al 1993) and the combination of a setron and dexamethasone can provide complete protection from emesis in 70–90% of cases (Roila et al 1996). There is evidence that this potentiating effect of dexamethasone is dose-dependent, with 20 mg dexamethasone being significantly better than 8 mg at controlling both emesis and nausea when combined with a 5HT3 receptor antagonist (control of vomiting achieved in 69% at 8 mg, 78% at 12 mg and 83% at 20 mg dexamethasone; control of nausea achieved in 61% at 8 mg, 66% at 12 mg and 71% at 20 mg dexamethasone) (Italian Group for Antiemetic Research 1998). In comparative studies equivalent efficacy and tolerability has been shown for ondansetron, granisetron and dolasetron (Italian Group for Antiemetic Research 1995a, Navari et al 1995) in controlling cisplatin-induced emesis.

For moderately emetogenic chemotherapy prophylactic treatment with 5HT3 receptor antagonists is appropriate; used alone or in combination with dexamethasone. In some places metoclopramide is still used, which may also be combined with dexamethasone. The combination of granisetron plus dexamethasone produced complete protection for 93% of patients compared with 70% of those treated with dexamethasone or granisetron alone (Italian Group for Antiemetic Research 1995b) and the protective effect of the combination persisted for three consecutive cycles (Italian Group for Antiemetic Research 1995c).

The 5HT3 receptor antagonists have been shown to be highly effective in controlling emesis induced by conditioning chemotherapy treatment or total body irradiation in patients undergoing BMT and are the first-line treatment for both adult and paediatric patients undergoing such therapies (Agura et al 1995, Belkacemi et al 1996).

Effective control of acute emesis contributes to prevention of delayed or anticipatory symptoms. Anti-emetic cover should be continued with a 5HT3 receptor antagonist plus dexamethasone after highly emetogenic therapy; in low-risk patients dexamethasone alone may be sufficient. If breakthrough vomiting occurs, then switching from one setron (ondansetron) to another (granisetron) has proved successful (Schnell 2003).

Evidence on radiotherapy-induced vomiting is scanty, but 5HT3 antagonists have been shown to be superior to prochloperazine and metoclopramide (Priestman et al 1993).

A crucial point to remember is that although nausea and vomiting can be treated it is usually better to adopt a prophylactic approach and give anti-emetics before treatment. Prophylactic anti-emetic treatment with a 5HT3 antagonist and dexamethasone is recommended by the American Society of Clinical Oncology (ASCO) and Multinational Association of Supportive Care in Cancer (MASCC) for all patients undergoing moderate to highly emetogenic chemotherapy or radiotherapy (Schnell 2003).

The latest development in anti-emetic therapy has been the development of a NK1 antagonist, aprepitant. This drug is yet to be licensed in some countries including the UK. Two phase III trials have been published in three papers (Hesketh et al 2003, Poli-Bigelli et al 2003, Warr et al 2003) which demonstrate superiority for the combination of a 5HT3 antagonist (ondansetron), aprepitant and dexamethasone over ondansetron plus dexamethasone (in study 1: complete control of vomiting on day 1 in 62.7% of the aprepitant arm compared with 43.3% in the ondansetron plus dexamethasone arm; in study 2 these results were

72.7% and 52.5% respectively). Nausea and emesis were also significantly better controlled on days 2 to 5 in both studies and there is evidence that aprepitant may be more useful in the delayed phase than the 5HT3 receptor antagonists (Van Belle et al 2002). Our understanding of the neuropharmacology of the emetic reflex would support a role for a combination of both of these antagonists in the optimal control of emesis and further investigations of the best dosing schedules may produce improvements in anti-emetic control.

Whichever anti-emetic is used, it must be tailored to the type of treatment being given, and to the susceptibility of the individual patient. Sedatives are often added to anti-emetic regimens to reduce anxiety; a sedative alone may be sufficient for patients receiving drugs of a very low emetogenic potential.

Attention must also be paid to controlling symptoms of nausea. Nausea is a subjective experience and it is unlikely that an external observer can be aware that a patient is nauseated unless the patient tells him/her. Some patients may be reluctant to report symptoms or may not mention nausea that is occurring at home. Efficient control of vomiting is not always accompanied by control of nausea and for some patients persistent nausea can be more distressing than vomiting (Hawthorn 1995). However, few studies have commented on the control of nausea and numerous methodological problems with measuring nausea mean that it is a neglected symptom.

Side effects of anti-emetics

A common problem with the dopamine receptor antagonist category of anti-emetics is extrapyramidal reactions (EPRs), which consist of restlessness, akisthisia (involuntary shaking of the limbs), torticollis (spasms of neck and facial muscles giving rise to twisting of the head) and oculogyric crises (spasm of the muscles causing eyeball movement). EPRs are possible side effects of haloperidol, droperidol, prochlorperazine, chlorpromazine and high-dose metoclopramide. More common in younger patients and especially children, they are dose-related (Bateman et al 1989) and may be treated with benztropine, benzhexol or procyclidine. A better tactic may be to avoid dopamine receptor antagonists where possible, by using for example a 5HT3 receptor antagonist. The side effects of the 5HT3 receptor antagonists are headache, dizziness, constipation and diarrhoea, and when they occur they are usually mild and manageable. However, nurses need to be aware of their potential occurrence so they can inform patients and initiate management strategies.

NON-PHARMACOLOGICAL

Since anxiety exacerbates emetic symptoms, any intervention that promotes relaxation can have a beneficial effect on emetic symptoms. Useful techniques are:

Table 17.2
Examples of anti-emetic regimens for chemotherapy or radiotherapy (not all of these anti-emetics are available worldwide)

Emetic potential of chemotherapy	Acute emesis	Delayed emesis
Very low	Lorazepam 1–2 mg po bd/tds	
Low	Prochlorperazine 12.5–25 mg iv q3-6 h	
	Metoclopramide 5–10 mg po tds	Dexamethasone 4 mg po tds for 3 days
Medium	Metoclopramide 30–100 mg iv + dexamethasone 4–8 mg iv	Metoclopramide 20 mg qds for 3 days + dexamethasone 4 mg po for 2 days
	Ondansetron 8 mg po bd	
	Granisetron 1 mg × 2 po or 2 mg po	
	Tropisetron 5 mg iv/po	
High/very high	Ondansetron 8 mg iv before chemo* then 8 mg iv × 2, 2–4 hours apart or 32 mg iv	Ondansetron 8 mg po bd up to 5 days + dexamethasone 8 mg po or im on day 2 and 3, 4 mg on day 4
	Oral ondansetron 8 mg bd	
	Granisetron 3 mg iv before chemo* repeated at 10 min interval up to 9 mg in 24 h	
	Tropisetron 5 mg iv before chemo*	Tropisetron 5 mg po up to 5 days
	Dolasetron 100 mg iv or po	
	Palonosetron 0.25 mg iv	
	Aprepitant 125 mg po od	Aprepitant 80 mg po once daily for 2 days
Radiotherapy		
Fractionated	Metoclopramide 10–20 mg q 6 h	
	Domperidone 20 mg po q 6 h	
	Ondansetron 8 mg po q 8 h	
TBI	Dexamethasone 6 mg iv 30 min prior to irradiation + ondansetron 6 mg iv	

*Add dexamethasone 8–20 mg od for highly emetogenic chemo or high-risk subject.
This information is taken from the literature. The manufacturer's data sheet should always be consulted for full information. N.B. Anti-emetic regimens containing dexamethasone are not used for individuals receiving high dose steroids as part of their cytotoxic regimen.

- relaxation
- progressive muscle relaxation (PMRT)
- hypnosis
- guided imagery
- systematic desensitisation
- therapeutic touch
- aromatherapy and massage.

The basis of many of these techniques is relaxation. Relaxation may be induced by placing the subjects in a soothing environment, playing gentle background music or using a commentary (Copley Cobb 1984). A more definite image may be introduced by using guided imagery. The therapist 'paints' a scene verbally so that the subject can visualise it in some detail; a simple cue can then allow the image to be recalled at a later date to aid relaxation (see Donovan 1980 for a complete script). In PMRT, patients are taught to tense the entire body and, moving slowly from feet upwards they actively relax each section of their body. Aromatherapy and massage both involve physical contact with the nurse or therapist. Touching can be important in reducing anxiety and opening up lines of communication (Byass 1988), and by 'formalising' such contact it can be carried out without invasion of an individual's personal space. Even where formal relaxation procedures are not employed a calm and soothing approach from the nurse can do much to help patients.

Generally speaking these techniques alone cannot control nausea and vomiting. However, they do make a valuable contribution to patient comfort and wellbeing; patients receiving supportive interventions have reported feeling more unafraid, in control, hopeful, powerful and relaxed (Troesch et al 1993).

Acupressure

Another supportive technique for controlling nausea and vomiting is acupuncture or more usually acupressure (pressing the acupuncture point rather than inserting a needle). The acupressure point for emesis, the Nei-Kuan or P6 point, is on the inside of the wrist, three finger widths above the crease of the wrist joint between the two visible tendons. This point can be pressed either with a finger or a wristband containing a small plastic stud positioned over the acupressure point. In 80 patients admitted for high-dose chemotherapy plus autologous peripheral blood stem cell transplantation, acupuncture at P6 offered no additional benefit over ondansetron (Streitberger et al 2003). However, clinical trials have shown some benefit for acupressure (Stannard 1989, Dundee & Yang 1990, Treish et al 2003), which is non-invasive and often appreciated by patients since it gives them some feeling of control over their situation – which may lower anxiety and have an indirect effect.

NURSING CONSIDERATIONS

When nursing patients who are likely to experience nausea and vomiting there are a few interventions that can help patient comfort:

- It is important to assess patients adequately before chemotherapy or radiotherapy is given. Patients who are particularly prone to vomiting or who will be receiving highly emetogenic treatment should be given anti-emetics prophylactically.
- Make sure that appropriate anti-emetics have been prescribed and are administered before treatment and on schedule afterwards.
- Position patients away from stimuli that may cause nausea and vomiting – the smell of food from the kitchens, other patients being sick, strong odours.
- Try to provide some privacy – most patients find being sick in public quite embarrassing. Screens or curtains are useful.
- Reassure the patient that it is normal – and quite acceptable – to be sick, but that there are treatments that they can be given to control symptoms.
- Have a vomit receiver and tissues to hand – but perhaps out of sight.
- Monitor whether anti-emetics are being successful. It may be useful to keep a chart to document the amount of emesis a patient is experiencing, but avoid constant questioning about nausea and vomiting – it could act as an emetic stimulus.
- If anti-emetics are inadequate, discuss this with the medical staff and consider changing dose, changing drug or adding supportive techniques.
- Anecdotally, fizzy drinks, especially soda water or ginger ale, can help to relieve nausea. Some people prefer flat ginger ale. Dry toast helps some people.
- Try to soothe/relax the patient by contact, verbal comments, music, etc. as appropriate.
- Where vomiting is prolonged the patient's fluid and electrolyte balance should be monitored as dehydration and electrolyte imbalance can be serious problems.
- If patients are being treated as day case or being discharged, make sure that they or their carer understands about delayed symptoms.

REFLECTION POINT Review the non-pharmacological strategies currently used within your clinical area. Are there strategies that could be developed further?

Patient education is always an important part of the nursing process. Anxiety will exacerbate symptoms, so a proper explanation of what is about to happen and investing time in trying to calm and reassure the patient is usually worthwhile. Nurses should be realistic, but not alarmist, about the likelihood of nausea and vomiting occurring. For radiotherapy patients it may be less frightening to be given a 'tour' of the radiotherapy apparatus before they are left alone in the treatment room.

Case study 17.1

Marion is a 37-year-old lady with a recurrence of non-Hodgkin's lymphoma. She was originally diagnosed 7 years ago and treated at another hospital. Marion gave a history of severe emesis during her previous chemotherapy regimen.

During pre-chemotherapy assessment Marion was very anxious concerning the recommencement of chemotherapy after her previous encounter when she had lost 2 stones in weight; which she attributed to nausea and vomiting. Marion also gave a history of emesis during pregnancy 12 years earlier. An anti-emetic regimen was discussed with

Marion, including the use of a 5HT3 receptor antagonist for 3 days followed by 7 days of metoclopramide together with the use of a relaxation tape (progressive muscle relaxation). Marion was taught the relaxation technique and was informed how to contact staff on the unit if she encountered any problems. She was given an outpatient appointment for 10 days post-treatment.

Marion experienced no vomiting during her chemotherapy and was very pleased with the anti-emetic regimen.

CONCLUSION

It is important for nurses to try and ameliorate emetic symptoms as much as possible for patient comfort and to aid compliance with treatment. Within the constraints of time it is important to try and provide a calm and soothing atmosphere. Anti-emetics should be monitored, given in the correct dose and on time. Prophylactic anti-emetics should always be given to those patients about to receive highly emetogenic procedures or who are at high-risk of developing nausea and vomiting. Day-case patients or those being discharged should have sufficient anti-emetics dispensed to cover the period when delayed symptoms may occur.

DISCUSSION QUESTIONS

1. What are the physiological processes of nausea and vomiting?

2. What are the main predisposing factors to nausea and vomiting in an individual with a haemato-oncological disorder?

3. Which anti-emetics are most effective in highly emetic drug regimes?

4. What would lead you to suspect that an individual is suffering anticipatory vomiting?

5. What pharmacological and non-pharmacological interventions would you use in an individual suffering from anticipatory vomiting?

References

Aapro M S, Selak E, Lichnitser M, Santini D, Mocciocchi A 2003 Palonosetron (PALO) is more effective than ondansetron (OND) in preventing chemotherapy-induced nausea and vomiting (CINV) in patients receiving moderately emetogenic chemotherapy (MEC). Results of a phase III trial. Proceedings of the American Society for Clinical Oncology 22:726

Agura E D, Brown M C, Schaffer R et al 1995 Antiemetic efficacy and pharmacokinetics of intravenous ondansetron infusion during chemotherapy conditioning for bone marrow transplant. Bone Marrow Transplant 16:213–222

Allwood M, Stanley A, Wright P 1997 The cytotoxics handbook, 3rd edn. Radcliffe Medical Press, Oxford

Andrews P L R, Davis C J 1993 The mechanism of emesis induced by anti-cancer therapies. In: Andrews P L R, Sanger G J (eds) Emesis in anti-cancer therapy. Mechanisms and treatment. Chapman Hall, London

Andrykowski M A, Gregg M E 1992 Development of anticipatory nausea: a prospective analysis. Journal of Consulting Clinical Psychology 53:447–454

Bateman D N, Darling W M, Boys R, Rawlins M D 1989 Extra-pyramidal reactions to metoclopramide and prochlorperazine. Quarterly Journal of Medicine 264:307–311

Belkacemi Y, Ozsahin M, Pere F et al 1996 Total body irradiation prior to bone marrow transplantation: efficacy and safety of granisetron in the prophylaxis and control of radiation-induced emesis. International Journal of Radiation Oncology Biology and Physics 36:77–82

Byass R 1988 Soothing body and soul. Nursing Times 84(24):39–41

Coates A, Abraham S, Kaye S B et al 1983 On the receiving end – patient perception of the side-effects of chemotherapy. European Journal of Clinical Oncology 19:203–208

Copley Cobb S 1984 Teaching relaxation to cancer patients. Cancer Nursing 7:157–161

Cunningham D, Dicato M, Verweij J et al 1996 Optimum anti-emetic therapy for cisplatin induced emesis over repeat courses: ondansetron plus dexamethasone compared with metoclopramide, dexamethasone plus lorazepam. Annals of Oncology 7:277–282

Del Favero A, Roila F, Tonato M 1993 Reducing chemotherapy-induced nausea and vomiting. Current perspectives and future possibilities. Drug Safety 9:410–428

Doherty K M 1999 Closing the gap in prophylactic antiemetic therapy: patient factors in calculating the emetogenic potential of chemotherapy. Clinical Journal of Oncology Nursing 3(3):113–119

Donovan M I 1980 Relaxation with guided imagery: a useful technique. Cancer Nursing 3:27–32

Dundee J W, Yang J 1990 Prolongation of the anti-emetic action of P6 acupuncture by acupressure in patients having cancer chemotherapy. Journal of the Royal Society of Medicine 83:360–362

Giffin A M, Butow P N, Coates A S et al 1996 On the receiving end V: patient perceptions of the side effects of cancer chemotherapy in 1993. Annals of Oncology 7:189–195

Gralla R J, Itri L M, Pisko S E et al 1981 Antiemetic efficacy of high-dose metoclopramide: randomized trials with placebo and prochlorperazine in patients with chemotherapy-induced nausea and vomiting. New England Journal of Medicine 3055:905–909

Hawthorn J 1995 Understanding and management of nausea and vomiting. Blackwell Science, Oxford

Hesketh P J, Beck T, Grunberg S M et al 1995 A proposal for classifying the emetogenicity of cancer chemotherapy (abstract). Seventh International Symposium, Multinational Association of Supportive Care in Cancer (MASCC), Luxembourg 20–23 September

Hesketh P J, Grunberg S M, Gralla R J et al 2003 The oral neurokinin-1 antagonist aprepitant for the prevention of chemotherapy-induced nausea and vomiting: a multinational, randomized, double-blind, placebo-controlled trial in patients receiving high-dose cisplatin – the aprepitant protocol 052 study group. Journal of Clinical Oncology 21:4112–4119

Italian Group for Antiemetic Research 1992 Ondansetron + dexamethasone vs metoclopramide + dexamethasone + diphenhydramine in prevention of cisplatin-induced emesis. Lancet 340:96–99

Italian Group for Antiemetic Research 1995a Dexamethasone, granisetron, or both for the prevention of nausea and vomiting during chemotherapy for cancer. New England Journal of Medicine 332:1–5

Italian Group for Antiemetic Research 1995b Ondansetron versus granisetron, both combined with dexamethasone, in the prevention of cisplatin-induced emesis. Annals of Oncology 6:805–810

Italian Group for Antiemetic Research 1995c Persistence of efficacy of three antiemetic regimens and prognostic factors in patients undergoing moderately emetogenic chemotherapy. Journal of Clinical Oncology 13:2417–2426

Italian Group for Antiemetic Research 1998 Double-blind dose-finding study of four intravenous doses of dexamethasone in the prevention of cisplatin-induced acute emesis. Journal of Clinical Oncology 16:2937–2942

Lindley C M, Bernard S, Fields S F 1989 Incidence and duration of chemotherapy-induced nausea and vomiting in the outpatient oncology population. Journal of Clinical Oncology 7:1142–1149

Mantovani G, Maccio A, Curelli L et al 1998 Comparison of oral 5-HT3 receptor antagonists and low-dose oral metoclopramide plus i.m. dexamethasone for the prevention of delayed emesis in head and neck cancer patients receiving high-dose cisplatin. Oncology Reports 5:273–280

Martin C G, Rubenstein E B, Elting L S, Jun Kim Y, Osoba D 2003 Measuring chemotherapy-induced nausea and emesis. Cancer 98:645–655

Merrifield K R, Chaffee B J 1989 Recent advances in the management of nausea and vomiting caused by antineoplastic agents. Clinical Pharmacy 8:187–199

Multinational Association for Supportive Care in Cancer 2004 Antiemetic guidelines. Endorsed June 1, 2004. www.mascc.org Accessed 12 Nov 2004

Navari R, Gandara D, Hesketh P et al 1995 Comparative clinical trial of granisetron and ondansetron in the prophylaxis of cisplatin-induced emesis. The granisetron study group. Journal of Clinical Oncology 13:1242–1248

Osoba D, Zee B, Pater J, Warr D, Latreille J, Kaiser L 1997 Determinants of postchemotherapy nausea and vomiting in patients with cancer. Journal of Clinical Oncology 15(1):116–123

Passik S D, Kirsh K L, Rosenfield B et al 2001 The changeable nature of patients' fears regarding chemotherapy: implications for palliative care. Journal of Pain and Symptom Management 21:113–120

Poli-Bigelli S, Rodrigues-Pereira J, Carides A D et al 2003 Addition of the neurokinin 1 receptor antagonist aprepitant to standard antiemetic therapy improves control of chemotherapy-induced nausea and vomiting. Results from a randomised, double-blind, placebo-controlled trial in Latin America. Cancer 97: 3090–3098

Priestman T 1988 Radiation-induced emesis. Clinician 6:40–43

Priestman T J, Roberts J T, Upadhyaya B K 1993 A prospective randomized double-blind trial comparing ondansetron versus prochlorperazine for the prevention of nausea and vomiting in patients undergoing fractionated radiotherapy. Clinical Oncology (Royal College of Radiologists) 5:358–363

Ritter Jr H L, Gralla R J, Hall S W et al 1998 Efficacy of intravenous granisetron to control nausea and vomiting during multiple cycles of cisplatin-based chemotherapy. Cancer Investigations 16:87–93

Roila F, Tonato M, Basurto C 1988 Antiemetic activity of high doses of metoclopramide in cisplatin treated cancer patients: a randomised double-blind trial of the Italian Oncology Group for Clinical Research. Journal of Clinical Oncology 5:141–149

Roila F, Tonato M, Basurto C et al 1989 Protection from nausea and vomiting in cisplatin-treated patients: high-dose metoclopramide combined with methyl prednisolone versus metoclopramide combined with dexamethasone and diphenhydramine: a study of the Italian Oncology Group for Clinical Research. Journal of Clinical Oncology 7:1693–1700

Roila F, Tonato M, Ballatori E, Del Favero A 1996 Comparative studies of various antiemetic regimens. Supportive Care in Cancer 4:270–280

Schnell F M 2003 Chemotherapy-induced nausea and vomiting: the importance of acute antiemetic control. The Oncologist 8:187–198

Stacher G 2002 Palonosetron. Current Opinion in Investigational Drugs 3:1502–1507

Stahl S M 2003 The ups and downs of novel antiemetic drugs, Part 1 Substance P, 5-HT, and the neuropharmacology of vomiting. Journal of Clinical Psychiatry 64:498–499

Stannard D 1989 Acupressure prevents nausea. Nursing Times 85(4):33–34

Streitberger K, Friedrich-Rust M, Bardenheuer H et al 2003 Effect of acupuncture compared with placebo-acupuncture at P6 as additional antiemetic prophylaxis in high-dose chemotherapy and autologous peripheral stem cell transplantation. Clinical Cancer Research 9:2538–2544

Treish I, Shord S, Valgus J et al 2003 Randomized double-blind study of the Reliefband as an adjunct to standard antiemetics in patients receiving moderately-high to highly emetogenic chemotherapy. Supportive Care in Cancer 8:516–521

Troesch L M, Rodehaver C B, Delaney E A, Yanes B 1993 The influence of guided imagery on chemotherapy-related nausea and vomiting. Oncology Nursing Forum 20:1179–1185

Van Belle S, Lichinister M R, Navari R M et al 2002 Prevention of cisplatin-induced acute and delayed emesis by the selective neurokinin-1 antagonists L-758, 298 and MK-869. Cancer 94:3032–3041

Warr D, Gralla R J, Hesketh P J et al 2003 The oral NK1 antagonist aprepitant for the prevention of chemotherapy induced nausea and vomiting: 2 randomized, double-blind, placebo controlled trials. Proceedings of ASCO 22:726

Zook D J, Yasko J M 1983 Psychological factors: their effect on nausea and vomiting experienced by clients receiving chemotherapy. Oncology Nursing Forum 10:76–81

Further reading

Copley Cobb S 1984 Teaching relaxation to cancer patients. Cancer Nursing 7:157–161
This article is useful because it actually provides concrete instructions for nurses on how to teach patients to relax, including a script for the reader to follow.

Hawthorn J 1995 Understanding and management of nausea and vomiting. Blackwell Science, Oxford
This book (which won an award in the BMA Medical Book Competition) is a comprehensive text on nausea and vomiting. It gives a complete account of the physiology of nausea and vomiting and discusses the pharmacology and use of anti-emetic drugs. It also contains a discussion of the

nursing approach to controlling nausea and vomiting, including alternative therapies. The book covers all types of nausea and vomiting but is more oriented towards oncology nurses.

MASSC guidelines – www.mascc.org
MASCC established an Anti-emetic Guideline Committee, an international group of 23 doctors and nurses with experience in the field of research and treatment of emesis. The group were divided into 10 working committees each of which conducted a survey and critical evaluation of the available information about different areas of emesis treatment (e.g. acute emesis highly emetogenic

chemotherapy, refractory emesis, rescue anti-emetic therapy, multiday chemotherapy, etc). The committees produced recommendations for optimal anti-emetic use in each circumstance, these guidelines were then voted upon and a 75% consensus of the whole group required before a guideline was adopted or changed. The result is recommendations for optimal anti-emetic use in different treatment settings.

Schnell F M 2003 Chemotherapy-induced nausea and vomiting: the importance of acute antiemetic control. The Oncologist 8:187–198

This article gives a good review of the 5HT3-receptor antagonists and emphasises the need for good prophylactic treatment of emesis. It can be downloaded free of charge from: http://theoncologist.alphamedpress.org/cgi/content/full/8/2/187

Chapter **18**

Oral care

Lynne Dickinson and Helen Porter

KEY POINTS
- Oral complications can be life-threatening.
- Assessment is an essential part of the oral care process.
- Oral care is an essential, skilled nursing intervention.
- Evidence-based protocols for effective oral care in the immunosuppressed individual are an indication of good practice.

INTRODUCTION

For the individual with a haematological cancer, oral problems can be the cause of immense pain and discomfort. Loss of function can occur and local infection may lead to systemic problems. Development of oral problems can initiate life-threatening complications such as systemic sepsis that may not be resolved with aggressive medical, nursing and dental interventions (Madeya 1996). Causality is multi-faceted, including the disease itself and the treatment with its specific side effects. A healthy mouth in terms of quality of life is highly relevant to the care of all patients, but in the case of a patient with cancer, the maintenance of oral health is integral to care (Rawlins & Trueman 2001). Individuals with haematological cancers develop oral complications more often than those with solid tumours (Madeya 1996). Oral care, therefore, is an essential, skilled nursing intervention. Nurses must be able to identify which clients are at risk of developing oral complications, adopt preventative measures, detect changes to the oral cavity early and initiate prompt appropriate therapy. An in-depth knowledge of all aspects of oral care is therefore required.

THE HEALTHY ORAL CAVITY

The oral cavity is lined by a mucous membrane consisting of three layers. The top layer is composed of stratified squamous epithelium, which covers a layer of loose connective tissue called the lamina propria. Within this layer there are blood vessels, sensory nerve endings, lymphatic vessels and smooth muscle fibres. The submucosa is a layer of loose connective tissue, which contains larger blood vessels, lymphatics, nerve fibres and exocrine glands. The basement layer, between the lamina propria and the submucosa, is where epithelial cells replicate (Martini 1992). It is estimated that the surface epithelial layer of the oral mucosa is replaced every 7–14 days. This rapid turnover of cells renders the epithelium prone to damage in treatments such as radiotherapy and chemotherapy (see Chapters 9 & 10). Within the oral cavity are the specialised structures of dentition, the tongue, and the salivary glands. In health, approximately 1000–1500 mL of saliva is produced daily. The oral cavity has a variety of functions, which can be acutely affected by haemato-oncology disorders, their treatment and other associated problems.

The functions of the oral cavity are:

● ingestion of food and water
● communication
● breathing (with nasal cavity) (Lippold & Winton 1972).

THE EFFECT OF HAEMATO-ONCOLOGY DISORDERS ON THE ORAL CAVITY

Haemato-oncology disorders can cause problems from local disease infiltration, immunosuppression, myelosuppression, and associated coagulopathies.

LEUKAEMIA

Neutropenia and thrombocytopenia render the client at risk from oral infection and bleeding. Spontaneous bleeding from the gums is a common feature at diagnosis. Gum hypertrophy and infiltration with leukaemic cells is a feature of acute myeloid, myelomonocytic and monocytic leukaemias (Hoffbrand & Pettit 1993), whereas individuals with acute promyelocytic leukaemia may develop disseminated intravascular coagulation (DIC) leading to bleeding problems (see Chapters 4 & 16).

LYMPHOMA

Loss of cell-mediated immune reactions may occur in lymphomas (Hoffbrand & Pettit 1993). Therefore, although individuals may not be neutropenic at diagnosis, their immune function will be impaired (see Chapter 6). Individuals may also have local infiltration of tissue with lymphoma. Where bone marrow involvement is evident, neutropenia and thrombocytopenia may occur.

MYELOMA

Deficient antibody production and neutropenia may lead to persistent infections. Abnormal plasma proteins interfere with platelet function and coagulation and may lead to bleeding. In patients with amyloid the tongue may become abnormally enlarged (see Chapter 5).

EFFECTS OF TREATMENT ON THE ORAL CAVITY

All treatments used in haemato-oncology can have an adverse effect on the oral cavity and improved treatments for cancer may go hand in hand with significant destruction of normal tissue (Kenny 1990). Until recently, mucositis was thought to be due to the effect of cytotoxic drugs or radiotherapy on rapidly dividing epithelial cells. However, newer evidence suggests that mucositis following chemotherapy and radiotherapy is a consequence of a series of complex biological interactions. Although these interactions are viewed as five phases, many of the interactions occur simultaneously rather than in a linear manner (Sonis et al 2004).

The five phases of mucosal injury are:

1. Initiation – the endothelial and connective tissues of the submucosa are damaged before epithelial damage occurs.

2. Up-regulation of genes and generation of messenger signals – damaged tissues generate oxidative stress stimulating production of a number of transcription factors and up-regulation of many other genes, causing apoptosis of stem cells in the basal epithelium.
3. Signalling and amplification – proinflammatory cytokines have a role in both direct and indirect signalling and amplification of mucosal injury.
4. Ulceration – epithelial apoptosis and necrosis result in ulceration and full-thickness mucosal damage.
5. Healing – stimulated by signals from the extracellular matrix, e.g. after haemopoietic stem cell transplant (HSCT), leucocyte recovery marks the healing phase (Rubenstein et al 2004, Sonis et al 2004).

However, even after mucosal healing has occurred, the mucosa is permanently altered and individuals are at increased risk of mucositis with subsequent cancer treatment (Sonis et al 2004).

CHEMOTHERAPY

Many cytotoxic drugs used in the treatment of haematological malignancies are associated with oral problems, most commonly mucositis (Knox et al 2000). Antimetabolites (e.g. cytosine arabinoside, methotrexate) and antitumour antibiotics (e.g. daunorubicin, doxorubicin) are most frequently associated with mucositis (Madeya 1996). High-dose melphalan often included in conditioning regimens before HSCT is also associated with high rates of mucositis (Wardley et al 2000). The extent of damage is generally dose-related. High-dose chemotherapy and continuous or frequently repetitive schedules, such as methotrexate, severely damage the mucosa (Cooley 2002). Clinically, oral mucositis is characterised by erythema, swelling and ulceration. The non-keratinised mucosa of the cheeks, the lips, the soft palate, and tongue are frequently affected (Raber-Durlacher 1999). Mucosal damage usually occurs 5–7 days after treatment and takes 2–3 weeks to heal in the non-myelosuppressed individual (Dose 1995). Indirect damage to the mucosa may also occur due to bone marrow suppression causing neutropenia, stomatitis and dental decay (Corbett 1997).

Xerostomia, described as dryness of the mouth caused by a reduction or absence of saliva, can also be caused by chemotherapy, although chemotherapy-associated salivary gland injury is usually transient.

RADIOTHERAPY

Radiotherapy may be administered locally, e.g. cranial, or to the whole body, e.g. TBI (total body irradiation) or whole nodal (see Chapter 10). Effects range from mild inflammatory changes to ulcerated bleeding mucosa. The severity of mucositis increases as the dose of radiation escalates (Shih et al 2003). The incidence of oral mucositis in patients receiving combination chemotherapy and radiotherapy can increase from 60% to 100% (Dose 1995). Fibrosis of the structures of the oral cavity with bone and dentition changes, including an accelerated rate of dental caries, a slow growth rate and decreased osteoclastic and osteoblastic activity may occur.

Radiation directed at the parotid or submandibular glands will result in a marked decrease in salivary flow. The severity of xerostomia is related directly to the dose of radiotherapy, and may be permanent in total doses over 6000 cGy (Shih et al 2003). Saliva regulates the pH of the oral cavity, controlling bacterial flora, lubricating the mucosa and cleansing the teeth. When the amount of saliva and consistency are changed, generalised oral disease can occur. Xerostomia may lead to functional changes, such as impaired taste, difficulty in forming a food bolus, local immunosuppression and speech problems.

EFFECT OF IMMUNOSUPPRESSION ON THE ORAL CAVITY

Immunosuppression resulting from either the disease process or treatment-induced myelosuppression will render the individual at risk from infection. The infection risk increases the longer the period of immunosuppression (Barton Burke et al 2001). Alteration in the normal microflora caused by salivary changes or systemic antibiotic or steroid therapy also increases the risk.

Local superimposed infection in the oral cavity may be bacterial, viral or fungal. Damage to mucosal integrity allows oral pathogens to enter the circulation and may lead to systemic sepsis and life-threatening infection. Infection may arise from existing commensal organisms or from introduced pathogens (Porter 1994). Common oral pathogens include bacteria, fungi and viruses.

Bacteria

In immunocompromised individuals 70% of severe bacterial infections are Gram-negative (*Pseudomonas aeruginosa*, Klebsiella, *Escherichia coli*), the remaining 30% are Gram-positive infections (*Staphylococcus aureus*, *Staphylococcus epidermidis*, Enterococcus).

Fungi

Candida albicans and Aspergillus are the most common fungal infections. Candida usually presents as pseudomembranous candidiasis, acute atrophic candidiasis, chronic hyperplastic candidiasis or candidal cheilosis (Ventafridda et al 1993).

Viruses

Herpes simplex and herpes zoster are characterised by single or multiple clusters of small vesicles (Madeya 1996) appearing commonly on the lips or in the mouth. Immunosuppression may cause reactivation of the latent virus in patients who have had previous infection.

OTHER CAUSES OF ORAL PROBLEMS IN THE HAEMATO–ONCOLOGY PATIENT

As well as the disease and its treatment there are a number of other factors that predispose an individual with a haemato-oncological disease to develop oral complications.

Graft-versus-host disease (GvHD) may be a significant problem in allogeneic transplantation (see Chapter 13). Oral GvHD occurs in over 80% of cases of chronic GvHD and resembles lesions in connective tissue disorders with mucosal erythema, atrophy, ulceration and lichen planus-like lesions (Schubert & Sullivan 1990).

Many of the drugs used in the treatment of haemato-oncological conditions will cause xerostomia. These include tricyclic antidepressants, antihistamines, anticholinergics, anticonvulsants, beta-blockers, diuretics, opiates and hypnotics. In the individual with xerostomia, vomiting can cause specific problems. The normal nausea and vomiting process ensures protection of the mucosa and dentition from the acidic contents of the stomach through increased saliva production. If there is no saliva to act as a buffer, the client becomes more susceptible to developing mucositis and dentition damage.

Reduced nutritional intake secondary to mucositis may increase the severity of the mucositis owing to decreased cellular renewal and migration (Madeya 1996). Vitamin deficiencies can also lead to oral problems. Riboflavin deficiency can lead to lesions in the mucocutaneous surfaces of the mouth (angular stomatitis, cheilosis and glottis) and vitamin C deficiency can lead to bleeding gums (DoH 1991).

Effect of mucositis on therapy

Systemic chemotherapy regimens may be altered as mucositis develops. Drug doses may be adjusted, omitted or delayed if there is significant mucositis. This may lead to less than optimal therapy with a potentially negative effect on the individual's prognosis. Patient education and participation in self-care are therefore crucial in ensuring that oral care is strictly maintained throughout the treatment process. Nurses have an important role in providing effective oral care and a health promotion role in teaching patients about the importance of oral care and assessment (Xavier 2000). Educating patients and encouraging them to minimise their risk factors may help in reducing the risk of oral complications, which in turn may improve their quality of life (Ohrn et al 2000).

ORAL ASSESSMENT

Assessment is an essential part of the oral care process and consensus appears to exist in relation to the benefits of oral assessment (Milligan et al 2001, Rawlins & Trueman 2001). An assessment of the oral cavity should be carried out prior to treatment commencing, in order to provide a baseline from which to measure change. Early assessment also increases the likelihood of early detection of treatable oral disease, appropriate pharmacological intervention or further referral (Sweeney 1998). Assessment tools can help nurses to identify the severity of oral complications and should be quick and easy to use (Porter 1992). Assessment tools may be descriptive or numerical. A number of tools have been developed to enable thorough assessment of the oral cavity. When choosing a tool, ease of use, applicability to the client population and proven reliability and validity are important factors to consider (McGuire 2003).

Numerous oral assessment tools are available in the literature, a number of which have been specifically developed for the haemato-oncology population. One example is the OAG (oral assessment guide) developed by Eilers et al (1988). This tool was developed in the bone marrow transplant setting and has shown itself to be useful in clinical practice by a number of authors (Graham et al 1993, Holmes & Mountain 1993, Feber 1995). It is a nurse-administered scoring system consisting of the following eight categories:

- voice
- swallow
- lips
- tongue
- saliva
- mucous membranes
- gingiva
- teeth or dentures.

The assessment tool allows a score of 1 to 3 for each category, with 1 being normal and 3 indicating severe problems.

REFLECTION POINT   What factors would you take into consideration when deciding on an oral assessment tool to implement in your ward/department?

AIMS OF ORAL CARE

Cooley (2002) describes the aims of oral care as to:

- keep the mucosa clean, soft, moist and intact
- keep the lips clean, soft, moist
- remove plaque and food substances without damaging the mucosal integrity
- prevent or treat oral discomfort and pain
- identify early and treat oral problems with the most appropriate equipment or treatments
- prevent bad breath and keep the mouth fresh.

GUIDELINES FOR GOOD PRACTICE

The administration of oral care can be subdivided into frequency of care, oral tools and oral agents and solutions. Unfortunately, there is still little research within the haemato-oncology setting to guide clinical practice. Nurses must identify the specific care needs of the individual and formulate a care plan to meet them. Changes in the oral cavity can occur rapidly and so the frequency of assessment and care must be adapted to the individual.

In England and Wales, oral hygiene currently has a high profile as one of the eight clinical benchmarks proposed as part of the nursing strategy 'Essence of care' document (DoH 2001). The main focus of this is to improve the quality of the fundamental and essential aspects of care (DoH 1999). Encouraging a collaborative approach to oral care promotes best practice through sharing, comparing and disseminating examples of high-quality care. The National Institute for Clinical Excellence publication 'Improving outcomes in haematological cancers' (NICE 2003) also encompasses oral care in the recommendation that guidelines are in place for the prevention and treatment of the side effects of chemotherapy.

The following guidelines reduce the potential for the development of oral complications.

ORAL ASSESSMENT

The oral cavity should be assessed at least daily using an assessment tool that has been tested for reliability and validity. Where severe mucositis develops this should be increased to twice daily. The appropriateness of the chosen assessment tool is paramount to the meaningfulness of the information obtained (Miller & Kearney 2001).

FREQUENCY OF CARE

There is no consensus within the literature on the recommended frequency of oral care. This stems from a lack of recent research and clearly indicates the need for further research into this essential aspect of care. Oral care should be performed at least four times a day, e.g. after meals and before going to sleep, reducing the potential for infection from micro-organisms (Krishnasamy 1995). Care should be increased to 2-hourly in patients with severe mucositis or xerostomia. Increasing the frequency of oral care has been shown to have a positive effect on the oral health of the patient (Miller & Kearney 2001).

ORAL CARE AGENTS

The literature suggests that the pharmacological treatment regimes for oral mucositis are well articulated but not always evidence-based (Evans

Table 18.1
Oral care agents

Agents	Action	Reference
Antifungal agents		
Amphotericin	Topical antifungal agent	Finlay 1995
Nystatin	Antifungal antibiotic	Campbell 1995
Miconazole	Topically acting azole, effective against candida and Gram-positive cocci	Wray & Bragg 1997
Itraconazole	Orally absorbed antifungal azole	Worthington et al 2001
Fluconazole	Orally absorbed antifungal azole	Brammer 1990
Antiviral agents		
Acyclovir	Inhibits herpes virus replication	Saral 1990
Cleansing/antimicrobial		
Chlorhexidine	Broad-spectrum antimicrobial activity, prevents dental plaque formation, sustained release from mucosal surfaces	Beck & Yasko 1993, Raybould et al 1994
Iodine	Antiseptic and antibacterial	Adamietz et al 1998
Protection of the mucosa		
Sucralfate suspension	Coating and protection of the mucosa	Franzen et al 1995, Cengiz et al 1999
Allopurinol	Provides mucosal protection	Loprinzi et al 1990, Nakmura et al 1996
Gelclair	Provides mucosal protection	De Cordi et al 2001, Innocenti et al 2002
Xerostomia		
Artificial saliva	Buffers acidity and lubricates the mucous membranes	Feber 1996, Little 1996, Haddad & Karimi 2002
Pilocarpine	A parasympathetic agent that stimulates remaining salivary gland function	Singal et al 1995, Hawthorne & Sullivan 2001
Miscellaneous		
Fluoride	Enhances remineralisation and inhibits bacterial metabolism	Cooke 1996
Saline	Aids in the formation of granulation tissue, promotes healing, non-irritant	Kennedy & Diamond 1997
Colony stimulating factors (G-CSF, GM-CSF)	Promotes mucosal healing	Kannan et al 1997, Rovirosa et al 1998

2001, Borbasi et al 2002). This emphasises the need for nurses to acquire the skills to critically appraise published research to determine the most appropriate patient care.

Care should be taken to choose the appropriate oral care agent for the specific need, e.g. antimicrobial (Table 18.1). In patients at risk of secondary infection, chlorhexidine gluconate (a bisguanidine) provides anti-plaque and broad-spectrum antimicrobial activity. Rawlins & Trueman (2001) suggest that solutions containing chlorhexidine are effective in reducing bacteria in 80% of patients. Chlorhexidine gluconate has also been intensely investigated to determine its benefits in relation to the prophylactic and therapeutic treatment of oral mucositis. However, randomised controlled trials have failed to support its use in the prophylaxis or treatment of oral mucositis occurring as a result of antineoplastic treatment (Wolfgang et al 2001, Clarkson et al 2004). Feber (1995) suggests that chlorhexidine should not be used before meals as it may cause temporary taste changes. Chlorhexidine is also known to stain teeth, although dentists can remove these stains.

Topical antifungal agents may also be of value but care must be taken to leave an interval of 30–60 minutes between administering chlorhexidine mouthwash and nystatin. Concurrent use renders nystatin ineffective (Gibson & Nelson 2000).

Many oral care agents have been investigated (Table 18.1). However, Rubenstein et al (2004) conclude that there is still insufficient robust research evidence to support the use of specific agents.

ORAL CARE TOOLS

A number of different oral care tools are described in the literature including the toothbrush, foam sticks, dental floss and gauze. It is, however, important to select the most suitable tool and this should be determined by its efficacy and potential to damage the gingiva. Where appropriate a toothbrush should be used as it is the best tool for removing debris and preventing plaque formation. The effectiveness of a small, soft toothbrush over other tools is well documented (Pearson 1996, Bowsher et al 1999, Evans 2001). Using a small soft brush also helps in preventing damage to the oral mucosa (Krishnasamy 1995). However, it may cause further discomfort for patients with severe mucositis (Holmes 1998).

The specific problems of thrombocytopenia and coagulopathy must also be considered when choosing between toothbrushes and other tools. Toothbrushing and dental flossing are not recommended in patients with thrombocytopenia (platelet count >50,000/mm^3) (Barker 1999). Using a gloved finger or foam swab may be more appropriate for patients for whom toothbrushing is precluded, e.g. in spontaneous bleeding or pain (Krishnasamy 1995). The use of the swabbed finger is not, however, recommended by Wood (2004) who suggests that this action may put nurses at risk.

If the toothbrush is used, care must be taken to ensure that the toothbrush is kept free from infection as toothbrushes have been shown to harbour organisms such as group A beta-haemolytic streptococci, staphylococci, candida and pseudomonas (Brook & Gober 1998). This can be achieved by ensuring that the toothbrush is thoroughly cleaned under running water after each use and allowed to dry.

Denture management is also an important part of oral care. Dentures can accumulate food debris and microbial plaque (Xavier 2000). However, varying advice exists on effective cleansing. Xavier (2000) suggests cleaning dentures with soap and water and soaking in clean water or a proprietary cleaner when not worn. Roberts (2000) suggests that once cleaned, dentures should be soaked in a proprietary solution. Feber (1995) also advocates cleansing with soap and water, but suggests that dentures should be soaked two to three times a week in a hypochlorite denture cleansing agent (e.g. Dentural or Steradent). Based on information produced by the British Dental Health Foundation (2004) dentures should be cleaned using a small- to medium-headed toothbrush or soft nailbrush using soap and water. The dentures should be soaked in a specialist cleaner for the time recommended by the manufacturer. Dentures should be removed at night or if they are causing patient discomfort, and stored in water to prevent warping or cracking.

PSYCHOLOGICAL IMPACT

The psychological importance of poor oral health should not be underestimated – the mouth plays a major role in communication through both speech and physical expression (Xavier 2000). When planning oral care, thought must be given to the psychological effects of oral problems. Mucositis can be an extremely distressing symptom, with both structural and functional effects. Dysfunction will effect patients' perception of body image and their sense of wellbeing.

REFLECTION POINT   Consider the effect that severe mucositis may have on a patient's sense of wellbeing and their body image.

PAIN RELIEF

The sensation of burning is often the first indication of mucositis and may be present without any visible abnormality. As mucositis progresses, the patient may experience severe pain. The degree of pain may vary throughout the day as the patient experiences different stressors such as eating, drinking and performing oral hygiene. The experience of pain will decrease compliance with mouth care and reduce the intake of food and fluids. Oral pain also has a detrimental effect on the patient's quality of life. Although the experience of oral pain is well documented, there is a dearth of information regarding guidance on appropriate, effective analgesia. The choice of analgesia may be limited by the side effects of drugs (e.g. bleeding with aspirin) and potential problems with routes of administration (e.g. risk of infection with per rectum analgesia in the myelosuppressed client and the risk of bleeding and bruising with skin punctures). In severe pain, intravenous opiates may offer relief.

Case study 18.1

Anne is a 35-year-old woman with Hodgkin's disease. She is in remission and has recently undergone high-dose chemotherapy with an autologous peripheral blood stem cell transplant. Anne had good oral hygiene techniques and visits her dentist regularly. The oral assessment guide (Eilers et al 1988) was used with Anne twice a day and she used a prophylactic regime of chlorhexidine mouthwash and topical antifungal mouthwash after meals and before going to sleep at night, allowing 30 minutes between the two mouthwashes.

Five days after her chemotherapy commenced, Anne developed severe mucositis, which was treated with Oramorph 1 hour before each meal, first thing in the morning and last thing at night. She was unable to brush her teeth due to pain and foam sticks and gauze swabs were gently used to clean her mouth every two hours. After a further 7 days Anne's mucositis improved, allowing her to commence a soft diet and clean her teeth with a soft toothbrush. The Oramorph was discontinued but continued use of chlorhexidine mouthwash was encouraged.

Oral care may also involve novel approaches in the management of mucositis. There is some evidence to suggest that using ice chips for 5 minutes prior to the administration of 5-fluorouracil (5FU) and for 25 minutes after is effective (Cansinu et al 1994). Cryotherapy, or rapid cooling of the oral cavity using ice, causes local vasoconstriction. This reduces the blood flow to the mucosa, which reduces the amount of 5FU taken up, thus reducing cellular damage. Although 5FU is predominantly used in gastrointestinal cancers, this method of prophylaxis has also been shown to have some efficacy in preventing melphalan-induced stomatitis (Meloni et al 1996).

REFLECTION POINT

Mr Jones is receiving craniospinal radiotherapy in conjunction with his induction chemotherapy for acute lymphoblastic leukaemia. What risk factors does he have for developing oral complications and what oral care should be initiated?

CONCLUSION

Delivery of effective oral care is a skilled nursing activity, involving assessment, goal setting, care delivery and evaluation (Porter 1994). The needs of haemato-oncology patients are complex but it is essential that oral care be given priority to prevent life-threatening complications and maintain quality of life. It is therefore essential to ensure that care delivered is evidence-based and that practice is continuously improved through audit and research.

DISCUSSION QUESTIONS

1. What are the physical manifestations of the different types of oral infections that you have seen?

2. What characteristics of the patient population on your ward/department make them at risk of developing oral complications?

3. What is the evidence base for the oral care protocol in your ward/department?

References

Adamietz I A, Rahn R, Bottcher H D, Schafer V, Reimer K, Fleisher W 1998 Prophylaxis with povidone-iodine against induction of oral mucositis by radiochemotherapy. Supportive Care in Cancer 6:373–377

Barker G J 1999 Current practices in the oral management of the patient undergoing chemotherapy or bone marrow transplantation. Supportive Care in Cancer 7:17–20

Barton Burke M, Wilkes G M, Inwersen K 2001 Cancer chemotherapy: a nursing process approach, 3rd edn. Jones and Bartlett, Boston

Beck S, Yasko J 1993 Guidelines for oral care, 2nd edn. Sage, Crystal Lake, IL

Borbasi S, Cameron K, Quested B, Olver I, Evans D 2002 More than a sore mouth: patient's experience of oral mucositis. Oncology Nursing Forum 29(7):1051–1057

Bowsher J, Boyle S, Griffiths J 1999 Oral care: a clinical effectiveness-based systemic review of oral care. Nursing Standard 3(37):31

Brammer K W 1990 Management of fungal infection in neutropenic patients. Haematology and Blood Transfusion 33:546–550

British Dental Health Foundation 2004 http://www.dentalhealth.org.uk/faqs/leafletdetail.php?LeafletID=11#faq217 Accessed 27 Oct 2004

Brook I, Gober A E 1998 Persistence of group A beta-hemolytic streptococci in toothbrushes and removable orthodontic appliances following treatment of pharyntonsillitis. Archives of Otolaryngology – Head and Neck Surgery 124(9):993–995

Campbell S 1995 Treating oral candidiasis. Nurse Prescriber 1(5):12–13

Cansinu S, Fedeli A, Fedeli S L, Catalano G 1994 Oral cooling (cryotherapy) an effective treatment for the prevention of 5-fluorouracil induced stomatitis. Oral Oncology European Journal of Cancer 30B:234–236

Cengiz M, Ozyar E, Ozturk D, Akyol F, Atahan I L, Hayran M 1999 Sucralfate in the prevention of radiation-induced oral mucositis. Journal of Gastroenterology 28(1):40–43

Clarkson J E, Worthington H V, Eden O B 2004 Interventions for prevention oral mucositis for patients with cancer receiving treatment. The Cochrane Database of Systematic Reviews. The Cochrane Library 2

Cooke C 1996 Xerostomia – a review. Palliative Medicine 10:284–292

Cooley C 2002 Oral health: basic or essential care? Cancer Nursing Practice 1(3):33–39

Corbett A 1997 Mouth care and chemotherapy. Paediatric Nursing 9(3):19–21

De Cordi D, D'andrea N, Giorgutti E, Martina S 2001 Gelclair: potentially an efficacious treatment for chemotherapy-induced mucositis. Abstract: Italian Tumour League 111 congress for professional oncology nurses, Conegliano, Italy

Department of Health 1991 Report on health and social subjects 41. Dietary reference values for food energy and nutrients for the United Kingdom: report of the panel on dietary values of the committee on medical aspects of food policy. HMSO, London

Department of Health 1999 Making a difference. Strengthening the nursing, midwifery and health visiting contribution to health. HMSO, London

Department of Health 2001 The essence of care: patient focused benchmarking for health care practitioners. HMSO, London

Dose A M 1995 The symptom experience of mucositis, stomatitis, and xerostomia. Seminars in Oncology Nursing 11(4):248–255

Eilers J, Berger A M, Peterson M C 1988 Developing, testing and application of the oral assessment guide. Oncology Nursing Forum 15(3):325–330

Evans G 2001 A rationale for oral care. Nursing Standard 1(43):33–36

Feber T 1995 Head and neck oncology nursing. Whurr, London

Feber T 1996 Mouth care for patients receiving oral irradiation. Professional Nurse 10(10):666–669

Finlay I 1995 Oral fungal infections. European Journal of Palliative Care 2(2 Suppl):4–7

Franzen L, Henrikson R, Littbrand B, Zackrisson B 1995 Effects of sucralfate suspension of mucositis during radiotherapy to malignancies in the head and neck region. A double-blind placebo controlled study. Acta Oncologica 34:219–223

Gibson F, Nelson W 2000 Mouth care for children with cancer. Paediatric Nursing 12(1):18–22

Graham K M, Pecoraro D A, Ventura M, Meyer C C 1993 Reducing the incidence of stomatitis using a quality assessment and improvement approach. Cancer Nursing 16(2):117–122

Haddad P, Karimi M 2002 A randomised, double-blind, placebo-controlled trial of concomitant pilocarpine with head and neck irradiation for prevention of radiation-induced xerostomia. Radiotherapy and Oncology 64(1):29–32

Hawthorne M, Sullivan 2001 Pilocarpine for radiation-induced xerostomia in head and neck cancer. International Journal of Palliative Nursing 6(5): 228–232

Holmes S 1998 Cancer chemotherapy: a guide for practice. Asset Books, Dorking

Holmes S, Mountain E 1993 Assessment of oral status: evaluation of three assessment guides. Journal of Clinical Nursing 2:35–40

Hoffbrand A V, Pettit J E (eds) 1993 Essential haematology, 3rd edn. Blackwell Science, Oxford

Innocenti M, Moscatelli G, Lopez S 2002 Efficacy of gelclair in palliative care patients with oral lesions: preliminary findings from an open pilot study. Journal of Pain and Symptom Management 24(5):456–457

Kannan V, Bapsy P P, Anantha N et al 1997 Efficacy and safety of granulocyte macrophage-colony stimulating factor (GM-CSF) on the frequency and severity of radiation mucositis in patients with head and neck cancer. International Journal of Radiation, Oncology Biology and Physics 37(5):1005–1010

Kennedy L, Diamond J 1997 Assessment and management of chemotherapy induced mucositis in children. Journal of Paediatric Oncology Nursing 14(1):164–174

Kenny S A 1990 Effect of two oral protocols on the incidence of stomatitis in hematology patient. Cancer Nursing 15(3):345–353

Knox J J, Puodziunas A L, Feld R 2000 Chemotherapy induced oral mucositis, prevention and management. Drugs and Aging 17(4):257–267

Krishnasamy M 1995 Oral problems in advanced cancer. European Journal of Cancer Care 4(4):173–177

Lippold A J C, Winton F R 1972 Hearing and speech. Human physiology. Churchill Livingstone, Edinburgh, pp 443–464

Little J 1996 Head and neck cancer: oral care during radiotherapy. Nursing Standard 10(22):39–42

Loprinzi C L, Cianflone S G, Dose A M et al 1990 A controlled evaluation of allopurinol mouthwash as prophylaxis against 5-fluorouracil induced stomatitis. Cancer 65:1879–1882

Madeya M 1996 Oral complications from cancer therapy: part 1 – physiology and secondary complications. Oncology Nursing Forum 23(5):801–807

Martini F 1992 Fundamentals of anatomy and physiology, 2nd edn. Prentice Hall, New Jersey

Meloni G, Capria S, Proia A, Trosolini S M, Mandelli F 1996 Ice pops to prevent melphalan induced stomatitis. Lancet 347:1691–1692

McGuire D 2003 Barriers and strategies in implementation of oral care standards for cancer patients. Supportive Care in Cancer 11:435–441

Miller M, Kearney N 2001 Oral care for patients with cancer: a review of literature. Cancer Nursing 24(4):241–254

Milligan S, McGill M, Sweeney M P, Malarkey C 2001 Oral care for people with advanced cancer: an evidence based protocol. International Journal of Palliative Care 7(9):418–426

Nakamura K, Natsugoe S, Kumanohoso T et al 1996 Prophylactic action of allopurinol against chemotherapy-induced stomatitis-inhibition of superoxide dismutase and proteases. Anticancer Drugs 7:235–239

National Institute for Clinical Excellence 2003 Improving outcomes in haematological cancers. NICE, London

Ohrn K E O, Wahlin Y B, Sjoden P O 2000 Oral care in cancer nursing. European Journal of Cancer Care 9:22–29

Pearson L S 1996 A comparison of the ability of foam swabs to remove dental plaque: implications for nursing practice. Journal of Advanced Nursing 23: 62–69

Porter H 1992 Oral care for bone marrow transplant patients. Nursing Standard 7(6):54–55

Porter H J 1994 Mouth care in cancer. Nursing Times 90(14):27–29

Raber-Durlacher J 1999 Current practices for management of oral mucositis in cancer patients. Supportive Care in Cancer 7:71–74

Rawlins C A, Trueman I W 2001 Effective mouth care for seriously ill patients. Professional Nurse 16(14): 1025–1028

Raybould T P, Carpenter A D, Ferretti G A, Brown A T, Lillich T T, Henslee J 1994 Emergence of Gram-negative bacilli in the mouths of bone marrow transplant recipients using chlorhexidine mouthrinse. Oncology Nursing Forum 21(4):691–695

Roberts J 2000 Developing an oral assessment and intervention tool for older people, part 2. Evidence based practice in relation to oral care agents and interventions. British Journal of Nursing 9(18): 2033–2240

Rovirosa A, Ferre J, Biete A 1998 Granulocyte macrophage-colony stimulating factor mouthwashes heal oral ulcers during head and neck radiotherapy. International Journal of Radiation, Oncology Biology and Physics 41(4):747–754

Rubenstein E B, Peterson D E, Schuber M et al 2004 Clinical practice guidelines for the prevention and treatment of cancer therapy-induced oral and gastrointestinal mucositis. Cancer 100(9 Suppl): 2026–2046

Saral R 1990 Management of acute viral infections. In: National Cancer Monographs No. 9. Consensus development conference on oral complications of cancer therapies: diagnosis, prevention and treatment. National Cancer Institute, Bethesda, pp 135–143

Schubert M M, Sullivan K M 1990 Recognition, incidence and management of oral graft versus host disease. In: National Cancer Institute Monographs No. 9. Consensus development of conference on oral complications of cancer therapies: diagnosis, prevention and treatment. National Cancer Institute, Bethesda, pp 135–143

Shih A, Miaskowski C, Dodd M, Stotts N, Macphail L 2003 Mechanisms for radiation-induced oral mucositis and the consequences. Cancer Nursing 26(3): 222–229

Singal S, Mehta J, Rattenbury H, Trealeaven J, Powles R 1995 Oral pilocarpine hydrochloride for the treatment of refractory xerostomia associated with chronic graft versus host disease. Blood 85:1147–1148

Sonis S T, Elting L S, Keefe D et al 2004 Perspectives on cancer therapy-induced mucosal injury: pathogenesis, measurement, epidemiology and consequences for patients. Cancer 100(9 Suppl):1995–2025

Sweeney M P 1998 Mouth care in nursing. Part 3: Oral care for the independent patient. Journal of Nursing Care Autumn: 7–9. Cited in: Milligan S, McGill M, Sweeney P, Malarkey C 2001 Oral care for people with advanced

cancer: an evidence-based protocol. Journal of Palliative Nursing 7(9):418–426

Ventafridda V, Ripamonti C, Sbanotto A, DeConno F 1993 Mouth care. In: Doyle D, Hanks G W C, McDonald N (eds) Oxford textbook of palliative medicine. Oxford Medical Publications, Oxford, pp 434–445

Wardley A M, Jayson G C, Swindell R et al 2000. Prospective evaluation of oral mucositis in patients receiving myeloablative conditioning regimens and haemopoietic progenitor rescue. British Journal of Haematology 110:292–299

Wolfgang J, Hejna M, Wenzel C, Zielinski C 2001 Oral mucositis complicating chemotherapy and/or radiotherapy: options for treatment. A Cancer Journal for Clinicians 51(5):290–315

Wood A 2004 Mouth care and ritualistic practice. Cancer Nursing Practice 3(4):34–39

Worthington H V, Clarkson J E, Eden O B 2001 Interventions for preventing oral candidiasis for patients with cancer receiving treatment. Cochrane Library, Issue 1, 2003

Wray D, Bragg J 1997 Pocket reference to oral candidosis. Science Press, London

Xavier G 2000 The importance of mouth care in preventing infection. Nursing Standard 14(18):47–51

Further reading

Borbasi S, Cameron K, Quested B, Olver I, Evans D 2002 More than a sore mouth: patients' experience of oral mucositis. Oncology Nursing Forum 29(7):1051–1057
An interesting article which explores patients' experiences of chemotherapy-induced oral mucositis

Buschel P C, Whedon M B 1995 Bone marrow transplantation. Administrative and clinical strategies. Jones and Bartlett, Boston
This text includes a comprehensive chapter relating to oral complications during bone marrow transplantation and gives advice on appropriate therapeutic intervention and assessment.

Coleman S 1995 An overview of oral complications of adult patients with malignant haematological conditions who have undergone radiotherapy or chemotherapy. Journal of Advanced Nursing 22(6):1085–1091

This article gives a comprehensive overview of complications of patients with haematological malignancies and relates the theory practice gap and therefore implications for practice.

Griffiths J, Boyle S 1993 Colour guide to holistic care: a practical approach. Mosby-Year Book Europe, London
An opportunity to see visual representations of oral complications.

Kwong K F 2004 Prevention and treatment of oropharyngeal mucositis following cancer therapy. Cancer Nursing 27(3):183–205
This article reviews the current research studies on the prevention and treatment of oropharyngeal mucositis following chemotherapy, radiotherapy, and bone marrow transplantation.

Chapter **19**

Nutritional issues

Ulu Mehmet

KEY POINTS

- Malnutrition is the most common secondary diagnosis in patients with cancer.
- Malnutrition is associated with a poor response to cancer therapy and reduced quality of life.
- Early nutritional intervention can help to optimise nutritional status.
- Adhering to food hygiene principles reduces the risk of food-borne infection.

INTRODUCTION

Malnutrition in cancer patients results from multifactorial events and is associated with an alteration of quality of life (Nitenberg & Raynaud 2000). It is the most common secondary diagnosis in patients with cancer and is a major prognostic indicator for poor response to cancer therapy and shortened survival (Wilson 2000). A variety of factors suggest that individuals with haematological cancers may be at increased risk of developing malnutrition. Maintaining or improving nutritional status is therefore vitally important. Early nutritional intervention can help to optimise nutritional status during the stress imposed by the disease and its treatment. This chapter discusses nutritional requirements and the importance of nutritional assessment and management.

FACTORS CONTRIBUTING TO MALNUTRITION

Numerous factors have been implicated in the development of malnutrition – their interrelationships are complex and unclear. Metabolic changes, reduced food intake, malabsorption, disease and treatment-related effects all impact on nutritional status.

EFFECTS OF DISEASE

Haematological cancers often produce symptoms that affect appetite, and the ability to prepare and eat food. Individuals with leukaemia may suffer from symptoms such as bleeding gums, and recurrent infection, severe fatigue and lethargy. In lymphoma, lymphadenopathy of the neck may affect chewing and swallowing; mesenteric lymphadenopathy may affect stomach capacity and satiety. In myeloma, nausea and vomiting may be a problem due to hypercalcaemia. Individuals also have further nutritional challenges to face from their treatment.

EFFECTS OF TREATMENT

Chemotherapy can cause a multitude of gastrointestinal (GI) symptoms including stomatitis, mucositis, nausea, vomiting, diarrhoea, constipation and infection. Decreased or viscous saliva and taste changes may also occur (see Chapter 9). GI pain can often occur as a result of treatment, e.g. vincristine is associated with severe constipation, bowel spasm and in extreme cases, paralytic ileus. Mucositis can also lead to GI pain.

Radiotherapy can lead to decreased saliva production, mucositis, stomatitis and enteritis, with malabsorption of nutrients (see Chapter 10). Other drugs such as antibiotics, antiviral and antifungal agents and some analgesics can also adversely affect nutritional status as they may cause nausea, vomiting and diarrhoea.

The high dose and combined therapies frequently given in haemato-oncology cause many side effects that affect food intake and may contribute to the development of malnutrition. Maintaining nutritional status is key to promoting positive outcomes from aggressive cancer therapies as a well-nourished patient is more likely to be able to withstand the effects of treatment.

METABOLIC CHANGES

An increased basal metabolic rate (BMR) has been suggested as one possible cause of malnutrition (Knox et al 1983). The disseminated nature of haematological cancers, frequent infections and associated pyrexia may be contributory factors to the increase in BMR. Whether metabolic changes are related to an alteration of the metabolism of the tumour or to a change in the metabolism of the host remains controversial. Differences in metabolism have also been found between different diseases, with individuals with leukaemia shown to be hypermetabolic and those with lymphoma hypometabolic (Humberstome & Shaw 1988).

Many individuals with haematological cancers experience reduced appetite – oral intake may be reduced at a time when metabolic needs are increased. The production of cytokines is thought to be the physiological mechanism behind appetite suppression and reduction in spontaneous food intake. Cytokines may contribute to anorexia and alter the way the liver metabolises proteins. Changes in metabolic pathways and metabolism driven by the proliferation of abnormal cells may also contribute to hypermetabolism.

ENERGY EXPENDITURE

In cancer patients generally, a heterogeneous picture of energy expenditure has been described with resting energy expenditure (REE) varying between less than 60% and more than 150% of that predicted (Barber et al 2000). However, it has been suggested that although resting energy expenditure is often increased, total energy expenditure may be unchanged due to an adaptive fall in physical activity (Barber et al 2000). The REE has also been observed to fall significantly as a result of the metabolic effect of chemotherapy on tumour metabolism. Chemotherapy and steroids have a specific effect of increasing energy expenditure in the host and this may account for some of the differences in REE (Delarue et al 1990). A variety of other factors also affect energy requirements, such as age, concurrent disease and temperature; it is therefore important to assess and monitor each patient individually.

Transplant

Energy expenditure may differ between autologous and allogeneic blood and marrow transplants (BMT) although consensus exists that energy requirements in BMT are 130–150% of predicted basal energy expenditure. Protein requirements are also elevated (Muscaritoli et al 2002).

When energy input is consistently less than energy output, through inadequate nutrient intake, ineffective use of nutrients or raised metabolic rate, the result is persistent erosion of body cell mass and muscle stores. The eventual changes in muscle function and strength result in decreased energy and strength (Wilson 2000). The risk of complications such as depression of the immune system also increases.

NUTRITIONAL REQUIREMENTS

Very few references regarding nutritional requirements specifically for patients with haematological cancers exist. However, a literature search revealed a 10–30% increase in energy requirements from basal metabolic rate for haemato-oncology patients (Lerebours et al 1988). Nutritional requirements are currently calculated for patients using the Schofield equation (Schofield 1985) and Elia Normogram (Elia 1990). These calculations are in the process of being updated by the Parenteral and Enteral Nutrition (PEN) group. In determining these calculations the age, sex and weight of the patient, disease state, activity and pyrexia are considered. As their use is somewhat open to interpretation, users require training. If time is limited, a quick simple guide for estimating calorie requirements is to calculate 25–35 kcal/kg body weight per day. Nutritional assessment is used to quantify nutritional status and to determine whether an individual is meeting their nutritional requirements.

NUTRITIONAL ASSESSMENT

Nutritional assessment aims to:

- assess current nutritional status and obtain information regarding adequacy of intake
- identify individuals who require nutritional support
- evaluate, by serial measurements, the efficacy of nutritional support.

Various nutritional assessment techniques are available but may be subject to factors that affect their accuracy.

Weight is affected by changes in fluid balance. Patients may appear to gain or lose several kilograms of weight in a few days due to the large volumes of fluids infused and problems with fluid retention. This is a particular problem in BMT patients. Fluid retention may also be exacerbated by hypoalbuminaemia. Patients who are not eating adequately often appear to *gain* weight. It is important that the patient is weighed at every admission as this should be a 'dry' weight and can be used as a comparison with successive weights taken weekly during all inpatient stays. Weights should be recorded when the patient attends for clinic or day unit appointments.

Weight loss – an unintentional weight loss of >10% of body weight in the previous 3–6 months suggests development of undernutrition, irrespective of the patient's current weight (Garrow et al 2000). This is particularly important for overweight individuals who although losing >10% of their body weight remain overweight and therefore may not be perceived as malnourished. For these individuals undergoing a stressful episode, e.g. chemotherapy, energy and protein requirements for maintaining body weight should be provided rather than basing requirements on ideal body weight.

Body mass index (BMI) has an important predictive value in terms of morbidity and mortality in those classified as underweight or obese (de Onis & Habicht 1996). BMI is calculated using the following equation:

$$BMI = \frac{weight\,(kg)}{height\,(m^2)}$$

BMI is interpreted as:

- <16: severely underweight
- 16–19: underweight
- 20–25: normal range
- 26–30: overweight
- 31–40: obese
- >40: morbidly obese.

These levels are, however, somewhat arbitrary and based on data derived from young healthy adults. BMI needs to be used with caution for patients who have a distorted fluid balance. Enforced immobility results in reduction of muscle mass, with subsequent weight loss, affecting BMI values. Furthermore, the use of height for BMI calculation fails to take into account loss of height with increasing age, or due to damage to the spine from osteoporosis or myeloma (Thomas 2001).

Biochemistry – several biochemical indicators can be used to assess nutritional status. These are, however, affected by treatment and disease. Albumin is a serum protein frequently used to assess nutritional status. However, it is a poor indicator of nutritional status with a long half-life of 21 days, providing a picture of nutritional status from 3 weeks previously. It is slow to show signs of depletion and repletion, even with appropriate levels of nutritional support. As with any serum protein, albumin levels are influenced by hydration status and various disease processes such as hepatic and renal failure. Albumin levels should be interpreted in association with C-reactive protein (CRP) levels (an acute phase protein increased in infection and disease). Raised CRP levels and low albumin levels are likely to indicate immune response to disease or infection, whereas hypoalbuminaemia with normal or low CRP indicates malnutrition. Albumin levels below the normal range may be indicative of longstanding inadequate intake (Gosling 1995).

Transferrin (and other short half-life proteins such as retinol binding protein (RBP) and thyroxine binding prealbumin (TBPA), haemoglobin and total lymphocyte count are all affected by treatment and disease. These are not therefore, reliable indicators of nutritional status in haemato-oncology patients.

Nitrogen balance studies provide one of the most valuable methods of determining whether the anabolic state has been achieved in response to nutritional support. Nitrogen is a component of the protein molecule and so this measurement gives an indication of protein status. Nitrogen (protein) intake is measured using dietary assessment. Nitrogen output is derived from the quantity found in the urine. It is usual to carry out estimates of nitrogen balance studies over three consecutive days, necessitating 3×24-hour urine collections (Taylor & Goodinson-McLaren 1992).

Skin-fold thickness measurements (SFT) involve pinching a fold of skin with a pair of skin-fold callipers. This gives an indication of total body fat. The most accurate estimates require measurements at a number of sites. These data can be used to evaluate body composition in patients with ascites and peripheral oedema who cannot be weighed. However, it takes time and practice to acquire a measurement technique that gives reproducible recordings. Measurements may differ substantially from those made on the same patient by different observers (Thomas 2001).

Mid-arm circumference (MAC) is a measurement of the circumference of the non-dominant arm midway between the shoulder and the elbow. This can be used as a simple determinant of muscle mass. MAC may be a better option than SFT as this involves only a measurement using a tape measure.

Mid-arm muscle circumference (MAMC) is an estimate of skeletal muscle mass derived from using a combination of the values obtained from skin-fold thickness and mid-arm circumference.

Biochemical impedance analysis (BIA) is based on the principle that lean tissue, with its high water and electrolyte content, is highly conductive to electrical current whereas fat tissue is more resistant. By measuring the change in voltage when a small current is passed through electrodes placed on specific parts of the body, a measure of total body water can be made. From this, estimates for body fat and lean tissue can be calculated. In practice these readings are affected by oedema, which is often present in haemato-oncology patients. Readings are taken from a meter with a digital readout, therefore skills of the operator are not as crucial compared with taking skin-fold thickness measurements.

Grip strength (hand dynamometry) measurements can be a useful indicator of muscle function – values below 85% of normal may indicate malnutrition. Readings are not affected by operator skill or fluid retention. Digital displays make readings easier to obtain.

Food charts are only as accurate as the information provided by the person filling them in. Lack of time or other priorities may mean that information provided is inaccurate or incomplete. Rough ideas of portion sizes eaten are very useful, e.g. a block of cheese the size of a matchbox. Information may be more accurate if the patient or a relative completes the food chart as they have more time to do this. If the patient is not confused and is well enough, a 24-hour dietary history may be taken. This consists of asking the patient to recall everything they have eaten the day before and documenting the information in as much detail as possible. Food charts or dietary histories provide information that can be used to assess calorie and protein intake.

In practice, a more accurate picture may be obtained by using a combination of some of the techniques described above. The simplest data to obtain are those of weight, height, and food intake. Serial measurements of weight, calorie intake and data obtained using the techniques described all help to determine whether nutritional goals are being met and the effectiveness of nutritional intervention.

NUTRITIONAL SCREENING TOOLS

In recent years various nutritional screening tools (NSTs) have been developed to help to assess an individual's risk of developing malnutrition. A scoring or grading system is applied to a number of indicators of nutritional status, such as changes in body weight, appetite, and dietary intake (Thomas 2001).

One difficulty with NSTs is that those that identify the nutritional risk with the greatest degree of accuracy tend to be the most complex to use. Furthermore, tools designed in the past were often only suitable for one care setting, e.g. hospital, community, or residential care. To ensure accurate results, tools need to have been tested for reliability and validity in the setting in which they are to be used. Screening tools must be valid and reliable. In practice, tools/techniques that are quick and easy to use are more likely to be accepted.

Much of the information required to assess the risk of malnutrition can be derived from asking four simple questions (Lennard-Jones et al 1995):

- Have you unintentionally lost weight recently?
- Have you been eating less than usual?
- What is your normal weight?
- What is your height?

Once the degree of nutritional risk has been determined it is necessary to establish any barriers to eating and initiate interventions to maximise intake.

REFLECTION POINT

Consider the following questions in relation to your own practice:

- Is everyone weighed on admission and at regular intervals during their hospital stay?
- Where is weight recorded?
- Are weight changes communicated to all members of the multidisciplinary team?
- Is a nutritional assessment screening tool used in your area?
- How often is assessment undertaken?
- Are you always aware of the amount and types of foods your patients are eating?
- When should nutritional assessment take place?

After reviewing the above points you may want to discuss this issue in more detail with your colleagues in order to determine an appropriate assessment schedule for your area.

MAXIMISING INTAKE

It is important to establish why individuals are not eating. Barriers to eating include:

- poorly controlled side effects of disease and treatment
- not liking the food on the main hospital menu
- individual dietary preferences, e.g. a vegetarian diet or religious food practices
- food texture may be a problem for individuals with a sore mouth or swallowing difficulties
- anxiety
- inability to sleep
- interruptions at meal times, e.g. drug rounds/ward rounds
- fasting for investigations.

Once the main barriers to eating have been established interventions can be initiated to improve intake. Interventions include:

- liaising with dietitian, catering staff
- examining practical issues that can be changed easily
- refer to other professionals if appropriate, e.g. occupational therapy (OT) for assessment for feeding aids
- liaising with other members of the multidisciplinary team to ensure good symptom control
- good oral hygiene to prevent infection (see Chapter 18)
- monitoring mucositis closely, especially during high-dose therapy
- early introduction of supplements/artificial nutritional support before weight loss occurs
- counselling – may help with emotional issues.

The individual's home situation should also be considered, especially if they live alone. Advice about the use of convenience foods and ensuring a good supply of store cupboard items may help to improve intake. Foods offered to the patient should be as energy-dense as tolerated. If possible, supplementation of foods will add to calorie intake. Specific interventions addressing the most common factors affecting food intake are summarised in Table 19.1.

When efforts to maximise food intake in this way have been exhausted and energy/protein intake is still inadequate for requirements, use of proprietary products may be necessary. Supplement drinks are available as milkshakes (ready to drink or powdered ones that are made up with fresh milk), fruit-juice style or glucose drinks. These are often very sweet so tolerance may be increased by chilling/freezing or diluting these drinks. They may also have an after-taste due to the mineral and vitamin content or due to the UHT (ultra heat treated) process. Supplements made up with fresh milk and ice cream may be better tolerated and also soothing if the mouth is sore. Other options include:

- pudding supplements – soft, with a high calorie/protein density; useful if the patient has difficulty swallowing solids or a sore mouth

Table 19.1
Nutritional interventions

Factors affecting food intake	Interventions
Anorexia and early satiety	– Offer small, frequent meals, e.g. 2-hourly – Offer food when the individual feels most hungry, e.g. at breakfast – Present meals attractively – Provide snack foods and supplements which are high in calories but low in quantity and which are attractively presented – Alcohol before meals may stimulate appetite (check first for drug interactions) – If possible encourage the patient to go into the fresh air for a walk – Increase calorific value of foods by adding milk, cream, butter, ice cream, sauces, mayonnaise, sugar or glucose to soups, cereals, puddings and drinks – Avoid drinks close to meal times, especially carbonated ones
Nausea and vomiting	– If cooking smells put the patient off eating, keep them away from the kitchen while a meal is being prepared – Offer cold meals or food from the freezer that only needs heating up – Avoid greasy, fatty fried foods – Suggest some dry food such as toast/crackers first thing in the morning – Avoid tight clothing – Taking a short walk before meals may help – Encourage eating and drinking slowly, and relaxing after meals – Avoid drinking at mealtimes, take drinks 1 hour after eating a meal
Taste changes	*If meat tastes unpleasant* – If the patient finds meat tastes strange or unpleasant, encourage chicken, fish, milk, eggs, cheese, beans or nuts. These foods also contain protein. Cold meat may taste more palatable. *If sweet foods seem too sweet* – Encourage more savoury foods instead – Choose unsweetened fruit juices and tinned fruit in natural juice. Keep supplements/milkshakes in the fridge and offer cold. – Add lemon juice to foods that taste sickly sweet *If foods have less flavour* – Use herbs in cooking – Add flavours to vegetables, e.g. small pieces of bacon, ham, onion or lemon juice – Use pickles or chutneys – Try marinating meat, poultry or fish before cooking, e.g. in wine, cider or fruit juice – Add condensed soups or sauce mixes to mince and casseroles *If a bitter or metallic taste is present* – Avoid foods and drinks containing saccharin (an artificial sweetener) – Try lemon juice in water as a mouthwash before meals – Sharp-tasting foods like fresh fruit, fruit juices and bitter boiled sweets are refreshing and leave a pleasant taste in the mouth – If the tongue is 'coated' it may make food taste unpleasant and might discourage eating. The tongue can be cleaned with a bicarbonate of soda solution – 1 teaspoon of bicarbonate in a pint of warm water. Use cotton wool dipped in this solution. *Care should be taken that the patient's oral intake is not deficient, e.g. all the protein foods are being avoided.*

table continues

Table 19.1
Nutritional interventions – Cont'd

Factors affecting food intake	Interventions
Sore mouth	– Avoid rough-textured foods such as toast or raw vegetables, which can be abrasive to the lining of the mouth – Encourage soft/moist foods; add plenty of sauces and gravy, milk, yoghurt, evaporated milk or cream to dishes – Avoid spicy hot or very dry foods; ice creams and cold puddings are soothing – Smooth, sieved textures may be easier to manage – Avoid very salty or spicy foods, e.g. curry, chilli or nutmeg – Dentures may be left out temporarily – Ensure good oral hygiene measures (see Chapter 18)
Dry mouth/sore throat	– As above, choose foods with plenty of sauces or gravy – Drink plenty of fluids, especially cold or fizzy drinks. Using a straw may help. Sip regularly. – Suck ice-cubes, ice-lollies, boiled sweets, i.e. fruit/acid drops – Fruit juices and squash may be frozen into cubes – Try drinks such as weak lemon tea or herbal teas – Artificial saliva sprays or pastilles may help – Ensure good oral hygiene measures (see Chapter 18)
Difficulty swallowing	– Soft/pureed foods may be easier to swallow, eat little and often, fortify food, e.g. add grated cheese to soup, supplement drinks/foods
Diarrhoea	– Try small frequent meals – Drink plenty of fluids. Avoid strong teas, coffee and alcohol.
Constipation	– Choose foods high in fibre, such as wholemeal bread, wholegrain cereals, fruit and vegetables, wholewheat crackers, digestive biscuits, brown rice and pasta, beans and pulses – Drink plenty of fluids – at least 8 cups daily – Take some light exercise daily, e.g. daily walk

- soup supplements – higher calorie/protein/vitamin and mineral content than ordinary soup
- powders – glucose polymers or protein powders may be added to soups, puddings and cereals to improve nutrient density.

FOOD SAFETY

The immunosuppression inevitably experienced by individuals with haematological cancers makes food hygiene and an awareness of foods that are high risk for food poisoning a high priority. Dietary restrictions with varying degrees of severity have been advocated for individuals with neutropenia. The purpose of these food restrictions is to:

- reduce exposure to classic food and water-borne pathogens, e.g. Salmonella and Listeria
- reduce exposure to opportunistic pathogens, e.g. aerobic Gram-negative bacteria.

Food restrictions include decreasing exposure to Gram-negative bacilli such as *E. coli*, as Gram-negative sepsis remains an important cause of morbidity/mortality in neutropenic patients. Some foods (salads, raw vegetables, fruit) are particularly associated with Gram-negative bacteria (e.g. Klebsiella and Pseudomonas). Patients, carers and health-care professionals require education about food hygiene, preparation and storage and avoiding 'high risk' foods, e.g. unpasteurised milk/diary products (particularly unpasteurised or blue-veined cheese), pâté, raw and soft boiled eggs, undercooked meat (particularly poultry), cook-chill foods and takeaway/restaurant food. Staff involved in food preparation should have a food hygiene certificate.

Great variation appears to exist throughout the UK regarding food safety restrictions for neutropenic patients. One audit of nutritional advice to BMT patients in the UK (Bibbington et al 1993) revealed that there was a wide variation in practice and although sterile diets (previously advocated for transplant recipients) were rarely used, low microbial diets were common. One quarter of BMT units used microbiological screening of food but there were no standards and little data available. Little appears to have changed in the last decade as more recently Smith & Besser (2000) carried out a survey of cancer centres in the UK and found that food restrictions and the definitions used for neutropenia were extremely variable.

Evidence supporting the effectiveness of food restrictions is, however, still required (Moody et al 2002). It is therefore beneficial to the patient to impose minimum restrictions, as they may be detrimental to food intake and result in:

- poor nutritional intake
- wastage/cost, i.e. individually packaged items
- negative psychological and social impact on the patient and family
- unnecessary anxiety and confusion.

Ideally the hospital catering department should provide meals for all patients. Family and friends should be discouraged from bringing cooked meals or chilled/frozen meals into hospital. However, if they wish to bring in extra food, it should be discussed with the dietitian/nurse in charge. Suitable items include long-life tinned and packet items, chocolate, biscuits, cake and fruit. Chilled items such as yoghurts should be transported in a cool bag, dated and kept in the fridge. There is a lack of clear evidence concerning the safety of yoghurt. Most yoghurt sold in the UK is 'live', in that it still contains some of the original culture. Consensus opinion from microbiologists, is that ordinary yoghurts are safer for haematology patients, but 'bio' or 'live' yoghurts, which contain an inoculation of pro-biotic bacteria, should be avoided, as the effect on an immunocompromised individual is not known (Hastings 2003).

Most importantly the principles of food hygiene should be adhered to. Ordinary ward food with minimum modifications, e.g. no salads, raw vegetables or other high-risk foods, should be offered to patients. Local policies regarding food and the neutropenic patient should be consulted.

Water safety

No clear guidelines exist for water. It is important to remember that the bacterial content of bottled water is likely to be higher than that of tap water. For this reason, bottled water should be treated as perishable food and once opened used as quickly as possible. Ice and ice-making machines may be subject to contamination, therefore manufacturers' guidelines should be followed.

Supplement drinks

Supplement drinks should be consumed within 4 hours of opening. Cartons should be date and time marked when opened.

If, despite all efforts, strategies to increase oral intake fail to maintain nutritional status, then artificial nutritional support may be required. Patients should be assessed for feeding if they have a low BMI (19 or less) or if they have lost 10% body weight, either since admission, or in the last 3 months.

ARTIFICIAL NUTRITIONAL SUPPORT

ENTERAL FEEDING

It is well accepted that if the gut is functioning nutritional support should be given via the enteral route. Feeding enterally aids maintenance of the structure and function of the gut. Direct nourishment of enterocytes helps to keep the junctions between cells from leaking and thereby prevents passage of pathogens from the gut into the blood stream. Enteral nutrition represents less of an infection risk than parenteral feeding and is also more cost-effective (Bird 2002).

Results from a randomised trial of parenteral versus enteral nutrition in allogenic BMT found a reduction in both pyrexia and hospital stay for those who were enterally fed (Young et al 1998). Furthermore, an audit of nutritional support in one bone marrow transplant unit in the UK demonstrated that it is possible to maintain nutritional requirements by enteral nutrition in 50% of the patients undergoing allogenic transplant (Todd et al 1999). However, a Cochrane review of nutritional support for BMT patients concluded that there was a lack of evaluable data to compare the effectiveness of enteral to parenteral nutrition (Murray & Pindoria 2002). Therefore choice of route is likely to be determined by the clinical team and individual patient characteristics.

Enteral feeding is not suitable for all patients. Factors to consider prior to initiating this method of feeding are:

- patient consent to tube insertion
- nausea and vomiting
- mucositis (it may be possible to predict this, i.e. when planning high-dose chemotherapy or specific agents that are high risk for endothelial cell damage)
- GI ulceration
- oral/throat pain or bleeding
- low platelet count
- malabsorption/diarrhoea
- gut function.

Patients are often reticent, anxious or completely object to having a feeding tube. Speaking to fellow patients or a clinical team member about their personal experiences of receiving enteral feeding and demonstrating a sample feeding tube can sometimes help. Emphasising the benefits of enteral feeding in maintaining nutrition and reducing the number of days in hospital may also be persuasive. Discussion of these issues in the earlier stages of treatment may be of benefit as patients are prepared long before enteral feeding becomes necessary and have time to think about the advantages and disadvantages. However, this has to be balanced with the enormous amount of information patients have to absorb in the early stages of their disease and treatment.

The timing of the insertion of a tube for the patient at risk of developing severe mucositis is important. Insertion should be considered after high-dose chemotherapy (and radiotherapy if part of the BMT regimen), i.e. the day after finishing conditioning chemotherapy or the day *after* transplant. Insertion on the actual day of transplant can be difficult as the preservative used for stem cells may cause nausea. The window of opportunity is therefore very small for a patient who may soon develop mucositis. The tube should remain in situ for as long as possible as it may not be possible to reinsert a tube if it is lost. Anti-emetic control should be reviewed prior to insertion.

Complications

Diarrhoea is often associated with feed administration, but there are often other causes or contributory factors, e.g. graft-versus-host disease (GvHD) can produce stools of a distinctive appearance (see Chapter 13), damage to the gut from chemo/radiotherapy, viral/bacterial infection, or a malabsorptive state such as ulcerative colitis. In tube-fed patients, evidence suggests that the most common cause of diarrhoea is antibiotic therapy (Keohane et al 1984). Diarrhoea caused by antibiotics can last for up to 2 weeks after the cessation of the antibiotics. The most likely mechanism is an alteration of the normal intestinal flora leading to superinfection with other, resistant organisms.

It is important to establish the appearance and volume of the diarrhoea as this may have a bearing on treatment. Volume may be difficult to collect/assess if the patient is incontinent or if diarrhoea becomes mixed with urine. At volumes over and above 500 ml in 24 hours, the effectiveness of enteral nutrition starts to decrease as absorption of nutrients from the gut is reduced.

Treatment of diarrhoea

Dietary fibre is known to have a modulatory effect on bowel function. Gut bacteria cause fermentation of fibre, leading to the production of short chain fatty acids (SCFA). SCFAs are used as an energy substrate by enterocytes, and act as a stimulus for colonic water and electrolyte absorption. Fibre-free feeds may result in impaired SCFA production so as to hinder colonic water and electrolyte absorption (Silk 1993). A trial of this type of feed may be carried out if the standard feed seems to be associated with diarrhoea.

Use of anti-diarrhoeal agents may be possible if stool samples are negative for infection. If diarrhoea is not well controlled and increasing in volume, it may be necessary to consider parenteral feeding in order to maintain nutritional status.

A lack of enteral intake for as little as 72 hours can result in gut atrophy and subsequent diarrhoea on refeeding. A minimal enteral intake equivalent to 10–15 ml/hour can prevent gut atrophy and this may be accomplished even in patients receiving parenteral nutrition. An elemental or semi-elemental feed may be indicated but the osmolarity of such feeds requires gradual introduction. Concentration and volume should be slowly increased over a few days (Weekes 1996).

Case study 19.1

Steve, a 21-year-old student recently diagnosed with acute lymphoblastic leukaemia, had lost one stone (6.35 kg) in weight in the 4 weeks prior to diagnosis. Both Steve and his parents were concerned about his weight loss. His parents tried to tempt him with his favourite foods, but Steve had no appetite. He was seen by the dietitian, who offered him alternatives to the hospital menu. She suggested that he try to eat small high-calorie snacks and asked him to trial some supplement drinks. His energy intake from the food chart was assessed and his nutritional requirements calculated. This information was explained to Steve.

Steve made a great effort to eat but the chemotherapy caused nausea, early satiety and a metallic taste – all of which was compounded by a dry mouth. As his weight was continuing to decrease, he was assessed for artificial nutritional support. It was possible to control his nausea using effective anti-emetics and a nasogastric tube was passed. Feeding initially supplied all of Steve's requirements, but as he began to be able to take food and supplements again, the feed administration was changed to overnight. When Steve was able to maintain his intake orally, the nasogastric tube was removed.

PARENTERAL FEEDING

In the past, problems with nausea, vomiting, mucositis and diarrhoea have led to the use of parenteral nutrition (PN) as first-line nutritional support. Although sometimes there may be no alternative, use of PN should be limited to essential cases only owing to the risks it represents to the patient. If the benefits outweigh the risks, it should be administered for at least 5 days. Approximately 5 days are needed for the hepatic enzyme systems that metabolise intravenous nutrients to become established. It is therefore wasteful to administer PN for less time than this (Taylor & Goodinson-McLaren 1992).

In order to make valid judgements and informed decisions about instigating PN it is beneficial to seek the advice of expert multidisciplinary team members or a clinical nutrition support team (clinician, biochemist, specialist nurse, dietitian and pharmacist) if one is available. These experts can provide assessment and advice on issues such as access, infection control and appropriate regimens.

Disadvantages of parenteral nutrition

As PN bypasses the gut, the cells of the gut are not stimulated to function, leading to gut atrophy. Further malabsorption may be caused as a result of gut endothelial cells with poor structure and function. Patients should be encouraged to continue some oral intake to help to maintain the structure and function of the gut.

PN is also an infection risk to an already immunocompromised patient. Existing infections could be exacerbated by the use of PN as it provides an energy substrate that can be utilised by bacteria. PN is also thought to have a negative effect on immunity (Pomposelli & Bistrian 1994). Most haemato-oncology patients have long-term, central venous catheters and catheter-related sepsis is the most common complication of PN (Burnham 1999). Good aseptic technique and ideally use of a dedicated line for PN will reduce the risk of infection. Poor techniques in manipulating equipment increase the risk of contamination and the number of manipulations should be kept to a minimum (Bird 2002).

Peripherally-inserted central catheters (PICC) can also be used for PN for periods of 6–9 months. PICCs are associated with a lower rate of infection possibly due to the antecubital fossa being less subject to bacterial infection as it is not as oily or moist as the neck/chest area (Department of Health 2001).

PN results in an extra metabolic load for the liver, whose function is already compromised by the effects of chemotherapy and other drug treatment. Any features of abnormal liver function must be thoroughly investigated in the light of the patient's current diagnosis, the treatment planned and given. However, an elevation in serum liver enzymes, caused by the induction of enzymes for the metabolism of PN substrate, is commonly seen at the beginning of parenteral feeding (Taylor & Goodinson-McLaren 1992). PN may add to problems with fluid overload and there may not be enough time in 24 hours of line use to administer the volume needed. Fluid volume can, however, be reduced by adding electrolytes such as potassium to the PN rather than administering it separately or using reduced volume PN.

Blood glucose should be carefully monitored due to the risk of hyperglycaemia, which may be associated with immunosuppression. PN contains a large amount of glucose, which stimulates insulin production. It is therefore important to try to 'wean' PN down slowly as abrupt cessation may lead to rebound hypoglycaemia. Blood glucose should be monitored regularly, e.g. every 6 hours for the first 24 hours, then discontinued if levels remain within the normal range. If blood glucose levels are abnormal, monitoring should continue. It may be necessary to commence insulin depending on glucose levels.

CONCLUSION

The many factors that may contribute to the nutritional status of the haemato-oncology patient have been highlighted. It is important to identify patients at risk of malnutrition early as there is a better chance of improving and maintaining nutritional status. Careful screening, monitoring and early referral for dietetic assessment and intervention are essential.

DISCUSSION QUESTIONS

1. What are the limitations of using weight and albumin to assess nutritional status?

2. If a patient cannot be weighed, how would you assess their nutritional status?

3. How can you ensure a patient who is malnourished is identified early?

4. If a nutritional screening tool is to be adopted, what criteria are important to consider?

5. What are the advantages and disadvantages of using enteral versus parenteral nutrition for the haemato-oncology patient?

6. When would it be appropriate to use enteral or parenteral nutrition?

References

Barber M D, Ross J A, Fearon K C H 2000 Disordered metabolic response with cancer and its management. World Journal of Surgery 24:681–689

Bibbington A, Wilson P, Jones M et al 1993 Audit of nutritional advice given to bone marrow transplant patients in the UK. Clinical Nutrition 12:230–235

Bird M 2002 Infection control during parenteral nutrition. Complete Nutrition 2(4):12–14

Burnham P 1999 Parenteral nutrition. In: Dougherty L, Lamb J (eds) Intravenous therapy in nursing practice. Churchill Livingstone, Edinburgh, pp 333–356

De Onis M, Habicht J P 1996 Anthropometric reference data for international use: recommendations from a World Health Organization Expert Committee. American Journal of Clinical Nutrition 64:650–658

Delarue J, Lerebours E, Tilley H et al 1990 Effect of chemotherapy on resting energy expenditure in patients with non-Hodgkin's lymphoma. Cancer 65:2455–2459

Department of Health 2001 Guidelines for preventing infections associated with the insertion and maintenance of central venous catheters. Journal of Hospital Infection 47(Suppl):S47–S67

Elia M 1990 Artificial nutritional support. Medicine International 82:3392–3396

Garrow G S, James W P T, Ralph A 2000 Human nutrition and dietetic practice. Churchill Livingstone, Edinburgh

Gosling P 1995 Albumin and the critically ill. Care of the Critically Ill 2:57–61

Hastings M 2003 Diet and the immuncompromised (personal communication: Dr M Hastings, University Hospital of Wales, Cardiff)

Humberstome D A, Shaw J H F 1988 Metabolism in hematologic malignancy. Cancer 62:1619–1624

Keohane P P, Attrill H, Love M, Frost P, Silk D B A 1984 Relation between osmolarity of diet and gastrointestinal side effects of enteral nutrition. British Medical Journal 288:678–681

Knox L S, Crosby L O, Feurer I D, Buzby G P, Miller C L, Mullen J L 1983 Energy expenditure in malnourished cancer patients. Annals of Surgery 197:152–162

Lennard-Jones J E, Arrowsmith H, Davison C et al 1995 Screening by nurses and junior doctors to detect malnutrition when patients are first assessed in hospital. Clinical Nutrition 14:336–340

Lerebours E, Tilley H, Rimbert A, Delarue J, Piguet H, Colin R 1988 Changes in energy and protein status during chemotherapy in patients with acute leukaemia. Cancer 61:2412–2417

Moody K, Charlson M E, Finlay J 2002 The neutropenic diet: what's the evidence? Journal of Pediatric Hematology/Oncology 24(9):717–721

Murray S M, Pindoria S 2002 Nutrition support in bone marrow transplant patients. Cochrane Review, Issue 2. Cochrane Library, Oxford

Muscaritoli M, Grieco G, Capria S, Iori A, Fanelli F 2002 Nutritional and metabolic support in patients undergoing bone marrow transplantation. American Journal of Clinical Nutrition 75:183–190

Nitenberg G, Raynaud B 2000 Nutritional support of the cancer patient: issues and dilemmas. Critical Reviews in Oncology-Haematology 34(3):137–168

Pomposelli J J, Bistrian B R 1994 Is total parenteral nutrition immunosuppressive? New Horizons 2(2):224–229

Schofield W N 1985 Predicting basal metabolic rate: new standards and review of previous work. Human Clinical Nutrition 44:1–19

Silk D B A 1993 Fibre and enteral nutrition. Clinical Nutrition 12(Suppl 1):S106–S113

Smith L H, Besser S G 2000 Dietary restrictions for patients with neutropenia: a survey of institutional practices. Oncology Nursing Forum 27(3):515–530

Taylor S, Goodinson-McLaren S 1992 Nutritional support: a team approach. Wolfe Medical, London

Thomas B (in conjunction with the British Dietetic Association) 2001 Manual of dietetic practice. Blackwell Science, Oxford

Todd A, Dickinson P, Frost G S 1999 The effect of enteral nutrition in allogenic bone marrow transplant patients on length of hospital stay, pyrexia, diarrhoea, nausea and vomiting. Abstracts of original communications. BAPEN, London

Weekes E 1996 Diarrhoea – if it's not the feed causing it, then what? Penlines (BAPEN) 9:6–7

Wilson R L 2000 Optimizing nutritional support for patients with cancer. Clinical Journal of Oncology Nursing 4(1):23–28

Young M, Stanford J, Walker D, Frost G 1998 Preliminary report on the efficacy of nasogastric feeding in allogeneic adult bone marrow transplant patients. Proceedings of the Nutrition Society 57(3):92A

Further reading

The texts cited below give further detail regarding the topics mentioned in the chapter. The first two are books used by dietitians and detail how nutritional assessment and requirements are obtained.

Garrow G S, James W P T, Ralph A 2000 Human nutrition and dietetic practice. Churchill Livingstone, Edinburgh

Thomas B (ed) in conjunction with the British Dietetic Association 2001 Manual of dietetic practice. Blackwell Science, Oxford

The following supplements provide up-to-date nutritional standards for BMT, oncology and palliative care.

Dugeut A, Bachmann P, Lallemand Y, Blanc-Vincent M P 2003 Summary of the standards, options and recommendations for malnutrition and nutritional assessment in patients with cancer (1999). British Journal of Cancer 89(Suppl 1):S92–S97

Nitenberg G, Bachmann P, Schneider S et al 2003 Summary of the standards, options and recommendations for palliative or terminal nutrition in adults with progressive cancer (2001). British Journal of Cancer 89(Suppl 1):S107–S110

Raynard B, Nitenberg G, Gory-Delabaere G et al 2003 Summary of the standards, options and recommendations for nutritional support in patients undergoing bone marrow transplantation (2002). British Journal of Cancer 89(Suppl 1):S101–106

Chapter **20**

Fertility issues

Evelyn Dannie

KEY POINTS

- Gonadal failure and sexual impairment are side effects of both chemotherapy and radiotherapy.
- Both men and women are affected.
- A number of strategies are available for maintaining fertility post-treatment.
- Patients should be advised of appropriate strategies prior to commencing treatment.
- Advice should be given on contraception during treatment.

INTRODUCTION

The use of high-dose chemotherapy/radiotherapy in the treatment of haematological malignancies results in a number of serious side effects that can potentially interfere with any of the body's cellular, anatomical, physiological, behavioural, social and reproductive functions (Sherins 1993). Normal reproduction in both sexes requires a complex interplay between the gonads and the hypothalamic pituitary and endocrine axis; the uterus must also be receptive to implantation and capable of growth in pregnancy. Tissue in the reproductive system vulnerable to damage from chemo/radiotherapy and these treatments can not only lead to sexual dysfunction but may affect embryo implantation and cause an increase in pregnancy complications (Salooja et al 2004).

Gonadal failure and sexual impairment are late side effects of blood and marrow transplant (BMT) (Kolb et al 1989, Vose et al 1992). Such late effects are often of low priority at the time of treatment but are permanent and inevitable consequences of high-dose alkylating agents and/or total body radiation (TBI) (Sanders et al 1983, Dannie et al 1994). The low priority afforded this side effect may previously have been related to the high mortality and morbidity rates associated with transplant procedures. However, with survival curves now showing a gradual rise (Gratwohl et al 1993, Marks et al 1993) quality of life post-BMT has become increasingly important and fertility is a major concern for survivors and their partners.

Infertility is important not only because of its long-term physical, psychological and emotional consequences but also because the prospect of infertility has led some patients to refuse the treatment most likely to cure their disease or it has adversely influenced their decision to enter clinical trials. This chapter reviews the effects of chemotherapy/radiotherapy on gonadal function and discusses strategies for reducing these effects and maintaining fertility post-treatment. The role of hormone replacement therapy (HRT) and specific nursing issues are addressed.

EFFECTS OF RADIOTHERAPY AND CHEMOTHERAPY ON GONADAL FUNCTION

RADIOTHERAPY

Males

Damage to the testes caused by radiotherapy is well documented. Spermatogenesis can be affected by even small doses of radiotherapy, resulting in oligo-azoospermia approximately 50 days post-treatment and much earlier with larger doses. Recovery of spermatogenesis depends on the total dose administered and the mode of administration, such as a single total dose or several fractionated doses. High doses result in permanent sterility, although there is some considerable variation in susceptibility between individuals (Speiser et al 1972, Lushbaugh & Casarett 1976, Chatterjee et al 1994, Grigg et al 2000). In one study of 32 men with leukaemia treated with TBI prior to BMT, only two recovered spermatogenesis 6 years after transplant (Sanders et al 1983). In contrast, of 72 men with aplastic anaemia without TBI in their preparative transplant regimes, 65% had normal sperm counts and some had fathered children naturally (Sanders et al 1988).

Females

Premature ovarian failure occurs commonly following radiotherapy. Gonadal toxicity varies between individuals and sensitivity is related to the dose, type and duration of treatment, age and the development stage of the germ cell (Gradishar & Schilsky 1989, Salooja et al 2004). Advancing age and TBI appear to be correlated to ovarian failure. Single doses of radiation will often induce menstrual irregularities in women of all ages. However, less than 60% aged between 15 and 40 will be infertile, whereas in those aged 40 and over 100% will be infertile (Baker et al 1972). The main characteristics of ovarian failure are:

- ovarian fibrosis
- primordial follicle destruction
- elevated follicle-stimulating hormone (FSH) and luteinising hormone (LH) levels
- low oestradiol levels
- amenorrhoea
- menopausal symptoms, including:
  - oestrogen deficiencies
  - hot flushes
  - vaginal dryness
  - vaginitis
  - dyspareunia
  - decreased libido
  - vaginal epithelial atrophy
  - vaginal stenosis
  - sexual dysfunction.

CHEMOTHERAPY

Several chemotherapeutic agents profoundly influence male and female gonadal function, particularly the alkylating agents. Some of these agents are shown in Table 20.1.

Effects of chemotherapy on males

Alkylating agents are more likely to induce permanent infertility than other cytotoxic agents (Wang et al 1980) and both the mature and immature testes are at risk (Shalet et al 1981, Charak et al 1990). The testes are very sensitive to chemotherapy, with the germinal cells within the seminiferous tubules being directly affected. Testicular biopsies in patients treated by chemotherapy show aplasia of the germinal epithelium with normal Sertoli's and Leydig's cells, which is reflected in a reduced sperm count with normal testosterone levels (Fairley et al 1972, Chatterjee et al 1994). The characteristics of gonadal dysfunction in men and commonly reported problems are listed below:

- testicular germ cell aplasia
- reduced testicular volume
- atrophic seminiferous tubules
- oligospermia
- azoospermia
- elevated FSH and LH levels
- testosterone deficiencies

Table 20.1
Chemotherapeutic agents
associated with infertility

Drugs	
Male	**Female**
Definite infertility	
Chlorambucil	Cyclophosphamide
Cyclophosphamide	Nitrogen mustard
Nitrogen mustard	Busulphan
Busulphan	L-Phenylalanine
Procarbazine	
Nitrosoureas	
Probable infertility	
Imatinib (Glivec)	Imatinib (Glivec)
Doxorubicin	Etoposide
Vinblastine	
Cisplatin	
Cytosine arabinoside	
Etoposide	
Unlikely infertility	
Methotrexate	Methotrexate
5-Fluorouracil	5-Fluorouracil
6-Mercaptopurine	6-Mercaptopurine
Vincristine	
Fertility risk unknown	
Bleomycin	Doxorubicin
	Bleomycin
	Vinca alkaloids
	Nitrosoureas
	Cisplatin
	Cytosine arabinoside

Adapted from Gradishar & Schilsky 1989

- permanent sterility
- depressed libido
- sexual dysfunction
- erectile difficulties
- premature ejaculation.

Effects of chemotherapy on females

A great number of different chemotherapeutic agents have been associated with ovarian failure (see Table 20.1). In addition to alkylating agents such as busulphan and cyclophosphamide (Udall et al 1972), combination therapy used for Hodgkin's disease causes permanent infertility in 70% of patients, regardless of age (Chapman & Sutcliffe 1981). Drugs such as etoposide have also been reported to cause ovarian toxicity (Choo et al 1985, Meirow & Nugent 2001). More recently the introduction of novel drugs such as imatinib to treat patients with chronic myeloid leukaemia (CML) has added to the fertility dilemma (Marrin 2002). Little is known of its effects on fertility and pregnancy but animal studies have shown it to be teratogenic (Hensley & Ford 2003)

As with radiation, the process of follicular growth and maturation of oocytes are affected; ovarian fibrosis results, with follicular destruction. This is clinically manifested by menstrual irregularity and eventual amenorrhoea, with increased levels of FSH and LH and lowered levels of oestradiol, resulting in symptoms of the menopause and sexual dysfunction (Quigley & Hammond 1979, Byrne et al 1992, Larsen et al 2003). Additionally chemotherapy and radiotherapy cause damage to the uterine endometrium and the ability of the endometrium to proliferate in response to hormonal stimulation may be lost. This may affect both embryo implantation and the ability to carry a pregnancy to full term (Gonen et al 1989, Rio et al 1994, Apperley & Reddy 1995).

The most important risk factor for ovarian failure is age at treatment (Fig. 20.1). Recovery of gonadal function is often reported in younger women but sadly only the occasional pregnancy (Sanders et al 1996). However, it appears that women who recover gonadal function will suffer the menopause at an earlier age than women in the normal population (Horning et al 1981, Meirow & Nugent 2001).

RECOVERY OF GONADAL FUNCTION AFTER HIGH–DOSE CHEMOTHERAPY/RADIOTHERAPY

Severe gonadal damage can be identified immediately after high-dose chemotherapy/radiotherapy, although recovery can occur with time (Giri et al 1992). The chance of recovery is influenced by a number of issues, including:

- sex of the recipient
- age at BMT
- nature and doses of drugs and irradiation.

Figure 20.1
A model of ovarian failure and possible recovery following chemotherapy/radiotherapy

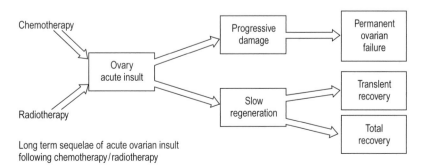

Long term sequelae of acute ovarian insult following chemotherapy/radiotherapy

Table 20.2
Factors affecting recovery of
gonadal function

Male	Female
Age	Pubertal status
Underlying disease	Age at diagnosis
Type of drugs used	Fertility status pre-treatment
Nature of the drug	Disease status
Total cumulative dose of chemotherapy	Nature, dose and duration of chemotherapeutic agents used at diagnosis
Duration of administration	Nature and dose of chemotherapeutic agent used in transplant conditioning
Site, dose, mode of administration and duration of radiotherapy	Dose, site and mode of administration of radiotherapy
	Type of transplant

After cyclophosphamide alone, 60–70% of male and female transplant patients had normal gonadotrophin levels 6 years post-BMT compared with only 20% of those whose conditioning regimens included TBI (Sanders et al 1983). However, it is important to note that normal gonadotrophin levels do not necessarily indicate a return of fertility (Chatterjee et al 1994).

Late recovery of spermatogenesis up to 14 years following treatment has been reported (Watson et al 1985). A number of factors are identified not only for causing infertility but also for influencing the chances of recovery of spermatogenesis. These are shown in Table 20.2.

REFLECTION POINT

The distressing short- and long-term side effects of chemotherapy/radiotherapy are further exacerbated by premature ovarian failure and infertility. Consider the consequences of gonadal failure in both males and females. How could you prepare, educate and support a patient and their partner at this time?

THE ROLE OF HORMONE REPLACEMENT THERAPY

The majority of women who develop ovarian failure will experience distressing menopausal symptoms. Some women also perceive loss of their femininity, resulting in lack of confidence, self-esteem and depression. Because of the rapidity of the onset of the menopause, 70% of women will suffer vasomotor symptoms as well as a number of other equally important and more permanent problems (Fig. 20.2) (Studd & Whitehead 1988, Dannie et al 1994).

In recent years hormone replacement therapy (HRT) has been recognised as a successful method of treating distressing menopausal symptoms. It is used routinely in women suffering ovarian failure as a result of chemotherapy/radiotherapy treatments. The aim of HRT is to restore oestrogen levels to near normal, minimising symptoms and short- and

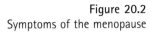

Figure 20.2
Symptoms of the menopause

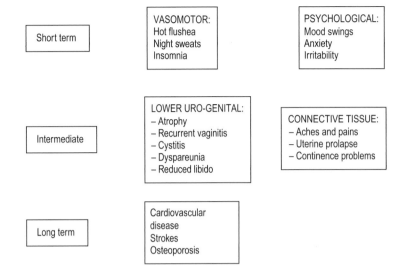

long-term sequelae such as osteoporosis, heart disease and cerebrovascular accidents. Additionally, it may help to improve uterine function, enabling endometrial proliferation in response to exogenous hormones for successful embryo transfer.

Treatment should commence at the onset of symptoms; for women who are asymptomatic gonadotrophin levels should be monitored and therapy begun when levels suggest ovarian failure. Menopausal symptoms such as night sweats may be similar to symptoms of CML and other haematological disorders. Therefore HRT must be commenced as soon as possible to prevent confusion between menopausal symptoms and signs of disease relapse (Goldman 1990, Chiodi et al 1991).

Premature menopause is associated with premature ageing. HRT can help to restore physical and mental wellbeing as well as reducing morbidity and mortality associated with osteoporosis and heart disease. It should be recommended for all suitable patients, and commenced as soon as possible. However, HRT is not suitable for all women. The side effects and contraindications can be just as distressing for some women as the symptoms of the menopause itself. It is therefore important that each woman is assessed individually and provided with full counselling and an explanation of the benefits and side effects.

A variety of differing preparations are available including oral, transdermal, subcutaneous and vaginal. The use of HRT varies widely between institutions and each patient must be assessed individually to determine the suitability of preparations and their associated risks. Products should be prescribed for maximum benefit, comfort and minimal risk. Careful follow-up is essential to monitor benefit, record side effects, and recommend different preparations as clinically indicated. Side effects and contraindications of HRT are shown in Table 20.3.

Table 20.3
Side effects and
contraindications for HRT

Common side effects of HRT	Contraindications for HRT
Breast tenderness	Breast cancer
Fluid retention	Known or suspected pregnancy
Leg cramps	Active liver disease/abnormal liver function
Nausea and vomiting	Endometrial cancer
Vaginal discharge	Vaginal bleeding of unknown cause
Gastro-intestinal symptoms	Venous thrombosis
Headache	Hypertension
Acne	Gallstones
Depression	Benign breast disease
Irritability	

Education for the woman and her family will encompass a number of issues but information given must be clear and simple. Nurses should be aware of the potential problems of treatment and its side effects. They should take the lead in initiating and encouraging discussion, as patients may be embarrassed to do so. The nurse's role should also encompass advice on physical, emotional and sexual wellbeing.

REFLECTION POINT

Consider the questions you might be asked by a woman who has been advised about the likelihood of premature menopause following treatment and is concerned about the effects these symptoms might have on her relationships. How would you respond to these questions?

STRATEGIES FOR MAINTAINING FERTILITY

Currently, gonadal failure cannot be prevented but a number of strategies are available to enable patients undergoing chemotherapy/radiotherapy the possibility of parenthood after treatment (Winston & Handyside 1993, Rio et al 1994). For men it is possible to cryopreserve sperm, for female patients it may not be as easy. A number of techniques have been used to preserve fertility during gonadotoxic treatment (Morris & Shalet 1990); these include embryo cryopreservation in women with a regular partner, and oocyte and ovarian cryopreservation as a possible future option for women without a regular partner and young girls.

Other strategies for maintaining fertility have included oophoropexy, which involves surgical intervention to place the ovaries midline behind the uterus (Sherins 1993), and the development of chemotherapy combinations to include dose limitation of alkylating agents which retain efficacy against the disease and less gonadal toxicity (Viviani et al 1985). Strategies for maintaining fertility post-treatment are:

- sperm banking
- testicular shielding
- embryo cryopreservation

- oocyte and ovarian cryopreservation
- oophoropexy
- dose limitation of alkylating agents
- substitution of drugs for less toxic substances
- combined oestrogen/progesterone contraceptive pill
- gonadotrophin-releasing hormone (GnRH) analogues.

Some of these strategies require delaying the commencement of chemotherapy; some require surgical intervention, taking account of the patient's general condition and disease status; others utilise different doses or toxicity of drugs in an attempt to reduce gonadal toxicity. However, whichever type of strategy is used, a substantial proportion of patients will remain at risk of infertility. Therefore the treatment option must be agreed by the patient, be effective against the disease and must not compromise the therapeutic outcome (Gradishar & Schilsky 1989, Apperley & Reddy 1995, Sonmezer & Oktay 2004).

Sperm banking

It is important that the patient is referred for sperm banking at the time of diagnosis as semen from men pre-treated for cancer or haematological cancers may reveal a low sperm count and inadequate sperm motility (Redman et al 1987, Anger et al 2004).

If possible, sperm should be stored on three separate occasions and at 48-hour intervals. Often patients have not been referred if they have already started treatment, because of the likelihood of obtaining an inadequate specimen. However, it appears that recent chemotherapy may not affect the quality of sperm, as sperm contained in an ejaculate began their maturation process 3 months earlier and are highly unlikely to be adversely affected by recent chemotherapy (Apperley & Reddy 1995). Theoretically patients can be referred early in their treatment, when their condition has been stabilised. However, these men must be counselled and prepared for the possibility of sperm counts being low and of poor quality, thereby reducing the chances of achieving a subsequent pregnancy (Apperley & Reddy 1995). The evidence for teratogenicity is severely limited and clearly the best approach is to refer the patient as early as possible after diagnosis (Whedon & Wujcik 1997).

Sperm banking should be offered to all men likely to suffer gonadal dysfunction. Those accepting the offer should be advised that successful pregnancy depends on the quality and quantity of sperm at the time of storage. If good-quality sperm is stored in sufficient quantities to permit six cycles of artificial insemination, there is a 45% cumulative chance of pregnancy. In contrast, storage of a single ejaculate of poor-quality sperm only offers, at best, a 20% chance (Scammel et al 1985).

Sperm banking has been widely available for some time and many men experiencing gonadal failure as a consequence of treatment will have sperm stored. Nevertheless, studies have shown that there are few requests to use frozen sperm. This may be partly attributable to those men who have already completed their families or those who are not completely recovered and have fears and concerns for the welfare of any subsequent child.

Figure 20.3
Typical pattern of treatment a
male patient with CML may
follow

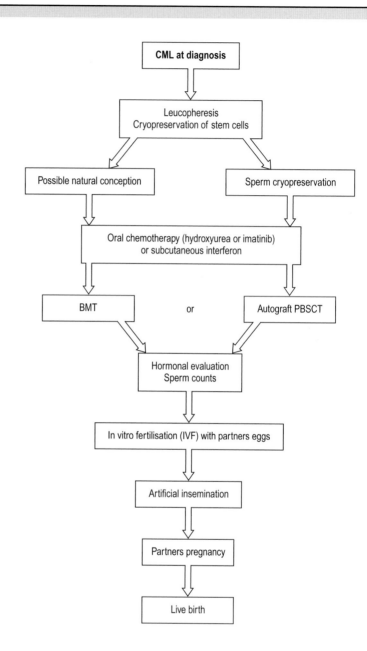

The ability to achieve pregnancy from frozen sperm is also low. This may be because sperm specimens were obtained from unsuitable candidates initially, including those having had previous intensive treatment (Friedman & Broder 1981) (Fig. 20.3).

Strategies for women

Women who develop ovarian failure as a consequence of chemotherapy/radiotherapy have three choices for motherhood. First, if they have a

Figure 20.4
Typical pattern of treatment a female patient with CML may follow

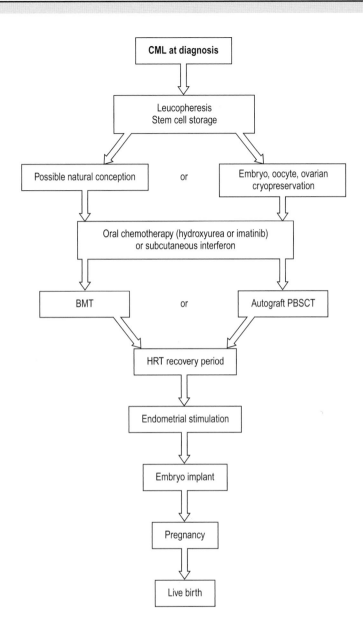

CML at diagnosis

Leucopheresis
Stem cell storage

Possible natural conception   or   Embryo, oocyte, ovarian cryopreservation

Oral chemotherapy (hydroxyurea or imatinib) or subcutaneous interferon

BMT   or   Autograft PBSCT

HRT recovery period

Endometrial stimulation

Embryo implant

Pregnancy

Live birth

regular partner and the commencement of treatment can be delayed, ovarian hyperstimulating oocyte collection, fertilisation and cryopreservation of embryos can be performed. If the start of treatment cannot be delayed, the second option involves fertilisation of donor eggs by their partner's sperm or donated embryos from an unrelated couple. The third option is the possibility of surrogacy. There are advantages and disadvantages to each approach. However, surrogacy is surrounded by emotional, legal and ethical problems, and is probably the least feasible option (Fig. 20.4).

Embryo cryopreservation

Women wishing to have embryo cryopreservation must undergo super-ovulation for at least one and possibly more menstrual cycles. This is usually achieved by using one of a variety of protocols to stimulate multiple follicle maturation (e.g. clomiphene alone or in combination with FSH or a GnRH agonist, e.g. buserelin). Eggs are not always retrieved using this procedure and it is not without risk. Women and their partners must therefore be well prepared and counselled before the procedure is undertaken.

If the procedure is successful, multiple oocytes can be harvested, enabling several embryos for cryopreservation. The ability to collect and fertilise good-quality oocytes depends on adequate ovarian function at the time of hyperstimulation and a number of other issues, including:

- advancing age
- fertility status pre-diagnosis
- underlying disease
- patient's general condition to enable the procedure
- impaired ovarian function due to prior exposure to chemotherapy
- successful superovulation technique
- failure to retrieve eggs
- time available
- more than one stimulation cycle necessary
- quality and quantity collected
- fertilisation and quality of embryos for storage.

Prior exposure to chemotherapy and increasing age will diminish successful collection cycles. A further problem for patients with malignant disease is the time needed for the procedure. Each ovarian hyperstimulation cycle requires 4 weeks. For some conditions, such as CML and Hodgkin's disease, this delay in commencing treatment may be reasonable; for others, including the acute leukaemias, it will not be feasible. Treatment may need to be administered before gametes can be harvested and stored, which may affect the quantity and quality of oocyte harvested and, consequentially, the chances of future pregnancies.

Fertilisation of donor eggs

An alternative when time is of the essence is fertilisation of donor eggs with the partner's sperm. Unfortunately, there is a waiting list for donor eggs and a limited supply. Most women undergoing a superovulation programme are understandably often reluctant to donate their eggs for fear of limiting their own chances of future pregnancies. Often family and friends are looked to for help in such situations, but this is not without emotional entanglement and such donors must be fully counselled of the risks involved. Another possible solution is the use of donated embryos from storage after a couple has completed their family. However, it is important to note that any offspring born from donated embryos will not be genetically related to the recipient couple, although they will be considered the parents under UK law (Human Fertilisation and Embryology Act 1994, 2004).

Pregnancy after treatment

Spontaneous pregnancies have been reported in patients treated for severe aplastic anaemia by BMT (Schmidt et al 1987, Salooja et al 2001), for cancer (Aisner et al 1993) and treated by autologous transplant (Salooja et al 1994, 2001). However, for those treated with TBI and BMT such pregnancies are rare (Lipton et al 1993).

The possible use of embryos after transplant is a highly charged ethical and emotional issue. To date there are two known cases of successful pregnancy after BMT utilising embryo implantation, the first with a fresh donor embryo (Rio et al 1994) and the second from a cryopreserved embryo prior to BMT for CML (Atkinson et al 1994).

A review of the published reports of pregnancies after BMT suggests an increased risk of both pregnancy and neonatal complications. In particular the incidence of eclampsia, pre-term labour and low birth-weight infants seems higher than normal (Hinterberger-Fischer et al 1991, Sanders et al 1993, 1996, Atkinson et al 1994, Apperley & Reddy 1995, Green et al 2002). Complications seen in pregnancy and neonates post-BMT are shown in Table 20.4.

Early clinical relapse, after delivery, has also been reported in some women treated by BMT for CML. These incidences of relapse may have occurred independently; however, it is thought that the immunosuppression associated with pregnancy may reduce the graft versus leukaemia (GVL) effect known to help suppression or eradication of residual disease post-BMT (Sanders 1983, Atkinson et al 1994, Rio et al 1994).

Another problem associated with embryo transfer is the increased risk of multiple pregnancy due to the increased number of embryos transferred at each session. The greater the number of embryos transferred, the higher the incidence of achieving a pregnancy. This is now a great concern of the Human Fertilisation and Embryology Authority (HFEA) who have imposed an upper limit of transferring three embryos at each replacement cycle.

Spontaneous abortion is also common in the first trimester of pregnancy utilising frozen embryos (Van-Steirteghem et al 1987). This risk is thought to increase with advancing age (Austin & Short 1986, Kelly et al 2004, Salooja et al 2004). Pregnancy and live birth rates have also been reported to be lower with cryopreserved embryos than those following fresh embryo transfer (HFEA 2004). Therefore it is essential that

Table 20.4
Complications seen in pregnancy and neonates post-BMT

Pregnancy	Neonates
Multiple pregnancy	Congenital abnormalities
Spontaneous abortion	Pre-term labour
Eclampsia	Low birth weight
Hypertension	Post-natal complications
Placenta praevia	Pulmonary complications
Placental insufficiency	Failure to thrive
Increased caesarean delivery	Increased susceptibility to malignancies
Disease relapse	

maximum numbers of good-quality embryos are stored to enable multiple attempts at transfer. This may not always be possible in patients awaiting chemotherapy and they must therefore be counselled about the chance of success to avoid disappointment in the future.

Case study 20.1

Gaynor was diagnosed with chronic myeloid leukaemia aged 22. She was 8 weeks' pregnant in her second pregnancy, the first having resulted in a spontaneous abortion at 5 weeks' gestation. Gaynor was not given chemotherapy to treat her leukaemia and her white cell count was controlled by leucopheresis. The pregnancy progressed normally and in August 1988 Gaynor delivered a normal healthy female infant weighing 3 kg. She was commenced on hydroxyurea and in 1989 decided she wanted another child. The pregnancy ended in spontaneous abortion at 7 weeks' gestation.

Bone marrow transplantation from her identical human leucocyte antigen (HLA) sibling was decided upon to treat her leukaemia; Gaynor and her partner chose embryo storage. Superovulation was induced, utilising buserelin and pergonal, and 24 eggs were collected. Normal fertilisation occurred with sperm from her husband, and the resulting 13 embryos were cryopreserved.

One year after diagnosis Gaynor received her allogeneic BMT. She recovered well with minimal graft-versus-host disease (GvHD). HRT was commenced 3 months after transplant, which controlled her menopausal symptoms but she experienced no menstrual bleeds.

Two and a half years after her transplant Gaynor and her partner decided to attempt a pregnancy. The first embryo transplant was attempted but exogenous endometrial stimulation with routine treatment failed. Gaynor was commenced on prolonged high-dose oestradiol to stimulate endometrial response. A year later a further embryo replacement cycle was attempted. Despite double-dose prolonged treatment the endometrium still failed to respond and at the patient's request embryos were transferred with progesterone support for endometrial maintenance.

Twenty-eight days following embryo transfer a twin pregnancy was confirmed. At 10 weeks' gestation one twin stopped developing. The remaining fetus continued to develop normally. Gaynor was closely monitored throughout by obstetricians and haematologists. The pregnancy and her haematological status continued normally until 34 weeks' gestation when during a routine antenatal visit Gaynor was found to have pre-eclampsia. She was admitted to hospital and underwent emergency Caesarean section being delivered of a live female infant weighing 1.9 kg.

Since delivery, Gaynor's CML has relapsed. She received lymphocytes from her sibling donor and remained in remission for some time. Sadly 15 years after a successful allogeneic SCT, Gaynor lost her life to secondary malignancies of breast and colon. Her children are healthy with normal development.

Oocyte and ovarian cryopreservation

Currently, embryo cryopreservation is the only strategy available to women post-BMT to have genetic offspring. This option is not offered to all patients, and it is especially limited to patients without a regular partner or premenarchal girls. For these patients, fertility options are less straightforward; in the future ovarian cryopreservation may offer further opportunities. Oocyte and ovarian cryopreservation are the subject of active laboratory research but are not yet available in clinical practice and should only be used for young girls, adolescents and when IVF is contraindicated (Gosden et al 1994, 1999, Revel & Schenker 2004). Additionally, ovarian cryopreservation involves a minor operative procedure, which may be contraindicated in the pancytopenic patient, and the ability to fertilise an oocyte appears to be profoundly affected by freezing (Gosden et al 1999).

The collection of oocytes requires at least one ovarian hyperstimulation cycle and should take place prior to the start of chemotherapy. This introduces a delay of approximately 4 weeks between diagnosis and treatment, which may be neither medically advisable nor acceptable to the patient and her physician (Apperley & Reddy 1995, Leibo 2004).

Ovarian tissue and the ability to collect oocytes should not be affected by the underlying disease, i.e. the ovaries should not contain malignant cells and impaired gonadal function should not be a feature of the disease at presentation. Again this procedure involves surgical intervention and may be contraindicated by the patient's general condition.

The advancement of research in this area is important. To date only two pregnancies from cryopreservation of oocytes have been reported (Chen 1986, Van Uem et al 1987). The complexity of the cryopreservation technique is thought to be owing to the oocyte's biological properties (Fabbri et al 2001, Boldt et al 2003, Revel & Schenker 2004). Some of the problems are now being addressed and it is likely that in the near future the technical difficulties will be overcome and the procedure will be offered to BMT recipients as the technique of choice for maintaining fertility, with a real likelihood of achieving a successful pregnancy and live birth (Hunter et al 1991, Apperley & Reddy 1995, Revel & Schenker 2004).

NURSING ISSUES

The success of fresh embryo transfer has helped many infertile couples to have children. However, such procedures raise a number of legal and ethical issues and procedures are controlled by legislation. In the UK, the HFEA provides guidance and direction to licensed units providing treatment for infertility, storage of embryos/gametes and research. Nurses need to be aware of these legal and ethical issues and to be able to address them with patients and their partners.

Counselling is the key element in the provision of an assisted conception service and is emphasised in the Warnock report (1985). Counselling involves helping couples to understand the various options open to them, including medical interventions, as well as coming to terms with disappointment and failure, possible relapse of their disease and the possibility of being outlived by their gametes. The availability of effective, informed, independent and involved counselling is essential, and if done with warmth and a genuine caring attitude will help reassure, build trust and confidence, and help the patient to feel cared for whatever the outcome (Edwards 1996).

The nurse's role in counselling is both supportive and educational, addressing fertility and sexuality issues (Puukko et al 1997). Time constraints on medical staff often mean that issues associated with sexuality are not discussed. Specialist nurses are, however, in a prominent position to identify problems, paving the way for more in-depth and genetic counselling by trained professionals.

The educative role of the specialist nurse is not an easy one. Up-to-date knowledge of current research and developments is necessary to be able to provide realistic, accurate information without giving false hope and to help to empower patients to make informed choices. Nurses need to be able to explain the investigations needed before treatment and the process and outcomes of treatment. Handled sensitively this information can help to alleviate many fears and worries. Provision of information is an important part of the nurse's role and professional integrity must be maintained. Continuing education is required to keep nurses well informed so that they in turn can inform, counsel, and educate, giving individuals a sense of control over their lives, in spite of the emotional, ethical and legal difficulties associated with assisted reproduction.

REFLECTION POINT

Strategies for maintaining fertility pre-treatment are time-consuming, costly and not easily available or accessible. Consider your unit's current policy relating to this issue. Should the service be offered to all suitable candidates? What are the main constraints in your institution? What is your role in patient education?

CONCLUSION

Gonadal failure and infertility are inevitable consequences of high-dose chemotherapy and TBI. Currently there are a number of strategies for maintaining fertility after treatment. However, these are not without their difficulties, and the issues require to be handled with care and sensitivity.

DISCUSSION QUESTIONS

1. What are the main strategies for maintaining fertility post-treatment and the factors affecting gonadal recovery post-BMT?

2. Which HRT preparations are commonly prescribed in your unit? What are their common side effects and their short- and long-term benefits and risks?

3. What supporting services are currently available in your unit for patients facing infertility? How accessible are these services?

4. What ethical, legal and emotional issues may be associated with assisted reproduction?

5. Central to the systemic approach to comprehensive and effective follow-up of patients post-transplant is the detection and treatment of potential complications at an early stage. How can nurses in your unit contribute to this in relation to fertility issues?

References

Anger J T, Gilbert B R, Goldstein M 2004 Cryopreservation of sperm: indication methods and results. Journal of Urology 170:1079–1084

Aisner J, Wienik P H, Pearl P 1993 Pregnancy outcome in patients treated for Hodgkin's disease. Journal of Clinical Oncology 11(3):507–512

Apperley J, Reddy N 1995 Mechanism and management of treatment related gonadal failure in recipients of high dose chemo-radiotherapy. Blood Reviews 19:93–116

Atkinson H G, Apperley J F, Dawson K, Goldman J, Winston R 1994 Successful pregnancy following allogeneic bone marrow transplantation for chronic myeloid leukaemia. Lancet i(344):199

Austin C R, Short R V 1986 Reproduction in mammals. In: Austin C R, Short R V (eds) Manipulating reproduction, vol 5, 2nd edn. Cambridge University Press, Cambridge

Baker J W, Morgan R L, Peckham R J, Smithers D W 1972 Preservation of ovarian function in patients requiring radiotherapy for para aortic and pelvic Hodgkin's disease. Lancet i:1307–1308

Boldt J, Cline D, McLaughlin D 2003 Human oocyte cryopreservation as an adjunct to IVF-embryo transfer cycles. Human Reproduction 18:1250–1255

Byrne J, Fears T, Gail M 1992 Early menopause in long term survivors of cancer during adolescence. Americal Journal of Obstetrics and Gynecology 166:788–793

Chapman R M, Sutcliffe B 1981 Protection of ovarian function by oral contraceptives in women receiving chemotherapy for Hodgkin's disease. Blood 58:849–851

Charak B, Gupta R, Mandrekar G 1990 Testicular dysfunction after cyclosphosphamide-vincristine-procarbazine-prednisolone chemotherapy for advanced Hodgkin's disease. A long-term follow up study. Cancer 65:1903–1906

Chatterjee R, Mills W, Katz M, McGarrigle H H, Goldstone A H 1994 Prospective study of pituitary-gonadal function to evaluate short-term effects of ablative chemotherapy or TBI with autologous marrow transplantation in post menarcheal women. Bone Marrow Transplantation 13: 511–517

Chen C 1986 Pregnancy after human oocyte cryopreservation. Lancet i:884–886

Chiodi S, Spinelli S, Cohen A 1991 Cyclic sex hormone replacement therapy in women undergoing allogeneic marrow transplantation: aims and results. Bone Marrow Transplant 8(Suppl 1):47–49

Choo Y C, Chan S Y, Wong L C, Ma H K 1985 Ovarian dysfunction in patients with gestational trophoblastic neoplasia treated with intensive courses of etoposide (VP16–213). Cancer 55:2348–2352

Dannie E, Apperley J, Lindsay K 1994 A study of the disease and its treatment on gonadal function in women with chronic myeloid leukaemia. Unpublished dissertation for BSc in Health Studies, University of Surrey

Edwards S D 1996 Nursing ethics. Macmillan Press, London

Fabbri R, Porcu E, Marsell T, Rocchetta G, Ventouroli S 2001 Human oocyte cryopreservation: new perspective regarding oocyte survival. Human Reproduction 16:411–416

Fairley F K, Barrie J U, Johnson W 1972 Sterility and testicular atrophy related to cyclophosphamide therapy. Lancet i:568–569

Friedman S, Broder S 1981 Homologous artificial insemination after long-term semen cryopreservation. Fertility and Sterility 35:321–324

Giri N, Vowels M R, Barr A L, Mamegham H 1992 Successful pregnancy after total body radiation and bone marrow transplantation for acute leukaemia. Bone Marrow Transplantation 10:93–95

Goldman J M 1990 Options for the management of CML. Leukaemia and Lymphoma 3:159–164

Gonen Y, Casper R F, Jacobson W, Blankier J 1989 Endometrial thickness and growth during ovarian stimulation. A possible predictor of implantation in IVF. Fertility and Sterility 52:446–450

Gosden R G, Baird D T, Wade J C, Webb R 1994 Restoration of fertility to oophorectomised sheep by ovarian autografts stored at −196 degrees C. Human Reproduction 9:597–603

Gosden R G, Picton H, Nugent D, Rutherford A 1999 Gonadal tissue cryopreservation. Clinical objectives and practical prospects. Human Fertility 2:107–114

Gradishar W J, Schilsky R L 1989 Ovarian function following radiation and chemotherapy for cancer. Seminars in Oncology 16(5):425–436

Gratwohl A, Hermans J, Neiderwieser D et al 1993 BMT for CML long term effects. Bone Marrow Transplantation 1(2):509–516

Green P M, Whitton J, Stovall M et al 2002 Pregnancy outcomes of female survivors of childhood cancer Survivor study. American Journal of Obstetrics and Gynecology 187:1070–1080

Grigg A, McLachlan R, Zaja J, Szer J 2000 Reproductive status in long term bone marrow transplant survivors receiving Busulphan-Cyclophosphamide (120 mg/kg). Bone Marrow Transplantation 26:1089–1095

Hensley M L, Ford J M 2003 Imatinib treatment: specific issues related to safety, fertility and pregnancy. Seminars in Hematology 40(Suppl 2):21–25

Hinterberger-Fischer M, Kier P, Kahls P et al 1991 Fertility, pregnancy and offspring complications after BMT. Bone Marrow Transplantation 199(7):5–9

Horning S J, Hoppe R T, Kaplan H S, Rosenberg S A 1981 Female reproductive potential after treatment for Hodgkin's disease. New England Journal of Medicine 304:1377–1382

Human Fertilisation and Embryology Authority (HFEA) 1994 Third Annual Report, Department of Health. HMSO, London

Human Fertilisation and Embryology Act (HFEA) 2004 Department of Health. HMSO, London

Hunter J E, Bernard A, Fuller B, Amso N, Shaw R W 1991 Fertilisation and development of the human oocyte following exposure to cryoprotectants, low temperature and cryopreservation: a comparison of two techniques. Human Reproduction 6:1460–1465

Kelly S, Rao D, Dean N, Tan L 2004 In vitro fertilisation and embryo banking. In: Tulandi T, Gosden R (eds) Preservation of fertility. Taylor & Francis, London, pp 101–110

Kolb H J, Bender-Gotze C, Haas R J 1989 Late effects in marrow transplanted patients' results of the AG-KMT Munich. Bone Marrow Transplantation 4(Suppl 3):31–35

Larsen E, Muller J, Rechnitzer C 2003 Diminished ovarian reserve in female childhood cancer survivors with regular menstrual cycles and basal FSH. Human Reproduction 18:417–422

Leibo S P 2004 Cryopreservation of mammalian oocytes. In: Tulandi T, Gosden R (eds) Preservation of fertility. Taylor & Francis, London, pp 141–155

Lipton J H, Derzko C, Fyles G 1993 Pregnancy after bone marrow transplantation. Three case reports. Bone Marrow Transplantation 11:415–418

Lushbaugh C C, Casarett G W 1976 The effects of gonadal irradiation in clinical irradiation: a review. Cancer 37(Suppl 2):1111–1125

Marks D J, Cullis J O, Ward K N 1993 Allogeneic bone marrow transplant for chronic myeloid leukaemia using sibling and unrelated donors. Annals of Internal Medicine 119:207–214

Marrin D 2002 Use of imatinib in CML: practical considerations. Haematologica 87:979–988

Meirow D, Nugent D 2001 The effects of radiotherapy and chemotherapy on female reproduction. Human Reproduction 7:535–543

Morris I D, Shalet S M 1990 Protection of gonadal function from cytotoxic chemotherapy and irradiation. Baillière's Clinical Endocrinology and Metabolism 4(1):97–118

Puukko L, Hirvonem E, Aalberg V, Hovi L et al 1997 Sexuality of young women surviving leukaemia. Archives of Diseases in Childhood 76:197–202

Quigley M M, Hammond C B 1979 Oestrogen-replacement therapy: help or hazard. New England Journal of Medicine 301:646–648

Redman J R, Bajorunas D R, Goldstein M C et al 1987 Semen cryopreservation and artificial insemination for Hodgkin's disease. Journal of Clinical Oncology 5:233–238

Revel A, Schenker J 2004 Ovarian tissue banking for cancer patients: is ovarian cortex cryopreservation presently justified? Human Reproduction 19(11):14–19

Rio B, Letur-Konirsch H, Ajchenbaum-Cymbalista F et al 1994 Full term pregnancy with embryos from donated oocytes in a 36 year old woman autografted for chronic myeloid leukaemia. Bone Marrow Transplantation 13:487–488

Salooja N, Chatterjee R, Macmillan A K et al 1994 Successful pregnancy in women following simple autotransplant for acute myeloid leukaemia with a chemotherapy ablation protocol. Bone Marrow Transplantation 13:431–435

Salooja N, Szydlo R, Socie G 2001 Pregnancy outcome after peripheral blood or bone marrow transplant: a retrospective survey. Lancet 358:271–276

Salooja N, Reddy N, Apperley J 2004 Vulnerability of the reproductive system to radiotherapy and chemotherapy. In: Tulandi T, Gosden R (eds) Preservation of fertility. Taylor & Francis, London, pp 39–64

Sanders J E, Buckner C D, Leonard J M et al 1983 Late effects on gonadal function after cyclophosphamide and total body irradiation and bone marrow transplantation. Transplantation 36:252–255

Sanders J E, Buckner C D, Amos D et al 1988 Ovarian function following marrow transplantation for aplastic anaemia or leukaemia. Journal of Clinical Oncology 6:813–818

Sanders J E, Buckner C D, Storb R, Doney K, Sullivan K, Witherspoon R 1993 Pregnancy outcome after bone marrow transplantation for AA or haematology malignancies. Experimental Haematology 21(Abstr 210):1067

Sanders J E, Hawley J, Levy W et al 1996 Pregnancy following high-dose cyclophosphamide with or without high-dose busulphan or total body irradiation and bone marrow transplantation. Blood 7:3045–3052

Scammel G E, White N, Stredronska J, Hendry W F, Edmonds D K 1985 Cryopreservation of semen in men with testicular tumour or Hodgkin's disease. Lancet ii:31–32

Schmidt H, Ehninger G, Dopfer R, Waller H D 1987 Pregnancy after bone marrow transplantation for severe aplastic anaemia. Bone Marrow Transplantation 2:329–332

Shalet S M, Hann I M, Lendon M, Morris-Jones P H, Beardwell C J 1981 Testicular function after combination chemotherapy in childhood for acute lymphoblastic leukaemia. Archives of Diseases in Childhood 56:275–278

Sherins R J 1993 Gonadal dysfunction. In: De Vita V T, Hellman S, Rosenberg S A (eds) Cancer: principles and practice of oncology, Vol 2, 4th edn. Lippincott, Philadelphia, pp 2395–2406

Sonmezer M, Oktay K 2004 Fertility preservation in female patients: a comprehensive approach. In: Tulandi T, Gosden R. (eds) Preservation of fertility. Taylor & Francis, London, pp 177–190

Speiser B, Rubin P, Casarett G 1972 Aspermia following lower truncal irradiation in Hodgkin's disease. Cancer 32:692–698

Studd J W W, Whitehead M I 1988 The menopause. Blackwell Scientific, Oxford

Udall P R, Kerr D N S, Tacchi D 1972 Amenorrhoea and sterility. Lancet i:693–694

Van-Steirteghem A C, Van der Abeel E, Braeckmans P, Camus M 1987 Pregnancy with a frozen-thawed embryo in a woman with primary ovarian failure. New England Journal of Medicine 317:113–116

Van Uem J, Siebzehnrubl E, Schuh B, Koch R, Trotnow S, Lang M 1987 Birth after the cryopreservation of unfertilised oocytes. Lancet i:752–753

Viviani S, Santoro A, Gangi G, Bonfante V, Bestetti O, Bonadonna G 1985 Gonadal toxicity after combination chemotherapy for Hodgkin's disease. Comparative results of MOPP vs ABVD. European Journal of Cancer & Clinical Oncology 21:601–605

Vose J M, Kennedy B C, Bierman P J 1992 Long term sequelae of autologous bone marrow or peripheral stem cell transplantation for lymphoid malignancies. Cancer 69:784–789

Wang C, Ng P R, Chan T K 1980 Effect of combination chemotherapy on pituitary-gonadal function in patients with lymphoma and leukaemia. Cancer 45:2030–2037

Warnock M 1985 A question of life. Basil Blackwell, Oxford

Watson A R, Rance C P, Bain J 1985 Long term effects of cyclophosphamide on testicular function. British Medical Journal 291:1457–1460

Whedon M B, Wujcik D 1997 Bone and marrow stem cell transplantation: principles, practice and nursing insights, 2nd edn. Jones and Bartlett, Boston

Winston R M L, Handyside A H 1993 New challenges in human in vitro fertilisation. Science 260:932–936

Further reading

Apperley J, Reddy N 1995 Mechanism and management of treatment-related gonadal failure in recipients of high dose chemo-radiotherapy. Blood Reviews 9:95–116

This article describes the normal reproductive function relevant to patients at risk of chemotherapy or radiotherapy-induced infertility. It gives a good overview of the mechanism by which fertility may be affected and preventative measures that may be employed. It also describes methods of IVF from stored gametes, and the legal and ethical aspects of assisted reproduction.

Barton C, Waxman J 1990 Effects of chemotherapy on fertility. Blood Reviews 4:187–195

This article reviews the effects of chemotherapy on gonadal function utilising single and combination therapy for a variety of malignant disorders. It also gives a brief overview of prevention strategies and management of gonadal failure.

HFEA Human Fertilisation and Embryology Act 1990 (2004) HMSO, London

This Act and its subsequent frequent reports give an in-depth description of the legal and ethical issues of assisted conception in respect to the units that are licensed to provide infertility treatment, storage of embryos and gametes and research involving embryos. It also states the rights of IVF treatment in patients with cancers and defines the status of the parties involved in donation and reception of embryos or gametes outlining the concerns for the welfare of any children and the prospective parents.

Puukko L, Hirvonem E, Aalberg V, Hovi L et al 1997 Sexuality of young women surviving leukaemia. Archives of Diseases in Childhood 76:197–202

This piece of research assesses the sexuality of young women surviving leukaemia. This is sensitively done and highlights the difficulties facing this group of patients. It concludes that while most have appropriate sexual development, vulnerability exists and early recognition of problems may help to treat effectively.

Revel A, Schenker J 2004 Ovarian tissue banking for cancer patients: is ovarian cortex cryopreservation presently justified? Human Reproduction 19(11):14–19

This article emphasises the difficulties in cryopreservation of female gametes. It discusses ovarian tissue banking as an experimental technology and its application for selected young female patients and where IVF is contraindicated.

Salooja N, Reddy N, Apperley J 2004 Vulnerability of the reproductive system to radiotherapy and chemotherapy. In: Tulandi T, Gosden R (eds) Preservation of fertility. Taylor & Francis, London, pp 39–64

This book gives a good overview and will help understanding of alternatives for preserving fertility and development of relevant technologies. The first three chapters discuss age and fertility and the vulnerability of the reproductive system to chemo/radiotherapy. The remaining chapters cover assisted reproductive techniques and new developments for cryopreservation as well as psycho/social, legal and ethical issues.

Studd J W W, Whitehead M I 1988 The menopause. Blackwell Scientific, Oxford

This book gives a good general overview of the physiological aspects of the menopause. It is sensitively written in respect to distressing menopausal symptoms, femininity issues and the short- and long-term side-effects, as well as the benefits and risks, of HRT.

Whedon M B, Wujcik D 1997 Fertility and sexuality issues. In: Blood and marrow stem cell transplantation, 2nd edn. Jones and Bartlett, Boston

This chapter written by nurses working in a BMT unit describes the inevitable consequences of chemotherapy/radiotherapy on gonadal function, and the resulting infertility and psychosexual issues. It also gives a good overview of how nurses may approach this sensitive subject with patients and their partners, and interventions that may be employed to improve sexual function.

Chapter 21

Sexuality and nursing practice

Marvelle Brown

CHAPTER CONTENTS

KEY POINTS
- Sexuality although linked to fertility is a separate entity.
- Nurses need to develop the necessary interpersonal skills to effectively discuss sexuality issues with patients.
- Utilising the PLISSIT model or an adaptation of it alongside establishing a comfort zone are important means of communicating about sexuality.
- Post-registration education programmes should effectively incorporate the theoretical underpinning of sexuality to provide the foundation for developing the skills and competencies required for addressing sexuality issues in nursing practice.

INTRODUCTION

This chapter addresses sexuality – a fundamentally challenging quality of life issue. Sexuality is a multifaceted, multidimensional phenomenon and should form an integral part of nursing assessment (Rafferty 1995, Hughes 1996). The impact of a cancer diagnosis and its treatment may well not place sexuality at the top of the agenda for health-care professionals, but regardless of race, gender, ethnicity and age, it is a significant aspect of life that many patients will want to explore at some point during their treatment. Sexuality is an important part of many patients' lives, and unlike fertility, sexuality is not destroyed but compromised by cytoreductive therapy.

Sexuality and fertility, although linked, are separate entities and need to be viewed in their own distinct manner. Attempts to define sexuality have been difficult, as it is heavily subjective, based on personal beliefs, values, experiences, culture, upbringing and personal sexual orientation. Some researchers in the past focussed on specific parts of sexuality: Platzer (1990) on sexual orientation, Baguley & Brooker (1990) on sexual dysfunction and Thompson (1990) on self-concept and body image. Unsurprisingly, such approaches have led to confusion regarding what sexuality is and how to address it in nursing practice. The Royal College of Nursing (RCN) (2000, p 2), has embodied a number of these concepts and formulated a generally clearer and useful definition:

> 'sexuality is an individual's self-concept, shaped by their personality and expressed as sexual feelings, attitudes, beliefs and behaviours, expressed through heterosexual, homosexual, bisexual or transsexual orientation'

Ultimately, sexuality is the embodiment of the physical, psychological and emotional facets of an individual that makes them unique. Sexuality is the basis on which individuals perceive themselves and how they want society to view them. Sexuality is expressed through body image, gender roles, patterns of affection, social and family roles and genital sex. This chapter reviews the key physiological and psychological effects of cancer treatment on sexuality and discusses how nurses can manage sexuality issues.

PHYSIOLOGICAL EFFECTS OF CANCER TREATMENT ON SEXUALITY

A positive interrelationship of physical, psychological, neurological and hormonal interactions, with an intact genitalia and a sound vascular system are crucially important for healthy sexual functioning. The sexual response involves five phases (Ofman & Auchincloss, 1992):

- desire (excitement)
- arousal (readiness)
- plateau (heighten)
- orgasm (reflex)
- resolution (satisfaction).

All the above are affected to a lesser or greater extent following cytoreductive therapy and specific problems affecting men and women are outlined.

PHYSIOLOGICAL EFFECTS IN WOMEN

In women, oocytes are formed prior to birth. No further oocytes are produced following birth, instead oocytes are lost through menses until natural menopause occurs in the late 4th or 5th decade. The fact that women do not produce new oocytes is a key factor in compromising reproductive ability following aggressive cancer treatment. If a woman has had problems with menses, e.g. irregular cycles, polycystic ovaries, prior to treatment, it will be extremely difficult for her to recover fertility post-treatment. Loss of oestrogen production due to primary ovarian failure and disturbance in the production of follicle-stimulating hormone (FSH) and luteinising hormone (LH) can lead to vaginal dryness, vaginal stenosis and vaginal atrophy. Vaginal ulcerations can also be a consequence of cancer treatment (Cancer BACUP 2004) (see Chapter 20 for further information on fertility).

These changes can have a negative impact on sexual desire (Barton et al 2004) and sexual response, and can cause dyspareunia (painful sexual intercourse). Additionally, genital numbness can reduce sexual arousal. The menopause is artificially induced by cancer treatment leading to a sudden drop in oestrogens, which causes a greater degree of discomfort in symptoms associated with the menopause, such as irritability, insomnia, vaginal dryness and, in particular, hot flushes.

Androgens are produced in the ovaries and adrenal glands, to encourage sexual desire and arousal in women. Ovarian dysfunction leads to a sudden drop in androgens, reducing libido. In natural menopause, the levels of androgens are generally unaffected, which enables women to continue to have sexual desire and become aroused. In medical menopause the sudden loss of ovarian function leads to a decrease in androgens and hence reduction in sexual desire.

Vaginal infections are very common in women undergoing chemotherapy, especially vaginal candidiasis. The potential for developing these infections is increased if steroids or powerful antibiotics are being taken.

Osteoporosis, another potential consequence of reduced oestrogen production, can also occur with the drugs used to ameliorate cancer. Drugs such as steroids are known to potentially cause osteoporotic problems. Difficulties with mobility and the existence of pain can affect the wellbeing of the patient, reducing their self-esteem and desire to have any sexual relationship.

A further potential problem is vaginismus, described as an: 'involuntary spasm of the muscles around the vagina, whenever the vulva is touched, either during sexual activity or medical examination. The result is dyspareunia' (Brooker 2002, p 453). Dyspareunia can occur as a problem in itself and is usually caused by pelvic irradiation, total body irradiation and reduction or loss of vaginal secretions, again due to reduced oestrogen production. A negative cycle can occur – the woman fears sexual intercourse, fear reduces vaginal secretions, reduced vaginal secretions potentially lead to dyspareunia. The need for early diagnosis of these problems to improve morbidities and enhance quality of life cannot be underestimated.

PHYSIOLOGICAL EFFECTS IN MEN

In men, the seminiferous tubules produce sperm – men continue to produce sperm and testosterone well into the 6th or 7th decades. Under the influence of follicle-stimulating hormone the spermatids become spermatozoa. The Leydig cells secrete testosterone under the influence of luteinising hormone (Smith & Babaian 1992). Following chemotherapy treatment, the germinal cells (Sertoli cells) are damaged, leading to oligospermia. Leydig cells are generally unaffected by chemotherapy and hence testosterone production is normal; FSH and LH are also usually normal. Total body irradiation destroys both the Sertoli and Leydig cells, leading to azoospermia and sterility. Reduction in testosterone levels due to chemotherapy can reduce libido.

Gynaecomastia (breast enlargement in men) can occur following treatment and persist for many weeks post-treatment. Failure to attain or retain an erection and premature ejaculation are not uncommon. Difficulty with retaining an erection quite commonly has psychological rather than physiological causes. Generally heightened anxiety levels can be a major factor in gaining an erection. Impotence is another potential problem, warranting specialist intervention.

Dry ejaculation may occur in some men who are able to have and maintain erections. In dry ejaculation, the semen passes into the bladder and not through the penis (Cancerbacup 2004). Cloudy urine following sexual intercourse occurs with dry ejaculations, due to semen in the urine.

GENERAL PROBLEMS FOR BOTH MEN AND WOMEN

Symptoms such as nausea, emesis, alopecia, fatigue, pain and weight loss commonly affect sexuality and sexual drive in both men and women. Some drugs used to manage the side effects of cancer treatment can also affect sexuality:

- Anti-emetics such as phenothiazines (dopamine antagonists), e.g. prochlorperazine, chlorpromazine, can cause difficulties in erection and ejaculation.
- Anxiolytics such as diazepam and lorazepam can reduce libido.
- Corticosteroids can be another contributory factor leading to irregular menses.
- Opioid analgesia can also reduce sexual desire.
- Other groups of drugs that can affect sexuality include anticonvulsants, antihypertensives and antidepressants (Reid et al 1989)

Patients who develop chronic graft-versus-host disease can have particular physiological effects, impacting on sexuality (Box 21.1).

> **Box 21.1   Effects of chronic graft–versus–host disease on sexuality**
>
> - Skin – hyperpigmentation, patchy alopecia, joint contractions
> - Gut – damage to the epithelial cells in the gut, compromises the absorption of nutrients, leading to weight loss or poor weight gain
> - Ocular damage* – due to cataracts; tear production from the lachrymal glands is reduced or stopped leading to dry, itchy eyes
> - Tremors* – loss of fine pincer movement
> - Somnolence* – intermittent drowsiness
> - Muscle wasting[†]
> - Muscle weakness[†]
> - Osteoporosis[†] – bone weakness
> - Hirsutism[†] – male distribution of hair in women
>
> *related to cyclosporin
> [†]related to steroids

PSYCHOLOGICAL EFFECTS OF TREATMENT ON SEXUALITY

Having a diagnosis of cancer and undergoing, in some cases, life-threatening treatment undoubtedly has a major psychological impact on the patient (see Chapter 23). Emotions such as anger, fear and frustration are not uncommon (Whedon et al 1995). Grieving over the potential loss of future plans, the fear of the unknown and the word 'cancer' can all make a patient feel that death is imminent.

Gender role re-definition may occur, with the patient possibly having to review how the family and finances will be managed whilst they are receiving and recovering from treatment. Financial pressures can have a negative impact on patients' sexuality.

Guilt can also affect sexuality, from a number of perspectives. Some patients from certain cultures or with particular religious beliefs may view their cancer as a punishment to be endured because they have committed some offence against God (Powe 1992). This can be of significance for elderly patients from particular ethnic minorities such as South East Asian and African communities.

Male partners of female patients may feel concerned about causing pain (in relation to sexual intercourse) and therefore their approaches to intimacy may change. Changes in intimacy can also occur because the patient does not feel attractive, is suffering fatigue and generally has no desire to be intimate. Fear of pain can heighten senses and add to the anxiety and stress around intimacy.

How we view ourselves and how we present ourselves to the world has an effect on our self-esteem and self-confidence. Price (1990 p 3) provides us with the concepts of: 'body reality (as the body is), body ideal (as it "should" be) and body presentation (as it shows and acts)'. Interwoven with these concepts are cultural, sociological and ethnic factors that underpin the body image. Generally, we all anticipate that we will go through the life cycle and we can anticipate that changes will occur (e.g. ageing). Chemotherapy/radiotherapy may speed up some of these changes (e.g. menopause); physical changes such as alopecia, scarring from a Hickman line or weight loss can significantly change an individual's appearance in a relatively short space of time. Such changes can affect the way individuals view themselves and how others view them (Jenkins & Price 1996). Unsurprisingly, altered body image can be the cause of distress and engender feelings of shame, inferiority or embarrassment (Heath 2002).

Regaining self-confidence is a significant milestone in recapturing sexuality. There is a positive correlation between altered body image, sexual intercourse, depression, stage of illness and the patient's level of self-confidence. The longer the cancer is in remission the more likely the patient is to regain their interest in sexual intercourse, with a corresponding enhancement in body image, reduction in depression and anxiety, and increase in self-confidence. Part of the development of self-confidence for some patients is the ability to return to work. Planning return to work should be part of the rehabilitation process. For those patients who were working prior to their diagnosis and treatment, being back at work helps to give back some normality to their lives and enables them to fulfil their role within the family, their relationship, or just for themselves. However, this can be a very challenging, Herculean time for some patients. A degree of stigma is still attached to the word cancer and patients may feel uncomfortable informing colleagues of their illness. Failure to gain promotion and lack of career mobility can be difficult hurdles individuals may have to overcome (Brown & Tai-Seale 1992).

Cancer diagnosis can place a tremendous strain on a relationship – relationship breakdowns are unfortunately not uncommon. If a relationship has been difficult, a cancer diagnosis can either recapture and solidify the relationship or can be the trigger causing relationship breakdown. Such a situation serves to further undermine the patient's sexuality and self-confidence.

NURSING PRACTICE AND SEXUALITY

Managing sexuality revolves around the acronym ASK: attitudes, skills, knowledge (Brown 2001). Before nurses can support and manage sexuality issues with patients, they need to be very comfortable about their own sexuality and have the ability to be non-judgemental in actions or inactions regarding sexuality (Gamel et al 1993).

Communication is fundamental to the ability to address sexuality with patients. Skills in attentive listening and being reflective with issues raised are fundamental skills to acquire (Burnard 1999, Nelson Jones 1999). It is essential that nurses develop the interpersonal skills to enable patients to understand how to minimise the effects of treatment on their sexuality. Nurses need to be able to speak to individuals using appropriate language and without embarrassment. An in-depth knowledge of how treatment may affect sexuality and the competence and confidence to address patients' concerns are paramount.

Empowering patients to recapture their sexuality should be an essential part of the rehabilitation process. Hughes (1996, p 1599) succinctly summarises Ferrell et al (1995), by making a poignant point when she states:

> '. . . one of the most negative influences on the social wellbeing of a survivor of marrow transplantation is the change in sexuality that health professionals *fail* [author's emphasis] to address.'

Furthermore, the RCN (2000, p 4) states that:

> '. . . nurses need to recognise that sexuality and sexual health is an appropriate area of nursing activity and that they have a professional and clinical responsibility to address it.'

Writing 'not applicable' in the sexuality section of nursing documentation is not uncommon and can be insulting to the patient.

Satisfactory sexual relationships play a key role in the recovery process and nursing research identifies sexuality as important – yet in practice sexuality and sexual health are poorly addressed (Shell 1995, Waterhouse 1996). Faulkner & Regnard (1994) identified that nurses had different levels of interaction with patients, particularly on sensitive issues and the question 'How are you?' is used to highlight the different levels of interaction (Table 21.1). Arguably, nurses do not go beyond level 1. Many nurses would not pick up on the hint, either because they do not actively listen or because they refuse to acknowledge that the patient wants to talk about something that is clearly of concern to them, leaving the patient feeling disheartened and uncomfortable.

Many authors, such as Kantz et al (1990), Lewis & Bor (1994) and Crounch (1999), have asked why it is difficult to communicate with patients on sexuality issues. Brown (2001) conducted an exploratory study and identified similar factors, alluded to by prior researchers (Box 21.2). This clearly demonstrates the need for nursing education still to address this issue at both pre-registration and post-registration level. Education should provide a safe arena for nurses to address their anxieties and concerns, and challenge attitudes and behaviours on this sensitive aspect of patient care.

Table 21.1
Levels of interaction
(Faulkner & Regnard 1994)

Level of interaction	Feeling expressed by the patient	Response to question: 'How are you?'
0	No feeling	'I'm fine'
1	Hint	'I suppose I'm okay'
2	Mention of feeling	'I'm worried about sex'
3	Feelings expressed	'I'm really worried about sex. I really want to have sex as soon as possible, but can I have sex and will it hurt?'

> **Box 21.2** Barriers to effective communication about sexuality for nurses (Brown 2001)
>
> - Lack of good interpersonal skills
> - Sensitivity of the subject
> - Taboo
> - Marital status of the patient
> - Gender difference between the patient and nurse
> - Age
> - Staff shortage
> - Cultural/ethnic difference between patient and nurse
> - Religion
> - Time
> - Embarrassment
> - Conversation not initiated by the patient
> - Lack of privacy
> - Prejudicial attitudes

Without doubt, sexuality is a sensitive subject, particularly as it is so personal and subjective. However, creating the right environment through privacy, building a rapport, developing trust and providing the opportunity to discuss issues of a personal nature can help the patient to feel comfortable about talking about sexuality issues, if they wish. Sensitive questioning and the right approach can reduce anxieties around the subject.

REFLECTION POINT

When carrying out a patient assessment do you discuss sexuality issues? If not, what are the reasons for not doing so? What do you need to do to develop your knowledge and skills in addressing sexuality?

Regardless of the age of the patient, sexuality is important. An assumption is often made that individuals beyond the age of 50 do not have any sexuality (Brown 2001, Heath 2002). Talking with younger patients or patients of the opposite sex can be challenging but not impossible (Brown 2003). Unless nurses have the motivation and interest to discuss sexuality issues with the patient, they will never get over any embarrassment they may have and will, instead, continue to deliver less than holistic care. If the subject is too difficult, it is incumbent on the nurse to ensure that the patient has access to relevant information and should refer appropriately.

Time is clearly a challenge in discussing sensitive issues, not least because of staff shortages and heavy workload pressures. However, time is necessary to enable the patient to discuss their concerns. Nurses can provide patients with written information and then plan to return at a specific time – giving patients the opportunity to read the information in their own time, digest that information, and formulate questions. This is a constructive way of overcoming time shortages. There is some excellent patient information from cancer charities on sexuality, which should be made available to patients as a reference source.

The marital status of the patient – married, co-habiting or single – is inconsequential. The opportunity to discuss concerns around sexuality should be offered and questions raised by the patient should be addressed.

Case study 21.1

During a routine follow-up, the husband of a 30-year-old patient 2 years post-BMT for chronic myeloid leukaemia broke down in tears. Following sensitive questioning, his wife revealed her total lack of interest in sex and that she slept in a separate bedroom. She had suggested to her husband that he could have extra-marital relations to satisfy his needs. It became clear in the discussion that she had vaginismus. They were referred to a specialist, with a successful outcome.

The PLISSIT model (Anon 1976) was used to form the RCN (2000) guidance on sexuality and sexual health, and provides a useful framework for initiating discussion about sexuality issues with the patient. Unpicking PLISSIT helps in understanding its usefulness in practice. To successfully use PLISSIT, nurses should aim to achieve ASK. Attitudes, levels of knowledge and interpersonal skills in communication are fundamental in undertaking assessment utilising PLISSIT.

P = permission

'Permission' encourages discussion and gives legitimacy to discuss aspects of sexuality that are important to the patient. This requires nurses to have good interpersonal skills, to help to put the patient at their ease and feel comfortable. It provides an arena for early identification of any problems – knowing that cancer affects sexuality gives the nurse the permission to ask questions. Similarly, it gives the patient permission to ask for help and not to fear embarrassed responses from nurses. It is always important to establish the patient's goals. Soon after diagnosis is made and treatment commenced, discussions on sexuality should start and continue throughout treatment (Lamb 1995). Nurses are in a unique position to initiate this discussion.

LI = limited information

This step helps to dispel any misconceptions or myths about treatment and its effects on sexuality. It enables accurate information to be given to the patient to allow them to make informed decisions and requires nurses to be knowledgeable about treatment effects and their effects on sexuality. It has been found that patients prefer to have information on sexuality from nurses rather than being referred to a specialist (Schover 1993).

SS = specific suggestions

Specific suggestions can include: finger dilation, use of vaginal dilators, use of foreplay, hand–foot massage, bathing together and 'planning ahead'. Vaginal narrowing can sometimes be helped by vaginal dilators, used in conjunction with a lubricant or contraceptive cream. Regular intercourse also helps to widen the vagina. There has been some suggestion that Viagra may be useful to raise sexual desire and arousal in women and possibly aid in achieving an orgasm (Cancer BACUP 2004). Viagra in men has been used to attain an erection, but is contraindicated in the presence of cardiac dysfunction. Making specific suggestions may be difficult for some nurses but should not be ignored. Nurses who lack confidence or knowledge to provide individuals with specific suggestions should ensure that the patient is able to access that information from other sources.

IT = intensive therapy

This step requires referral for expert specialist support. Depending on the problem, the referral may be to a clinical psychologist, sex therapist or genitourinary specialist.

REFLECTION POINT

What advice can you give about reducing vaginal dryness? Do you have enough knowledge to advise on erectile dysfunction? If not, where can you access this information?

To utilise PLISSIT in the practice setting, both the nurse and the patient need to be in what could be termed the 'comfort zone'. This is about providing privacy, establishing a trusting relationship and ensuring confidentiality. It is essential that the nurse does not show signs of boredom or over-react. For example, a patient who is homosexual and asks the question: 'When can I have sex with my partner?' should not be met with a shocked response.

There is a need to develop and build a rapport with the patient – moving from less sensitive to more sensitive issues helps to build that rapport. In this environment, useful information can be ascertained from the patient in a non-threatening way. An example of such an approach can be found in McPhetridge (1968). A set of questions such as:

- Has the cancer or its treatment interfered with you being a mother/father, husband/wife/partner?
- Has cancer or its treatment changed the way you see yourself as a man/woman?
- Has cancer or its treatment caused any change in your sexual function/sex life since you left hospital?

The first two questions do not mention sex, but the answers could indicate any concerns regarding sexuality issues in a way that is not embarrassing to either party.

Contraception should always be advised regardless of the gender of the patient for at least 2 years whilst they are undergoing chemotherapy/radiotherapy. Anecdotal evidence suggests that contraception should continue 2 years post-treatment to reduce teratogenic damage to the fetus. Female patients who use the contraceptive pill should be advised that emesis and diarrhoea reduce contraceptive efficacy.

Barrier methods used effectively can be useful and, in conjunction with a spermicidal cream, can help to moisten the vagina. Anecdotal evidence has suggested that female partners of male patients have complained of vaginal irritation following sexual intercourse whilst their partner has been on chemotherapy, hence the use of condoms or Femidom will reduce that discomfort. If the patient wants to have sexual intercourse but experiences pain, suggesting a lubricant or a change of position could be helpful.

OTHER MEASURES TO ENHANCE SEXUALITY

Hair loss can adversely affect body image and sexuality; wearing a good-quality wig can help to boost self-confidence. The effect of hair loss for adolescent boys cannot be underestimated. It is sometimes taken for granted that hair loss is not such a significant problem for males as it is for females; however, adolescent years are image-forming and hair is as important to boys as it is to girls – their feelings about alopecia should be discussed with them.

Gentle exercise has been indicated as being helpful in restoring well-being owing to the release of endorphins. Exercise can also help to reduce fatigue (a common debilitating symptom), which is cumulative and long-term, reducing desire or a positive view of self (Winningham et al 1994, Tompkins-Stricker et al 2004). Keeping a diary of activities can help individuals to identify how to plan their day and begin to give them some degree of control (see Chapter 22).

Pain can be soul-destroying and increases feelings of anxiety and tiredness. Effective analgesia, and, if appropriate and safe to offer, complementary therapy could be encouraged to increase the quality of life.

Providing dietary and nutritional advice is important for several reasons: first, to aid recovery from cancer treatment and to help to replenish lost nutrients through emesis, diarrhoea and nausea; second, maintaining or increasing body weight can help to give a more positive body image and therefore help with enhancing sexuality.

It is important to remind the patient and their partner that hugging, holding hands and kissing are as important as sexual intercourse in improving self-confidence and maintaining intimacy.

That nurses need to appreciate and understand the cultural, religious and ethnic issues of their patient population that impact on sexuality is also fundamental. A male nurse for example calling orthodox Muslim women 'darling' or 'dear' would be inappropriate behaviour.

CONCLUSION

All patients – regardless of age, gender, marital status, religion, race, ethnicity – must be given the opportunity to discuss issues around sexuality. The challenge is for nurses to acquire, develop and continue to enhance their skills, confidence and competence in this vitally important aspect of the patient's life. Sexuality is difficult but not impossible to discuss – time taken to enhance skills in this aspect of care would be hugely beneficial to the patient.

DISCUSSION QUESTIONS	1. How do attitudes to sexuality affect the way care is delivered in your workplace?
	2. What support is available to help patients with sexuality issues, in both the voluntary and health sector?
	3. How can you and your colleagues integrate sexuality into your nursing assessment?

References

Anon J 1976 The P-LI-SS-IT models. Journal of Sex Education Therapy 2:1–15

Baguley I, Broker C 1990 Schizophrenia and sexual functioning. Nursing Standard 4(39):34–37

Barton D, Wilwerding M B, Hill A M 2004 Libido as part of sexuality in female cancer survivors. Oncology Nursing Forum 31(3):599–609

Brooker C 2002 Churchill Livingstone Dictionary of Nursing, 18th edn. Churchill Livingstone, Edinburgh

Brown H G, Tai-Seale M 1992 Vocational rehabilitation of cancer patients. Oncology Nursing Forum 8(3): 190–201

Brown M 2001 Nurses attitudes towards talking about sexuality with haemato-onclogy patients. Unpublished thesis. Thames Valley University, London

Brown M 2003 Psychological impact of undergoing bone marrow transplant for sickle cell disease: parents and childrens' experiences. Unpublished thesis. Thames Valley University, London

Burnard P 1999 Counselling skills for health care professionals. Stanley Jones, Gloucester

Cancer BACUP 2004 Some solutions to sexual problems caused by cancer and its treatment. http://www. cancerbacup.org.uk/resourcessupport. Accessed January 2005

Crounch S 1999 Sexual health 1: sexuality and nurses' role in sexual health. British Journal of Nursing 8(9):601–606

Faulkner A, Regnard C 1994 Talking to cancer patients and their relatives. Oxford University Press, Oxford

Ferrell B M, Dow K, Leigh S, Ly J, Gulasekaram P 1995 Quality in long-term cancer survivors. Oncology Nursing Forum 22(6):915–922

Gamel C, Davies B, Hengevald M 1993 Nurses' provision of teaching and counselling on sexuality a review of the literature. Journal of Advanced Nursing 18:1219–1227

Heath H 2002 Sexuality in later life. In: Heath H, White I (eds) The challenge of sexuality in health care. Blackwell Science, Oxford

Hughes M 1996 Sexuality issues: keeping your cool. Oncology Nursing Forum 22(10):1597–1600

Jenkins D, Price B 1996 Dementia and personhood: a focus for care? Journal of Advanced Nursing 42(1):84–90

Kantz D D, Dickey C A, Stevens M N 1990 Using research to identify why nurses do not meet established sexuality nursing care standards. Journal of Nursing Quality Assurance 43(3):63–78

Lamb M A 1995 Effects of cancer on the sexuality and fertility of women. Seminars in Oncology Nursing 11:120–127

Lewis S, Bor R 1994 Nurses knowledge and attitudes towards sexuality and the relationships of these with nursing practice. Journal of Advanced Nursing 20:251–259

McPhetridge I 1968 Nursing history: one means to personalized care. American Journal of Nursing 68:68–75

Nelson Jones R 1999 Introduction to counselling skills. Sage, London

Ofman U S, Auchincloss S S 1992 Sexual dysfunction in cancer patients. Current Opinions in Oncology 4:605–613

Platzer H 1990 Sexual orientation: improving care. Nursing Standard 4(39):31–34

Powe B 1992 Cancer fatalism among elderly Caucasian and African-Americans. Seminars in Oncology Nursing Forum 8(3):202–211

Price B 1990 Body image: nursing concepts and care. Prentice Hall, London

Rafferty D 1995 Putting sexuality on the agenda. Nursing Times 91(17):28–32

Reid J, Cubin P, Whiting B 1989 Lecture notes on clinical haematology. Blackwell Science, Oxford

Royal College of Nursing 2000 Sexuality and sexual health in nursing practice. RCN, London

Schover L R 1993 Sexual rehabilitation after treatment for prostate cancer. Cancer 7:1024–1030

Shell J 1995 Do you like the things that life is showing you? The sensitive self-image of the person with cancer. Oncology Nursing Forum 22(6):907–911

Smith D B, Babaian R J 1992 The effects of treatment for cancer on male fertility and sexuality. Cancer Nursing 15(4):271–275

Thompson J 1990 Sexuality: the adolescent and cancer. Nursing Standard 6(4):26–28

Tompkins-Stricker C, Drake D, Hoyer K A, Mock V 2004 Evidence based practice for fatigue management: exercise as an intervention. Oncology Nursing Forum 31(5):963–976

Waterhouse J 1996 Nursing practice related to sexuality: a review and recommendations. Nursing Times 1(6):412–418

Whedon M, Stearns D, Mills L E 1995 Quality of life of long term adult survivors of autologous bone marrow transplantation. Oncology Nursing Forum 22(2):1527–1544

Winningham M L, Nail L M, Burke M B et al 1994 Fatigue and the cancer patient experience. The state of knowledge. Oncology Nursing Forum 21:31–36

Further reading

Crounch S 1999 Sexual health 2: an overt approach to sexual education. British Journal of Nursing 8(10):669–675

Useful article to aid self-assessment on sexuality and provides a template for lecturers to incorporate sexuality into the curriculum.

Heath H, White I (eds) 2002 The challenge of sexuality in health care. Blackwell Science. Oxford

A very comprehensive insight with practical applications on sexuality issues.

Kelsey S 2005 Improving nurse communication skills with the cancer patient. Cancer Nursing Practice 4(2):27–29

This article stresses the significance of effective communication and provides examples of various approaches to communication.

Chapter 22

Fatigue

Shirley Crofts

KEY POINTS
- Fatigue is the most commonly reported symptom of cancer and cancer therapy.
- Severe fatigue is reported more frequently by individuals with haematological cancers than by those with solid tumours.
- Fatigue is a multidimensional, subjective experience.
- The impact of fatigue is often misperceived by health-care professionals.
- Fatigue is often poorly addressed by health-care professionals.
- Further research examining causes, effects and effective interventions for fatigue specifically related to haematological cancers is required.

INTRODUCTION

In recent years fatigue has become recognised as an extremely common problem for people with cancer, impacting significantly on quality of life and interfering with normal daily activities. Multiple disease- and treatment-related factors have been implicated in the occurrence, severity and prevalence of cancer-related fatigue. It is perceived to be multidimensional and can be described in terms of perceived energy, mental capacity, and psychological status.

Research into cancer-related fatigue is gaining momentum but the phenomenon remains incompletely understood. Much of the fatigue research has been undertaken with women with breast cancer or with mixed groups of cancer patients, some of which include individuals with haematological cancers (mainly lymphomas). However, a small number of studies focus on fatigue associated with bone marrow transplant (BMT) and haematological cancers. Individuals with haematological cancers are often treated with high-dose, multimodal or biological therapies that are thought to increase the severity and prevalence of fatigue (Ream & Richardson 1999). Severe fatigue also tends to be more frequent in individuals with haematological cancers (Cleeland & Wang 1999) and fatigue is shown to persist in survivors of BMT following completion of treatment (Knobel et al 2000). An understanding of fatigue, its impact and management is therefore crucial to haemato-oncology nurses. This chapter outlines the causes and effects of fatigue and explores assessment and management strategies.

DEFINING FATIGUE

Fatigue is a universal experience (Valdres et al 2001). Most people will have experienced fatigue at some point in their lives. However, for most healthy individuals it is a short-lived experience with rapid onset and short duration, usually follows exertion and is relieved by rest (De Jong et al 2002). Cancer-related fatigue is a different experience affecting the totality of the individual, which does not improve with rest or sleep and is frequently of an extended nature (Ancoli-Israel et al 2001). It is poorly defined and understood, and is a subjective experience which patients express in a variety of ways, using terms such as tired, weak, exhausted, weary, worn-out, lethargic, fatigued, depressed, unable to concentrate, bored, sleepy, heavy, or slow. Likewise, health professionals struggle to describe fatigue, using terms such as asthenia, fatigue, lassitude, prostration, exercise intolerance, lack of energy, and weakness.

Various definitions of fatigue have been offered. Holley (2000) suggests that cancer-related fatigue has a more rapid onset, is more intense, longer lasting and interferes with normal functioning. The difference between general fatigue and cancer-related fatigue is demonstrated by the struggle cancer patients have completing everyday tasks.

Stone et al (1998, p 1670) highlight the multidimensional aspects of fatigue and define fatigue as a: 'subjective state characterised by feelings of weariness and decreased capacity for physical or mental work. There is an objective decrease in physical or mental performance with repeated or prolonged activity'. Miaskowski & Portenoy (1998, p 1) illustrate the chronic nature of cancer-related fatigue and define it as: 'a prolonged debilitating fatigue that is persistent or relapsing lasting weeks, and is not anticipated to end soon. The tiredness of fatigue is not helped by rest'. However, this definition ignores the specific, subjective experience of fatigue and the feelings associated with it.

Following a concept analysis, Ream & Richardson (1996, p 527) suggested 'cancer-related fatigue is a subjective, unpleasant symptom, which incorporates total body feelings ranging from tiredness to exhaustion creating an unrelenting overall condition, which interferes with individuals' ability to function in their normal capacity'. Patients complain of having no energy and find it difficult to do even simple everyday tasks. This definition appears to have been accepted widely in the fatigue literature, although Atkinson et al (2000, p 152) have more recently defined fatigue as: 'an unusual persistent, subjective sense of tiredness related to cancer or cancer treatment that interferes with usual functioning'.

Although these definitions differ, there does appear to be some consensus that cancer-related fatigue is subjective, multidimensional, prolonged, unrelieved by rest and affects the ability to complete normal everyday activities.

PREVALENCE OF FATIGUE

Fatigue is a common symptom at diagnosis for many individuals with lymphomas and chronic myeloid leukaemia (Savage et al 1997, Wang et al 2002). It is also the most commonly reported symptom of cancer and cancer therapy (Portenoy et al 1994a, Miaskowski & Portenoy 1998). Prevalence estimates of fatigue experienced by cancer patients during radiotherapy and chemotherapy range from 60% to 96% (Devlin et al 1987, Irvine et al 1991, Smets et al 1993, Vogelzang et al 1997).

Severe fatigue has been reported more frequently by patients with haematological cancers than by patients with solid tumours (Cleeland & Wang 1999). However, studies demonstrating the prevalence of fatigue in individuals with haematological cancers are limited. One study demonstrated severe fatigue in 61% of individuals with acute leukaemia, 47% with chronic leukaemia and 46% with non-Hodgkin's lymphoma (NHL) (Wang et al 2002). Fatigue has also been shown to persist after completion of treatment. A further study of Hodgkin's disease survivors found that fatigue persisted for 6 months or longer in 26% of participants with older patients (aged 60–74 years) reporting the highest levels (Loge et al 2000).

Other studies have examined the prevalence of fatigue following BMT for a variety of haematological cancers including lymphoma and chronic myeloid leukaemia (Andrykowski et al 1990, Belec 1992, Molassiotis & Morris 1999, Knobel et al 2000, So et al 2003). The length of time post-BMT varies between studies and ranges from 2 months to 11.5 years post-transplant (Knobel et al 2000). Prevalence rates range from 15% to 79%. Other studies examining quality of life following BMT or in survivors of haematological cancers have also found fatigue to be one of the most common side effects (Bush et al 1995, Molassiotis et al 1995, 1996, Molassiotis 1999).

While further research is required to determine the prevalence of fatigue in individuals with haematological cancers, these studies indicate that fatigue is a significant problem and one that may persist for a lengthy period of time after completion of treatment.

CAUSES OF FATIGUE

There is a paucity of research examining the causes of fatigue in haematological cancers specifically. However, numerous factors are known to contribute to fatigue in individuals with cancer generally. Causative factors include biological, physiological, psychological and situational aspects. However, relationships between these factors, their role in the development of fatigue and the biological mechanisms of fatigue are complex and remain incompletely understood.

BIOLOGICAL AND PHYSIOLOGICAL CAUSES

Various underlying mechanisms related to cancer itself have been implicated as causes of fatigue including the release of substances from malignant cells, most notably cytokines or antibodies (Portenoy & Itri 1999). Cytokines such as interleukin (IL1) and tumour necrosis factor (TNF) produced by the tumour have been linked with structural or functional abnormalities in muscle tissue including muscle loss and changes in contractility (Baracos et al 1983, Bruera & MacDonald 1988, St Pierre et al 1992).

Increased metabolic processes as a result of tumour growth and imbalance in energy intake and expenditure frequently encountered in cancer and its treatment have also been suggested as causes of fatigue (Richardson 1995, Gutstein 2001). Pathophysiological mechanisms associated with malnutrition, cachexia and infection are also thought to be related to these processes.

Cancer treatments such as radiotherapy and chemotherapy inducing cell lysis and necrosis of the tumour mass with subsequent release of intracellular products and metabolites have also been suggested as causes of fatigue (Richardson 1995). The type of treatment may also impact on fatigue. In one study more than 75% of patients receiving chemotherapy and 65% of patients receiving radiotherapy experienced fatigue (Stone 2002). Fatigue is also known to be a dose-limiting side effect of biological therapies such as interferon alpha, commonly used in the treatment of some haematological cancers (Cortes et al 1996). High-dose and combination treatments have also been shown to increase fatigue (Fobair et al 1986, Woo et al 1998) and these findings are particularly relevant to individuals with haematological cancers who are likely to receive these treatments.

Fatigue is a well-documented side effect of anaemia – an almost inevitable consequence of haematological cancers and their treatment. Combined with cardiorespiratory and muscular changes, anaemia can significantly reduce work capacity; therefore patients require a higher degree of effort to perform their usual tasks. The resulting increments in metabolic rate and energy consumption produce tiredness and fatigue with normal daily activities. To reduce fatigue, patients may avoid physical exertion and reduce their activity level. The resulting physical inactivity induces muscle wasting and so further reduces performance. A vicious cycle of inactivity and fatigue is thus created (Dimeo et al 1999).

Other factors associated with fatigue include age, gender, cultural influences, type and stage of disease, endocrine, gonadal and biochemical changes such as low albumin levels (Cortes et al 1996, Knobel et al 2000, De Jong et al 2002, Wang et al 2002, So et al 2003). However, findings vary between studies and remain inconclusive. Concurrent illness, medications such as opioids, sedatives and blood transfusions, and other symptoms such as pain, nausea, and sleep disturbance are also associated with fatigue – although the cause and effect relationship between symptoms has yet to be established and further research is required (Gaston-Johansson et al 1999, Jacobsen et al 1999, Bower et al 2000, Ancoli-Israel et al 2001, Wang et al 2002).

PSYCHOLOGICAL CAUSES

Psychological theories of fatigue have been linked with stress. The reticular activating system (RAS) is involved in the stress response. Stimulation of RAS controls thinking, perception and consciousness and when RAS is inhibited fatigue is thought to result (Aisters 1987). Inhibition of RAS can occur in two ways: as a result of lowered sensory input due to such things as immobility or isolation leading to passive inhibition, or activity is reduced due to chronic stimulation resulting from pain or anxiety and leading to active inhibition (Aisters 1987).

Fatigue has also been conceptualised as a response to the continual stress inflicted by multiple physiological, psychological and situational factors related to the disease and its treatment (Aisters 1987). Energy stores are thought to be depleted as the individual, with no opportunity to restore energy, copes with these stressors on a continual basis. It is suggested that the initial reaction to stress is alarm in which stress hormones are released and the organism aroused (Selye 1976). Over time these reserves are depleted but to prevent this happening the parasympathetic nervous system activates the conservation withdrawal system, which causes feelings of fatigue to inhibit physical activity.

Attentional fatigue

Fatigue is frequently associated with difficulties in concentrating, directing attention, remembering things, keeping dates straight or solving problems (Curt et al 2000). This is often referred to as attentional fatigue

(Cimprich 2003). The ability to focus attention requires mental effort, and thus has limited capacity. Prolonged demands requiring directed attention can lead to fatigue, with subsequent loss of concentration (Cimprich 2003). Individuals may feel easily overwhelmed, and have difficulty organising their daily activities and meeting deadlines. Activities that were once automatic may require greater effort than usual.

Attentional fatigue may be caused by use of ineffective coping strategies to endure high levels of stress over a prolonged period of time. Blesch et al (1991) suggest that the mental effort required to cope with the intense and competing demands imposed by a diagnosis of cancer may lead to attentional fatigue.

Conversely, impaired cognitive function and mood disorders may also cause fatigue. Fatigue, anxiety and depression frequently co-exist. Depression is a common problem, with the overall rate of major depression in cancer patients being two to three times that of the general population (Valentine & Meyers 2001). One of the symptoms of depression is fatigue, and chronic fatigue may be one of the causal factors of depression (De Jong et al 2002). The relationships between these symptoms and cause and effect mechanisms are unclear. It is, however, suggested that depression and fatigue may both result from identical biological factors (Hayes 1991). It is also possible that patients associate increased fatigue with a deterioration in their condition, which subsequently results in increased anxiety and depression.

It is clear that fatigue is a multifactorial phenomenon and individuals with haematological cancers are likely to have multiple causal factors throughout the course of their disease and treatment.

TIMING OF FATIGUE

Studies have investigated the timing of fatigue particularly in relation to cancer treatments. Following chemotherapy, no standard pattern of fatigue can be identified and it appears to be dependent on factors such as diagnosis, chemotherapy regimen and method of drug administration (Richardson et al 1998). Different patterns identified include fatigue dramatically increasing with the start of chemotherapy while the level of fatigue remains fairly constant over treatment cycles (Jacobsen et al 1999), an increased level of fatigue 48 hours after receiving chemotherapy (Berger 1998, Schwartz 2000), then reducing mid-cycle, suggesting a roller-coaster pattern (Berger & Farr 1999).

Some patients receiving radiotherapy have reported increased prevalence and intensity in fatigue over time (Morrow et al 2002), suggesting the cumulative effects of the radiation therapy were related to the experience of fatigue. However, this is not consistent across all studies. Molassiotis (2000) found a pattern of highs and lows occurring every 3–4 days with lows corresponding with subsequent sessions of radiotherapy and fatigue persisting after treatment.

Fatigue has been shown to increase over the course of allogeneic BMT for breast cancer, although results were not statistically significant (Hann et al 1999). It is not known whether similar patterns of fatigue are experienced by individuals treated with BMT for haematological cancers.

This brief overview of studies would suggest that the onset and timing of fatigue in relation to treatment varies. Although there is little doubt that fatigue is a significant problem for many patients both during and after treatment, further research specific to haematological cancers and BMT is required.

EFFECTS OF FATIGUE

Fatigue can be all encompassing, affecting all aspects of life (Table 22.1). The effects interact with each other and generally are self-reinforcing, making fatigue difficult to change and treat. Fatigue impacts negatively on quality of life equal to or in excess of that of pain (Vogelzang et al 1997). It has been ranked as the symptom most affecting quality of life (Curt et al 2000) and been associated with decisions to delay or refuse treatment (Nerenz et al 1982).

Physical fatigue results in a decrease in energy levels, physical performance and activities, and reduces the ability to undertake the tasks of daily living. It also impacts on social and behavioural activities such as taking exercise, shopping, socialising and spending time with friends (Curt et al 2000). Fatigue has been found to impair walking ability, normal work and enjoyment of life in patients with acute leukaemia to a much greater extent than those with chronic leukaemia or NHL (Wang et al 2002). Employment status may also be affected, with individuals stopping work altogether, claiming disability allowance or using unpaid leave as a result of fatigue (Curt et al 2000). Fatigue also impacts on caregivers who may be forced to take time off work, take unpaid leave or even stop work completely because of their relative's fatigue (Curt et al 2000, Stone et al 2003).

Table 22.1
Effects of fatigue

Physical	Psychological	Social
Weakness	Sadness and depression	Difficulties in caring for the family
Somnolence	Irritability	
Need to rest	Impaired thinking	Unable to socialise
Trouble starting and finishing tasks	Mood disturbance	Unable to do household chores
Anorexia	Loss of control	Unable to work
Difficulty walking more than short distances	Hopelessness	Difficulties with preparing food
Difficulty climbing stairs	Loneliness	
Difficulty in caring for self, and dependency on another person	Isolation	Difficulties in interpersonal relationships and intimacy with partner
Shortness of breath	Lack of concentration	
Pain	Unable to enjoy life	
	Anxiety	

Fatigue has been found to be more strongly associated with psychological distress than symptoms such as nausea and vomiting (Nerenz et al 1982). Decreased motivation or interest and feelings of sadness, frustration and irritability may occur (Curt et al 2000). The combined effects of fatigue on activities of daily living and psychological wellbeing have been found to further compromise quality of life (Molassiotis 1999).

Fatigued individuals with acute leukaemia have reported greater impairment of mood, thinking abilities and relationships than those with chronic leukaemia or NHL (Wang et al 2002). Prolonged fatigue of over 6 months' duration has also been shown to result in higher levels of anxiety in individuals with Hodgkin's disease (Loge et al 2000). Perhaps not unsurprisingly, severe fatigue towards the end of treatment with allogeneic BMT for breast cancer has been associated with an increase in depressive symptoms and anxiety (Hann et al 1999). However, further research is required to establish whether this pattern of anxiety and depression is also experienced by those undergoing allogeneic BMT for haematological cancers.

PERCEPTIONS OF HEALTH-CARE PROFESSIONALS

The impact of fatigue on patient's lives is generally underestimated by health-care professionals, despite the increasing literature on the topic (Vogelzang et al 1997, Miller & Kearney 2001). Vogelzang et al (1997) found that although patients and oncologists agreed on the presence of significant fatigue in 75% of patients they disagreed on its importance – 61% of patients reported that fatigue affected their life more than pain, whereas 61% of oncologists believed that pain was the greater problem. Conversely, health-care professionals have been found to overestimate the impact of fatigue on some aspects of patients' lives (Stone et al 2003).

One explanation for these differences in opinion is that patients do not report fatigue to health-care professionals. Reasons for non-reporting include patients perceiving that fatigue is something to be endured as a normal part of cancer treatment, that nothing can be done to treat it, not wanting to complain to the doctor, not wanting to take medication for treating fatigue and failure on the part of health-care professionals to offer any interventions for fatigue (Passik et al 2002, Stone et al 2003). Treatment of fatigue is therefore frequently neglected (Vogelzang et al 1997, Stone et al 2003). These findings clearly indicate the importance of communication and involving individuals in the identification and assessment of their problems. Health-care professionals should take the initiative in discussing fatigue with patients – holistic assessment is the first step in addressing these issues.

ASSESSMENT

As fatigue is a subjective sensation, it should be assessed using self-report measures (Stone 2002). An increasing number of fatigue scales are

Box 22.1   Examples of assessment instruments measuring the psychological aspects associated with fatigue

- The profile of mood status (Short form) (POMS-SF) (McNair et al 1992)
- Symptom checklist SCL-90 (Yoshitake 1971)
- Fatigue scale from the Profile of Mood States (POMS-F) (McNair et al 1992)

Box 22.2   Examples of assessment instruments measuring the physical aspects of fatigue

- Symptom Assessment Scale (SAS) (Sutherland et al 1988)
- The Memorial Symptom Assessment Scale (MSAS) (Portenoy et al 1994b)

becoming available – this in itself often makes it difficult to decide which scale is the most appropriate. The choice of the instrument depends on the purpose for which the information is required. Some scales are unidimensional and measure fatigue severity (Portenoy & Itri 1999). Unidimensional instruments tend to focus on either psychological or physiological aspects and were not developed specifically to measure fatigue (Boxes 22.1 and 22.2). Multidimensional scales are broader and measure symptom quality and severity of fatigue. Examples of fatigue assessment scales are shown in Table 22.2.

Unidimensional scales are faster to complete and score, suggesting that they may be more suitable for clinical practice but as they only focus on one aspect they may not provide all the required information. A good measure needs to be multidimensional as fatigue is a complex phenomenon influenced by both physical and psychological factors. To gain an accurate picture of the impact of fatigue the assessment tool needs to encompass all these different aspects.

Assessment of fatigue by nurses has been found to be poor in clinical settings, with minimal documentation and poor review (Miller & Kearney 2002). Assessment tools are not widely used (Knowles et al 2000, Miller & Kearney 2001, 2002). Knowles et al (2000) suggest that this may be because most fatigue scales have been developed for research purposes and their degree of usefulness in clinical practice has yet to be determined. To be useful in practice a questionnaire needs to be capable of being completed within a few minutes and easily scored so results are readily available. Any assessment instrument also needs to be reliable and valid. However, development of reliable and valid measurement instruments is compromised by the lack of agreement on a definition of cancer-related fatigue (Richardson & Ream 1998). Further research is required to identify an assessment tool that is useful in

Table 22.2
Fatigue assessment scales

Scale	Description
Fatigue subscale of functional assessment of cancer therapy (FACT-F) (Yellen et al 1997)	13-item unidimensional questionnaire. 5-point Likert scale.
Revised Piper fatigue scale (PFS) (Piper et al 1998)	22-item multidimensional questionnaire. Four subscales: behavioural/severity, affective meaning, sensory and cognitive/mood. 11-point numerical rating scale.
Fatigue symptom inventory (FSI) (Hann et al 1998)	13-item multidimensional questionnaire. Three subscales: intensity, duration and interference with daily living. 11-point numerical rating scale.
Brief fatigue inventory (BFI) (Mendoza et al 1999)	9-item unidimensional questionnaire measuring fatigue intensity. Three items on severity and six items on interference with daily living. 11-point numerical rating scale.
Multidimensional fatigue inventory (Smets et al 1995)	20-item multidimensional questionnaire. Five subscales: general fatigue, physical fatigue, reduced activity, reduced motivation and mental fatigue. 5-point Likert scale.

practice. However, without a reliable assessment tool it is difficult to accurately assess the severity of fatigue experienced by an individual.

An alternative approach to assessment is the use of patient diaries. Patients record in the diary their level of fatigue each day, either in their own words or, more commonly, by using a simple rating scale to record the severity of fatigue. Richardson et al (1998) highlighted the value of this technique in capturing the patterns of fatigue in cancer patients and suggest that only by establishing the intensity and variation of fatigue can individualised interventions be planned.

REFLECTION POINT   Cancer-related fatigue is all encompassing for the patient and impacts on all aspects of their life. Any management strategy needs to address the individual's total situation. Small changes in one area may reap big changes in other areas. Consider how fatigue is assessed and managed in your area of practice.

MANAGEMENT AND TREATMENT OF FATIGUE

Individuals with cancer frequently perceive fatigue is not well managed with very few being offered any symptomatic relief or treatment by health-care professionals (Curt et al 2000, Stone et al 2000). The most common advice given in these studies was to increase rest and relaxation. Blood transfusion, nutritional advice and drug treatments were also recommended. However, no attention was given to correcting any underlying aetiologies or co-morbidities (Curt et al 2000).

For the person with a haematological cancer, fatigue is likely to be a chronic problem without return to earlier levels of functioning (Aisters 1987). Treating fatigue and improving functioning wherever possible are therefore vital. Reversible causes of fatigue such as pain, anorexia, infection, anaemia, depression, difficulties with sleeping and dyspnoea should be identified and treated (Mock 2001, Coackley et al 2002).

REVERSIBLE CAUSES OF FATIGUE

Anaemia

Blood transfusions can improve wellbeing in the short term and may quickly improve feelings of shortness of breath and fatigue. The effects may last between 2–6 weeks depending on whether chemotherapy is also given during this time. For patients with non-myeloid malignancies, subcutaneous erythropoietin (a naturally occurring hormone that acts as a haematological growth factor) given 1–3 times a week can achieve a longer lasting and more consistent rise in haemoglobin levels (Glaspy et al 1997, Demetri et al 1998, Gabrilove et al 1999). Consequently reduced levels of fatigue and improvements in energy levels and quality of life result.

Erythropoietin has only been investigated in the management of chemotherapy-related anaemia, and its role in the wider management of cancer-related fatigue has not yet been evaluated. It is unclear which patients would benefit most from therapy, or whether blood transfusion would be equally efficacious. Use of erythropoietin remains restricted due to the high perceived cost of treatment, most economic studies suggesting it is not cost-effective (Marchetti & Barosa 2004). However, economic evaluations are limited and further research is needed (Bokemeyer et al 2004).

Thyroid dysfunction

Hypothryroidism may occur as a consequence of total body irradiation used in conditioning treatment for BMT (see Chapter 13) and is easily corrected by the administration of thyroxine.

Interferon

Interferon is part of the treatment regime for several haematological cancers but can contribute to fatigue. Stopping interferon will stop the neurochemical insult that is the primary cause of symptoms experienced. However, an inability to tolerate interferon would necessitate a change in treatment.

Antidepressant therapy

Depression in cancer patients is often underdiagnosed and undertreated (Portenoy & Itri 1999). Antidepressants with more activating characteristics (i.e. fluoxetine, bupropion) may be good choices for depressed patients with significant fatigue because in addition to treating depression their stimulant properties counteract fatigue (Valentine & Meyers 2001).

Corticosteroids

Small doses of steroids have been used to increase energy in individuals with cancer although their effectiveness in treating fatigue has not been evaluated in clinical trials. Prednisolone and dexamethasone are most widely used. In clinical practice they are often prescribed for their non-specific effects on appetite, mood and energy levels (Stone 2002).

COPING WITH FATIGUE

Many individuals with cancer feel that fatigue is just something they have to live with and little can to be done to control it (Stone et al 2000). Aisters (1987) suggests that the goal of nursing care is the promotion of patient's adaptation or adjustment to the condition. Helping individuals to adjust is an important concept in haemato-oncology and emphasis should be placed on empowering patients to take control of their lives through education and the facilitation of self-care and independence. Assisting individuals to develop coping strategies for fatigue is likely to contribute to individual feelings of wellbeing and may help to promote adaptation. However, it should be noted that most suggested interventions used for fatigue have not been thoroughly evaluated.

Providing information and education about illness, treatment and side effects can help to improve coping and reduce stress. If patients know to expect fatigue, they are likely to be less distressed when it occurs and better prepared to cope (Mock 2001). Providing information that enables the patient to view symptoms as a normal part of their treatment rather than a sign of disease progression has been shown to be beneficial (Johnson et al 1988).

INFORMATION AND EDUCATION

Nurses have a vital role in helping individuals to cope with fatigue by providing information and support. However, Miller & Kearney (2002) found that leaflets and information sheets on fatigue were rarely used or available. They suggested that one potential explanation for this is that nurses do not feel adequately trained in the area of fatigue management. It is therefore vital that both nurse education and increasing the provision of written information are addressed as a matter of urgency if patient support is to be improved.

Advice on diet and nutrition may help to improve nutritional status and thereby also help to reduce fatigue. Advice may include avoiding substances that contribute to fatigue such as narcotics, sleeping pills, alcohol and caffeine (Aisters 1987). A multidisciplinary approach to fatigue management is therefore important.

REDUCING EMOTIONAL STRESS

Reducing emotional stress and anxiety may also help to reduce fatigue. Interventions that may decrease stress and anxiety and promote coping include counselling, relaxation, reframing, meditation, time management, support group participation, guided imagery, distraction and hypnosis (Mock 2001). Psychotherapeutic interventions may also help to reduce fatigue by reducing reliance on catastrophising and promoting adaptive coping strategies (Mock 2001). Diversional activities such as games, reading, crafts or participation in sport may help to promote relaxation (Mock 2001).

REDUCING ATTENTIONAL FATIGUE

Relaxation training may help to develop sustained attention. Attentional fatigue may also be helped by restorative therapy. Cimprich (1993) suggests that activities relating to regular natural environment experiences, such as gardening, sitting in a park or bird-watching helped to improve concentration and problem solving. These activities may not be very practical in a haemato-oncology inpatient setting. However, many individuals have windows in their hospital rooms. Encouraging them to observe what is happening in the outside world through the window for short periods of time each day may help to improve attention span and concentration.

Increasing numbers of haemato-oncology patients are being treated as day cases or outpatients and such restorative activities may be of benefit to them. However, for an activity to have restorative qualities it needs to catch the interest easily, involve a change from usual routines and be enjoyable (Cimprich 2003). The challenge for haemato-oncology nurses is to help individuals to find such an interest.

ENERGY CONSERVATION

Energy conservation and activity management are frequently suggested as means of coping with fatigue. Common suggestions to conserve energy include taking naps, going to bed earlier, keeping busy to take your mind off fatigue (Mock 2001). However, these suggestions should be used with caution as taking naps during the day may compromise the quality of night-time sleep and further contribute to fatigue (Ancoli-Israel et al 2001). Decreasing physical activity is a natural response to fatigue. Yet, over time this leads to reduced functional capacity and a decrease in ability to tolerate exercise and normal activity, which in turn increases fatigue (Mock et al 1997). While resting is important, it needs to be combined with practical strategies such as setting priorities in activities and roles, delegating tasks and exercise (Mock 2001).

Completing a diary will help individuals to work out when they have most energy. This information can then be discussed with nurses to plan an activity/rest programme that meets their individual needs and conserves energy while using available energy effectively. Times of peak energy should be used efficiently, e.g. preparing meals in the morning when people often have most energy. A planned routine frees the person from non-essential decisions that consume time and energy (Mock 2001). Activities need to be spaced out and rest periods can be scheduled at critical points such as before or after meals. Building and drawing on support systems are important as delegating tasks such as shopping can conserve energy (Mock 2001). However, it must be remembered that what one patient finds useful may be of no benefit to another.

Case study 22.1

Barbara is a 72-year-old lady recently diagnosed with myeloma who is being treated with 4 days of melphalan every 4–6 weeks. However, her haemoglobin is falling with each course of melphalan and she is feeling totally exhausted. She spends most of her time at home sitting in a chair, as she has no energy to help her husband around the house. She complains of being unable to sew or read and feels very low in mood.

At her last visit to the hospital Barbara's haemoglobin level was 7.6 g/dL and she was feeling quite hopeless about her situation. Barbara was transfused with 3 units of packed cells. It was also suggested that she kept a diary to help establish when she has more energy with a view to increasing her involvement in the house or doing a task that gives her some pleasure. Barbara was relieved to find out there might be something that could be done to improve her fatigue. Keeping the diary helped her to feel that she was gaining back some control over her life and this helped her to feel more hopeful for the future.

EXERCISE

There is evidence to suggest that individuals with cancer may benefit from exercise behaviours similar to those advocated for the general public (Coleman et al 2003). Lower levels of activity appear to show a positive relationship with fatigue. Regular exercise has also been shown to improve mood states and reduce depression and anxiety by increasing endorphins and improving sleep quality.

Exercise is one of the few tested interventions that have reliably demonstrated the ability to decrease fatigue levels in patients receiving cancer therapy (de Jong et al 2002). Exercise has been shown to increase the distance that individuals can walk after treatment and, in comparison to a control group, significantly improve patterns of fatigue, anxiety, depression and sleeping difficulties (Mock et al 1997).

These results need to be interpreted with caution as most studies have focussed on breast cancer patients and for the most part have included relatively fit people. However, a small study has been undertaken with individuals with myeloma (Coleman et al 2003). Results indicate that an exercise programme for patients receiving aggressive treatment may be feasible and effective in reducing fatigue. However, further studies of the benefits of exercise on fatigue levels need to be undertaken with people with haematological cancers. Physical condition and appropriateness of exercise for individuals needs to be discussed with the multidisciplinary team before exercise is recommended.

Interventions for fatigue need to be developed for individual patients. A multimethod programme is likely to be the most effective including information and education, energy conservation, planned activity and exercise, stress reduction strategies and nutritional counselling (Knowles et al 2000).

Case study 22.2

Tom is a 40-year-old man with CML. Before he was diagnosed he was a soldier and a keen sportsman. He has just undergone an allograft involving both total body irradiation and high-dose chemotherapy. He is recovering well post-transplant but is very worried and frustrated by low energy levels. At times he displays angry outbursts. What could you do to help him?

CONCLUSION

Fatigue is a common problem for patients with cancer and one that is often not well addressed by health-care professionals. It is an aspect of practice that requires further development in both practice and research. Research is required to determine the extent of the problem for those with haematological cancers and the effectiveness of management strategies including exercise programmes. However, accurate assessment, correction of reversible contributing factors, information and education, advice and support on energy conservation and using the natural restorative environment may help to reduce fatigue. Managing fatigue requires a multidisciplinary approach; however, numerous opportunities exist for nurses to lead practice development initiatives and act as key facilitators in developing integrated fatigue management programmes.

DISCUSSION QUESTIONS

1. What are the fatigue-related educational needs of haemato-oncology nurses?

2. What information do patients and their caregivers require about fatigue?

3. How could assessment and management of fatigue be improved?

References

Aisters J 1987 Fatigue in the cancer patients: a conceptual approach to a clinical problem. Oncology Nursing Forum 14(6):25–30

Ancoli-Israel S, Moore P J, Jones V 2001 The relationship between fatigue and sleep in cancer patients: a review. European Journal of Cancer Care 10(4):245–255

Andrykowski M A, Altmaier E M, Barnett R L et al 1990 The quality of life in adult survivors of allogenic bone marrow transplantation: correlates and comparisons with matched renal transplant recipients. Transplantation 50:399–406

Atkinson A, Barsevick A, Cella D et al 2000 National Comprehensive Cancer Network Practice guidelines for cancer related fatigue. Oncology 14(11A Suppl 10):151–161

Baracos V, Rodermann H, Dinarello C, Goldber A 1983 Stimulation of muscle protein degeneration and prostaglandin E_2 release by leukocytic pyrogen (interleukin-1). New England Journal of Medicine 308:553–558

Belec R H 1992 Quality of life: perceptions of long term survivors of bone marrow transplantation. Oncology Nursing Forum 19:31–37

Berger A M 1998 Patterns of fatigue and activity and rest during adjuvant breast cancer chemotherapy. Oncology Nursing Forum 25(1):51–62

Berger A M, Farr L 1999 The influence of daytime inactivity and nighttime restlessness on cancer-related fatigue. Oncology Nursing Forum 26(10):1663–1671

Blesch K S, Paice R W, Wickham R et al 1991. Correlates of fatigue in people with breast and lung cancer. Oncology Nursing Forum 18:81–87

Bokemeyer C, Aapro M S, Courdi A et al 2004. EORTC guidelines for the use of erythropoietic proteins in anaemic patients with cancer. European Journal of Cancer 40(15):2201–2216

Bower J E, Ganz P A, Desmond K A et al 2000 Fatigue in breast cancer survivors; occurrence, correlates and impact on quality of life. Journal of Clinical Oncology 18(4):743–753

Bruera E, MacDonald R N 1988 Asthenia in patients with advanced cancer. Journal of Pain and Symptom Management 3:9–14

Bush N E, Haberman M, Donaldson G, Sullivan K M 1995 Quality of life of 125 adults surviving 6–18 years after bone marrow transplantation. Social Science and Medicine 40:479–490

Cimprich B 1993 Developing an intervention to restore attention in cancer patients. Cancer Nursing 16:83–92

Cimprich B 2003 An environmental intervention to restore attention in women with newly diagnosed breast cancer. Cancer Nursing 26(4):284–293

Cleeland C S, Wang X S 1999 Measuring and understanding fatigue. Oncology 13:91–97

Coackley A, Hutchinson T, Saltmarsh P et al 2002 Assessment and management of fatigue in patients with advanced cancer: developing guidelines. International Journal of Palliative Nursing 8(8):381–388

Coleman A E, Coon S, Hall-Barrow J et al 2003 Feasibility of exercise during treatment for multiple myeloma. Cancer Nursing 265(5):410–419

Cortes J, Kantarjian H, O'Brien S et al 1996. Results of interferon-alpha therapy in patients with chronic myelogenous leukaemia 60 years of age and older. American Journal of Medicine 100(4):452–455

Curt G A, Breitbart W, Cella D et al 2000 Impact of cancer-related fatigue on the lives of patients: new findings from the Fatigue Coalition. The Oncologist 5:353–360

de Jong N, Courtens A M, Abu-Saad H H et al 2002 Fatigue in patients with breast cancer receiving adjuvant chemotherapy: a review of the literature. Cancer Nursing 25(4):283–297

Demetri G D, Kris M, Wade J et al 1998 Quality of life benefit in chemotherapy patients treated with epoietin alfa is independent of disease response or tumour type: results from a prospective community oncology study. Journal of Clinical Oncology 16:3412–3425

Devlin J, Maguire P, Phillips P et al 1987 Psychological problems associated with diagnosis and treatment of lymphomas. British Medical Journal 295:953–957

Dimeo F C, Stieglitz R D, Novelli-Fischer U et al 1999 Effects of physical activity in the fatigue and psychological status of cancer patients during chemotherapy. Cancer 85(10):2273–2277

Fobair P, Hoppe R, Bloom J, Cox R, Varhese A, Speigel D 1986 Psychosocial problems among survivors of Hodgkin's disease. Journal of Clinical Oncology 4:805–814

Gabrilove J L, Einhorn L, Livingston R B et al 1999 Once weekly dosing of epoietin alpha is similar to three times weekly dosing in increasing haemoglobin and quality of life. Proceedings of American Society of Clinical Oncologists 18(57a):2216

Gaston-Johansson F, Fall-Dickson J M, Bakos A B et al 1999 Fatigue, pain and depression in pre-auto transplant breast cancer patients. Cancer Practice 7(5):240–247

Glaspy J, Bukowski R, Steinberg D et al 1997 Impact of therapy with epoietin alfa on clinical outcomes in patients with nonmyeloid malignancies during cancer chemotherapy in community oncology practice. Journal of Clinical Oncology 15(3):1218–1234

Gutstein H B 2001 The biologic basis of fatigue. Cancer 92(6 Suppl):1678–1683

Hann D M, Jacobsen P B, Azzarello L M et al 1998 Measurement of fatigue in cancer patients: development and validation of the Fatigue Symptom Inventory. Quality of Life Research 7(4):301–310

Hann D M, Garovoy N, Finkelstein B et al 1999 Fatigue and quality of life in breast cancer patients undergoing autologous stem cell transplantation: a longitudinal comparative study. Journal of Pain and Symptom Management 17(5):311–319

Hayes J 1991 Depression and chronic fatigue in cancer patients. Primary Care 18:327–339

Holley S 2000 Cancer related fatigue – suffering a different fatigue. Cancer Practice 8(2):87–95

Irvine D, Vincent L, Bubela N et al 1991 A critical appraisal of the literature investigating fatigue in the individual with cancer. Cancer Nursing 14:188–199

Jacobsen P B, Hann D M, Azzarello L M et al 1999 Fatigue in women receiving adjuvant chemotherapy for breast cancer: characteristics, course and correlates. Journal of Pain and Symptom Management 18(4):233–242

Johnson J, Nail L, Lauver D et al 1988 Reducing the negative impact of radiation therapy on functional status. Cancer 61:46–51

Knobel H, Loge J H, Nordøy T et al 2000 High level of fatigue in lymphoma patients treated with high dose therapy. Journal of Pain and Symptom Management 19(6):446–456

Knowles G, Borthwick D, McNamara S et al 2000 Survey of nurses' assessment of cancer related fatigue. European Journal of Cancer Care 9(2):105–113

Loge J H, Abrahamsen A F, Ekeberg Ø, Kaasa S 2000 Fatigue and psychiatric morbidity among Hodgkin's disease survivors. Journal of Pain and Symptom Management 19(2):91–99

Marchetti M, Barosa G 2004 Clinical and economic impact of epoietins in cancer care. Pharmacoeconomics 22(16):1029–1045

McNair D, Lorr M, Droppleman L 1992 Profile of mood states manual, revised edn. Education and Industrial Testing Service, San Diego

Mendoza T R, Wang X S, Cleeland C S et al 1999 The rapid assessment of fatigue in cancer patients: use of the Brief Fatigue Inventory. Cancer 865(5):1186–1196

Miaskowski C, Portenoy R K 1998 Update on the assessment and management of cancer-related fatigue. Principles and Practice of Supportive Oncology Updates 1(2):1–10

Miller M, Kearney N 2001 Nurses' knowledge and attitudes towards cancer-related fatigue. European Journal of Oncology Nursing 5(4):208–217

Miller M, Kearney N 2002 Institutional management of cancer-related fatigue: a comparison of clinical specialities. European Journal of Oncology Nursing 6(1):45–53

Mock V 2001 Fatigue management: evidence and guidelines for practice. Cancer 92(6 Suppl):1699–1707

Mock V, Dow K H, Meares C J et al 1997 Effects of exercise in fatigue, physical functioning, and emotional distress during radiation therapy for breast cancer. Oncology Nursing Forum 24(6):991–1000

Molassiotis A 1999 A correlational evaluation of tiredness and lack of energy in survivors of haematological malignancies. European Journal of Cancer Care 8(1):19–25

Molassiotis A 2000 Fatigue patterns in Chinese patients receiving radiotherapy. Recent Advances and Research Updates 1(2):81–88

Molassiotis A, Morris P 1999 Quality of life in patients with chronic myeloid leukaemia after unrelated donor bone marrow transplantation. Cancer Nursing 22(5):340–349

Molassiotis A, Boughton J H, Bourgoyne T et al 1995 Comparison of the overall quality of life in 50 long-term survivors of marrow transplantation. Journal of Advanced Nursing 22:509–516

Molassiotis A, van den Akker O B A, Milligan D W et al 1996 Quality of life in long-term survivors of marrow transplantation: comparison with a matched group receiving maintenance chemotherapy. Bone Marrow Transplantation 17:249–258

Morrow G R, Andrews P L R, Hikok J T et al 2002 Fatigue associated with cancer and its treatment. Supportive Care in Cancer 10:389–398

Nerenz D R, Leventhal H, Love R R 1982 Factors contributing to emotional distress during cancer chemotherapy. Cancer 50:1020–1027

Passik S D, Kirsh K L, Donaghy K et al 2002 Patient-related barriers to fatigue communication: initial validation of the Fatigue Management Barriers Questionnaire. Journal of Pain and Symptom Management 24(5):481–493

Piper B F, Dibble S L, Dodd M J et al 1998 The revised Piper Fatigue Scale: psychometric evaluation in women with breast cancer. Oncology Nursing Forum 25(4):677–684

Portenoy R K, Itri L M 1999. Cancer-related fatigue: guidelines for evaluation and management. The Oncologist 4:1–10

Portenoy R K, Thaler H T, Kornblith A B et al 1994a Symptom problems, characteristics and distress in a cancer population. Quality of Life Research 3:183–189

Portenoy R K, Thaler H T, Kornblith A B et al 1994b The Memorial Symptom Assessment Scale: an instrument for the evaluation of symptom prevalence, characteristics and distress. European Journal of Cancer 30A:1326–1336

Ream E, Richardson A 1996 Fatigue: a concept analysis. International Journal of Nursing Studies 33(5):519–529

Ream E, Richardson A 1999 From theory to practice: designing interventions to reduce fatigue in patients with cancer. Oncology Nursing Forum 26(8):1295–1303

Richardson A 1995 Fatigue in cancer patients: a review of the literature. European Journal of Cancer Care 4(1):20–32

Richardson A, Ream E 1998 Recent progress in understanding cancer-related fatigue. International Journal of Palliative Nursing 4(4):192–198

Richardson A, Ream E, Wilson-Barnett J 1998 Fatigue in patients receiving chemotherapy. Patterns of change. Cancer Nursing 21:17–30

Savage D G, Szydlo R M, Goldman J M 1997 Clinical features at diagnosis in 430 patients with chronic myeloid leukaemia seen at a referral centre over a 16 year period. British Journal of Haematology 96:111–116

Schwartz A L 2000 Daily fatigue patterns and effects of exercise in women with breast cancer. Cancer Practice 8(1):16–24

Selye H 1976 The stress of life. McGraw-Hill, New York

Smets E M, Garssen B, Schuster-Uitterhoeve A L et al 1993 Fatigue in cancer patients. British Journal of Cancer 68(2):220–224

Smets E M, Garssen B, Bonke B et al 1995 The Multidimensional Fatigue Inventory (MFI): psychometric qualities of an instrument to assess fatigue. Journal of Psychosomatic Research 39(3):315–325

So W K, Dodgson J, Tai J W 2003 Fatigue and quality of life among Chinese patients with haematologic malignancy after bone marrow transplantation. Cancer Nursing 26(3):211–219

Stone P 2002 The measurement, causes and effective management of cancer related fatigue. International Journal of Palliative Nursing 8(3):120–128

Stone P, Richards M, Hardy L 1998 Fatigue in patients with cancer. European Journal of Cancer 34(11): 1670–1676

Stone P, Richardson A, Ream E et al on behalf of the Cancer Fatigue Forum 2000 Cancer related fatigue: inevitable, unimportant and untreatable? Results of a multi-centre patient survey. Annals of Oncology 11: 1–5

Stone P, Ream E, Richardson A et al 2003 Cancer-related fatigue – a difference of opinion? Results of a multicentre survey of healthcare professionals, patients and caregivers. European Journal of Cancer Care 12:20–27

St Pierre B, Kasper C, Lindsey A 1992 Fatigue mechanisms in patients with cancer: effects of tumor necrosis factor and exercise on skeletal muscle. Oncology Nursing Forum 19:419–425

Sutherland H J, Walker P, Till J E 1988 The development of a method of determining oncology patients' emotional distress using linear analogue scales. Cancer Nursing 11:303–308

Valdres R U, Escalante C, Manzullo E 2001 Fatigue – a debilitating symptom. Nursing Clinics of North America 36(4):685–694

Valentine A D, Meyers C A 2001 Cognitive and mood disturbance as causes and symptoms of fatigue in cancer patients. Cancer 92(6 Suppl):1694–1698

Vogelzang N J, Breitbart W, Cella D et al 1997 The fatigue coalition patient, caregiver and oncologist perceptions of cancer-related fatigue: results of a tripart assessment survey. Seminars in Haematology 34:4–12

Wang X S, Giralt S A, Mendoza T R et al 2002 Clinical factors associated with cancer-related fatigue in patients being treated for leukaemia and non-Hodgkin's lymphoma. Journal of Clinical Oncology 20(5):1319–1328

Woo B, Dibble S L, Piper B F et al 1998 Differences in fatigue by treatment methods in women with breast cancer. Oncology Nursing Forum 25(5):915–920

Yellen S B, Cella D F, Webster K et al 1997 Measuring fatigue and other anaemia related symptoms with the Functional Assessment of Cancer Therapy (FACT) measurement system. Journal Pain and Symptom Management 13(2):63–74

Yoshitake H 1971 Relation between the symptoms and the feelings of fatigue. Ergonomics 14:175–186

Further reading

Cimprich B 2003 An environmental intervention to restore attention in women with newly diagnosed breast cancer. Cancer Nursing 26(4):284–293

This article offers advice on how to make major changes in attentional fatigue using very simple methods. It seems applicable to all areas of fatigue and may be useful to both nurses and patients.

Chapter **23**

Psychological issues

Mandy Ellis, Clare Woodcock, Elizabeth Rawlings and Linda Bywater

KEY POINTS

- Psychological distress is common in patients with haematological cancers.
- The psychological impact of a haematological cancer affects the patient and each member of their family.
- Nurses play a key role in minimising psychological effects and enhancing coping.
- Promoting psychological wellbeing should be a focus of clinical practice.

INTRODUCTION

As previous chapters have indicated, haematological cancers are often of acute onset with a diagnosis made shortly after symptoms occur. Symptoms can be very general and frequently do not hint at the seriousness of the underlying condition. The diagnosis itself must be considered a major traumatic event and the patient is subsequently bombarded with complex information regarding their disease, its treatment and clinical trials while undergoing an array of medical interventions. Making treatment decisions can be challenging and bewildering for patients in this situation, especially as in many cases treatment needs to be instigated very quickly, resulting in unpleasant side effects and periods of hospitalisation. Following treatment a patient's future remains uncertain and the long-term effects of treatment may persist.

In view of this process of events, patients and their families are required to develop strategies to enable them to make decisions and cope with their situation. Some of these strategies will be more successful than others and unsuccessful adjustments may result in psychological morbidity (Nezu et al 1999). The way in which an individual makes decisions and copes with any stressful stimulus will depend on their personality, previous experience, social network and the nature of the stimulus. This chapter outlines psychological issues, discusses some of the factors affecting psychological morbidity and suggests how nurses can attempt to provide care that takes account of psychological issues.

STRESS AND STRESS RESPONSES

Throughout their lives individuals have to deal with events and stressful situations. Stress is the perception that events being experienced are injurious to physical or psychological wellbeing (Atkinson et al 2000). Stressors are by their nature traumatic, uncontrollable, unpredictable or involve change or conflict. The diagnosis of a haematological cancer fulfils nearly all of these characteristics and can be considered a major stressor. Some of the adverse effects of stress are (Atkinson et al 2000):

- anxiety
- depression
- aggression
- cognitive impairment.

Anxiety is the emotional response to excessive stress and is characterised by worry, apprehension, fear, tension and a feeling of isolation (Atkinson et al 2000). In its most extreme form it can result in panic attacks with associated palpitations, arrhythmias, hyperventilation and dizziness.

Depression is associated with negative thinking, having no feelings of hope, being unable to derive any pleasure from life. Once again it leads to social isolation, lack of concentration, apathy, the inability to relate to others and loss of concentration. It can lead to withdrawal, regression and ultimately suicide (Valente & Saunders 1997).

Other stress responses include anger and aggression when someone perceives that they are being blocked from achieving their goals. If the source of the stress cannot be addressed, these responses may be misdirected towards others. Stress can also hamper concentration, memory and cognitive ability and may be manifested as a lack of concentration, an inability to make decisions and a poor memory; these can be exacerbated by insomnia, which is common in people under psychological pressure.

Individuals are exposed to numerous stressors when faced with a life-threatening illness and attempt to adapt by using coping mechanisms.

COPING

Watson et al (1988) identified five broad coping styles in adjustment to cancer that can be helpful in understanding individual reactions to diagnosis:

1. denial/avoidance
2. fighting spirit – I am not going to let this beat me
3. acceptance/fatalism – this is something I am just going to have to live with
4. helplessness/hopelessness – there is nothing I can do
5. anxious preoccupation.

Some of these coping styles are considered more successful than others in protecting against psychological morbidity, e.g. fighting spirit. Denial can be both a positive and negative coping mechanism. Temporary denial of life-threatening illness may provide time to enable individuals to adapt and come to terms with their condition and prognosis. Denial can therefore be necessary to maintain psychological health in times of stress (Morley 1997). Nurses should acknowledge and understand such denial, which is often short in duration and usually moves on to a state of acceptance (Morley 1997). However, protracted denial can cause practical problems as appropriate planning for the future may be hampered (Murray-Ross et al 1992).

A helpless/hopeless response is associated with the development of depression whereas anxious preoccupation is thought to reinforce existing anxiety (Little et al 1998).

Factors that influence positive coping include learned behaviour from previous experience, marital satisfaction, religious resources, good problem-solving abilities and higher educational attainment (Dunkel-Schetter et al 1992, Nezu et al 1999, Weihs et al 1999, Gall et al 2000, Bourjolly & Hirschman 2001).

Social support is also thought to positively influence coping and includes: general socialising providing distraction, increasing self-esteem, receiving advice and the feeling of being loved. As an integral part of social support next-of-kin play a vital role in enhancing coping for patients with cancer (Lobchuk & Degner 2002).

HOPE

Hope and coping are closely related. Hope is the expectation of achieving realistic future goals of significance to the individual (Dufault & Martocchio 1985). Hope can be focussed on long-term goals such as survival or short-term targets such as being able to achieve a task or improve symptom control. Hope has been identified by patients as one of the most important elements when living with cancer (Ballard et al 1997). The level of hope held by patients has been found to be stable and unrelated to prognosis or the cancer experience (Nowotny 1991, Ballard et al 1997, Herth 2000). Facilitating the maintenance of realistic hope in some way, irrespective of individual circumstances, is therefore clearly very important in maintaining psychological health.

SPIRITUALITY

Many people have some fundamental spiritual belief that is often used by individuals to help them to cope with cancer. Living with cancer often increases an individual's awareness of their spiritual self (Taylor 2003).

> 'Faith can provide a framework for finding meaning and perspective through a source greater than self. Faith provides a sense of control over feelings of helplessness along with the natural social support of community.'
>
> (Weaver et al 2001, p 2)

Studies have indicated that there is a positive correlation between hope, coping, quality of life and family life in patients and their families who have a faith (Swensen et al 1993, Ballard et al 1997, Weaver et al 2001). Spiritual resources used to cope with illness include prayer – individually, with others, or being prayed for (Soderstrom & Martinson 1987, VandeCreek et al 1999). However, spirituality involves the attempt to find meaning from a situation and may or may not involve defined religious beliefs.

DECISION–MAKING

Nurses may play quite a unique role in supporting patients in this respect. By building dialogue with their patients, nurses can begin to understand how patients view themselves as individuals, what is important to them, and how their relationships with others may affect their decisions and their ability to then live with those decisions during their treatment and beyond.

REFLECTION POINT
Decision-making is rarely a simple rational response to purely factual information – think of all the factors that may affect even simple everyday decisions in your own life.

In very intense or even life-threatening situations many factors may influence patients' choices. Bywater & Atkins (2001) demonstrate that decisions to undertake very complex haematological treatments such as bone marrow transplant can be based upon a wide variety of contextual factors and idiosyncratic reasoning. How health-care professionals present treatment information can also, sometimes inadvertently, affect patients' decisions. Getting to know patients and helping them to think through information in the context of their own lives can therefore be an important aspect of good psychological care and support.

Of course, this type of support does not end with decision-making. Increasing numbers of patients are surviving haematological cancers and the focus of patient care now encompasses the psychological care and support of patients throughout their treatment and longer-term survival.

FACTORS AFFECTING PSYCHOLOGICAL MORBIDITY

DISEASE

Psychological symptoms may result from the underlying disease. Lymphoma and leukaemia can affect the central nervous system, leading to confusion, poor concentration or agitation. Acute confusion may result from electrolyte imbalance such as hypercalcaemia in patients with myeloma. Physiological causes of psychological symptoms must be investigated, as these symptoms should resolve quickly with effective treatment.

DIAGNOSIS

Adapting to a diagnosis of a haematological cancer is, quite clearly, a traumatic process. The acute onset of some haematological cancers leads to a rapid commencement of treatment and individuals have little opportunity to adjust to their situation. They are also bombarded with information that is difficult to assimilate due to its complexity and unfamiliarity.

People carry with them beliefs about a cancer diagnosis. For many the diagnosis of a haematological cancer is a death sentence (Woods et al 1989) and they may find it difficult to formulate any realistic hope of a positive outcome. Fear and anxiety is a normal response to such a diagnosis and patients are likely to feel vulnerable and out of control. Some patients will attempt to regain control by seeking as much information as possible, others will avoid engagement in this way, preferring to delegate responsibility to professionals or family members (Link et al 2004). This period is the beginning of the adaptation process. The manner in which the diagnosis is given to a patient is likely to enhance or hinder this adaptation process (Cancer Services Collaborative 2004) – the role of nurses in delivering significant news is crucial.

TREATMENT

Following diagnosis the patient becomes immersed in the bewildering environment of the hospital where they have to adjust to a new lifestyle and a new language. Health-care workers often underestimate the amount of unfamiliar terms used when talking to patients. Individuals have instantly exchanged the familiar and controllable with the unfamiliar and uncontrollable, leading to high levels of anxiety.

REFLECTION POINT   Take some time to observe care being carried out in your clinical area. How often are terms used that may be unfamiliar to patients? You may find this exercise quite revealing.

Treatment itself produces an array of physical symptoms that impede the patient's ability to adapt to their circumstances. Common treatment-related symptoms associated with chemotherapy, e.g. nausea and fatigue, can have a devastating impact on quality of life and affect cognitive function. Other factors that can affect the psychological response to treatment include alterations in body image, challenges to identity, pain and anticipatory nausea and vomiting.

Steroid–induced psychosis

High-dose steroids commonly used in the treatment of many haematological cancers can produce a range of psychological symptoms. In most cases these are mild effects such as:

- insomnia
- agitation
- mood swings
- memory impairment
- psychomotor retardation
- euphoria.

However, in some cases patients may develop severe psychosis, indicated by depression, mania, paranoia or hallucinations (Watson 1991). These patients need urgent psychiatric assessment, as they are at risk of self-harm.

Females are more susceptible to psychiatric toxicity from steroids with incidence being strongly dose-related, particularly when the drugs are given in a single dose (Lewis & Smith 1983). Symptoms are usually acute in onset and become evident within 2 weeks of treatment commencing. In most cases the symptoms are reversible and will subside as the dose is reduced. As steroids cannot be stopped abruptly, haloperidol is useful to ameliorate symptoms without causing excessive sedation.

Although severe psychiatric problems are rare, many patients will experience minor symptoms. Nurses need to make a careful assessment of patients' symptoms, observing for signs of agitation, euphoria and sleeplessness. Providing patients with information about the more common effects can help them to make sense of how they feel and reduce anxiety; it is particularly relevant to ensure that relatives are alerted to potential changes in mood, so that they are aware of what to expect and can communicate significant problems to the clinical team.

Anticipatory nausea and vomiting

With the development of better pharmacological control, vomiting may be a less common effect of treatment. However, nausea is exacerbated by anxiety and remains a significant problem (Roscoe et al 2000, Matteson et al 2002). Owing to the effect of anxiety on nausea, approaches to emetic control need to address psychological issues. Anxiety associated with treatment can be manifested as anticipatory nausea and vomiting, and can be triggered by visits to the hospital or smells associated with their treatment (see Chapter 17).

Pain

Pain can be a common problem in this group of patients, and may be acute, resulting from specific procedures or disease processes, or chronic, as experienced by many suffering from myeloma. Psychological factors can interact with physical factors and there is a close correlation between levels of pain experienced and anxiety (Turk & Fernandez 1991). Anxiety heightens the activity of the sympathetic nervous system, resulting in muscle tightening and the release of pain-producing substances. It is clear, therefore, that effective pain control should focus on analgesia coupled with anxiety-reducing strategies.

It has been shown that providing patients with some control over their symptom management can be very successful (Holdroyd et al 1984). Bone marrow transplant patients with mucositis are commonly given intravenous morphine infusions, frequently using a patient-controlled analgesia device (PCA). However, a systemic review of the literature concluded that although PCAs are commonly used, there is no significant benefit over continuously infused morphine – although when a PCA is used, the amount of morphine used by the patient is less (Clarkson et al 2003).

Fatigue

Fatigue is an almost universal consequence of treatment for cancer; the psychological effects of fatigue that have been reported are feelings of uselessness, reliance on others affecting role perceptions, frustration and depression (see Chapter 22).

CHALLENGES TO IDENTITY

Our identity is a complex amalgam of our personality, background, experiences, self-image, role and values (Handy 1989). It is what defines us as individuals and includes the image we project and that which we keep hidden. The diagnosis and treatment of cancer challenges this identity on many levels and can lead to poor adjustment, resulting in a decline in quality of life or leading to psychological morbidity.

Many patients are parents and illness will inevitably disrupt family life as well as affect the role of a parent who is sick. Parents attempt to protect their children from the effects of the illness but this can drain them of the energy to cope with their disease (Schumacher & Meleis 1994). In a study by Elmberger et al (2002) focussing on fathers dealing with haematological cancers, the men saw themselves transformed from being strong and capable to weak and ill. Some changes in role were considered positive as fathers spent more time at home and were forced to re-evaluate their priorities in a way they found more rounded. Many families will experience financial difficulties as hospital appointments disrupt work patterns.

Case study 23.1

Peter is a 16-year-old who is having a matched, unrelated bone marrow transplant. His mother is staying with him in his room. At times Peter has found this reassuring but he has also found his mother's constant presence frustrating. His home is approximately 60 miles away from the hospital. His father, as well as working full-time, is responsible for the care of Peter's younger siblings. Peter's father and siblings are only able to visit at weekends. Peter has lots of school friends but is unable to see them. Some contact is maintained via the telephone. Peter is however finding these calls difficult, as some of his friends don't seem to know what to say to him.

Periods of neutropenia prevent individuals from mixing in large crowds and fear of infection may inhibit participation in usual activities. Those undergoing bone marrow transplant are often isolated for many weeks, and in some centres are advised to limit contact with family and friends. Studies have shown that this has an adverse effect on psychological wellbeing (Winters et al 1994, Gaskill et al 1997). Patients may experience loss of control, loss of independence and loss of role – the degree to which these are experienced has been shown to be influenced by the patients' physical wellbeing (Hengeveld et al 1988). Nurses can help patients to maintain a sense of control by giving them simple choices, e.g. furniture placement (Collins et al 1989).

A sensitive approach to managing the inpatient environment can help to preserve patients' individuality. Encouraging patients to maintain their usual routines and providing assistance when necessary will help them to feel better about themselves. Optimising privacy may also be important, and may be achieved by employing such simple measures as knocking before entering a patient's room. With the continuing evolvement of bone marrow transplant techniques, the need for complete isolation is being reconsidered in many centres, which may help to reduce the psychological impact of transplant.

Body image

One of the most obvious and frequently discussed psychological challenges is the alteration in body image that can result from a cancer diagnosis and subsequent treatment. Having cancer can alter the way someone feels about their body – in effect they can lose trust in it, it becomes hostile to them. An individual's body image informs the way they feel about themselves and the way they perceive others feel about them. It is closely linked to self-esteem and an adverse change in body image is likely to have an effect on how patients view themselves (Bello & McIntire 1995).

As body image is a perception of ourselves, so it may or may not be affected by actual changes in appearance (Bello & McIntire 1995). Factors that determine the effect of physical changes on appearance depend upon an individual's coping mechanisms and, crucially, their social support (Price 1990). Dewing (1989) identifies some of the stages a patient may go through when experiencing challenges to their body image:

- impact – the initial shock and anger
- retreat – a period of mourning for the loss
- adaptation – the patient can confront their problem, leading to acknowledgement and reconciliation.

Factors affecting body image

The disease itself may cause weight loss, pallor, bruising and the inability to carry out normal activities owing to pain or fatigue. Further factors include physical and psychological effects of treatment. Chemotherapy may require the presence of a central venous catheter, situated in intimate areas of the body, particularly around the breast area in women. The catheter serves as a constant reminder of illness, can make people feel squeamish and affect an individual's feeling of attractiveness to their partner (Daniels 1995).

Other side effects of treatment can have a negative influence on body image, the most obvious being alopecia. Freedman (1994) states that 'the loss of hair as a symbol of loss of self creates an alienation from the self and from others'. Indeed some patients have commented that when they look in the mirror they no longer recognise themselves. Hair loss can occur rapidly making adjustment difficult. Other treatment effects include weight gain and hirsutism associated with steroid therapy, dry skin, rashes, mucositis and diarrhoea.

Additional factors can exaggerate the physical changes that occur – patients who are feeling nauseated, fatigued or depressed are less able to make the most of their appearance. It is important that these physical symptoms are effectively managed, for example, through medication, education and support. Hospitalisation can interrupt the patient's usual hygiene or beauty routine and the sharing of hospital rooms and bathrooms affects privacy.

Any combination of these factors may reduce the patient's self-confidence and ability to engage in their normal social environment. The patient's ability to adjust to physical changes will depend on their general coping ability and the quality of their social network. However, nurses can assist patients through the stages identified by Dewing (1989), by providing good information at the start of treatment and support and empathy as physical changes occur. Commenting on positive aspects of a person's appearance is a simple way of increasing their self-esteem.

Sexuality

Sexuality is an integral part of identity that may be affected by a haematological cancer. Lamb (1996) estimated that 90% of cancer patients experience some problems associated with sexuality. Clearly an altered body image will have an effect on sexuality and treatment for haematological cancers may have an effect on sexual function such as loss of libido, impotence or vaginal fibrosis or dryness. Many patients will find these issues difficult to discuss in their consultations – gentle questioning may allow patients to discuss any concerns in this area.

Partners can feel inhibited from engaging in sexual activity for fear of causing harm to the patient, e.g. dislodging a central venous catheter or causing infection. This can lead to feelings of rejection and a further loss of self-worth. Once again the provision of good information and support can alleviate these effects as well as optimising communication (see Chapter 21).

Fertility

Treatment for haematological cancers may affect fertility and may have long-term consequences that will impact on quality of life and sexuality (see Chapter 20).

Case study 23.2

Charles, a 50-year-old man, has recently been diagnosed with acute myeloid leukaemia. He has a central venous catheter in situ and is receiving chemotherapy. Charles has noted the following changes to his body image:

- Hair loss. Charles is finding this difficult to cope with. He does not want to wear a wig, and has found it hard to find a hat that he is happy with. Charles reports that people whom he doesn't know react differently to him as

they make incorrect assumptions regarding his appearance.
- Central venous catheter. For Charles this serves as a constant reminder of his illness. He finds it difficult to look at and is unwilling to learn how to care for it at present.
- Sexuality. Charles is happily married and whilst in hospital has found it difficult to have privacy, including time alone with his wife. His wife is anxious not to pass on any infection to him and doesn't know how intimate they can be.

SURVIVORSHIP

Once treatment is completed, the patient has to undergo another period of adjustment. They need to re-establish their role and it is often at this point that the impact of their experience needs to be worked through – unfortunately this coincides with the time when they have less contact with hospital staff and previous sources of support. In spite of this, most will be able to pick up their lives and gradually the period of illness will fade. However, follow-up appointments, even years later, can stimulate a surge of anxiety as they are reminded of their illness and the fear of relapse is brought into sharp focus (Barraclough 1994).

REFLECTION POINT   Consider how a patient may feel on completion of treatment. What anxieties may they experience?

For many patients 'Survival is not simply the end of the story, it is the beginning of another, often troubled story' (Little et al 2000, p 502). As patients successfully complete their journey through treatment, it is important that they are given access to help and support to deal with the transition to survivorship; independent support groups may be particularly helpful at this time.

A significant group of patients will be living with long-term effects of their treatment. Physical changes in their appearance can be permanent – patients who have suffered alopecia may find that their hair grows back differently, scars from central lines can serve as permanent reminders of treatment, and chronic graft-versus-host disease often has an impact on an individual's appearance. Despite these physical changes current research suggests that quality of life is not adversely affected (Andrykowski et al 1995, Molassiotis 1997).

The fear of relapse may dominate some patient's lives with any symptom taking on great significance (Benner & Wrubel 1989). It is important to refer such patients for psychological support to enable them to regain some normality in their lives.

A significant issue facing families of those with haematological cancers is the search for potential sibling donors (see Chapter 24). In most cases siblings are extremely keen to volunteer to be screened as they see this as a way in which they can help their brother or sister (Christopher 2000). Those who are not matched can feel that they have let their sibling down. In families where relationships have broken down between siblings the donor search can be very traumatic and it is best to involve family mediators at the earliest opportunity.

PSYCHOSOCIAL CARE

Psychosocial care aims to lessen the emotional and social impact of cancer on patients and their families by reducing anxiety levels and improving adjustment (Watson 1991). There is also a requirement to detect psychological, psychiatric or social morbidity and ensure treatment is made available. Psychological techniques encourage the expression of feelings, promote a sense of control and allow patients to participate in their treatment.

The National Institute for Clinical Excellence (NICE) (2003) guidelines 'Improving Outcomes in Haematological Cancers' recognise the importance of providing psychosocial care with particular reference to the role of the clinical nurse specialist (CNS). This document recommends that the CNS has specific training in counselling, to combine specialist clinical skills and knowledge with the ability to support patients through the process of treatment and follow-up.

The provision of good psychosocial care has been shown to be beneficial to patients by reducing both psychological distress and physical symptoms through increasing quality of life, enhancing coping, and reducing levels of pain and nausea (Baider et al 2001), with a consequent reduction on demands for hospital resources (Watson 1991).

ASSESSMENT

Assessment is the first step in providing good psychological care. In order to assess the psychological status of patients it is important that nurses optimise the environment to maximise the exchange of information. This can be challenging in a busy ward or day clinic. The principle of assessment is to gain an understanding from the patient's perspective of their feelings and emotions. The use of open questions can elicit the most useful information regarding the individual's psychological status, coping strategies and support network. Gathering such information takes time; patients will often not reveal their greatest anxieties in the first discussions.

Psychosocial assessment should take cognisance of known risk factors for developing psychological morbidity including the individual's coping style, number of stressful life events, perceived loss of control, economic pressures and level and quality of social support.

When psychological wellbeing causes concern, it may be appropriate to use a formal assessment tool to gain more insight, e.g. the Hospital Anxiety and Depression Scale, a self-administered questionnaire with 14 questions (Zigmond & Snaith 1983). A score greater than 8 on either scale is indicative of a pathological state of either anxiety or depression. This scale has been well validated and widely used and serves as a useful tool for assessing patients.

INTERVENTIONS

A number of interventions are discussed below that can be used to diminish psychological symptoms.

Pharmacological treatments

Anxiolytics provide immediate relief from the feelings of anxiety; they are suitable treatments for short-term relief from symptoms until the stressor has passed or to allow for the return of effective problem solving. Anxiolytics are addictive if taken for an extended period, it is therefore important to ensure the underlying cause of the anxiety is addressed. Antidepressants have a role in the treatment of patients with haematological cancers under the supervision of a psychiatric service.

Counselling

Counselling aims to enable individuals to gain insight into their situation and develop problem-solving strategies. In some departments patients have access to professional counsellors but provision remains patchy and usually only the highest risk patients or those already displaying adjustment problems receive help. Nurses are in the unique position to provide support to all patients by using effective communication skills. However, time needs to be prioritised if this is to be successful.

Complementary care

Complementary care is viewed as treatment that runs alongside conventional medicine and helps to relieve stress and anxiety common to patients with cancer (McGinnis 1990). A range of techniques can be employed; these can be divided into two main groups – psychological and physical therapies.

Psychological therapies are aimed at helping people to cope with feelings of stress, anxiety and depression. They include relaxation techniques, stress management, visualisation and meditation. All these techniques can be learnt by patients and their family, and promoted by nurses, thereby increasing feelings of control and empowerment

Physical therapies usually involve professional therapists and include reflexology, massage, shiatsu, acupuncture and hypnotherapy. The benefit of these therapies tends to be short term as they are aimed at relieving symptoms, thereby reducing anxiety. However, they are reliant on the intervention of professional therapists rather than helping individuals to develop coping techniques.

Increasingly, patients are enquiring about the use of complementary therapies as a way of managing their symptoms and helping them to gain some sense of control over their treatment. One study found that 70% of cancer patients had considered using complementary therapies (Downer 1994). Therefore nurses need to ensure that they are aware of the role of complementary therapies and how they can be accessed as part of patient/family care.

Information

Good information and education provides individuals with a degree of control and reduces feelings of hopelessness (Fawzy et al 1995). Individual requirements for information vary widely and may be at odds with that desired by their friends and relatives. Some people clearly do not want much information and this can cause tension with health-care professionals' responsibility to ensure that patients give informed consent to treatment.

The Cancer Services Collaborative (CSC) 'Improvement Partnership' has recently published a framework to improve communication with cancer patients (CSC 2004). In the past, many patients have not received enough information to enable them to make decisions about their care. It is recommended that organisations should provide every patient and their carer with as much information as they need at each stage of their cancer journey (CSC 2004, NICE 2004). Information should be in an appropriate format and at a level that they can understand.

Patients who are feeling anxious will find it difficult to remember and process complex information. Information may need to be repeated many times and given in digestible chunks. Supporting verbal information with written information enables the patient to learn at their own pace but is no substitute for good verbal communication, which enables the patient to respond, ask questions, and feel the support of another person.

Having a family member with cancer also puts families under enormous pressure. Family members have to adjust to changes in roles, the stress response of the patient and the trauma of witnessing a loved one undergoing distressing treatments and side effects (see Chapter 24). Information requirements of family members may differ from those of the patient, however, and confidentiality issues must be borne in mind. Relatives may find support groups very useful and should be given details of how to contact such organisations (see Appendix).

Delivering significant news

The manner in which significant news is given can either assist individuals' adaptation or inhibit it. NICE (2003) recommends that staff undergo training to improve their skills in this area. Several factors need to be considered when planning to convey significant news to a patient:

1. Preparation – the individual conveying the news should ensure that they think through what they are going to say and there is time available.
2. Location – it is important to optimise the environment for the meeting so that it is comfortable, quiet and affords privacy.
3. Verbal communication – information should be given clearly, avoiding unfamiliar terminology. It is vital to assess the patient's requirement for additional information as too much or too little information can increase stress and anxiety (Osuna et al 1998).
4. Non-verbal communication – the information giver should sit in close proximity to the patient, maintain eye contact and have an open stance.
5. Active listening – the patient should be given the opportunity to respond to the news and have their feelings acknowledged, this can be achieved though paraphrasing what the patient says.
6. Closure – bringing the meeting to a close but providing the patient with the opportunity for a follow-up meeting and some written information to support what they have been told.

REFLECTION POINT

Try and remember an occasion when breaking significant news was done well. Why was this? Then try and remember a time when it didn't go well and why this was the case.

Patients report that health-care professionals are often focussed on imparting information rather than providing support and they are given little opportunity to respond (Ford et al 1996). The therapeutic effect of caring or 'being there' should not be underestimated and is a core element of nursing (Dunniece & Slevin 2000). Encounters with health professionals considered 'caring' have been shown to increase patients' feelings of wellbeing, sense of security and acceptance, and produce an internal sense of healing (Halldorsdottir & Hamrin 1997).

Use of touch

The use of touch can be very therapeutic but should be used sensitively as not everyone likes being touched. Bottorff et al (1995) describe two types of touch – comforting and connecting. Comforting touch is particularly effective in times of distress where it can help to reassure and calm patients and their family. Connecting touch is more commonly used when patients are not distressed as a way of reinforcing a connection with the patient/family. The hands, arms, back or legs are the most common sites utilised when offering comforting touch. Touch associated with connecting touch is usually light and shorter in duration and focussed on the hand or arm (Bottorff 1993).

Support groups

There has been a growth in support groups in recent years (Adamsen & Rasmussen 2001). Support groups come in all shapes and sizes and aim to meet different needs. Many of these groups have been established at local level to fulfil a particular need, such as patients in one centre deciding to join together to fill perceived gaps in the service provided by the treatment centre. Most often the identified gaps are in information and support. Support groups are informal and may or may not involve health-care professionals. Increasingly such groups are being organised at national level to provide telephone advice, support and written information, and to raise public awareness. These groups also play an important role in informing government policy.

Several studies have been carried out to investigate the benefits of involvement in support groups. Participants appear to gain mental strength, feel less isolated and learn more effective coping mechanisms (Gray et al 1997). They have also been shown to increase participants' activity levels, strengthen their self-perception and increase self-confidence (Adamsen & Rasmussen 2001). Hatch & Kickbusch (1983) felt that the primary role of support groups was to provide a framework for social networking, as they fulfil needs that family and friendship networks are unable to cope with sufficiently. Participation in support groups can also allow individuals to feel normal within the group, where they feel abnormal outside of it. Yet Bauman (1999) sounds a note of caution, suggesting that these groups may encourage individuals to become very inward-looking, resulting in over-dependence on the group and its members thus impoverishing other personal relationships. On balance, however, these groups do provide a vital role for some patients and relatives and contact details should be made available to allow people to make their own decisions about their benefits.

CONCLUSION

Nurses play an important role in supporting patients with haematological cancers and their families. By using good communication skills, and being aware of and utilising available resources nurses can help individuals to cope with diagnosis, treatment, adjusting to a new lifestyle, living with uncertainty and maintaining quality of life. To be effective it is essential that nurses recognise that each person is an individual going through a unique experience. During this experience, individuals have ongoing psychological needs that may change frequently. Recognising these needs and identifying the appropriate support and care can minimise psychological distress and enhance coping.

DISCUSSION QUESTIONS

1. An individual's coping strategy may be determined by several factors. In your nursing care, do you need to be aware of all factors?

2. Does an individual need to 'come to terms' with their illness? What does this actually mean?

3. Can you remember a patient who was in denial? How did you care for them and how did this make you feel?

4. Is there a role for the counsellor/psychologist/psychiatrist in the care of individuals with haematological cancers? If so, when and how would you decide that an individual was 'not coping' and needed support?

References

Adamsen L, Rasmussen J M 2001 Sociological perspectives on self-help groups: reflections on conceptualisation and social processes. Journal of Advanced Nursing 35(6):909–917

Andrykowski M A, Bruehi S, Brady M J, Henslee-Downey P J 1995 Physical and psychosocial status of adults one year after bone marrow transplantation: a prospective study. Bone Marrow Transplant 15(6): 837–844

Atkinson R L, Atkinson C A, Smith E E, Bem D J, Nolen-Hoeksema S 2000 Hilgard's introduction to psychology, 13th edn. Harcourt, Orlando

Baider L, Peretz T, Hadani P E, Koch U 2001 Psychological intervention in cancer patients: a randomised study. General Hospital Psychiatry 23:272–277

Ballard A, Green T, McCaa A, Logsdon C 1997 A comparison of the level of hope in patients with newly diagnosed and recurrent cancer. Oncology Nursing Forum 24(5):899–904

Barraclough J 1994 Cancer and emotion: a practical guide to psycho-oncology, 2nd edn. Wiley, Chichester

Bauman Z 1999 In search of politics. Polity Press, Cambridge

Bello L K, McIntire D 1995 Body image disturbances in young adults with cancer – implications for the oncology clinical nurse specialist. Cancer Nursing 18(2):138–143

Benner P, Wrubel J 1989 The primacy of caring: stress and coping in health and illness. Addison Wesley, Wokingham

Bottorff J L 1993 The use and meaning of touch in caring for patients with cancer. Oncology Nursing Forum 20(10):1531–1538

Bottorff J L, Gogag M, Engelberg-Lotzkar M 1995 Comforting: exploring the work of cancer nurses. Journal of Advanced Nursing 22(6):1077–1084

Bourjolly J N, Hirschman K B 2001 Similarities in coping strategies but differences in sources of support among African American and white women coping with breast cancer. Journal of Psychosocial Oncology 19:17–38

Bywater L, Atkins S 2001 Factors influencing patients' decisions to undergo BMT from a sibling or matched unrelated donor. European Journal of Oncology Nursing 5(1):7–17

Cancer Services Collaborative 'Improvement Partnership' 2004 Improving communication in cancer care. www.modern.nhs.uk/cancer/5629/Cancer%20Comms %20Sept04.pdf Accessed Dec 2004

Christopher K A 2000 The experience of donating bone marrow to a relative. Oncology Nursing Forum 27:693–700

Clarkson J E, Worthington H V, Eden O B 2003 Interventions for preventing oral mucositis for patients with cancer receiving treatment. The Cochrane Database of Systemic Reviews, Issue 3 Art No: CD000987. DOI: 10.1002/14651858.

Collins C, Upright C, Aleksich J 1989 Reverse isolation; what patients perceive. Oncology Nurses Forum 16:675–679

Daniels L E 1995 The physical and psychosocial implications of central venous access devices in cancer patients: a review of the literature. Journal of Cancer Care 4:141–145

Dewing J 1989 Altered body image. Surgical Nurse 2(4):17–20

Downer S 1994 Pursuit and practice of complementary therapies by cancer patients receiving conventional treatment. British Medical Journal 212:86–89

Dufault K, Martocchio B C 1985 Hope: its spheres and dimensions. Nursing Clinics of North America 20:379–391

Dunkel-Schetter C, Feinstein L G, Taylor S E, Falke R I 1992 Patterns of coping with cancer. Health Psychology 11:79–87

Dunniece U, Slevin E 2000 Nurses' experience of being present with a patient receiving a diagnosis of cancer. Journal of Advanced Nursing 32(3):611–618

Elmberger E, Bolund C, Lutzen K 2002 Men with cancer: changes in attempts to master the self-image as a man and as a patient. Cancer Nursing 25(6):477–485

Fawzy F I, Fawzy N W, Arndt L A, Pasnau R O 1995 Critical review of psychosocial interventions in cancer care. Archives of General Psychiatry 50:100–113

Ford S, Fallowfield L, Lewis S 1996 Doctor–patient interactions in oncology. Social Science and Medicine 42(11):1511–1519

Freedman T G 1994 Social and cultural dimensions of hair loss in women treated for breast cancer. Cancer Nursing 17(4):334–341

Gall T L, Miguez de Renart R M, Boonstra B 2000 Religious resources in long-term adjustments to breast cancer. Journal of Psychosocial Oncology 18:21–37

Gaskill D, Henderson A, Fraser M 1997 Exploring the everyday world of the patient in isolation. Oncology Nursing Forum 24(4):695–700

Gray R E, Fitch M, Davis C, Phillips C 1997 Interviews with men with prostate cancer about their self-help group experience. Journal of Palliative Care 13:15–21

Halldorsdottir S, Hamrin E 1997 Caring and uncaring encounters with nursing and healthcare from the cancer patient's perspective. Cancer Nursing 20(2): 120–128

Handy C B 1989 Understanding organisations. Penguin, Middlesex

Hatch S, Kickbusch I (eds) 1983 Self-help and health in Europe: new approaches in health care. World Health Organization, Copenhagen

Hengeveld M, Houtman R, Zwaan F 1988 Psychological aspects of bone marrow transplantation: a retrospective study of 17 long-term survivors. Bone Marrow Transplant 3:69–75

Herth K 2000 Enhancing hope in people with a first recurrence of cancer. Journal of Advanced Nursing 32(6):1431–1441

Holdroyd K A, Penzien D B, Hursey K G et al 1984 Change mechanisms in EMG feedback training: cognitive changes underlying improvement in tension headache.

Journal of Consulting and Clinical Psychology 52:1039–1053

Lamb M 1996 Sexuality and the cancer patient. Gynaecological Oncology Nursing 6(3):38–45

Lewis D A, Smith R E 1983 Steroid-induced psychiatric syndromes: a report of 14 cases and a review of the literature. Journal of Affective Disorders 5:319–332

Link L B, Robbins L, Mancuso C A, Charlson M E 2004 How do those patients who try to take control of their disease differ from those who do not? European Journal of Cancer Nursing 13:219–226

Little M, Sayers E, Paul K, Jordens C 2000 On surviving cancer. Journal of the Royal Society of Medicine 93(10):501–502

Little M, Jordens C F, Paul K, Montgomery R, Philipson B 1998 Liminality: a major category of the experience of cancer illness. Social Science and Medicine 47: 1485–1494

Lobchuk M M, Degner L F 2002 Patients with cancer and next of kin response comparability on physical and psychological symptom well-being: trends and measurement issues. Cancer Nursing 25(5):358–374

Matteson S, Roscoe J, Hickok J, Morrow G R 2002 The role of behavioural conditioning in the development of nausea. American Journal of Obstetrics & Gynecology 186(5 Suppl):S239–243

McGinnis L S 1990 Alternative therapies. Cancer 67:1788–1792

Molassiotis A 1997 Psychosocial transitions in the long term survivors of bone marrow transplant. European Journal of Cancer Care 6(2):100–107

Morley C 1997 The use of denial by patients with cancer. Professional Nurse 12(5):380–381

Murray-Ross D, Petteet J R, Madeiro C et al 1992 Difference between nurses' and physicians' approach to denial in oncology. Cancer Nursing 15(6):422–428.

National Institute for Clinical Excellence 2003 Improving outcomes in haematological cancers. NICE, London

National Institute for Clinical Excellence 2004 Improving supportive and palliative care for people with cancer: the manual. NICE, London

Nezu C M, Nezu A M, Friedman S H et al 1999 Cancer and psychosocial distress: two investigations regarding the role of social problem solving. Journal of Psychosocial Oncology 16:27–40

Nowotny M 1991 Every tomorrow, a vision of hope. Journal of Psychosocial Oncology 9(3):117–126

Osuna E, Perez-Carceles M D, Estaban M A, Luna A 1998 The right to information for the terminally ill patient. Journal of Medical Ethics 24:106–109

Price B 1990 A model for body image care. Journal of Advanced Nursing 15:585–593

Roscoe J A, Morrow G R, Hickok J T, Stern R M 2000 Nausea and vomiting remain a significant clinical problem: trends over time in controlling chemotherapy-induced nausea and vomiting in 1413 patients treated in community clinical practices. Journal of Pain & Symptom Management 20(2):113–121

Schumacher K, Meleis A 1994 Transitions: a central concept in nursing. IMAGE Journal of Nursing Scholarship 26(2):119–127

Soderstrom K E, Martinson I M 1987 Patients' spiritual coping strategies: a study of nurse and patient perspectives. Oncology Nursing Forum 14: 41–46

Swensen C H, Fuller S, Clements R 1993 Stages of religious faith and reactions to terminal cancer. Journal of Psychology and Theology 21:238–245

Taylor E 2003 Spiritual needs of patients and their family caregivers. Cancer Nursing 26(4):260–266

Turk D C, Fernandez E 1991 Pain and cancer: a cognitive-behaviour perspective. In: Watson M (ed) Cancer patient care: psychosocial treatment methods. Cambridge University Press, Cambridge, pp 15–44

Valente S M, Saunders J 1997 Diagnosis and treatment of major depression among people with cancer. Cancer Nursing 20(3):168–177

VandeCreek L, Rogers E, Lester J 1999 Use of alternative therapies among breast cancer outpatients compared with the general population. Alternative Therapies in Health and Medicine 5(1):71–76

Watson M (ed) 1991 Cancer patient care: psychosocial treatment methods. Cambridge, Cambridge University Press

Watson M, Greer S, Young J, Inayat Q, Burgess C, Robertson B 1988 Development of a questionnaire to measure adjustment to cancer: the MAC scale. Psychological Medicine 18:203–209

Weaver A J, Flannelly L T, Flannelly K J, VandeCreek L, Koenig H, Handzo G 2001 A 10 year review of research on chaplains and community based clergy in 3 primary oncology nursing journals: 1990–1999. Cancer Nursing 24(5):335–340

Weihs K, Enright T, Howe G, Simmens S J 1999 Marital satisfaction and emotional adjustment after breast cancer. Journal of Psychosocial Oncology 17:33–49

Winters G, Miller C, Maracich L, Compton K, Haberman M 1994 Provisional practice: the nature of psychosocial bone marrow transplant nursing. Oncology Nursing Forum 21:1147–1154

Woods N F, Lewis F M, Ellison E S 1989 Living with cancer – family experiences. Cancer Nursing 12(1):28–33

Zigmond A S, Snaith R P 1983 The HAD scale. Acta Psychiatrica Scandinavia 67:361–370

Further reading

Bottorff J L, Gogag M, Engelberg-Lotzkar M 1995 Comforting: exploring the work of cancer nurses. Journal of Advanced Nursing 22(6):1077–1084
This article examines how comforting strategies can play a major role in helping cancer patients cope with their illness and treatment.

Kruijver I P M, Kerkstra A, Bensing J M, van de Wiel HBM et al 2000 Nurse–patient communication in cancer care. A review of the literature. Cancer 23(1):20–31
This paper examines the importance of nurses' communication skills when caring for patients with cancer.

Link L B, Robbins L, Mancuso C A, Charlson M E 2004 How do those patients who try to take control of their disease differ from those who do not? European Journal of Cancer Nursing 13:219–226
This article describes a study of patient's psychological adjustment to cancer related to the type of coping strategies used along with beliefs about control.

Chapter 24

Addressing the needs of families

Daniel Kelly

KEY POINTS

- Families have a key role to play in supporting patients with haematological cancers. However, they also have their own support and information needs.
- Family units are socially and culturally defined. Non-traditional, multi-generation or distantly located families may become the norm.
- Haematological cancers raise specific concerns for families, such as their role in donation of bone marrow or stem cells. This may place an extra burden on members who may already be experiencing anxiety about their loved-one's diagnosis.
- The supportive care needs of families and friends should be considered across the cancer trajectory. The burdens placed on individuals will change as the patient progresses through treatment.
- Professionals should appreciate that families may require practical support, such as financial assistance, to cope with the demands of cancer.

INTRODUCTION

This chapter considers the supportive care needs of spouses, partners, family members and friends of those receiving active treatment or supportive care in haemato-oncology settings. Research will be used to illustrate the range of needs that are likely to be experienced by these 'lay' caregivers. The terms 'family' or 'caregiver' are used interchangeably throughout the chapter to include all those who are considered important to the patient – whether they are related or not. The issues raised in the chapter are relevant for nurses working in a rapidly evolving specialty that must take into account the physical, emotional and social needs of patients. Holistic philosophies of nursing care have long advocated that the needs of those closest to the patient are important to consider. It is only recently, however, that research studies have been able to clarify the nature of the family's needs in the context of cancer care. Plant, for example, explored the impact of cancer on the family and suggests (Plant 2001, p 86):

> 'Family relationships are dynamic and the diagnosis of cancer in one member will resonate throughout the whole social group, changing the relationship with the person who has cancer and with one another . . . The close family and friends of someone with cancer will experience distress. However, the extent of this distress is difficult to gauge.'

It is natural for families to react in a protective way when a member is diagnosed with an illness that is certainly serious, and may even be life-threatening, as is the case with a haematological cancer. The challenge for professionals is to respond appropriately and to help to focus this protective instinct to benefit the patient.

CARING ACROSS THE ILLNESS TRAJECTORY

From the point of diagnosis onwards the different phases of care are characterised by particular concerns – each of these impacts on families in different ways (Lesko 1993). For instance, during the initial diagnostic phase everyone involved is likely to feel some degree of shock and disbelief. Information will be sought, as well as clarification of treatment options. Underpinning such activity will be an anxiety about the likelihood of achieving cure. This is illustrated by the following quote relating to bone marrow transplant (BMT) (Haberman 1995, p 28):

> 'BMT patients live by the numbers, the mathematical odds of surviving BMT or experiencing BMT complications, as a way to impose order on the BMT experience and to give meaning to the protracted suffering that accompanies this aggressive therapy.'

The diagnostic phase will be superseded by concerns about the significance of pre-treatment tests and procedures. A concern of particular importance for families at this time may be the search for a matched donor.

REFLECTION POINT How is information about the diagnosis and treatment shared with patients and families in your service? Can you think of any ways in which this could be improved?

The diagnostic and pre-treatment phases are likely to be characterised by high levels of activity as well as feelings of anticipation and hope that a successful outcome will be achieved. In such a situation it may sometimes be difficult for families or partners to accept that other aspects of life should also continue outside of the hospital. A natural reaction is to gather round the individual in order to offer encouragement and support about the challenges ahead. As induction regimens are introduced, the first side effects will inevitably be encountered that will rely on professional expertise to be controlled effectively. This is also an important time to establish a relationship of trust with caregivers or close family members.

Families have an important contribution to make in supporting the patient in all phases of care; however, they will also need to feel included and valued by the professional health carers in order to do so. Educating families about side-effect management, for instance, may help to ensure compliance with routines such as mouth care when the patient themselves may lack motivation.

Obviously the diagnostic and pre-treatment phases are highly important times for the individual patient as well as their family as they are expected to assimilate a sometimes-bewildering range of unfamiliar information. They will also be facing the first of many body image changes – such as having peripheral or central venous lines inserted. During this time people are starting to assume the patient role and have to learn to accommodate this new persona alongside their own personal, social and professional lives.

BECOMING A PATIENT

The process of becoming a patient has been described by a number of authors, including the sociologist Talcott Parsons (1951) who coined the term 'sick role'. Essentially this suggests that people are only allowed to adopt the patient role if they agree to be treated by expert medical professionals, to accept the care offered and to resume normal social responsibilities when they are well enough. In return, they can expect to receive care from experts and to be excused from normal responsibilities (such as paid work). However, there is also the expectation that they will comply with medical advice and accept the required treatment. As well as the individual patient, however, families also have to adapt to a new identity that includes having a member who has received a serious diagnosis. The family must learn to adapt to life with this new identity and to cope with the disruptions and changes that will result.

The theory of the sick role is also highly relevant in haemato-oncology settings as the conditions involved are serious and require treatments that may be aggressive. For many people this will require them to give up their independence, to agree to stay in hospital for long periods at a time and to accept a number of unpleasant procedures and treatments – including protective isolation (Collins et al 1989). Sontag (1977) talked about this process of adaptation to illness as moving from 'the kingdom of the well' into 'the kingdom of the sick'. Undoubtedly, family and friends also undergo a similar form of transition and may need help to cope with this unfamiliar new world that they find themselves in. Importantly, it will be families and friends who will also provide uniquely important sources of support and encouragement at such times – as well as maintaining the all-important link with the 'kingdom of the well'. Bringing in food, reading material, music or games as well as news from the outside world can help to punctuate the unrelenting boredom associated with long hospital stays (Holloway et al 1999).

TREATMENT AND BEYOND

As treatment continues into the induction phase and perhaps a transplant procedure, the individual has to adapt to a more dependent role when they become susceptible to infections and other side effects. Professionals should be aware of the beneficial support that family or friends can continue to provide at these times. When long periods of hospitalisation or isolation are required, it is important to be aware of the need to overcome feelings of loneliness, boredom and anxiety (Holloway et al 1999). Families and friends are one of the most important resources available to help to address these issues. Professionals will be too preoccupied with clinical tasks to be able to offer distraction or social interactions to the same extent.

With such a valuable contribution to make it is important to emphasise that these 'invisible' members of the team will have their own unique support needs that should also be recognised. Patients and caregivers have reported feeling excluded and confused when they were not included in decision-making about cancer treatment choices (Steinhauser et al 2000). Research conducted some time ago suggests that four salient family needs emerged as particularly important – these included the need for information, the need for hope, the need to ventilate feelings and the need for interventions to be directed towards the patient. These findings seem especially relevant in terms of how families can adapt given support, time and appropriate information:

> 'One of the most important premises in family system theory is that the family is capable of taking in information, changing, and growing throughout the course of patient's illness . . . Nursing interventions that were directed toward giving to the patient and family were rated very high, regardless of phase of living with cancer . . .'
>
> (Lewandowski & Jones 1998, p 321)

The treatment phase will also impact on those family caregivers who find themselves in a situation over which they have little control. Family members and friends gradually may assume the role of carer for someone who, previously, had been an independent figure within their home or social circle. For this reason families and friends should be expected to feel anxious and uncertain when first offering help to the patient. They may need to be reassured that it is fine just to sit quietly and read while the person sleeps, for example, rather than always feeling the need to hold a conversation. Children may also find themselves having to reassure or comfort a parent. Friends may experience the need to offer words of support but feel unsure about the best way to do so.

At the same time those involved will also be aware that they risk losing their loved one, despite the arduous treatments and side effects they are experiencing as a result of treatment. The role of the professional at this time is to acknowledge the different support needs of those who, in turn, are helping the patient to deal with their situation. This need not involve formal 'counselling'. Instead, simply taking the time to find out how someone is coping may make the difference between the caregiver feeling abandoned or acknowledged in his or her difficulty. The concept of *family nursing* is relevant in this regard (Flanagan 2001). In essence family nursing is defined as (Flanagan 2001, p 177):

> 'An approach to care increasingly discussed within the practical and academic nursing literature . . . Family nursing is a model of care distinct from family-centered or family-focused care, as the family itself is seen as the unit of care rather than the context of care.'

This approach has important implications for nurses working in haemato-oncology settings. It may involve a formal assessment of the family, for instance, which could include questions on family history and life events, as well as functional assessments of communication patterns and health awareness (Whyte 1997). With such objective information about the way the family functions, professionals may be better equipped to deliver support, information or advice.

Clark & Gwin (1993) examined the needs of families in relation to their psychosocial responses to cancer. They reviewed a number of formal assessment tools that can be used to assess the characteristics of families and how they function. Such a formal approach may not be appropriate for everyday clinical situations, however, and professionals should be aware that specialist interventions may be needed if families are not coping well with particular aspects of the disease and treatment experience. This may be especially important for families with co-existing risk factors such as a history of previous mental illness, multiple adverse events or unresolved relationship problems (Clark & Gwin 1993). It should also be remembered that families may also be worried about the inherited risk of developing cancer and may require advice on this issue (Arden-Jones & Eeles 2001).

Whilst this is an important point, the tempo of practice in haemato-oncology settings also must be borne in mind when providing information or support to families or friends. Anyone who has been a visitor in a BMT unit will probably have perceived staff appearing busy and pre-occupied with a number of highly technical tasks (dealing with infusions, ordering blood products or recording observations, for example). In such a context it may be very daunting to approach a professional to ask for what may feel like an insignificant piece of information. By addressing the needs of caregivers within the plan of care for the patient, these issues are much more likely to be given the importance they merit. They are also likely to be addressed at an appropriate time in a situation more conducive to effective communication, such as a quiet room or office.

The emotional responses of the patient as treatment progresses may be mirrored by those closest to them. Feelings may fluctuate between optimism, anger, denial, despair and apparent acceptance of the situation. Appreciating the psychological reactions of patients, families and friends at such times may help health professionals to feel prepared to offer care and support in ways that are likely to be well received. Professional caring involves behaviours and attitudes that respond to spoken as well as unspoken needs; however, personally focussed caring usually differs from professional caring in the way it is expressed (Kelly 1998). The quality of personal caregiving has been compared to professional caring roles (Kelly 1998, p 732):

> 'Qualities implicit in the lay caring relationship such as commitment and the personalisation of task-oriented activities have, in turn, been used as markers to measure the quality of professional caring. Whilst the lay carer may exhibit desirable caring behaviors due to kinship or friendship, the nurse must somehow nurture these attitudes whilst operating in a professional role within the institutional setting.'

This point emphasises an important difference between personal and professional caring roles. Nurses or other professionals cannot be expected to demonstrate the same level of concern for patients as would their family or friends. Indeed it might be considered inappropriate if they did. Instead, it is important to value personal approaches of caring and to support families and friends when they make this contribution in clinical settings. It is also important to recognise and to thank families for their commitment and support of the patient – especially in busy technical environments such as haemato-oncology settings. Importantly, personal caregivers also recognise when professionals appear uncaring in their reactions towards their loved ones. This should prompt professionals to be aware of the manner in which we sometimes routinise the care of those who are facing life-threatening situations (Taylor 1992).

Plant (2001, p 90) examined the impact of cancer on families and friends and explained their reactions to cancer:

> 'Buffering or protecting the person who has cancer from painful information and experiences is common. The most extreme form of this might be for the family to try to prevent the individual from knowing their diagnosis. This now happens infrequently, although families may still wish to protect the person from knowing the full extent of the severity of their illness and may not pass on any additional information that they may have from health professionals.'

Appreciating what families and friends are going through can help to explain protective behaviours, even if they seem to go against what professionals feel 'ought' to be done or said.

UNDERSTANDING FAMILY/CAREGIVER EXPERIENCES

The impact of a diagnosis of a haematological cancer extends beyond the individual patient to those most important to them. Awareness of supportive care for caregivers requires that the concept of 'family' be accepted as a highly fluid one that mirrors social and cultural norms as well as individual lifestyles and cultures. Plant's research (2001) emphasised that siblings, parents, friends and colleagues can all be expected to experience some degree of distress as a result of learning of a cancer diagnosis in someone close to them. This can evoke feelings of shock, fear, protectiveness, anger and injustice, as well as the desire to help. These reactions may be magnified when younger people are involved. The process of donation and the final phase of care are two points in the BMT trajectory that require specific consideration when seeking to understand the specific needs of families or other caregivers.

There are also practical concerns that families will have to address when a member undergoes treatment for cancer. Taking time off work to visit, for example, may impact on their careers or workload. The financial burden of travelling to hospital may also need to be considered, and the input of social services may be required in low-income families who are facing money problems as a result. This is especially important, as specialist cancer centres may be some way from the family's base. Such issues may be highlighted at the nursing assessment but should also be borne in mind as the treatment phase progresses and conflicting demands begin to impinge on those closest to the patient.

THE NEEDS OF DONORS

The involvement of siblings or other family members in the donation of bone marrow cells may offer their loved one the chance of a cure. Whilst this may at first seem a highly positive way to offer practical help in a desperate situation, feelings of fear or disappointment may also be evoked should the transplant be unsuccessful. The support needs of those close to the patient at this time need to be appreciated before health professionals can address them effectively.

Research by Munsenburger et al (1999) helps to provide some insight into the emotional and physical demands of donation. The study suggested that the search for a donor is an important phase of care, as it will involve the family directly in medical procedures. As a result it is likely to evoke feelings of hope as well as anxiety. Additional reactions may include having to accept that the least 'preferred' family member may turn out to be the most biologically compatible. As the researchers point out (Munzenberger et al 1999, p 59):

'When the name of the most biologically compatible donor is subsequently announced, the reactions depend on whether this choice is in accordance with the individual's *a priori* designation in the family.'

This means that individuals may find themselves in the spotlight when they would prefer not to carry such responsibility. Similarly, families may sometimes prefer certain family members to play a more central role in the transplant process than their biological make-up allows. One of the participants in the above study (a 34-year-old unmarried manual worker) spoke of how difficult he found it to be named as the donor:

'The hardest part was being told I was the donor. I fretted about it. There were nights when I couldn't sleep and I began to cry . . .' (Munzenberger et al 1999)

The study also suggested that the donation was associated with a sense of obligation and duty. It was a moral decision based on the fact that the person in danger had to be helped. Misunderstandings about the donation process, however, were also identified. One female donor worried that she might become sterile as a result of the donation of peripheral stem cells. Another confused 'growth factors' with 'growth hormones'.

The lead-up period to donation was also significant as individuals talked about preparing themselves both physically and mentally for the event. Afterwards they talked about feeling fatigued as well as mentioning vague symptoms associated with the injection of growth factors:

'I felt there was something terribly wrong with my body . . . I felt as if I was in an abnormal state . . . as if I no longer mastered my body, as if there was something very wrong inside me . . .' (Munzenberger et al 1999)

In the face of a life-threatening condition the donation of cells is a powerfully symbolic event. Two of the female participants in the above study spoke of it as a life-giving event:

'I gave life to my children and now I give life to my brother . . .' (Munzenberger et al 1999)

There was also a close bond established between donor and recipient that was expressed in the following way:

'He and I we are just like a single person . . .' (Munzenberger et al 1999)

However, other issues may also arise during the donation process. For instance, donors may discover concurrent medical conditions that they were not aware of or they may fail to appreciate the poor outcome that the recipient may still face (Williams et al 2003). Donation is a complex issue that requires careful preparation to prepare both donor and recipient for what may be involved, as well as all possible outcomes. Those family members, such as siblings, may need particular attention to ensure that their information and support needs are met (Morrison et al 1998).

What support is available to donors in your service? Can you list some ways in which you might improve the information or support needs of donors? What sources of advice or financial help might you use to develop this aspect of practice?

THE AFTERMATH OF TREATMENT

As mentioned earlier, haemato-oncology settings are usually busy settings where relatives and friends may often feel rather helpless when surrounded by so much high-tech equipment. With time, however, they are likely to become accustomed to the surroundings and to seek ways of personalising the care setting in order to make their loved one's experience more bearable. Nurses have argued for attention to be paid to the environment of care in order to minimise feelings of vulnerability experienced by patients and their caregivers in highly technical health-care settings (Cooper & Powell 1998). This type of intervention should not be minimised, especially when it is known that patients undergoing bone marrow transplants can feel isolated and depressed (Molassiotis 1995).

Parents, siblings, friends and colleagues, however, may also require support to cope with the threat of imminent loss. Holistic approaches to cancer care require us to be aware of this issue. The relatively high mortality associated with haematological cancers suggests that more attention should be paid to the needs of caregivers in the end-of-life phase of care (Kelly et al 2000). One of the specific difficulties facing palliative care services in haematological settings, however, is knowing the best time to intervene. It is sometimes very difficult to know when 'active' treatment should be withdrawn, or when further blood product support is no longer justified. Family members may seem to be intuitively aware that a particular treatment is failing, yet they continue to offer support and encouragement:

> 'People can go through years and years of hoping that someone close to them might live, but knowing in the end they are going to die. I don't know how nurses and relatives can cope with that really. They just get on with things and have to get on . . .'
>
> (Smith & Gray 2000, p 67)

Decisions often have to be made very quickly about the withdrawal of active therapy and the instigation of palliative interventions. Families and caregivers may prefer to be involved in such discussions and will find it easier to do so if they have already established trusting relationships with the professionals involved. If treatment is failing, then the time remaining should be recognised as increasingly valuable for the individual and their family and friends who may wish to concentrate on personal and spiritual concerns in a more focussed way. Caregivers can be encouraged to be as involved in physical caring, such as bathing and feeding, as the person's condition allows. However, they are also likely to need support to move beyond feelings of intense disappointment, loss and sadness to make the final days of their loved one's life as special as possible.

Whilst there is lack of research into end-of-life care in haemato-oncology, insights can be drawn from other areas of practice. Dunne & Sullivan (2000), for example, carried out a study with a number of families to describe their experiences of witnessing a loved one's death in an acute hospital setting. Families described the hospital environment as feeling 'rushed and hurried', with loved ones being moved around the ward as the need for acute beds required. Acute care settings were mainly characterised by an emphasis on curative treatments, with little possibility of avoiding the many rules and routines that shape hospital life. Concerns were also expressed about privacy and overwhelming helplessness about the situation. Recommendations from the study included the need to educate all grades of staff about palliative care and to appreciate the needs of those who are facing the imminent loss of someone dear to them.

Case study 24.1

Ray is a 35-year-old man with high-grade B-cell lymphoma diagnosed five months ago following a fit whilst he was on holiday in Spain. He returned to the UK and was commenced on chemotherapy but reacted very badly, with severe nausea, vomiting and neutropenia. He began to lose weight almost immediately. Nasogastric feeding was started two weeks ago but his condition has continued to deteriorate to his present weight of 40 kg.

Ray has been married twice and has two children from each marriage. He owns property in both the UK and Spain but has never made a will. His mother is alive and he has an extended family of three sisters and several nephews and nieces.

The medical staff have always advised Ray and his wife and family that chemotherapy could be restarted when his condition allowed; however, he was noted to have deteriorated further during a recent ward round. Ray now appeared to be experiencing pain on movement and it was agreed that the advice of the palliative care team was needed.

John, a Clinical Nurse Specialist from the team, came to assess Ray the following day and suggested the prescription of oral morphine to make Ray more comfortable. The medical staff agreed to speak to the family, leaving John alone to speak to Ray about his situation. Previously this had been difficult, as the family had always insisted on staying in the room. Ray seemed to realise that he was deteriorating, and when the option was discussed, asked to be referred to a hospice close to his family rather than his own home in London. He felt this would make it easier for them to visit as he was most worried about being alone. He also asked John about making a will as soon as possible. John telephoned the hospice situated near Ray's family that agreed to accept a referral on this basis. John also involved the Trust's Patient Advocacy and Liaison Service (PALS) to help Ray to access a solicitor before his condition deteriorated any further. The medical staff agreed that he was still in sound mind to do so. With his family present Ray also asked that his nasogastric feeds be stopped before he was transferred to the hospice. On making the referral John emphasised that Ray's family would need support to adapt from a situation where treatment and cure were being emphasised to one where symptom relief and end-of-life care were now the focus.

A number of research studies also provide information on caregiving behaviours (although once again there has been a lack of research into this issue in the context of haemato-oncology). Nijboer et al (1998), for instance, suggest that those most likely to be involved in caregiving roles are female, with those from lower socioeconomic groups experiencing poorer health outcomes themselves as a result. Many of the studies on caregiving that have been conducted involve frail elderly populations, or families experiencing the care of a member with mental illness. There is a need to promote more studies that examine family issues in the context of today's society and the changing nature of what we even understand 'a family' to be.

Situations involving cancer may provoke existential concerns in caregivers who may begin to evaluate their own future in line with their loved one's fate. This may result in an alteration of life goals or priorities and staff may find themselves involved in such conversations at unexpected times. Those actually undergoing bone marrow transplant will have ongoing physical, social and emotional needs that will continue to change with time. Those expected to 'stand by' and witness what happens can be expected to experience some degree of stress as a result (Stetz 1987).

REFLECTION POINT

How are family members supported in your area of practice when their loved one's condition fails to respond to treatment? Can you suggest any ways of enhancing this aspect of care?

When treatment is successful, there are also issues of rehabilitation and recovery to be considered. Common to many other cancer patient groups, those who survive haematological conditions may experience fears of recurrence and a preoccupation with their health status (Schag & Heinrich 1990). There may also be difficulties in terms of personal and sexual relationships, as well as fatigue, mood changes and other psychosocial problems (see Chapters 22 & 23). More practical concerns may also arise for families as a result of financial worries and employment related difficulties (Pearce et al 2001). When considered in this way, it can be seen that families have much to offer that complements the technical expertise of the professionals involved in haemato-oncology care. In order to offer support, however, families and friends will also need their own unique needs to be met effectively.

CONCLUSION

This chapter has emphasised the impact of a serious haematological cancer on the family. Whether an individual recovers and returns to normal life, or whether they will die regardless of treatment interventions, they will do so with the help of their family and friends. To this extent the individuals who support the patient should be considered key to the delivery of effective supportive care in haemato-oncology. This chapter has argued that bone marrow transplant settings may not be particularly conducive to family care, as they are usually busy, highly technical environments that can seem very alien to patients and families. Complex machinery and isolation procedures serve to further emphasise the seriousness of the diagnosis. Professionals may also appear too preoccupied to be disturbed with what may feel like insignificant or unimportant concerns (Winters et al 1994).

Family-focussed care stems from an awareness of the needs of families and the contribution they make to effective and humane care. Formal tools for assessing family coping do exist, and professionals should be aware of their existence. However, it is unrealistic to suggest that they will be necessary in the majority of clinical situations. Instead, a feature of holistic practice is to ensure that the information and support needs of families are considered and incorporated into the overall plan of care. Without this it is difficult to imagine how the needs of culturally diverse, non-traditional and multi-generational families can be met in the busy reality of haemato-oncology settings.

Despite the use of aggressive treatment, cancer care will always be characterised by uncertainty about the final outcome. Everyone in this situation has to find a way of coping with such uncertainty and it may be easier to focus on a successful outcome to justify the side effects of treatment. This is likely to result in a number of emotional support needs that professionals should be aware of as they develop expertise in highly technical care (Kelly et al 2000). The threat of loss of a loved one may evoke a range of reactions in families including feelings of helplessness, anxiety and anger (Plant 2001). Inevitably, professionals may unwittingly become the focus for negative as well as positive feelings. By understanding what a family is going through such responses may be better appreciated. A final point to emphasise is that families and friends can play a uniquely valuable role in promoting care that really is patient-centred.

DISCUSSION QUESTIONS

1. There have been many changes to family life in the West over the past 50 years. Mothers are more likely to work, for instance, and children may choose to move away from the parental home to seek employment. Some families may also be considered 'non-traditional' (such as same-sex couples) with friends occupying a more central role than siblings. What might be the impact of such changes when a family member is diagnosed with a haematological cancer?

2. Family members may provide valuable psychosocial support to patients undergoing treatment for haematological cancers. However, they will also require advice, support and information to do so. What do you

DISCUSSION QUESTIONS – CONT'D

think are the unmet needs of families in your own area and how could this aspect of your service be improved?

3. Tensions that exist within all families may be magnified when a member is diagnosed with cancer. Frustration may be directed towards professionals when delays occur, or when the response to treatment is disappointing. Other factors may compound these difficulties (such as language barriers or existing interpersonal tensions between family members that emerge at times of stress). What communication skills might be employed to help families to cope in such situations?

References

Arden-Jones A, Eeles R 2001 Hereditary cancer. In: Corner J, Bailey C (eds) Cancer nursing. Care in context. Blackwell, Oxford, pp 297–313

Clark J, Gwin R 1993 Psychosocial responses of the family. In: Groenwald S, Hansen Frogge M, Goodman M et al (eds) Cancer nursing. Principles & practice. Jones & Bartlett, London, pp 468–484

Collins C, Upright C, Aleksich J 1989 Reverse isolation: what patients perceive. Oncology Nursing Forum 16:675–679

Cooper M, Powell E 1998 Technology and care in a bone marrow transplant unit: creating and assuaging vulnerability. Holistic Nursing Practice 12:57–68

Dunne K, Sullivan K 2000 Family experiences of palliative care in the acute hospital setting. International Journal of Palliative Nursing 6:170–178

Flanagan J 2001 Clinically effective cancer care: working with families. European Journal of Oncology Nursing 5:174–179

Haberman M 1995 The meaning of cancer therapy: bone marrow transplant as an exemplar of therapy. Seminars in Oncology Nursing 11:23–31

Holloway I, Smith P, Warren J 1999 Patients experienced a lack of control over their time in hospital. Journal of Clinical Nursing 7:460–466

Kelly D 1998 Caring and cancer nursing: framing the reality using social science theory. Journal of Advanced Nursing 28:728–736

Kelly D, Ross S, Gray B, Smith P 2000 Death, dying and emotional labour: problematic dimensions of the bone marrow transplant nursing role? Journal of Advanced Nursing 32:952–960

Lesko L 1993 Psychiatric aspects of bone marrow transplantation: Part 1: Special issues during pre-transplant assessment and hospitalization. Psycho-Oncology 2:161–185

Lewandowski W, Jones S 1998 The family with cancer. Nursing interventions through the course of living with cancer. Cancer Nursing 11:313–321

Molassiotis A 1995 Quality of life following bone marrow transplantation. Nursing Times 91:38–39

Morrison A E, Green R H, Watson D M, Franklin I M 1998 Evaluation and eligibility of HLA sibling donors for stem cell/bone marrow donation. Transfusion Medicine 8:215–220

Munzenberger N, Fortanier C, Macquart-Moulin G et al 1999 Psychosocial aspects of haematopoietic stem cell donation for allogeneic transplantation: how families cope with this experience. Psycho-Oncology 8:55–63

Nijboer C, Tempelaar R, Sanderman R, Triemstra M, Sprujit R, van der Bos G 1998 Cancer and caregiving: the impact on the caregiver's health. Psycho-oncology 7:3–13

Parsons T 1951 The social system. Routledge & Kegan Paul, London

Pearce S, Kelly D, Stevens W 2001 'More than just money' – widening the understanding of the costs involved in cancer care. Journal of Advanced Nursing 33:371–379

Plant H 2001 The impact of cancer on the family. In: Corner J, Bailey C (eds) Cancer nursing. Care in context. Blackwell, Oxford, pp 86–100

Schag C, Heinrich R 1990 Development of a comprehensive quality of life measurement tool: CARES. Oncology 4:135–138

Smith P, Gray B 2000 The emotional labour of nursing: how students and qualified nurses learn to care. A report on nurse education, nursing practice and emotional labour in the contemporary NHS. South Bank University, London

Sontag S 1977 Illness as metaphor. Penguin, London

Steinhauser K E, Clipp E C, McNeilly M, Christakis N A, McIntyre L M, Tulsky J A 2000 In search of a good death: observations of patients, families and providers. Annals of Internal Medicine 132:825–832

Stetz K 1987 Caregiving demands during advanced cancer: the spouse's needs. Cancer Nursing 10:260–268

Taylor B 1992 From helper to human: a reconceptualisation of the nurse as a person. Journal of Advanced Nursing 17:1042–1049

Whyte D 1997 Explorations in family nursing. Routledge, London

Williams S, Green R, Morrison A, Watson D, Buchanan S 2003 The psychosocial aspects of donating blood stem cells: the sibling donor perspective. Journal of Clinical Apheresis 18:1–9

Winters G, Miller C, Maracich L, Compton K, Haberman M 1994 Provisional practice: the nature of psychosocial bone marrow transplant nursing. Oncology Nursing Forum 21:1147–1154

Further reading

Clark J, Gwin R 2000 Psychosocial responses of the family. In: Groenwald S et al (eds) Cancer nursing. Principles & practice. Jones & Bartlett, London

This chapter provides a full review of methods for assessing families in cancer care situations. Although primarily drawing on American models of services, it provides a useful overview of many issues facing families (such as adaptation, relationships, assessment criteria and supportive interventions).

Murray M, Miller T, Fiset V, O'Connor A, Jacobsen M J 2004 Decision support: helping patients and families to find a balance at the end of life. International Journal of Palliative Nursing 10:270–277

This is an example of a piece of research carried out by nurses to enhance the role that patients and families can play in decision-making at the end of life. A framework is proposed for use in clinical settings that draws on assessed needs, decision support and evaluation of decision-making. A worksheet is also provided to guide professionals through the screening, probing and planning process for decision-making. Whilst this approach may not be feasible in all situations, the article provides insight into the ways that families and patients can be encouraged to request additional information and support when important decisions are being made (such as the withdrawal of treatment in haemato-oncology settings).

Nicholson Perry K, Burgess M 2002 Communication in cancer care. British Psychological Society/Blackwell, Oxford

This book provides a practical and concise summary of the impact of cancer and those it affects. It offers a useful summary of common situations, such as breaking bad news, and strategies for handling them using appropriate communication skills. Case studies are used to illustrate key points.

Plant H 2001 The impact of cancer on the family. In: Corner J, Bailey C (eds) Cancer nursing. Care in context. Blackwell, Oxford

This book chapter provides a useful overview of a research study that examined the experiences of family members caring for someone with cancer. Insights into the ways that families adjust to a cancer diagnosis in many different ways, and the impact that cancer treatment may have on those closest to the person are provided. Communication within the family is also addressed, as are feelings of helplessness that some individuals experience when a member is diagnosed with cancer. The research also indicates that some families may feel excluded from care, despite the many advances that have been made to make cancer services more 'family friendly'.

Chapter **25**

Social issues

Alexander Molassiotis

KEY POINTS
- Survivorship is viewed as living with, through and beyond cancer.
- Surviving a haematological cancer may result in an altered perspective on life and change relationships.
- Survivorship is related to individual adjustment to life after a cancer diagnosis.
- Psychological, physical and social difficulties may affect quality of life after bone marrow transplant.
- Nurses have an important role in the social and vocational integration of patients.

INTRODUCTION

Limited literature on social issues dealing exclusively with haemato-oncology patients exists and within this chapter inferences are drawn from other cancer studies that include small numbers of haemato-oncology patients. The more extensive literature on quality of life issues in bone marrow transplant (BMT) survivors is presented in detail. Common patient problems including fatigue, sexual dysfunction and cancer-related employment discrimination are examined and recommendations for nursing practice are outlined.

Research about social issues in cancer is limited, as nursing research has focussed mainly on biophysical issues of cancer and its treatments. There are several explanations for this lack of research:

- physical cancer-related problems and treatment complications place social issues in a secondary position
- pessimistic views and misconceptions about long-term survival
- minimal funding of research dealing with social issues in cancer patients
- time constraints and staff shortages
- lack of basic training or language barriers for multicentre studies in Europe (Molassiotis 1997, Fliedner 2002).

However, nursing interest in quality of life, long-term adjustment and psychosocial issues is high. These issues are identified as priorities for future research in both stem cell and bone marrow transplant (Haberman 1997), and also rank among the top ten oncology nurses' research priorities in the USA and in Europe (Oberst 1978, Degner 1987, Molassiotis 1997, Browne et al 2002) but also in paediatric haematology-oncology (Soanes et al 2003). These research priorities may reflect professional nursing attitudes that involve a multidimensional model of physical, psychological, social and spiritual care.

SURVIVORSHIP ISSUES

The concept of survivorship is relatively new in cancer nursing practice. Crude markers of survival, such as surviving for 5 years after an initial diagnosis of cancer, being in remission, needing no treatment or being cured from cancer, dominated the survival literature several decades ago but are now insufficient to describe survivorship. Nowadays, survivorship is viewed as a dynamic process, involving not only a disease-free life, but living with, through and beyond cancer (Herbst 1995). Certainly such a point of view is extremely important for nursing practice, as it can be used as a reflective model of care that could improve the humane and holistic way we treat and care for our patients. Breaden (1997) also describes in her phenomenological study that surviving cancer may be a process structured according to the everyday experiences and living in time, with different aspects of living (or being alive) characterising each part of the ongoing process of survivorship.

Shanfield (1980), Mullan (1985) and Dow (1990) described the process of surviving cancer and named the different stages 'seasons of survival'. Four main seasons are identified:

1. *Surviving the diagnosis and treatment* predominantly refers to the initial cancer treatment. Most of the cancer nursing research deals with this season, as great attention is focussed on physical complications of the disease and treatment and their nursing management.
2. *Extended survival* refers to the time after treatment, where patients go through a 'wait-and-see' period. During this season, fear of relapse is

the main feature (Carpenter et al 1989, Welch-McCaffrey et al 1989, Dow 1990).

3. *Surviving with uncertainty* – that is, dealing with the unknown. Avoidance of long-term plans and taking life as it comes dominate this season.

4. *Permanent survival*, where the likelihood of recurrence or relapse is so small that the disease is considered permanently arrested, and patients try to re-start their lives.

Bushkin (1993) stated that to survive is to learn to live, because the skills and attributes of survivorship are learned rather than innate. Haemato-oncology nurse specialists are in a unique position to enhance such skills in individuals and improve their psychosocial adjustment, either by promoting new health behaviours that can prevent additional risks (Rose 1989) or by teaching new coping skills and introducing social rehabilitation in long-term survivors.

Many individuals perceive post-treatment wellness as being 'normal' (healthy) or being the way they were before the cancer diagnosis. Dow (1990) disagrees, and states that getting well does not mean getting back to normal, because lives can be drastically changed by cancer. This is another important consideration in planning care. Many individuals have high expectations from their lives after treatment that, in some cases, will lead to frustration. The nursing role is to help to prevent such unnecessary frustration by providing accurate information and discussing with patients their outlook on life, future plans, perspectives and expectations.

Surviving a haematological malignancy may produce a sense of vulnerability, change in life priorities, heightened appreciation of life and fear of relapse and death. It may also involve changes in social relationships, relationships with health-care professionals, adjustment to physical complications, alterations in social support systems, isolation, and sexual and psychosexual problems. Finally, it may cause employment discrimination, insurance problems, uncertainty and emotional stress (Shanfield 1980, Welch-McCaffrey et al 1989, Haberman et al 1993, Ferrell et al 1995, Molassiotis et al 1995a). Further qualitative work suggests that when patients with leukaemia are confronted with their life-threatening situation from diagnosis to treatment to survival, they bring together their present values and life-long patterns of dealing with adversity in order to make sense of their experience (Xuereb & Dunlop 2003).

Survivorship is closely related to how patients adjust to everyday life after a diagnosis of cancer – physically, psychologically and socially. The degree of and perception of adjustment is described by another multidimensional concept, quality of life (QoL).

REFLECTION POINT   What assessment data do you think you need to collect in order to meet patients' survivorship needs? What might these needs be?

QUALITY OF LIFE

There is no universal definition of QoL. It has been described as:

- satisfaction with physical, psychological, social, functional, material and structural aspects of life (Hörnquist 1982)
- a global evaluation of an individual's satisfaction with life (Szalai 1980)
- shaped by physical symptoms, treatment toxicity, body image, mobility, mental state, interpersonal relationships, spiritual, financial, cultural, political and philosophical issues (Caplan 1987).

REFLECTION POINT   What do you think are the factors that contribute to the quality of life of your patients?

Few studies examine QoL exclusively in patients with haematological cancers: most include only some patients with leukaemia or lymphomas in their samples (Greaves-Otte et al 1991, Ferrell et al 1995). Despite achievements in the treatment of Hodgkin's disease (HD) and leukaemias in adults and children, psychosocial aspects of the illness seen as significant issues affecting QoL have been neglected (Yellen et al 1993). A recent review of 21 studies with haemato-oncology patients suggests that acute myeloid leukaemia has a substantial negative impact on their quality of life, with the worse time being soon after diagnosis and during treatment; however, long-term survivors tend to recover in most areas of life, with the exception of sexual dysfunction, which continues to be an impaired domain of life (Redaelli et al 2004).

QoL has been associated with a positive attitude to life, which is dependent on interpersonal relationships and autonomy by individuals with leukaemia (Bertero & Ek 1993). Security, support, respect, information and conversation were related to interpersonal relationships and autonomy. Additionally, eight core concepts have been reported as defining QoL by long-term BMT survivors (Ferrell et al 1992a):

- having family and relationships
- being independent
- being able to work/financial success
- having a heightened appreciation for life
- being normal
- being healthy
- being alive
- being satisfied and fulfilled with life.

These themes were also confirmed in a later qualitative study of chronic myeloid leukaemia BMT survivors (Molassiotis & Morris 1998). Three life areas of high importance in leukaemia and lymphoma patients were reported in another study: family, health and marriage. These seemed to be considerably more important than all other life areas examined (Montgomery et al 2002).

QUALITY OF LIFE IN BONE MARROW TRANSPLANT SURVIVORS

Several studies, using a wide range of outcome variables, address psychosocial issues related to QoL in BMT survivors. However, earlier studies, especially those before 1991, suffered from methodological difficulties with small sample sizes, limited quantification of outcome variables, failure to conceptualise QoL, retrospective study designs and unsuitable control groups. These weaknesses have been addressed in more recent studies. However, these methodological limitations should be considered when reviewing studies.

Both physical and psychological problems have been reported as affecting QoL post-BMT. Hengeveld et al (1988) found that many patients felt unprepared for the emotional and sexual problems they faced immediately after discharge. Their daily lives were hampered by illness-related physical complications, sexual problems, infertility and/or failure to return to employment. However, despite these problems, the majority of participants reported positive changes in their personality, outlook on life and social relationships. These results should be viewed with caution as the reliability of the study is not reported, although other studies also report positive changes on life following BMT, including great spiritual wellbeing and appreciation of life (Ferrell et al 1992b, Haberman et al 1993, Molassiotis & Morris 1998). Furthermore, strong family relationships were found to be related with improved psychosocial adjustment in BMT survivors (Molassiotis et al 1997), suggesting that families can provide much needed support to patients. It is interesting that in the latter study most patients mentioned at least one nurse as their support provider, highlighting the important role nurses have in the psychosocial adjustment of patients.

Other studies examining QoL in BMT survivors have found physical status and employment issues to be the main concerns (Belec 1992). Experiencing physical difficulties, losing relationships, having unfulfilled goals and being financially distressed worsened QoL (Ferrell et al 1992a). Additionally, subjects had considerable difficulty in re-establishing their lives, dealing with the physical complications of BMT, adjusting to their social environment and returning to work. Dealing with physical symptoms, family and friends and work/education issues, together with altered body image, were the most distressing aspects of their adjustment (Haberman et al 1993). Finally, problems with health and functioning had the most negative impact on QoL (Ferrell et al 1992b, Gaston-Johansson & Foxall 1996).

Younger age, a higher level of physical functioning, greater social support and self-esteem have all been found to be predictors of better

QoL (Baker et al 1994). Furthermore, more physical symptom distress had been reported following allogeneic BMT than after autologous BMT (Molassiotis et al 1995b, 1996).

Length of time post-transplant also has an impact on QoL. In one study 67 allogeneic BMT patients demonstrated maximum physical dysfunction 90 days post-BMT, but their functioning returned to pre-transplant levels 1 year later. After 2 years 68% had returned to full-time work/education, increasing to 91% after 4 years (Syrjala et al 1993). In a further study, most of the 162 adults (mean time post-BMT 5 years) and 50 children (mean time post-BMT 6 years) were doing well in the domains of QoL examined, with younger age being associated with better adjustment (Schmidt et al 1993). Approximately three-quarters of the study subjects had returned to employment, although a minority of respondents reported difficulties with sleeping or sexual activity.

Conversely a prospective study of allogeneic BMT patients showed that many experienced long-term problems of physical, emotional, occupational and cognitive functioning with little change over time (Andrykowski et al 1989). It is interesting that comparison of BMT and renal transplant patients revealed few differences between the two groups in post-transplant QoL, with both groups reporting impaired QoL following transplant (Andrykowski et al 1990).

Physical problems (e.g. fatigue, appearance or trouble eating), psychological problems (e.g. fears about future or anxiety) and community reintegration problems (e.g. difficulty returning to previous social roles, dealing with stigma or employment difficulties) were reported in a qualitative study of 84 patients 1 year after BMT (Baker et al 1999). Furthermore, BMT patients for acute myeloid leukaemia seem to have more physical problems, worse sexual and social relationships, or more impaired professional and leisure activities than intensive consolidation chemotherapy patients (Watson et al 2004). Mild to moderate cognitive impairment was also shown in 60% of a sample of BMT patients, with areas affected being selective attention and executive function, information processing speed, verbal learning, or verbal and visual memory (Harder et al 2002).

Such quality of life data is important for nurses, as they can prepare patients to cope better with the effects of the treatments and can provide accurate information to patients, leading to higher levels of quality care. It should be noted here that the majority of studies agree that most patients are able to cope with adverse effects (short- and long-term ones), with only a minority of patients needing more formal support.

More recently caregivers' quality of life has been highlighted as an important concept to explore, as often they have a critical influence on patient adaptation, and may require ongoing assistance themselves in order to maintain their primary support role (Boyle et al 2000).

MARITAL PROBLEMS

Marital problems have been reported in several studies. Wasserman et al (1987) found that lymphoma patients had higher divorce rates when compared with healthy others of a similar age and race in the USA. Furthermore, survivors of childhood cancer have been found to be more reluctant than sibling controls to marry, and have fewer children, irrespective of reproductive difficulties (Tooter et al 1987). Yellen et al (1993) found that HD survivors avoid intimate relationships for fear of an uncertain future and those already in a relationship often have difficulty communicating their disease-related concerns. Several studies have shown that patients' spouses often experience depression, distress and sexual difficulties when dealing with their partners' illness (Schmale et al 1983, Kissane et al 1994). Another study showed that couples were less committed to each other after the diagnosis of cancer, suggesting that marital commitment started to shift after the diagnosis from one based on each other as people to a commitment based on factors other than the spouse as a person, fitting the description of anticipatory grief (Swensen & Fuller 1992). However, other studies have shown that marital relationships strengthened after the diagnosis of HD (Hannah et al 1992). Some couples may be in need of more formal support and couples therapy has previously been shown to be beneficial (Mohr et al 2003, Kuijer et al 2004, Manne et al 2004).

SEXUAL FUNCTIONING

BMT survivors often become infertile due to aggressive chemotherapy and total body irradiation. Sexual difficulties are common (Lee et al 2001). Males more often experience impotence and females somatic symptoms (i.e. dyspareunia). Both may experience altered body image, decreased sexual satisfaction and low sexual desire (Auchincloss 1991, Mumma et al 1992, Molassiotis et al 1995a, 1996). Cancer patients, in general, have worse sexual functioning (in terms of desire, satisfaction with sexual life, somatic symptoms or body image) compared to sexually active young adults from the general population (Molassiotis 1998). These experiences limit their QoL. Thus, nursing interventions should be directed toward sexual/psychosexual rehabilitation. Sperm/ova banking before chemotherapy and/or radiotherapy may help BMT recipients (see Chapter 20).

If psychosexual problems exist, psychosocial/psychiatric support may improve the patients' QoL. In the UK psychosocial support is patchy and further resources are required. Patients at greater risk of psychosexual dysfunction (i.e. unmarried or younger patients) should receive therapy at an early, or preventative stage (Molassiotis et al 1995a, 1996).

Case study 25.1

Eight months after treatment for acute myeloid leukaemia with a BMT, a 28-year-old man wrote a letter to the unit's Sister asking for her advice about the impotence he was experiencing. He stated that, although his wife was very understanding and was not putting any pressure on him, he felt 'embarrassed and incomplete'. He asked what was wrong with him. He also wrote that he did not mention this problem to his consultant, as he was 'too shy'. He visited the unit at his follow-up clinic appointment 2 weeks later and some issues were discussed with him. Further to this, an investigation of his sexual hormonal levels was ordered, revealing that the hormonal levels (serum follicular stimulating hormone, luteinising hormone, testosterone) were within the normal range. Physiological dysfunction was therefore unlikely. An alternative explanation was impotence as a result of extreme stress and difficulties related to his post-treatment period. Together with his wife, he agreed to see a sex therapist. Two months later he called in the unit to thank the Sister and tell her that his problem no longer existed.

EFFECTS ON ACTIVITIES OF DAILY LIVING

Individuals treated with maintenance chemotherapy have reported a poorer QoL than those treated with BMT (Molassiotis et al 1996); however, 64.8% reported their QoL as good to excellent. Activities like shopping or climbing stairs were impaired among some patients in both groups, with social and domestic adjustment being most compromised when compared with healthy adults. In their study of lymphoma survivors, Wallwork & Richardson (1994) noted that patients' social activities decreased. Despite the small sample size, the authors reported that although many patients' lives had changed they adjusted their lives to accommodate these changes. Wallwork & Richardson called this 'subtle survivorship'.

FATIGUE

Fatigue seems to be the main problem in long-term survivors of haematological malignancies. Some studies estimate that 25–35% of patients with leukaemia and lymphomas report moderate to severe fatigue (Molassiotis et al 1996, Molassiotis & Morris 1998) while other studies suggest it may affect as many as 78.6% of patients (Molassiotis & Morris 1999). Fatigue in the latter study was predicted as a result of the combined effects of anxiety, presence of pain and infections. Additionally, in a group of patients with haematological cancers, lack of energy and tiredness (used as descriptors of fatigue) could be predicted by the combined effects of psychosocial and physical symptoms (i.e. shortness of breath, headaches, difficulty concentrating or social maladjustment) – suggesting that the concept of fatigue is multidimensional (Molassiotis 1999). Studies suggest that presence of fatigue (as well as emotional disorders) correlates highly with lower scores in quality of life assessments (Zittoun et al 1999).

However, fatigue research is relatively recent and many questions remain. Its prevalence and impact on patients' lives requires that nurses be aware of it, assess it regularly and test different interventions to combat it. Such interventions include periods of inactivity, sleep, exercise and stress management programmes, rearranging activities to conserve energy or manipulating the environment to allow undisturbed time for rest and sleep (Irvine et al 1991). Anecdotal data and clinical observations also link fatigue to periods of febrile illness, and alleviating fever may be helpful in decreasing fatigue (see Chapter 22).

More recently fatigue has been associated with the presence of anaemia in patients with haematological cancers. Anaemia affects a number of other areas of quality of life, such as dyspnoea or decreased motivation (Littlewood & Mandelli 2002). A large investment in the area over the past few years has resulted in the introduction of a new supportive care medication, epoetin alfa. Studies consistently show that administration of epoetin alfa produces statistically significant and clinically relevant improvements in quality of life (Turner et al 2001, Littlewood et al 2003), with those patients presenting with mild-to-moderate anaemia achieving the greatest improvements (Straus 2002).

Attentional fatigue manifesting as difficulties with concentration, memory and insomnia are frequently reported in QoL studies (Wallwork & Richardson 1994, Molassiotis et al 1996, Molassiotis 1999). Unless treated this can lead to social withdrawal, inability to work, maladjustment and even suicide. Nurses should assess such problems regularly and accurately. Training in the recognition and assessment of such symptoms may be necessary. Planned interventions should be flexible to meet each patient's needs.

Case study 25.2

A 33-year-old nursing sister received a BMT after failing to respond to conventional treatment for paroxysmal nocturnal haemoglobinuria. Approximately 1 month after BMT she developed symptoms thought to be indicative of graft-versus-host disease (GvHD). She was also complaining of short-term memory problems, episodes of crying and insomnia. She did not have a sustained depressive affect and refused antidepressants, which were also contraindicated because of her liver dysfunction. She was referred to the Psychological Medicine Department. However, she did not keep her appointment.

Later she was admitted to hospital with an acute psychotic episode. Her mental state had severely deteriorated since her last clinic visit. She had also attempted suicide. Her liver dysfunction made it difficult to prescribe medication and she was provided with 24-hour psychiatric nursing. Symptoms eventually subsided and prior to discharge her mental state showed an improvement. A week later she was admitted to hospital with further physical problems but mentioned that she still had short-term memory problems. A few months later she started work as a part-time nurse teacher and eventually a full-time one. However, she had problems coping with work, possibly due to her short-term memory loss. Her family were also concerned about her and she was referred to the hospital psychiatrist. Before the appointment she committed suicide.

The scenario described in case report 25.2 highlights the need for regular assessment and appropriate support (Molassiotis & Morris 1997). Nurses should provide patients and their families with realistic expectations for the chronic phase after treatment and assist them with realistic goal setting. Teaching and reinforcement of patients' health-promoting activities may lessen their health concerns. Supporting families could help to keep them together during the stressful and difficult times occurring throughout their disease experience. Encouraging patients to use their own coping mechanisms or teaching them to use effective coping skills may improve their adjustment. Counselling is important for patients and their families as it enhances social support and allows them to give vent to their feelings. Cognitive-behavioural interventions can improve long-term QoL, although different patients may need different types of interventions (i.e. progressive muscle relaxation, meditation or psycho-educational techniques).

DISCRIMINATION IN EMPLOYMENT AND FINANCIAL ISSUES

A major component of QoL is the vocational adjustment of cancer survivors. Although many studies have reported work-related problems in survivors of haematological cancers (Fobair et al 1986, Carpenter et al 1989, Greaves-Otte et al 1991, Wingard et al 1991, Molassiotis et al 1995b, 1996), many methodological inconsistencies exist, complicating the interpretation of results.

Despite methodological limitations, employment discrimination is a major problem for cancer survivors, further compromising their QoL and social adjustment. Fobair et al (1986) reported that, among 403 survivors from HD, up to 42% had problems in their workplace. Job problems included denial of insurance (11%), denial of other benefits (6%), denial of a job offer (12%), termination of employment following treatment (6%), conflict with supervisors and co-workers (12%) and rejection by the military (8%). A recent study with chronic myeloid leukaemia survivors also reported that over 10% of the sample had increased problems with co-workers as a result of their illness (Molassiotis & Morris 1999). HD survivors in another study perceived that their careers had been compromised as a result of their illness (Cella & Tross 1986). Survivors interviewed by Koocher & O'Malley (1982) reported job refusals, being denied benefits and conflict with supervisors. Furthermore, 76% of 422 cancer patients surveyed indicated that they were working at the time of diagnosis; this number decreased to 56% after diagnosis (Rothstein et al 1995).

REFLECTION POINT   Why might employers be reluctant to employ cancer survivors?

Individuals with leukaemia and lymphoma, along with those with lung and head and neck cancers and those aged over 45 years, have been shown to have lower return-to-work rates than other cancer survivors (van der Wouden et al 1992, Berry 1993). In a further study, 26% of patients with haematological cancers receiving maintenance chemotherapy (n = 73) and 19.3% of BMT patients (n = 91) had not returned to work an average of 40 months post-initial treatment or BMT, respectively (Molassiotis et al 1996). Although a major limitation in such a finding is that employment type and status before treatment was unknown, data show that unemployment after cancer diagnosis requires further attention, possibly through vocational rehabilitation services.

Reports of unemployment in other studies of BMT survivors range from 15% (Wolcott et al 1986) to 50% (Hengeveld et al 1988). Job discrimination in long-term BMT survivors has been shown to be independently associated with lack of and loss of employment (Wingard et al 1991). In the previous study, job discrimination was reported even among those who had been working, as 57% of subjects reporting substantial discrimination were employed full-time. Furthermore, a large study of 566 survivors in two rehabilitation centres showed that, in general, most patients seem either to resort to early retirement or are able to resume their occupational activity without special occupational training (Weis et al 1994). This same study demonstrated that medical rehabilitation had a negligible influence on vocational integration of cancer patients. In agreement with other reports, blue-collar workers returned less frequently to their former places of work, being more likely to take early retirement. Type of occupation has been found to be the main determinant of whether patients were employed after diagnosis (Rothstein et al 1995).

It is surprising that survivors of haematological or other types of cancers are discriminated against in their employment, as most of them are able to resume their previous work and are very willing to return to work, except those who experience physical complications from their disease or treatment. Cancer survivors appear to have similar productivity rates to other workers (Wheatley et al 1974). Several myths contribute to employment discrimination, including cancer is a death sentence (i.e. banks deny loans, assumption of short-term life), cancer is contagious and cancer survivors are an unproductive drain on the economy, as employers are afraid that insurance premiums will increase (Hoffman 1989).

Unemployment and employment discrimination, together with expenses associated with travelling to oncology centres for treatment, may have a negative impact on patients' financial status. Studies indicate that HD survivors may experience negative socioeconomic effects. Factors enhancing this negative effect include being male, earning less than US$15000 (£8,250) per year, being unemployed or unmarried, having had serious illnesses since treatment completion and being less educated (Kornblith et al 1992). Unfortunately such studies have yet to be conducted in the UK.

REFLECTION POINT What measures would you take to enable one of your patients to obtain and/or continue work?

CONCLUSION

BMT survivors often experience problems with physical health, sexual functioning, unemployment and dysfunction in social adjustment. Positive changes with social relationships also occur. However, more rigorous research with patients with haematological cancers is needed.

Nurses working in haematological oncology can play an important role in the social and vocational integration of their patients. Nurses can serve as their patients' advocates by making realistic assessments of patients' capacities and guiding them towards appropriate resources, such as employment counsellors, social workers, support groups and government agencies (Hoffman 1989). The existence of legislation of equal opportunities for all individuals with a cancer history is an important step in decreasing employment discrimination, and professional nursing bodies could advocate for this (i.e. the Royal College of Nursing in the UK or the Oncology Nursing Society in the USA). Further, nurses can assist their patients to plan a return-to-work schedule, as they can understand and assess the nature of the relationship between the patient's work responsibilities and the effects of treatment (Berry 1993). Being supportive, listening, assessing patients' needs and abilities, planning long-term care services and referring patients to other appropriate agencies can enhance patients' QoL and contribute to an easier patient transition from the sick role to post-cancer social integration and psychosocial adjustment.

DISCUSSION QUESTIONS

1. What assessment data would you need to collect from a long-term survivor of leukaemia or lymphoma? What would be the priorities in your care planning?

2. How could the specialist haemato-oncology nurse enhance the adjustment of his/her patients and support their families? Discuss individual interventions based on evidence.

3. What measures are you taking in your practice to assess and treat fatigue and sexual dysfunction in your patients?

4. Is there a role for a mental health nurse in the care of haemato-oncology patients?

5. How can the family be involved in the care of their relative? What are the objectives of such an involvement?

6. How could you increase awareness about social care among your colleagues?

References

Andrykowski M A, Henslee P J, Barnett R L 1989 Longitudinal assessment of psychosocial functioning of adult survivors of allogeneic bone marrow transplantation. Bone Marrow Transplantation 4:505–509

Andrykowski M A, Altmaier E M, Barnett R L, Otis M L, Gingrich R, Henslee-Downey P J 1990 The quality of life in adult survivors of allogeneic bone marrow transplantation. Transplantation 50:399–406

Auchincloss S S 1991 Sexual dysfunction after cancer treatment. Journal of Psychosocial Oncology 9:23–42

Baker F, Wingard J R, Curbow B et al 1994 Quality of life of bone marrow transplant long-term survivors. Bone Marrow Transplantation 13:589–596

Baker F, Zabora J, Polland A, Wingard J 1999 Reintegration after bone marrow transplantation. Cancer Practice 7(4):190–197

Belec R H 1992 Quality of life: perceptions of long-term survivors of bone marrow transplantation. Oncology Nursing Forum 19:31–37

Berry D L 1993 Return-to-work experience of people with cancer. Oncology Nursing Forum 20:905–911

Bertero C, Ek A C 1993 Quality of life of adults with acute leukaemia. Journal of Advanced Nursing 18: 1346–1353

Boyle D, Blodgett L, Gnesdiloff S et al 2000 Caregiver quality of life after autologous bone marrow transplantation. Cancer Nursing 23(3):193–205

Breaden K 1997 Cancer and beyond: the question of survivorship. Journal of Advanced Nursing 26(5):978–984

Browne N, Robinson L, Richardson A 2002 A Delphi study on the research priorities of European oncology nurses. European Journal of Oncology Nursing 6(3):133–144

Bushkin E 1993 Signposts of survivorship. Oncology Nursing Forum 20:869–875

Caplan K C 1987 Definitions and dimensions of quality of life. In: Aaronson N K, Beckmann J (eds) The quality of life of cancer patients. Raven Press, New York, pp 1–9

Carpenter P, Morrow G, Schmale A 1989 The psychosocial status of cancer patients after cessation of treatment. Journal of Psychosocial Oncology 7:95–103

Cella D F, Tross S 1986 Psychological adjustment to survival from Hodgkin's disease. Journal of Consulting and Clinical Psychology 54:616–622

Degner L 1987 Priorities for cancer nursing research: a Canadian replication. Cancer Nursing 10:319–326

Dow K H 1990 The enduring seasons in survival. Oncology Nursing Forum 17:511–516

Ferrell B, Grant M, Schmidt G M et al 1992a The meaning of quality of life for bone marrow transplant survivors. Part 1: The impact of bone marrow transplant on quality of life. Cancer Nursing 15:153–160

Ferrell B, Grant M, Schmidt G M et al 1992b The meaning of quality of life for bone marrow transplant survivors. Part 2: Improving quality of life for bone marrow transplant survivors. Cancer Nursing 15:247–253

Ferrell B R, Dow K H, Leigh S, Ly J, Gulasekaram P 1995 Quality of life in long-term cancer survivors. Oncology Nursing Forum 22:915–922

Fliedner M C 2002 Research within the field of blood and marrow transplantation nursing: how can it contribute to higher quality of care? International Journal of Hematology 76(Suppl 2):289–291

Fobair R, Hoppe R T, Bloom J, Cox R, Varghese A, Spiegel D 1986 Psychosocial problems among survivors of Hodgkin's disease. Journal of Clinical Oncology 4:805–814

Gaston-Johansson F, Foxall M 1996 Psychological correlates of quality of life across the autologous bone marrow transplant experience. Cancer Nursing 19:170–176

Greaves-Otte J G W, Greaves J, Kruyt P M, van Leeuwen O, van der Wouden J C, van der Does E 1991 Problems at social re-integration of long-term cancer survivors. European Journal of Cancer 27:178–181

Haberman M 1997 Nursing research in blood cell and marrow transplantation. In: Whedon M B, Wujcik D (eds) Blood and marrow stem cell transplantation, principles, practice and nursing insights, 2nd edn. Jones and Bartlett, Boston, pp 497–505

Haberman M, Bush N, Young K, Sullivan K M 1993 Quality of life of adult long-term survivors of bone marrow transplantation: a qualitative analysis of narrative data. Oncology Nursing Forum 20:1545–1553

Hannah M T, Gritz B R, Wellisch D K 1992 Changes in marital and sexual functioning in long-term survivors and their spouses: testicular cancer versus Hodgkin's disease. Psycho-Oncology 1:89–103

Harder H, Cornelissen J J, Van Gool A R, Duivenvoorden H J, Eijkenboom W M, van den Bent M J 2002 Cognitive functioning and quality of life in long-term adult survivors of bone marrow transplantation. Cancer 95(1):183–192

Hengeveld M W, Houtman R B, Zwaan F E 1988 Psychological aspects of bone marrow transplantation: a retrospective study of 17 long-term survivors. Bone Marrow Transplantation 3:69–75

Herbst S 1995 Survivorship: redefining the cancer experience. Oncology Nursing Forum 22:527–532

Hoffman B 1989 Cancer survivors at work: job problems and illegal discrimination. Oncology Nursing Forum 16:39–43

Hornquist J O 1982 The concept of quality of life. Scandinavian Journal of Social Medicine 10:57–61

Irvine D M, Vincent L, Bubela N, Thompson L, Graydon J 1991 A critical appraisal of the research literature investigating fatigue in the individual with cancer. Cancer Nursing 14:188–199

Kissane D W, Block S, Burns W I, McKenzie D, Posterino M 1994 Psychological morbidity in the families of patients with cancer. Psycho-Oncology 3:47–56

Koocher G P, O'Malley J E 1982 The Damocles syndrome: psychosocial consequences of surviving childhood cancer. McGraw-Hill, New York

Kornblith A B, Anderson J, Cella D F 1992 Hodgkin's disease survivors are at increased risk for problems in psychosocial adaptation. Cancer 70:2214–2224

Kuijer R G, Bram P, Buunk G, de Jong M, Ybema J F, Sanderman R 2004 Effects of a brief intervention program for patients with cancer and their partners on feelings of inequity, relationship quality and psychological distress. Psycho-Oncology 13(5):321–334

Lee S J, Fairclough D, Parsons S K et al 2001 Recovery after stem-cell transplantation for hematologic diseases. Journal of Clinical Oncology 19(1):242–252

Littlewood T, Mandelli F 2002 The effects of anemia in hematologic malignancies: more than a symptom. Seminars in Oncology 29(3 Suppl 8):40–44

Littlewood T J, Nortier J, Rapoport B et al 2003. Epoetin alfa corrects anemia and improves quality of life in patients with hematologic malignancies receiving non-platinum chemotherapy. Hematological Oncology 21(4):169–180

Manne S, Babb J, Pinover W, Horwitz E, Ebbert J 2004 Psychoeducational group intervention for wives of men with prostate cancer. Psycho-Oncology 13(1):37–46

Mohr D C, Moran P J, Kohn C et al 2003 Couples therapy at end of life. Psycho-Oncology 12(6):620–627

Molassiotis A 1997 Nursing research within bone marrow transplantation in Europe: an evaluation. European Journal of Cancer Care 6:257–261

Molassiotis A 1998 Measuring psychosexual functioning in cancer patients: psychometric properties and normative data of a new questionnaire. European Journal of Oncology Nursing 2:194–205

Molassiotis A 1999 A correlation evaluation of tiredness and lack of energy in survivors of haematological malignanacies. European Journal of Cancer Care 8:19–25

Molassiotis A, Morris P J 1997 Suicide and suicidal ideation after marrow transplantation. Bone Marrow Transplantation 19:87–90

Molassiotis A, Morris P J 1998 The meaning of quality of life and the effects of unrelated donor bone marrow transplants for chronic myeloid leukemia in adult long-term survivors. Cancer Nursing 21(3):205–211

Molassiotis A, Morris P J 1999 Quality of life in patients with chronic myeloid leukemia after unrelated donor bone marrow transplantation. Cancer Nursing 22(5):340–349

Molassiotis A, van den Akker O B A, Milligan D W, Boughton B J 1995a Gonadal function and psychosexual adjustment in male long-term survivors of bone marrow transplantation. Bone Marrow Transplantation 16:253–256

Molassiotis A, Boughton B J, Burgoyne T, van den Akker O B A 1995b Comparison of the overall quality of life in 50 long-term survivors of autologous and allogeneic bone marrow transplantation. Journal of Advanced Nursing 22:509–516

Molassiotis A, van den Akker O B A, Milligan D W et al 1996 Quality of life in long term survivors of marrow transplantation: comparison with a matched group receiving maintenance chemotherapy. Bone Marrow Transplantation 17:249–258

Molassiotis A, van den Akker O B A, Boughton B J 1997 Perceived social support, family environment and psychosocial recovery in bone marrow transplant long-term survivors. Social Science and Medicine 44:317–325

Montgomery C, Pocock M, Titley K, Lloyd K 2002 Individual quality of life in patients with leukaemia and lymphoma. Psycho-Oncology 11:239–243

Mullan F 1985 Seasons of survival: reflections of a physician with cancer. New England Journal of Medicine 313:270–273

Mumma G H, Mashberg D, Lesko L M 1992 Long-term psychosexual adjustment of adult leukemia survivors: impact of marrow transplantation versus conventional chemotherapy. General Hospital Psychiatry 14:43–55

Oberst M T 1978 Priorities in cancer nursing research. Cancer Nursing 1:281–290

Redaelli A, Stephens J M, Brandt S, Botteman M F, Pashos C L 2004 Short and long-term effects of acute myeloid leukemia on patient health-related quality of life. Cancer Treatment Reviews 30(1):103–117

Rose M 1989 Health promotion and risk prevention: application for cancer survivors. Oncology Nursing Forum 16:335–340

Rothstein M A, Kennedy K, Ritchie K J, Pyle K 1995 Are cancer patients subject to employment discrimination? Oncology 9:1303–1306, 1311–1312, 1315

Schmale A M, Morrow G R, Schmitt M H et al 1983 Well-being of cancer survivors. Psychosomatic Medicine 45:163–169

Schmidt G M, Niland J C, Forman S J et al 1993. Extended follow-up in 212 long-term allogeneic bone marrow transplant survivors. Transplantation 55:551–557

Shanfield S 1980 On surviving cancer: psychological considerations. Comparative Psychiatry 21:128–134

Soanes L, Gibson F, Hannan J, Bayliss J 2003 Establishing nursing research priorities on a paediatric haematology, oncology, immunology and infectious diseases unit: involving doctors and parents. European Journal of Oncology Nursing 7(2):110–119

Straus D J 2002 Epoetin alfa as a supportive measure in hematologic malignancies. Seminars in Hematology 39(4 Suppl 3):25–31

Swensen C H, Fuller S R 1992 Expression of love, marriage problems, commitment, and anticipatory grief in the marriages of cancer patients. Journal of Marriage & the Family 54(1):191–196

Syrjala K L, Chapko M K, Vitaliano P P, Cummings C, Sullivan K M 1993 Recovery after allogeneic marrow transplantation: prospective study of predictors of long-term physical and psychosocial functioning. Bone Marrow Transplantation 11:319–327

Szalai A 1980 The meaning of comparative research on the quality of life. In: Szalai A, Andrews F M (eds) The quality of life, comparative studies. Sage, Beverly Hills, pp 7–21

Tooter M A, Homes G E, Homes F F 1987 Decisions about marriage and family among survivors of childhood cancer. Journal of Psychosocial Oncology 5:59–68

Turner R, Anglin P, Burkes R et al 2001 Epoetin alfa in cancer patients: evidence-based guidelines. Journal of Pain & Symptom Management 22(5):954–965

van der Wouden J C, Greaves-Otte J G, Greaves J, Kruyt P M, van Leeuwen O, van der Does E 1992 Occupational reintegration of long-term cancer survivors. Journal of Occupational Medicine 34:1084–1089

Wallwork L, Richardson A 1994 Beyond cancer: changes, problems and needs expressed by adult lymphoma survivors attending an out-patients clinic. European Journal of Cancer Care 3:122–132

Wasserman A L, Thompson E I, Williams J A, Fairclough D L 1987 The psychological status of childhood/adolescent Hodgkin's disease. American Journal of Diseases in Childhood 141:626–631

Watson M, Buck G, Wheatley K et al 2004 Adverse impact of bone marrow transplantation on quality of life in acute myeloid leukaemia patients; analysis of the UK Medical Research Centre AML 10 Trial. European Journal of Cancer 40(7):971–978

Weis J, Koch U, Kruck P, Beck A 1994 Problems of vocational integration after cancer. Clinical Rehabilitation 8:219–225

Welch-McCaffrey D, Hoffman B, Leigh S, Loescher L, Meyskens F 1989 Surviving adult cancers. Part 2: psychosocial implications. Annals of Internal Medicine 111:517–523

Wheatley G M, Cunnick W R, Wright B P, van Keuren D 1974 The employment of persons with a history of treatment for cancer. Cancer 33:441–445

Wingard, J R, Curbow B, Baker F, Piantadosi L 1991 Health, functional status and employment of adult survivors of bone marrow transplantation. Annals of Internal Medicine 114:113–118

Wolcott D L, Wellisch D K, Fawzy I F, Landsverk J 1986 Adaptation of adult bone marrow transplant recipient long-term survivors. Transplantation 41:478–484

Xuereb M C, Dunlop R 2003 The experience of leukaemia and bone marrow transplant: searching for meaning and agency. Psycho-Oncology 12(5):397–409

Yellen S B, Cella D F, Bonomi A 1993 Quality of life in people with Hodgkin's disease. Oncology 7:41–45

Zittoun R, Achard S, Ruszniewski M 1999 Assessment of quality of life during intensive chemotherapy or bone marrow transplantation. Psycho-Oncology 8(1): 64–73

Further reading

Andrykowski M A 1994 Psychosocial factors in bone marrow transplantation: a review and recommendations for research. Bone Marrow Transplantation 13: 357–375
This article presents a critical analysis of all the existing literature at the time on the psychosocial issues of bone marrow transplantation. It highlights the important findings as well as the limitations of some studies. It also gives valuable directions for future research.

Auchincloss S S 1989 Sexual dysfunction in cancer patients: issues in evaluation and treatment. In: Holland J C, Rowland J H (eds) Handbook of psycho-oncology. Oxford, Oxford University Press
This chapter provides detailed information on research into sexuality and cancer patients and highlights important considerations in the assessment and measurement of sexual dysfunction and different treatment options, based on individual requirements.

Bradley C, Bednarek H L 2002. Employment patterns of long-term cancer survivors. Psycho-Oncology 11(3):188–198
This is one of the few papers dealing directly with the topic of work adjustment and employment in cancer survivors. They report results from a cross-sectional survey of 253 cancer survivors of mixed diagnosis carried out in the USA. A number of problems are reported, including employment discrimination, although the authors concluded that the ability of cancer patients to continue employment was optimistic.

Cella D, Webster K A 1999. Quality of life and treatment value in the management of hematologic malignancies. Seminars in Oncology 26(5 Suppl 14):34–42
This is a review article of QoL studies in patients with haematological malignancies, attempting to put such data in context with therapeutic benefit and treatment value.

de Haes J C J M, van Knippenberg F C E 1985 The quality of life of cancer patients: a review of the literature. Social Science and Medicine 20:809–817
Although not a recent article, it is very well written and provides a good background on definitions about quality of life, its assessment and methodological issues.

Greenberg D B, Kornblith A B, Herndom J E 1997 Quality of life for adult leukemia survivors treated on clinical trials of cancer and leukemia group B during the period 1971–1988. Cancer 80:1936–1944
This is a large study of QoL in leukaemia survivors an average of 5 years post-treatment. It identified predictors of greater psychological distress, including less education, younger age, poor family function, medical problems post-treatment and anticipatory distress during chemotherapy treatment. It also provides a post-traumatic stress disorder model for leukaemia survivors.

Little M, Paul K, Jordens C F C, Sayers E-J 2002
Survivorship and discourses of identity. Psycho-
Oncology 11(2):170–178

This article is an interesting philosophical paper around
cancer survivorship and the sense of identity in order to
more fully understand the experience of the survivor.
Identity may be composed of memory, embodiment and
continuity, and authors discuss how the extreme experience
of threat can affect identity.

Maunsell E, Brisson C, Dubois L, Lauzier S, Fraser A 2000
Work problems after breast cancer: an exploratory
qualitative study. Psycho-Oncology 8(6):467–473

This qualitative work with breast cancer survivors adds to
the work reported above by Bradley & Bednarek (2002) and
sheds more light around employment problems and
difficulties, exploring the experiences of patients in depth.

Molassiotis A 1997 A conceptual model of adaptation to
illness and quality of life for cancer patients treated
with bone marrow transplants. Journal of Advanced
Nursing 26:572–579

This article investigates the theory behind stress and
adaptation, and proposes a new theoretical framework of
assessment and interventions in patients with
haematological malignancies in relation to their quality of
life.

Nail L M, Winningham M L 1995 Fatigue and weakness
in cancer patients: the symptoms experience. Seminars
in Oncology Nursing 11:272–278

This article distinguishes fatigue and weakness and reviews
symptom management for both. The limited research on
fatigue and the development of interventions are discussed
as well as the implications for nursing practice.

Chapter 26

Palliative care

Helen Balsdon

KEY POINTS

- Haemato-oncology and palliative care have not always sat comfortably together.
- Palliative care is applicable from early in the course of the illness.
- Accurate multidisciplinary systematic assessment is vital to good palliative care.
- Patients and relatives should be fully informed and involved in making choices and decisions about care.

INTRODUCTION

Haemato-oncology and palliative care have not always sat comfortably together. There are a number of different reasons for this. Many haematological cancers are potentially curable and haemato-oncology is frequently associated with highly technical, curative treatment. This has been perceived as incompatible with the concept of palliative care, which has historically been associated with end-of-life care. Furthermore, the transition from curative treatment to palliative and terminal care can occur rapidly with some haematological cancers, e.g. acute leukaemias, leaving little or no time to initiate palliative care. Perceptions of palliative care are, however, changing, with the emphasis on symptom management, supportive care and quality of life starting at diagnosis and continuing throughout the course of a disease. This change of emphasis to support throughout the disease experience is particularly helpful in potentially curable haematological cancers.

Other haematological cancers are chronic diseases that individuals may live with for a number of years, although ultimately many are not curable. Supportive and palliative care are therefore required to manage symptoms and enhance quality of life. The extent to which palliative care is incorporated into haemato-oncology is unknown as there is a lack of research in this area. However, it appears that an increasing number of multidisciplinary haemato-oncology teams are developing core palliative care skills and involving specialist palliative care services in the care of patients from diagnosis onwards.

This chapter considers a number of common palliative care themes including:

- what palliative care is and how its guiding principles can be applied
- the differences between general and specialist palliative care
- how nurses can use specialist palliative care teams to their best advantage both in hospital and primary care settings
- practice issues associated with providing palliative care in a haemato-oncology setting.

Management of haematological cancers, their treatment and interventions to control symptoms and improve quality of life are considered, along with some of the challenges these may pose for nurses. Other aspects of care such as provision of information and education and the palliative care knowledge and skills required by haemato-oncology nurses are also discussed.

PALLIATIVE CARE AND ITS GUIDING PRINCIPLES

To understand how palliative care can be incorporated into haemato-oncology it is important to understand what palliative care is. The World Health Organization (WHO 2002) defines palliative care as:

'an approach that improves the quality of life of patients and their families facing the problems associated with life-threatening illness, through the prevention and relief of suffering by means of early identification and impeccable assessment and treatment of pain and other problems, physical, psychosocial and spiritual.'

This definition refers to the holistic approach of palliative care and its guiding principles and reflects the need to introduce palliative care early in a pathway of care. This approach is recognised as beneficial as problems at the end of life often have origins earlier in a disease trajectory (WHO 2002).

The principles of palliative care provide a framework for care by considering the physical, psychological, social and spiritual needs of patients and their family. Palliative care:

- provides relief from pain and other distressing symptoms
- affirms life and regards dying as a normal process
- intends neither to hasten nor postpone death
- integrates the psychological and spiritual aspects of patient care
- offers a support system to help patients to live as actively as possible until death
- offers a support system to help the family to cope during the patient's illness and in their own bereavement
- uses a team approach to address the needs of patients and their families, including bereavement counselling, if indicated
- will enhance quality of life, and may also positively influence the course of illness
- is applicable early in the course of illness, in conjunction with other therapeutics that are intended to prolong life, such as chemotherapy and radiation therapy, and includes those investigations needed to better understand and manage distressing clinical complications (WHO 2002).

The importance of involving patients and their families in decisions about their treatment and care, equity of access to the best possible symptom control and support and being able to die in the place of their choice is also advocated (National Institute for Clinical Excellence (NICE) 2004). These principles are applicable to any patient in any health-care setting.

The 2002 WHO definition and principles of palliative care and the NICE (2004) palliative and supportive care guidance highlight how the focus of palliative care has changed in recent years. Traditionally, palliative care has been associated with care of the dying; however, recently, increased emphasis has been placed on supportive care combined with both active treatment and palliative care principles, from diagnosis onwards, to ensure that individuals receive the best possible care.

The NICE 2004 palliative and supportive care guidance is aimed at cancer services but can be applied to any group of patients requiring palliative care. The guidance aims to define the service models needed to ensure that patients and carers received the very best support to help them to cope with a diagnosis of cancer and its treatment. Topics covered by the document include coordination of care, user involvement, communication, informational, psychological, social and spiritual support services, and general and specialist palliative care. The document provides guidance on best practice and has the potential to drive the development of palliative care services throughout the UK.

Palliative care has been used extensively in cancer nursing in the past and continues to have a significant role. However, just as haemato-oncology has rapidly moved forward in terms of new treatments and supportive care in the last decade, palliative care has also had many successes and developments. The role of palliative care is increasingly being recognised in chronic disease management, such as cardiac failure, and potentially curable diseases, including many haematological conditions.

Palliative care is provided by two groups of health-care professionals: general and specialist. All health-care professionals should have the knowledge and skills to provide comfort and support to those requiring palliative care – general palliative care is therefore the responsibility of everyone. According to Davies & Higginson (2004) palliative care principles should be an integral part of care. Palliative care specialists are, however, required to provide expert advice and help with complex care needs and combinations of symptoms. Palliative care specialists have extensive experience and have undertaken specialist education and training in the speciality and include consultants in palliative medicine and specialist palliative care nurses (National Council for Hospice and Specialist Palliative Care Services 2002 – NB now known as the National Council for Palliative Care). Palliative care specialists tend to be found within hospice settings or specialist palliative care teams based in hospitals or primary care.

One of the most common challenges in haemato-oncology is determining when palliative care should be introduced. This can occasionally be a source of conflict between different professional groups perhaps because to many people palliative care is still strongly associated with terminal care. In haemato-oncology, palliative care is often now introduced at diagnosis (Booth & Bruera 2003). Doctors have found this approach 'helpful' for patients undergoing intensive haematology treatments such as intensive chemotherapy or blood and marrow transplantation (Perkins & Closs 2003).

Introducing a specialist palliative care team at the time of a diagnosis of a haematological cancer can offer many benefits to the patient and their family, and the haematology team caring for them. For the patient and their family palliative care at this stage can offer:

- additional support as they come to terms with their diagnosis
- assistance with development of individual coping strategies
- practical assistance in dealing with the social implications of living with a life-threatening illness, such as financial issues (some patients may be unable to work for some time whilst undergoing treatment)
- advice on methods to control any distressing symptoms being experienced either as a consequence of the disease or its treatment.

The haemato-oncology team can also benefit as this additional resource can help to support and guide them in the management of complex symptoms, supportive treatments and decision-making.

Consider a patient newly diagnosed with a haematological cancer that you have cared for. What were the physical, psychological, social and spiritual needs of the patient and their family? When was specialist palliative care introduced and what assistance was offered to the patient, their family and you?

Involving a specialist palliative care team early in a patient's experience can also have benefits if the emphasis of care changes from curative to palliative or terminal care. Changes in an individual's blood picture and response to curative treatment can happen very rapidly, particularly in acute leukaemia, and managing the transition between curative and palliative care is challenging for all those involved (Jeffery & Owen 2003). The suddenness of this change can be confusing for patients and their families, as there is often limited or no time to come to terms with a changed prognosis. Health-care professionals may also find the rapid deterioration in an individual's condition difficult to cope with.

Nurses often feel uncomfortable raising the topic of palliative care with patients at this stage because of its associations with death. Equally, patients often feel uncertain of this new development because they feel that the team treating them is no longer interested in them or because they have a strong relationship with the treating team they see no reason to change or see other health-care professionals. If the patient and their family have already met the specialist palliative care team, this transition can often be more effectively managed.

PRACTICE ISSUES

ASSESSMENT

The importance of systematic and accurate assessment is vital to good palliative care and ensuring the needs and concerns of patients and their families are both identified and addressed. NICE (2004) recommend that all health-care professionals involved in the care of a patient and family in every care setting are expected to undertake a comprehensive assessment of need at key time points in the care pathway. They must take appropriate action to ensure patients and their families have access to the services required to help them meet identified needs. The key time points include: at diagnosis, at the commencement of, during and at the end of treatment, at relapse, and when death is approaching (NICE 2004).

Holistic assessment aims to ensure a smooth transition of care across organisational boundaries, ensure patients are able to access the right service at the right time and promote effective use of resources.

Nurses play a key role in assessment. Haemato-oncology nurses regularly assess patient wellbeing and needs, ensure patients and family needs have been identified, and that appropriate actions are taken to assist them in their daily lives in and outside the hospital. It is also important to ensure that the multidisciplinary team is involved in assessment. This may include haemato-oncology and specialist palliative care teams, physiotherapists, occupational therapists, therapy radiographers, faith leaders (e.g. hospital chaplain or local minister), general practitioner and other members of the primary health care team.

NICE (2004) recommends that assessment should encompass the following elements:

- information
- communication
- involvement in decision-making
- physical symptoms
- psychological, social and spiritual support
- rehabilitation
- complementary therapies
- self-management and peer support
- family and carer support, including bereavement support (if applicable)
- involvement in service design and delivery.

It also seems sensible to add education needs to this list. Education is a vital part of promoting self-care and empowering the patient and family to participate in decision-making. The education needs of a patient and their family will change throughout the care pathway and health-care professionals need to be able to assess these needs alongside other identified needs to ensure a truly holistic approach.

NICE (2004) also recognises that patients have a central role to play in assessment and recommends that health-care professionals ask them how they are feeling and involve them in assessing their own needs while enabling them to express their wishes and concerns. McGrath (2001) would also advocate for carers to be involved in the process, given the close partnerships often seen in haemato-oncology.

Systematic assessment can take many forms and includes talking to the patient and their family, asking questions and using one of the wide range of formal assessment tools available. Irrespective of the approach taken it is essential to communicate the findings to everyone involved in an individual's care and ensure a care plan is devised detailing how the multidisciplinary team will address their identified needs, wishes and concerns. Poor communication between team members may result in poorly controlled symptoms and psychological and spiritual distress – nurses have a crucial role in ensuring coordination of care.

KNOWLEDGE AND SKILLS DEVELOPMENT

Knowledge and skills development in palliative care incorporates many core competencies that can be used in any clinical setting including: communication skills, assessment skills, symptom control, managing psychological distress and use of advanced care planning tools such as the 'care of the dying' care pathway (Ellershaw & Wilkinson 2003).

Many palliative care skills can be learnt in the workplace with the support of clinical supervision or other methods that enhance reflective practice. Highly specialist multidisciplinary palliative care teams can also support and guide learning. Equally there are a variety of educational opportunities that can aid the development of this knowledge and associated skills.

REFLECTION POINT

What palliative care knowledge and skills do you currently have and what do you need to develop to become an expert haemato-oncology nurse with generalist palliative care knowledge and skills?

DISEASE MANAGEMENT AND SYMPTOM CONTROL

Haematological cancers include acute and chronic leukaemias, lymphomas, myeloma and myelodysplastic syndromes. Treatment for these diseases involves aggressive therapies including intensive chemotherapy, radiotherapy, biotherapies and blood and marrow transplantation (see Chapters 9, 10, 11 & 13). Treatment intent varies depending on the disease, the age of the patient, their performance status and, of course, the wishes of the patient and their families. Treatment intent can be viewed as a continuum; at one end is the intent to cure and at the opposite end is the aim to control the disease and/or its symptoms for as long as possible. However, regardless of treatment intent, maintaining a good quality of life is paramount.

All treatments have potential risks and benefits. These need to be considered by all involved – the multidisciplinary team, the patient and their family. The aim of any treatment will be to get the best possible outcome for the patient using a treatment that will have minimal side effects and a low risk of death. However, given the aggressive nature of the treatments used it is inevitable that patients will experience side effects and, despite increasingly successful treatments, many patients will die as a result of their disease or treatment.

Clinical trials

A large number of haematology patients are treated in the context of a clinical trial. Many trials in haematology are national studies comparing the best-known treatments. Other, more experimental trials may be open to patients if these best treatments fail. Palliative care is highly appropriate if the patient is in a very experimental trial because the introduction of clinical trials often comes at a time when there is a transition from cure to palliation; known curative treatments have failed and newer treatments where benefits are not yet known are used in an attempt to control a disease and understand more about it. It is not uncommon for patients to experience side effects from these treatments and/or distressing symptoms associated with their disease whilst taking part in a clinical trial. Therefore access to good symptom control and support is essential.

SYMPTOM MANAGEMENT

Symptom management is a key component of palliative care and can be used throughout an individual's illness experience irrespective of the stage of a disease. It is important to remember that inadequate symptom control can impair quality of life (Valente 2004). Haemato-oncology patients often have complex combinations of side effects frequently associated with the increased intensity of treatments. These combinations of side effects can be challenging to manage and can have a huge impact on the patient and their family in terms of physical and psychological wellbeing and may influence decision-making about continuing with treatment (McGrath 2001, Perkins & Closs 2003). It is therefore essential to manage symptoms effectively whilst taking an individualised holistic approach to assessment, planning, intervention and evaluation. Specialist palliative care teams can assist with the management of complex symptoms and offer continuing support to all.

The principles of good symptom management are impeccable assessment, find the cause, be proactive, treat a symptom promptly, prescribe and administer regularly, reassess repeatedly but only make one change at a time (Spathis 2003). Common symptoms experienced by haemato-oncology patients include:

- anaemia
- infection
- bleeding problems
- nausea and vomiting
- dry mouth
- sore mouth
- nutritional problems
- fatigue
- constipation
- anxiety and depression.

Each of these symptoms can be caused by the disease or its treatment and can be debilitating as they affect daily activities such as eating, drinking and sleep.

A wide range of interventions can be used in symptom management including transfusion, antibiotics, enteral feeding, emotional support, information and/or education, encouragement to eat, drink or keep active, providing uninterrupted time to facilitate sleep, providing a fan to keep cool or medications. The effectiveness of interventions should always be evaluated – simply repeating the assessment is one means of measurement. However, it is important to leave an adequate amount of time for the intervention to take effect before reassessment is undertaken.

MANAGEMENT OF ONCOLOGICAL EMERGENCIES

Haemato-oncology patients may also experience oncological emergencies including:

- major haemorrhage
- neutropenic sepsis
- superior vena cava obstruction
- hypocalcaemia
- spinal cord compression.

Each of these can be life-threatening and require emergency assessment and treatment. Nurses need to be aware of the potential development of such emergencies and be alert to any early warning signs. Thorough assessment, combined with good communication and monitoring of patients may be helpful in detecting the onset of these conditions early. Diagnosis involves blood and possibly radiological investigations. Treatment and interventions include antibiotics, transfusion, radiotherapy and surgery (see Chapters 5, 6, 15 & 16 for further information on these conditions). All of these conditions can be frightening to patients and their families and so the provision of emotional support and information are vital.

Prevention is always better than cure and patients should be advised on self-care measures they can use to try and avoid or prevent infections or bleeding (see Chapters 15 & 16). Active interventions may also be used, for example a patient may be given regular platelet transfusions to prevent bleeding. These are often routinely used when a patient is undergoing treatment and the full blood count is measured regularly to ensure that such interventions are given promptly if they are required. If there is a risk of bleeding, transfusion of blood components may still be appropriate for an individual receiving palliative care. However, the level of intervention is based upon the symptoms being experienced, the aim of treatment, how the symptom presents, e.g. emergency situation, the risks and benefits of interventions, and the wishes of the patient and their family as opposed to the values of the laboratory results (Twycross & Wilcock 2001).

COMMUNICATION

Communication can be challenging at the best of times, especially during a transition between curative and palliative or terminal care. How such significant news is broken often influences how individuals adapt and cope. Breaking significant news is difficult and it is essential that the conversation is held in a quiet environment, free from interruptions and in a sensitive manner.

Some patients and their families, when faced with significant news, will ask for more interventions or treatments. In these circumstances it can be difficult for medical staff to say no and they must ensure that the patient and family understand all the advantages and disadvantages associated with the different care and treatment options (Saunders et al 2003). This helps patients to make their own decisions about whether or not to continue treatment. Saunders et al (2003) suggest that individuals will often decide for themselves what is futile treatment and the decision will depend on what they are trying to achieve and the chances of success (Saunders et al 2003). These issues often need to be discussed many times for patients to come to some degree of acceptance of the situation and decide what they want.

Specialist palliative care teams deal with such situations frequently and have a great deal of experience in facilitating conversations and supporting the treatment teams. They may be able to advise on how best to approach the conversation. It is often useful to plan the breaking significant news discussion in advance as this can help to create the right environment, for example by ensuring that there are no inappropriate interruptions, there is time to talk and listen, and the right people are present, i.e. carers. It can also be useful for the health-care professionals involved to establish what issues are to be discussed and how they will be presented. This enables individuals to get things straight in their own minds first and to discuss any possible questions that may be asked, issues that may arise or expectations that may come to light.

Many health-care professionals are afraid that they will say something wrong. However, it is difficult to define what the wrong thing may be. In many cases listening is often more important than talking. The patient and family may experience a grieving process before the actual death and just being there and listening can be all that is needed. Many patients and their families will talk during this stage. Knowing when to talk and when to listen is hard and often comes with experience. Communication skills courses can be helpful but all skills require frequent and continued practice to become expert. Practising active listening, identifying and, more importantly, acting on the cues given by patients and their families can be helpful in skills development.

Fostering hope is recognised as an important aspect of palliative care and can be forgotten when breaking bad news. Hope has been strongly associated with coping, adaptation and quality of life (Farren et al 1995, Felder 2004) and is thought to offer a reason for continuing life and to ease dying (Hickey 1986). Hope can be fostered in a variety of ways including:

- providing support
- allowing the patient and carer to express their feelings, hopes and expectations for the future
- supporting and encouraging individuals to focus on realistic goals and expectations
- actively listening
- offering information which facilitates choice and decision-making
- good symptom control
- encouraging sense of self-worth
- facilitating religious/spiritual practice (Farren et al 1995, Mirando 2005).

The communication skills associated with breaking significant news can be difficult to learn. Valuable ways of learning such skills include: watching and learning from experts, practising in safe environments such as in a classroom or with colleagues and reflecting on situations experienced, considering what went well, what did not go well or was hard to manage, and what could be done to improve a similar situation in future. Haemato-oncology nurses need to develop communication skills in sensitive listening, giving information, engagement with patients and carers, communicating significant news, explaining complex treatment options and exploring uncertainty. With these skills a haemato-oncology nurse should be able to accurately assess patients, discuss changes in the emphasis of care, have confidence in their own ability to support the patient and carer and act as an advocate.

ETHICAL DILEMMAS

A number of ethical dilemmas may arise in haemato-oncology during palliative or terminal care. These include withdrawing or stopping treatment, end-of-life issues and resuscitation decisions (see Chapter 27 for further discussion of ethics). These can be challenging for everyone involved, especially when there is no right or wrong answer.

One recurring question is 'When should these decisions be made? Saunders et al (2003) distinguish between withholding treatment in an emergency situation and withdrawal of care in a managed environment. In practice it is much easier to make these decisions in a managed environment as opposed to an emergency situation. However, this still poses challenges and requires effective and open communication from everyone involved.

Providing the patient and their family with opportunities to discuss their wishes regarding treatment in the event of a sudden or unexpected deterioration in their condition and documenting outcomes clearly can aid decision-making in emergency situations and reduce the stress for everyone involved. Discussing these issues requires insight and sensitivity but health-care professionals working in haemato-oncology need to develop the skills and confidence to initiate such conversations.

A further issue relates to who makes the decision to withhold treatment – the medical team or the patient? Everyone involved is likely to find such a decision difficult. Patients and their families may require nurses to act as their advocate and help to explain the implications of continuing with or withdrawing treatment and communicate their decisions to the doctors. Nurses may find such a role difficult as they often know the patient well and tend to have their own values and beliefs on such issues. Doctors often find it difficult to estimate prognosis, predict death and make a decision to stop treatment if there is even a remote chance of success (Saunders et al 2003). Relatives may also have wishes that need to be considered. However, the ultimate decision should rest with the patient.

It is important to identify what the patient understands and what their wishes are. This will help to clarify whether the patient is coming to terms with the change of events and any aims and expectations they may have. Smith (2000) suggests that for terminally ill patients it is not only quality of life that is important but also the concept of a good death.

Steinhauser et al (2000) identifies the important factors for a good death as: the control of symptoms, preparation for death, the opportunity for closure or sense of completion of life and a good relationship with health-care professionals, thus emphasising the need for effective open communication.

Think of an end-of-life discussion that you have been involved in. What were the wishes of the patient, family, doctors and the nurses? How were these considered when addressing the subject? What was good and what was bad? What could have improved the way this was managed?

ENVIRONMENT

It is vital that patients are cared for in the most appropriate environment by the most appropriate health-care professionals at every stage of the disease trajectory. During treatment patients are usually cared for in a setting that is most appropriate for management of their disease. For example, patients with acute leukaemia receive most of their treatment and care in an acute inpatient setting whereas lymphoma patients are largely treated in day-case and outpatient settings.

However, palliative and terminal care may not always be provided in the most appropriate care setting and the majority of people with haematological cancers die in hospital. Providing palliative and terminal care in an acute hospital setting can be difficult, especially if the transition from curative treatment occurs rapidly. The environment is often highly technical and one Australian study found that as the patients' condition deteriorated, the use of technology increased (McGrath 2001). Patients' lives frequently ended in an intensive care unit or in chaotic and undignified resuscitation attempts. McGrath (2001) identified that caregivers found this high technological environment very stressful when the patient was dying, particularly as the increased use of technology prevented them from getting physically close to their loved one. The potential for long-term negative consequences for caregivers was also identified (McGrath 2001). This emphasises the need to ensure that patients and their carers are fully informed and involved in decisions about treatment, use of technology and preferred place of care in palliative and terminal situations.

Regardless of where care is provided access to an extended multidisciplinary team and support is essential. Support may be provided by the haemato-oncology team, the primary health-care team and/or specialist palliative care services. Irrespective of who is involved in providing care it is vital that care is coordinated and cohesive. Robust communication channels need to be established between secondary and primary care to facilitate this. It is essential that patients are consulted about their wishes and a comprehensive needs assessment undertaken to ensure they have the resources they require at the right time. A number of tools and frameworks are now available to help to improve palliative care and communication across professional and organisational boundaries. These tools and frameworks have been strongly recommended in a number of Government documents (e.g. Department of Health 2000, NICE 2004).

Case study 26.1

Jack, a 61-year-old male with acute myeloid leukaemia, has recently completed four cycles of intensive chemotherapy. He was admitted to a haemato-oncology ward having been found to have a falling full blood count during a routine follow-up appointment. He was accompanied by his wife.

Jack underwent a number of investigations including full blood count, a bone marrow aspirate and trephine biopsy and a physical examination. In addition to these examinations he also had detailed assessments from both medical and nursing teams. It was found that his acute myeloid leukaemia had relapsed. He was feeling relatively well other than experiencing a mild fatigue and emotional distress associated with the current turn of events and fears about the future.

The haemato-oncology team discussed how and when to tell him this news and the treatment options that he was to be offered. They agreed to tell him immediately and the consultant haematologist and a nurse met with Jack and his wife, in a side room, and broke the news of his relapse. Treatments options were discussed and Jack and his wife were encouraged to discuss the issues and ask questions.

Jack and his wife were left alone for a short time following this discussion. The nurse visited them later and was able to reiterate what had been said and talk through the options available to them and the practicalities that each option involved. They agreed that Jack and his wife would be referred once again to the specialist palliative care team (they had previously met the hospital-based team when he was originally diagnosed and had seen them regularly for support, advice and guidance regarding financial benefits and advice on symptom control during treatment) and the community specialist palliative care services.

The couple decided that Jack would have supportive treatment and care only. In the first instance this was to include blood and platelet transfusions and prophylactic medications such as antibiotics and mouthwashes. They also wanted Jack to be at home. It was agreed that he would stay in overnight to receive blood and platelet transfusions and be discharged the following day. It was agreed that his GP would coordinate care following discharge but that Jack would attend the day-case unit for transfusions as and when required. During his short stay Jack was seen by the specialist palliative care team who provided additional support, discussed the services that would be available to him following discharge and his concerns about death and dying.

All the discussions, referrals and actions taken during this time were documented in the multidisciplinary 'care of the dying' records that had been devised by the specialist palliative care team. Jack was discharged home to the care of his GP the following day. The GP planned to visit that day and a member of the community specialist palliative care team would visit the couple at home the following day.

During the next few weeks Jack received two blood transfusions before his condition deteriorated and he and his wife decided to stop all treatment. The specialist palliative care team and primary health-care team worked together to control his symptoms and care for him. He died peacefully at home a few days later with his family present.

TOOLS AND FRAMEWORKS AIMING TO IMPROVE PALLIATIVE CARE PROVISION

MACMILLAN GOLD STANDARDS FRAMEWORK

The Macmillan Gold Standards framework (GSF) is a national framework devised by and used in primary care. It aims to improve the organisation and quality of palliative care in the community (Thomas 2005). The GSF is implemented through general practices and is thought to improve communication with patients and their family, and between the health-care professionals involved in caring for them. Teamwork, continuity of care, anticipatory planning, symptom control and support for the patient and their family are also facilitated through implementation of the framework. Use of the GSF may enable the primary care team to ensure that patients and families receive all their support and care in the community rather than being admitted to hospital. Haemato-oncology nurses should be proactive in communicating with the primary care team to ensure a smooth transition from secondary to primary care. A sound knowledge of locally available, round-the-clock, palliative care services is also essential in facilitating this transition.

THE LIVERPOOL INTEGRATED CARE PATHWAY FOR THE DYING PATIENT

The Liverpool integrated care pathway for the dying patient is an evidence-based framework that assists health-care professionals to deliver high-quality care to dying patients and their relatives and has been highlighted as a beacon of good practice (Ellershaw & Wilkinson 2003). It aims to support 'generalists' to provide palliative care. The framework supports improvements in end-of-life care by facilitating multidisciplinary communication and documentation – including comfort and symptom control measures, psychological and spiritual issues, communication with the patient and their family, and communication with other health-care professionals. The pathway is being used across the UK and is very applicable in haemato-oncology.

PREFERRED PLACE OF CARE ASSESSMENT TOOL

The preferred place of care assessment tool (Storey et al 2003) can be used to record the patient and carers' wishes in relation to their place of care and ultimately their place of death. Patients' views should be reviewed at different stages in their trajectory of care. This tool may be very appropriate for use in palliative haemato-oncology patients who may wish to be treated closer to home, for example in a local district general hospital or hospice, or at home.

The different tools and frameworks have many commonalities. They all require patients to be involved in decision-making and their choices are placed at the centre of treatment and care. They also promote proactive planned care as opposed to reactive care. Patients and families need time to prepare for death (Saunders et al 2003). However, despite the best efforts of health-care professionals, acute situations sometimes arise that can interfere with this process – leading to a distressing and undignified end. Using a tool to assist early decision-making, in either hospital or primary settings, may offer patients time to prepare and plan for death and possibly prevent inappropriate or unwanted actions being taken in an acute or emergency situation.

In addition to these impacts on patient care the tools also enable nurses and other health-care professionals to determine their own learning and education needs in relation to palliative care. This information can then be used to plan education provision.

REFLECTION POINT   What tools and frameworks are used to support palliative care for patients in your area? If you are unaware of any tools or frameworks currently in use, speak to the specialist palliative care team to find out more about the tools available and any plans to implement these in your area.

EFFECTS ON HEALTH-CARE PROFESSIONALS

It can be very difficult for health-care professionals to care for a patient who has been given significant news about their disease and its treatment. In an inpatient haemato-oncology setting there may be several such patients at any one time. Often these patients have been in and out of the environment for a long period of time and have built up close relationships with the health-care professionals involved in their care. Such a situation can be very stressful for everyone, especially if the time between significant news being communicated to the patient and their family and death is short. Stressors include poor communication between health-care professionals, the patient and their family, or conflicting views on what is best for the patient, failure to stop treatment or close relationships between the patient and health-care professionals. However, this is by no means an exhaustive list and there may be more than one of these factors in play at any time.

If unexpected and unpredictable events occur leading to an undignified or distressing death, health-care professionals have to remain calm while providing whatever care and treatment is necessary and comforting and supporting both the patient and their family. However, professionals can often feel guilty in such situations and feel that they should have done more. This is not usually the case but such situations can have a lasting impact – health-care professionals also require support.

Strategies such as clinical supervision, which encourages the individual to reflect on the situation, and debriefing sessions may provide the opportunity for staff to learn from each other, reflect on situations and learn from the experience in a positive way. This proactive approach has the potential to reduce stress in this work environment (see Chapter 28).

CONCLUSION

Haemato-oncology nurses frequently encounter situations where palliative care is appropriate. This may be for a newly diagnosed haematology patient, a patient requiring symptom control during intensive chemotherapy or transplantation, or for a patient entering the palliative or terminal phase of their disease. Applying palliative care in the haemato-oncology setting can be challenging but the benefits for patients and their families are enormous.

DISCUSSION QUESTIONS

1. How can the needs of individuals requiring curative treatment and the needs of those requiring palliative care be integrated in your workplace?

2. For some individuals the transition between curative treatment and terminal care may progress very rapidly. Are there any actions that could be implemented to improve the care given to patients and relatives at this time?

References

Booth S, Bruera E (eds) 2003 Palliative care consultations: haemato-oncology. Oxford University Press, Oxford

Davies E, Higginson I J (eds) 2004 Better palliative care for older people. World Health Organization, Copenhagen

Department of Health 2000 The NHS cancer plan: a plan for investment, a plan for reform. Department of Health, London

Ellershaw J, Wilkinson S 2003 Care of the dying. A pathway to excellence. Oxford University Press, Oxford

Farren C J, Herth K A, Popovish J M 1995 Hope and hopelessness: critical clinical constructs. Sage, London

Felder B 2004 Hope and coping with cancer diagnoses. Cancer Nursing 27(4):320–324

Hickey S 1986 Enabling hope. Cancer Nursing 9(3): 133–137

Jeffery D, Owen R 2003 Changing the emphasis from curative care to active palliative care in haematology patients. In: Booth S, Bruera E (eds) Palliative care consultations: haemato-oncology. Oxford University Press, Oxford, pp 153–176

McGrath P 2001 Caregivers' insights on the dying trajectory in haematology oncology. Cancer Nursing 24(5): 413–421

Mirando S 2005 Palliative care. In: Kearney N, Richardson A (eds) Nursing patients with cancer: principles and practice. Churchill Livingstone, Edinburgh, pp 821–848

National Council for Hospice and Specialist Palliative Care Services 2002 Definitions of supportive and palliative care. Briefing paper 11. Cited in National Institute for Clinical Excellence (2004) Improving outcomes guidance for palliative and supportive care. HMSO, London

National Institute for Clinical Excellence 2004 Improving outcomes guidance for palliative and supportive care. HMSO, London

Perkins P, Closs S 2003 Palliative care for patients undergoing intensive chemotherapy. In: Booth S, Bruera E (eds) Palliative care consultations: haemato-oncology. Oxford University Press, Oxford, pp 75–88

Saunders Y, Ross J R, Riley J 2003 Planning for a good death: responding to unexpected events. British Medical Journal 327:204–206

Smith R A 2000 A good death: an important aim for health services and us all. British Medical Journal 320: 129–130

Spathis A 2003 The essentials of symptom control in haemato-oncology. In: Booth S, Bruera E (eds) Palliative care consultations: haemato-oncology. Oxford University Press, Oxford, pp 111–135

Steinhauser K E, Christakis N A, Clipp E C et al 2000 Factors considered important at the end of life by patients, family, physicians, and other care providers. JAMA 284:2476–2482

Storey L, Smith C, Overill S, Walker S E, Aldridge J 2003 Place of death: Hobson's choice or patient choice? Cancer Nursing Practice 2(4):33–38

Thomas K 2005 Gold Standards Programme, NHS End of Life Care Programme. http://www.

goldstandardsframework.nhs.uk/docs/gsf/
introduction_to_gsf.pdf Accessed June 2005
Twycross R, Wilcock A 2001 Symptom management in
advanced cancer, 3rd edn. Radcliffe Medical Press,
Abingdon

Valente S 2004 End of life challenges: honouring autonomy.
Cancer Nursing 27(4):314–319
World Health Organization 2002 National cancer control
programmes: policies and managerial guidelines, 2nd
edn. World Health Organization, Geneva

Further reading

**McGrath P 2001 Caregivers' insights on the dying
trajectory in haematology oncology. Cancer Nursing
24(5):413–421**

An insightful article discussing the demands made on
caregivers at the end of life.

Chapter **27**

Ethical issues

Colin Thain

KEY POINTS
- Ethics pervades all aspects of health care.
- There are no neat solutions to ethical problems arising in practice.
- The four ethical principles – respect for autonomy, beneficence, non-maleficence, justice – can be used to analyse ethical issues arising in practice.

INTRODUCTION

All areas of health care potentially raise issues of an ethical nature, and haemato-oncology is no different. This chapter examines the nature of some of these issues, beginning with why nurses need to be involved in examination of ethics, and how decisions can be made when faced with a situation that raises ethical concerns. This involves some consideration of ethical theories and principles, using examples to illustrate the nature of the decisions themselves, and discussion of how the situations can be resolved. As with much in ethics, the chapter does not offer neat and easy conclusions, but provides the reader with a means to consider problems or dilemmas faced in clinical practice, which may ultimately lead to the ability to participate in resolving the issues faced.

WHAT IS ETHICS?

Ethics is the study of the science of morals. For many, this involves decisions about how to act in a given situation, although some see it as being more about how people should live their lives, and what it means to be a good person. In Western philosophical thought, two dominant streams of ethical thinking, deontology and utilitarianism, have emerged. These theories have had a powerful influence on our conception of morality, although they represent very different approaches to conceptualising the moral life and moral decision-making.

The relationship between these theories and how we act as people and as health-care practitioners is not always clear, however. Edwards (1996) provides a structure for how everyday clinical decisions are underpinned by moral theories such as deontology and utilitarianism.

UTILITARIANISM

Utilitarianism is one of a group of ethical theories (termed consequentialist theories) that view the morality of actions according to their consequences. That it is to say, judgements as to the rightness or wrongness of an action are made on the balance of the outcomes of those actions, in terms of the benefits and harms that accrue. In utilitarian theory, the right action is the one that maximises overall good – the good in this case being happiness (Pettit 1991). Expressed in this way, it is difficult to see how anyone could disagree with utilitarianism: maximising good would seem to be a laudable aim, and we can see how this resonates in decisions about how to allocate health-care resources, which are often couched in terms of achieving greatest benefit.

However, a number of criticisms of utilitarianism have been raised: for example, it has been accused of being too demanding because it requires us always to *maximise* utility (Beauchamp & Childress 2001); and it is notoriously difficult to predict the outcomes of our actions (Edwards 1996). Further discussion of these criticisms, and others, is beyond the scope of this chapter, but interested readers should consult texts identified as further reading. Nevertheless, utilitarianism's focus on overall good has made a significant contribution to ethical discourse in health care (Beauchamp & Childress 2001).

DEONTOLOGY

Deontological theories view right actions as those based in duty – though these moral duties are not to be confused with professional duties such as those outlined in the Code of Professional Conduct (NMC 2002). In contrast to utilitarianism, the rightness of actions is determined without regard to their consequences – some actions are definitely morally right or wrong. A common example is that we have a moral duty to tell the truth, and therefore it is morally wrong to lie. Deontological theories typically have a number of such duties with which we are required to comply in order to act morally.

A key element of deontology as elucidated originally by Kant, is what he terms the categorical imperative, which states that a person should only perform an act if she is prepared to allow that everyone else should act that way in similar circumstances – in short, do unto others as you would have them do unto you (Edwards 1996). A person cannot act morally while exempting him or herself, or any other group, from a moral rule.

As with utilitarianism, a number of criticisms have been levelled at deontological theories. Key among them is that deontology does not tell us what to do when duties conflict: for example, if we have a duty to tell the truth, and a duty not to do harm, what should we do if telling the truth will result in harm? One of the strengths of deontology, though, is that it does seem to chime with human instincts – most individuals feel that some things are just wrong.

WHY ETHICS?

The short answer to this question, as Seedhouse (1998, p 36) suggests, is that health care is a moral endeavour. By this, he means that 'work for health is equivalent to acting morally', and that ethics (Seedhouse uses the terms ethics and morals interchangeably, as do many others) pervades all aspects of health care. Seedhouse argues that this must be the case because all health work is concerned with preventing or removing obstacles to people's potential to live fulfilled lives, and that this is also the true nature of moral endeavour. The two are related because ethics considers how to act in the presence of others, and health care involves intervention in human lives. Thus, ethics in health care is not simply about dramatic questions such as 'Should euthanasia be permitted?'

Johnstone (2002) similarly argues that all aspects of nursing have an ethical dimension, noting that no nursing action occurs in a moral vacuum. Thus, she argues, even apparently trivial actions on the part of nurses can have a significant impact on the welfare and moral interests of others, a point also made by Edwards (1996).

Indeed, it could be argued that ethical concerns are raised regularly in our daily lives, although we may not make conscious decisions when faced with them. This sort of everyday decision-making, however, is materially different from what needs to be done in many clinical situations. Much of the work of nurses crosses into intimate areas that are not normally part of everyday social interaction. Thus everyday ethics, which as Seedhouse notes is largely reactive, is insufficient to guide professional practice. For this reason it is important that nurses systematically engage with the study of ethics.

THE FOUR ETHICAL PRINCIPLES

Beauchamp & Childress (2001) suggest that ethical problems in health care can be analysed by attending to four basic principles:

- respect for autonomy
- non-maleficence
- beneficence
- justice.

This approach to the analysis of ethical problems has now become well established. These principles are to be understood as *prima facie* in nature, that is to say, each is considered binding unless in conflict with another principle. Where such conflict occurs, decisions about right actions are made by balancing the respective weights of the competing principles, and determining what should be done 'all things considered' (Beauchamp & Childress 2001, p 15). There is no mechanism for doing this, however; no over-riding principle as in utilitarianism. To reach a decision requires the exercise of judgement or, as Gillon (1994) puts it, 'attention to scope'.

AUTONOMY

The principle of respect for autonomy means respecting the decisions of autonomous persons, but also respecting them as persons. This further means that if health professionals wish to over-rule a patient's autonomous decision, they must have justification for doing so – the onus is on the professional to show why this is necessary. A number of implications flow from this principle, including that professionals should tell patients the truth, protect confidential information and obtain consent before carrying out interventions. In some conceptions of this principle, it also conveys a duty to assist patients to overcome dependence and to promote a greater degree of control (Beauchamp & Childress 2001). To some, respect for autonomy seems to have become the over-riding ethical principle in health care, possibly driven in part by the increasing focus on consumerism in our society. However, Beauchamp & Childress (2001), and other proponents of the four principles approach such as Gillon (1994) and Edwards (1996), are at pains to emphasise that no one principle is supreme, so at times it may be permissible to over-rule a patient's autonomous decision.

NON-MALEFICENCE

Non-maleficence means seeking to avoid inflicting harm on others. Whilst such a principle is in accordance with a maxim that health professionals should do no harm, it is a difficult principle to observe. Edwards (1996) asserts that harms can take a number of forms, and should not be taken simply to mean physical harms associated with assaults. Interpreted in this way, it becomes clear that health professionals often inflict harms on patients in the course of their work. Even relatively trivial interventions could result in harm – for example, taking someone's blood pressure may cause discomfort, even mild pain, which could be construed as harms. In treating haematological cancers, administering chemotherapy is likely to cause nausea, vomiting, myelosuppression and other effects, which are clearly harms. Intervention is still justified, however, on the basis that the aim of the treatment is cure of the patient's disease, which is deemed to be a good that outweighs the harms.

BENEFICENCE

The principle of beneficence implies an obligation to act for the benefit of others. This obligation is specifically identified in the NMC Code of Professional Conduct as a requirement to 'protect and support the health of individual patients and clients' and '. . . the wider community' (NMC 2002, para. 1.2). Although the principles of beneficence and non-maleficence are often interpreted as two sides of the same coin, Edwards (1996) explains that this is a mistake. An obligation to do good is more demanding than one to refrain from doing harm. As Edwards (1996) rightly notes, patients entering hospital, for example, expect not only to be protected from harm, but also to be made better (however we define it). It should also be noted that sometimes the obligation to benefit patients may mean we should not intervene (e.g. not instigate treatment in a patient who is terminally ill).

JUSTICE

The fourth principle is that of justice. In the field of health care, this is interpreted as an obligation to treat people fairly, which also implies that we should be impartial. According to Beauchamp & Childress (2001), a minimal requirement of justice is that equals must be treated equally; a corollary of this is that unequals should be treated unequally. This appears uncontentious, but the devil is in the detail – what characteristics must individuals equally possess to be treated equally? It could be argued, for example, that we should all have equal access to health care, but a second glance would tell us that this cannot be right – those in urgent need of treatment for a life-threatening condition should surely be treated before those with relatively minor complaints. Equality of access, however, is an issue that currently taxes Government: the setting up of the National Institute for Clinical Excellence (NICE) and the development of the Clinical Outcomes Guidelines (NICE 2003) are examples in tackling the 'postcode lottery' in cancer care. Justice also means, of course, that discrimination on grounds of characteristics such as sex, race or religious beliefs is wrong, and the Code of Professional Conduct (NMC 2002, para. 2.2) makes specific reference to this.

The four principles approach has been strongly criticised (Gert et al 1997, Seedhouse 1998). Amongst the criticisms levelled are that the approach lacks substance, that it offers no guidance on resolving conflict between principles, that it is sterile and boring, and that no justification is provided for the four principles themselves. Beauchamp & Childress (2001) concede that there is no mechanism for resolving conflict between principles in their framework, but argue that far from being a fault, this is a strength of their approach. They argue that such conflict and ambiguity are just part of the moral life, and an approach which incorporates an algorithm for decision-making yielding unequivocal answers is unrealistic. More detailed discussion of the strengths and weaknesses of principalism, as it has been termed, is beyond the scope of this chapter, but for those interested, consultation of texts in further reading will be useful. However, even critics of the approach do concede its usefulness in some respects (e.g. Seedhouse 1998, Campbell 2003).

ISSUES IN HAEMATOLOGICAL ONCOLOGY PRACTICE

Ethical issues arising in practice may often be the result of conflict between ethical principles, although it is not accurate to portray all ethical issues in this way. Nurses may become aware of concerns of an ethical nature because they are unsure of how to act in a particular situation, or because there is a clash between a treatment decision and an individual nurse's own values and beliefs, for example. However nurses become aware of such concerns, the four principles framework can be used to illuminate the different factors at play in a situation, enabling them to be viewed from different standpoints and discussed among the various parties to the situation in order to reach a decision on how to proceed.

It is worth reiterating Seedhouse's (1998) point that all health-care work is moral endeavour, and thus ethical decision-making is intrinsic to the work of all health-care professionals. Often this does not cause undue concern, and issues can be resolved easily and quickly (BMA 2004), but it is nevertheless important to remember the ethical dimension of practice. For example, a nurse may say to a patient that she needs to check his blood pressure, and he holds his arm out for her to perform the procedure. Even in this relatively minor incident there are ethical factors at play – it involves requesting and gaining consent to perform the procedure, and examination of this quickly reveals that it is more than just agreement with what the nurse wants. Some illustrative cases are now examined, some real, some imaginary, that serve to highlight the sorts of situations that can arise in practice.

A TRAGIC CASE

Case Study 27.1 relates the well-known case of Child B, Jaymee Bowen.

Case study 27.1

R v Cambridge Health Authority, ex parte B (a minor) (1995) 23 BMLR 1 (CA)

Jaymee Bowen was diagnosed with non-Hodgkin's lymphoma in 1990, aged six, and with acute myeloid leukaemia in 1993. She went into remission following chemotherapy, and received a bone marrow transplant in 1994. However, she relapsed 9 months later, and the view of the paediatric oncologists was that further intensive chemotherapy and a second BMT had about a 1% chance of success. They therefore reached the conclusion that palliative care was the best treatment option for Jaymee. However, her father refused to accept this, and instead sought other opinions from within the UK and abroad. These indicated a more optimistic outlook, and Mr Bowen asked the local Health Authority (HA) to authorise treatment under a leukaemia specialist in London, which they declined to do. They supported the view of the paediatricians that this was an experimental treatment with little evidence to support its use in this case. The HA also refused to fund private treatment for Jaymee.

Mr Bowen brought legal proceedings against the HA which ultimately failed in the Court of Appeal. However, the publicity generated by media coverage of the case led to an anonymous donor offering to fund treatment, and Jaymee underwent chemotherapy in a private hospital, resulting in her going into remission. Following this, the doctor concerned decided against proceeding with a second BMT, and instead undertook an experimental procedure, donor lymphocyte infusion (DLI). Jaymee's treatment finished in July 1995, and she was able to return to school. The HA took over the cost of her continuing care. However, she developed complications, and died in May 1996, some 16 months after first relapsing.

This case is complex and raises a number of ethical issues. Much of the media coverage at the time treated it as an issue about funding of treatment, suggesting that the HA's refusal to fund treatment was made on purely financial grounds. The debate became centred on rationing in the NHS, which was not really the essence of this particular case (Ham & Pickard 1998). Although the HA did consider financial aspects, and was of the opinion that such a use of resources would be 'inequitable' (Ham & Pickard 1998, p 13), a justice-based view, the central issue was the interests of the child. Nevertheless it is important to realise that rationing is always present in the NHS, and that decisions about which treatments to fund have to be made. One aspect of the structure of the NHS that the media coverage highlighted is that decisions about which treatments to fund are often left to managers to take at a local level when in fact they are often political decisions that should be taken by Government.

In English law, a child is usually deemed not to have the capacity to make decisions about treatment, these normally being taken by a parent. It is presumed that a parent's decision will be taken in the best interests of the child. However, the paediatricians also felt that they were required to act in Jaymee's best interests, and that consideration of these meant that proceeding with a second BMT was wrong. Clearly there was a desire for Jaymee to live, but this was tempered by the likely costs involved to her in trying to achieve this. Their clinical experience suggested that a second transplant was likely to do more harm than good – at the time, no child had survived a second transplant, and the side effects were burdensome. This can be viewed as a consequentialist form of argument, but one that also seeks to weigh the principles of beneficence and non-maleficence. This was the advice they gave the HA, and on which the refusal to fund treatment was taken (Ham & Pickard 1998). However, it should be noted that the other consultants contacted by Jaymee's father had a different view of the likely harms and benefits. Mr Bowen's case was based on the idea of the 'rule of rescue', which states that there is an obligation to intervene in cases where life is threatened (Ham 1999), regardless of utilitarian or distributive justice considerations. However, there is no requirement to treat when such treatment is viewed as 'futile'. This was clearly the view of the paediatricians in the case, whose opinion was that there was no effective treatment available, and therefore palliative care was the appropriate choice.

Jaymee herself was not party to the decisions made because her father wished to protect her from the seriousness of her situation (Ham & Pickard 1998). Her paediatricians would have liked to involve Jaymee as she was a very mature 10-year-old. It does appear, though, that her views would have been similar to those of her father since she indicated, while unaware of her situation, that she would have made just the choice that her father was making on her behalf (Ham & Pickard 1998).

This case can rightly be described as 'tragic', and is an example of the difficult dilemmas that can arise in haemato-oncology, when there may be uncertainty about the best form of treatment for a patient, or about the outcome. It also highlights the strong emotions that can be generated by ethical decision-making. In the end, Jaymee did not have a second BMT, but chemotherapy and DLI (then very much an experimental treatment). She did live longer than her paediatricians had expected, and was well enough to go back to school for a while.

CONSENT

Consent is a key issue in modern health care, after hundreds of years when it was barely considered (Beauchamp 1997). Until relatively recently, health-care interventions were paternalistic in nature: professionals (almost exclusively doctors) decided what treatments were best for patients, and informed those patients what was required of them. With illnesses such as cancers, it was often the case that patients were not even told their diagnosis, doctors having decided that it would be more harmful to inform them, as they would not be able to cope. Such an approach was founded on the principle of non-maleficence, since it clearly involved trying to protect the patient from a perceived harm. At no stage, however, were patients consulted as to whether they would actually perceive being given such information as a harm – patients were largely passive in the face of professional expertise.

Such an approach is no longer considered acceptable. Some of this is related to changes in professional outlook and ethical reflection, but much is probably due to societal factors such as the increase in individualism and consumerism in Western liberal democracies (Thain 2002). Consent is one of the key means of respecting an individual's autonomy. As such it plays a fundamental role in ensuring patients remain able to make their own decisions about how they are treated.

In order for an individual's consent to be valid, certain key conditions must be present. The patient must:

- be competent to take a decision
- have received sufficient information
- not be acting under duress (DoH 2001a).

It is also important that consent is viewed as a process in which dialogue between patient and professional takes place, rather than as a one-off event concerned with completing documentation (DoH 2001a).

Adults are presumed to be competent to take decisions unless it can be demonstrated otherwise. Suspicion may be raised about an individual's competence in decision-making where, for example, they have a mental illness, or they disagree with a professional's recommendation in relation to treatment, but of themselves these are not sufficient to deem a person to lack competence. Decisions can be valid even if they appear irrational, for example (BMA 2004). The case *Re: C* [1994] firmly established that mental illness need not be a barrier to patients making decisions about their care and treatment. Much legal and ethical discussion has taken place about what constitutes sufficient information on which to base a decision, and who should judge this. However, it is clearly important that professionals take time to explain procedures and treatments, answer patients' questions and ensure that they understand what is involved. To do this effectively requires well-developed communication skills, including listening skills, not just presenting the patient with a set of facts. The last condition means that consent must be freely given, and not the result of pressure being put on the patient. If this is not the case, consent will not be valid as it will not reflect the aims and values of the chooser (Brock 1993).

Where adults are unable to make decisions for themselves, it is important to realise that no other person, even a close relative, can give consent on their behalf (DoH 2001b). The decision taken must be on the basis of what is in the patient's best interests, and care must be taken to fully consider what those interests are. They are not to be considered synonymous with best medical interests. An example is provided in Case Study 27.2.

Case study 27.2

Superintendent of Belchertown v Saikewicz
Mass. 370 NE 2d 417 (1977)

Joseph Saikewicz was 67, and had lived in
institutions for over 40 years. He had a very low
IQ, and could communicate only through gestures
and grunts, and responded only to gestures or
physical contact. His health was generally good
until he was diagnosed with acute myelomonocytic
leukaemia. Chemotherapy could induce remission
in 30–50% of cases, although results were worse
in the over-60s. He could not have understood the
nature of such treatment, or have dealt with the
resulting side effects and discomfort. Without
chemotherapy, he could have expected to live for
several weeks. The courts in Massachusetts, where
the case took place, decided that treatment was
not in his best interests, judging that the potential
benefits (in terms of longer life) were outweighed
by the pain and suffering likely to be caused to a
man who could have no understanding of what
was happening. In this case, therefore, non-
maleficence outweighs beneficence.

REFLECTION POINT

Do you agree with this decision? Justify your answer with reference to
moral principles. Should we not seek to preserve life? Could this decision be
viewed as discriminating against people who are born with mental
incapacities?

REFUSAL OF TREATMENT

Any consent process must include the option to refuse consent – a
request that did not include the option to say 'no' would surely be
viewed with suspicion (DoH 2001a). However, refusal of treatment may
sometimes go against what the health professional considers to be in the
patient's best interests. Respecting the patient's autonomy, though,
would suggest that if there is no reason to suppose that the patient is
non-autonomous, then the patient's decision should be respected. This
does not mean, of course, that any refusal on the part of a patient should
be simply accepted as the end of the matter. There can still be dialogue
between patient and professional, and it is important that this is continued. It is important, too, that the patient's reasons for refusal are ascertained. It may be that the patient is labouring under a misapprehension
as to the nature of the proposed treatment, and when reassured or corrected, the patient will give consent. Nevertheless, it is always important
to remember that a patient can refuse any proposed treatment (apart
from in certain well-defined circumstances), provided that they are competent to make such decisions. In English law, this position has been
confirmed in a number of cases.

However, most patients would want some safeguards against making
choices that were clearly of harm to them. This is another reason why it
is important to view consent as a process rather than a one-off event. By
having a dialogue with the patient, professionals can gain an understanding of what the patient is seeking in terms of treatment and out-

comes. The patient can then be given information about treatments available, and the likely outcomes of having or refusing the treatment. Ultimately, it is for patients to decide what is in their best interests, and therefore whether to accept treatment.

If a patient does refuse treatment, to what extent can professionals question the patient or try to persuade a change of mind? Whilst it may be acceptable to ask why treatment is being refused, the patient is under no obligation to justify that decision. There must surely be limits on what can be done to persuade the patient to alter such a decision – repeated attempts could be construed as browbeating, and therefore coercive, thus invalidating any consent obtained.

Case study 27.3

Refusal of blood transfusion

David, a 30-year-old patient newly diagnosed with lymphoma, is a Jehovah's Witness. He makes clear to the team that he would not accept blood products as part of his treatment, as this would conflict with his religious beliefs. The team members explain to David the problems associated with this, including the likelihood of becoming anaemic, or suffering bleeds that could be life-threatening without transfusions of platelets and/or red cells. However, he is still adamant that he should not receive blood component transfusions. Two questions potentially arise: should the patient receive chemotherapy, given that this is likely to mean myelosuppression and a need for blood component support; and secondly, what should be done in an emergency situation, such as David experiencing life-threatening haemorrhage? (The question of how staff should deal with this situation could also be added.)

The second of these questions mirrors what has been called the 'standard' Jehovah's Witness case (Gillon 2003a). It is generally considered a 'standard' case because it provides a clear example of conflict of ethical principles. The principle of respect for autonomy would suggest that the patient's wishes must be respected, and the use of transfusions avoided – even where this is likely to result in death. It might be argued that the strictures of their faith mean that Jehovah's Witnesses cannot be considered autonomous, but this argument would be difficult to sustain and

would be tantamount to disrespecting a person's faith because of disagreement with what it entails. This could be seen as discriminatory, although it must be acknowledged that there are facets of people's faiths that in the UK are not permitted, such as multiple marriage.

The right to refuse blood transfusion by Jehovah's Witnesses has been enshrined in law. The case of *Re T* [1992], which involved refusal of blood products, established that a competent adult has the right to refuse treatment, whatever the reason, or even for no reason whatsoever. The key point here is whether the patient is competent to make a decision, but if he is, then his decision, if it is freely made, must be respected.

If, after discussion with staff, David is adamant about his refusal, understanding the potential problems that might ensue, his decision must be respected. Chemotherapy may be more risky as a result, but this would not really be a reason not to proceed. There are examples of Jehovah's Witnesses who have been successfully treated for haematological cancer without the use of blood component support (e.g. Laszlo et al 2004).

Should an emergency occur, it could be argued that staff should intervene to save David's life – indeed that they have a duty to do so and, if this requires blood components to be administered, then this should be done. There is a defence of necessity when acting in emergency situations, but this would be sustainable only where it is unclear what the individual's wishes are. Where it is known that a patient is a Jehovah's Witness, it

Case study 27.3 – Cont'd

would be incumbent on staff to ascertain his wishes regarding blood components and, if these are refused, it would not be permissible to give this form of treatment. To do so would clearly breach the principle of respect for autonomy, however well intentioned the intervention might be. It would also be a breach of law under the Human Rights Act, and is likely to be viewed as battery.

Of course such situations are difficult for staff. The inclination would be to act from a perceived duty to save lives, or on the principle of beneficence, but respect for autonomy is asserted here as the dominant principle. Additionally, as

Gillon (2003b) notes, the patient has made his own assessment of harms and benefits that would accrue, and made his decision accordingly. This case can be viewed as a clash of ethical principles: of respect for autonomy against beneficence (when we would wish to intervene to do good by preserving life) and non-maleficence (when we would want to intervene to prevent harm, in this case death). It may also be viewed as a clash of values, where professionals may have a different set of values and beliefs from the patient. It is important, though, that practitioners do not seek to impose their own value systems on patients.

REFLECTION POINT
Consider Case Study 27.3. What do you think should be done here? How do you think you would feel if you were nursing this patient?

BONE MARROW DONATION

Donation of tissues is viewed as a supererogatory (or heroic) act. It is regarded as voluntary and selfless, and superficially at least would appear to give little cause for concern. People may become donors simply because it is the right thing to do, or they feel that they have a duty to do what they can. However, several factors do need to be considered.

Donation is not without risks (see Chapter 13). The nature of these risks needs to be made clear to the potential donor, and any concerns discussed, as part of the process of consent. This is a fundamental aspect of consent, as discussed above, and it is important that the donor understands the nature of these risks before agreeing to the procedure.

The procedure itself is not really for the donor's benefit, although benefits may accrue in the form of good feelings about oneself, or the fact that a loved one is able to survive a fatal disease.

Consent for the procedure also needs to be voluntary. What if a potential donor does not wish to donate? This is the person's right, but how free will that person be to refuse consent? What would the reaction of the rest of the family be, if the patient is a brother or sister, for example? Such factors raise the question of whether a related donor can ever give valid consent. Of course most potential donors are only too happy to give, but it is nevertheless worth considering a situation in which consent is not forthcoming. Brazier (2003) notes that an American court refused to order a competent potential donor to submit to donation, and it seems likely that courts in this country would take a similar view.

Case study 27.4

Re Y (Mental Incapacity: Bone Marrow Transplant) [1996] 2 FLR 791

Y was a 26-year-old woman with severe learning difficulties. Her 36-year-old sister was diagnosed with myelodysplastic syndrome, and it was proposed that her best chance of cure was a bone marrow transplant, with Y as donor, if suitable. Application was made to the court for a declaration to allow performance of a blood test to determine Y's suitability to be the donor, and, if necessary, bone marrow harvest. The court heard that Y was very close to her mother, and that the sister's death was likely to have a bad impact on the mother, who was not in good health. Y's mother was also likely to have to look after her grandchild if Y's sister died, which would mean her visits to see Y would be drastically curtailed. Additionally it was noted that Y's bone marrow would regenerate, so any adverse effects were likely to be temporary. The court allowed the blood test and marrow harvest, on the grounds that they were in Y's best interests. However, particular attention was paid to the close family bonds and the relatively low risk levels involved, making it an exceptional decision. The court also indicated that subsequent similar cases would require application to a court for a declaration for such a procedure.

Note that even a blood test required permission from the court, as it was not of direct benefit to Y.

REFLECTION POINT Can a non-therapeutic intervention such as this really be said to be in the best interests of a non-competent adult? Should family members be compelled to donate regenerable tissues, such as bone marrow, for relatives? What are the ethical arguments for and against? What if the potential donor is unable to give consent, as in Case Study 27.4?

CLINICAL TRIALS

Clinical trials have been identified as key to advancing treatment and improving survival rates in all forms of cancer (DoH 2000). However, they do raise a number of ethical concerns. The research governance framework (DoH 2001c) makes it clear that trials must be subject to independent review by research ethics committees (RECs). The BMA (2004) outlines a set of general principles that will apply to research and innovative treatments, including clinical trials. While informed consent is prominent amongst these, along with voluntariness, truth-telling and effective communication, it is notable that they are also concerned with issues such as the balance of benefits and burdens, confidentiality and keeping all professionals involved with patients informed about the research. RECs will be particularly concerned about the balance of benefits and burdens, particularly since in clinical trials the new treatment may not benefit the individual. RECs will also scrutinise the information provided to participants, inclusion and exclusion criteria, and arrangements for obtaining consent. They will be anxious to see that there is honesty about what participants can expect to happen, and that there is no sense of patients being deceived or coerced into taking part. These are clearly essential means to respecting the autonomy of participants.

REFLECTION POINT

REFLECTION POINT   What would you do if a patient on a clinical trial told you she had no idea why she was on the trial?

It is also important that the nature of any risks is conveyed to the patient when deciding whether they wish to participate in a trial. This must be when the patient is weighing up factors in making this decision with respect to a treatment that may not be of direct benefit to them. Indeed Doyal (1997) argues that doctors have a stronger duty to communicate information about risks in clinical trials than in other aspects of clinical practice, and the same logic must surely apply to other professionals involved.

RECs, in examining benefits and burdens as they apply to participants in trials and seeking to protect their welfare, are clearly focussing on principles of beneficence and non-maleficence. The BMA (2004) also makes clear that justice also ought to be a consideration. This means finding ethical ways of involving people in trials who cannot give consent for themselves, and ensuring that groups are not excluded from trials on spurious grounds. An example of the latter might be people who cannot speak English – it is entirely possible to produce and relay information to people in their own language if necessary, although this should be done in a culturally sensitive manner. To exclude such people from entry to a trial, perhaps because it is more difficult to produce the necessary information, and then extrapolate the trial results to what might be a different ethnic group, is surely ethically dubious.

Finally, it is important to note that, when investigating a new drug or treatment regime, there should be genuine uncertainty about whether it is better than existing treatment. If this is not the case, then the trial is likely to be unethical, since it would involve denying some patients a treatment that is already known is better for them, or subjecting them to a treatment known to produce poorer outcomes. However, it is also the case that trials should not be ended prematurely on the basis of early trends suggesting superiority of one form of treatment – this may be a transient effect that disappears as the trial continues. Careful consideration needs to be given to abandoning a trial at such early stages, as this may ultimately lead to patients being given poorer treatment in the long run.

CONCLUSION

This chapter has really only scratched the surface of ethics in haematological oncology. It is undoubtedly the case that readers will be able to think of issues and cases from their own practice that are equally challenging. It is also likely that what has been discussed has raised more questions than have been answered. This, unfortunately, is often the case with ethics. However, it is hoped that the chapter has provided some insights into ethical decision-making. While it might be argued that the cases discussed, and the decisions that have to be taken, are the domain of doctors, and nurses need not get involved, this surely cannot be sustained. Nurses *must* be involved – they nurse these patients, and will continue to do so whatever decisions are made; and they will have to continue to support relatives and friends of patients, and answer their questions. Far better that nurses are able to analyse these situations, and express their perspective, thus contributing to the decision-making process and sharing the burden of the decisions.

DISCUSSION QUESTIONS

1. What is the nurse's role in informed consent and decision-making in relation to treatment options?

2. What are the ethical considerations for sibling donors?

3. What are the ethical problems arising most commonly in your area of practice?

References

Beauchamp T L 1997 Informed consent. In: Veatch R M (ed) Medical ethics, 2nd edn. Jones and Bartlett, Sudbury, MA

Beauchamp T L, Childress J F 2001 Principles of biomedical ethics, 5th edn. Oxford University Press, Oxford

Brazier M 2003 Medicine, patients and the law, 3rd edn. Penguin, London

British Medical Association (BMA) 2004 Medical ethics today: the BMA's handbook of ethics and law, 2nd edn. Ethics Department, BMJ Books, London

Brock D W 1993 Life and death: philosophical essays in medical ethics. Cambridge University Press, Cambridge

Campbell A V 2003 The virtues (and vices) of the four principles. Journal of Medical Ethics (Festschrift edition) 29(5):292–296

Department of Health 2000 The NHS cancer plan: a plan for investment. A plan for reform. DoH, London

Department of Health 2001a Good practice in consent implementation guide: consent to examination or treatment. DoH, London

Department of Health 2001b Reference guide to consent for examination or treatment. DoH, London

Department of Health 2001c Research governance framework for health and social care. DoH, London

Doyal L 1997 Informed consent in medical research: journals should not publish research to which patients have not given fully informed consent – with three exceptions. British Medical Journal 314: 1107–1111

Edwards S D 1996 Nursing ethics: a principle-based approach. Macmillan, Basingstoke

Gert B, Culver C M, Clouser K D 1997 Bioethics: a return to fundamentals. Oxford University Press, Oxford

Gillon R 1994 Medical ethics: four principles plus attention to scope. British Medical Journal 309:184

Gillon R 2003a Introduction: four scenarios. Journal of Medical Ethics (Festschrift edition) 29(5):267–268

Gillon R 2003b Ethics needs principles – four can encompass the rest – and respect for autonomy should be 'first among equals'. Journal of Medical Ethics (Festschrift edition) 29(5):307–312

Ham C 1999 Tragic choices in health care: lessons from the Child B case. British Medical Journal 319: 1258–1261

Ham C, Pickard S 1998 Tragic choices in health care: the case of child B. King's Fund, London

Johnstone M J 2002 A reappraisal of everyday nursing ethics. In: Daly J, Speedy S, Jackson D, Darbyshire P (eds) Contexts of nursing: an introduction. Blackwell, Oxford

Laszlo D, Agazzi A, Cinieri S et al 2004 Tailored therapy of adult acute leukaemia in Jehovah's Witnesses: unjustified reluctance to treat. European Journal of Haematology 72:264–267

National Institute for Clinical Excellence 2003 Improving outcomes in haematological cancer: the manual. NICE, London

Nursing and Midwifery Council 2002 Code of professional conduct. NMC, London

Pettit P 1991 Consequentialism. In: Singer P (ed) A companion to ethics. Blackwell, Oxford

R v Cambridge Health Authority, ex parte B (a minor) [1995] 23 BMLR 1 (CA)

Re C (Adult: Refusal of Treatment) [1994] 1 All ER 819

Re T (Adult: Refusal of Medical Treatment) [1992] 4 All ER 649

Re Y (Mental Incapacity: Bone Marrow Transplant) [1996] 2 FLR 791

Seedhouse D 1998 Ethics: the heart of health care, 2nd edn. Wiley, Chichester

Superintendent of Belchertown v Saikewicz Mass. 370 NE 2d 417 [1977]

Thain C W 2002 An examination of some issues in consent in bone marrow transplantation. Unpublished MA dissertation, Keele University

Further reading

Beauchamp T L, Childress J F 2001 Principles of biomedical ethics, 5th edn. Oxford University Press, Oxford

The classic text, though it can be heavy going, and very North American in outlook (understandably).

Edwards S D 1996 Nursing ethics: a principle-based approach. Macmillan, Basingstoke

Good introductory text. Straightforward in approach, and applied to nursing.

Gillon R 1986 Philosophical medical ethics. Wiley, Chichester

A concise, clear and very readable discussion of ethics in health care, although it is quite old and therefore does not incorporate some more recent court cases and changes to law and practice. Nevertheless, it covers most issues. Very pro-Four Principles approach.

Ham C, Pickard S 1998 Tragic choices in health care: the case of child B. King's Fund, London

An interesting discussion of the Jaymee Bowen case.

Kuhse H 1997 Caring: nurses, women and ethics. Blackwell, Oxford

An excellent, and very readable, discussion of ethics in nursing, and something of a rallying cry to nurses to get involved in decision-making.

Picoult J 2004 My sister's keeper. Hodder, London

This fictional account of a child conceived to be a donor for her sister raises some very real issues. Well worth reading.

Seedhouse D 1998 Ethics: the heart of health care, 2nd edn. Wiley, Chichester

A different approach, but stimulating and thought-provoking. Very critical of the Four Principles approach, and offers an alternative way of framing ethical issues.

Chapter 28

Staff support and retention

Timothy Jackson

CHAPTER CONTENTS

KEY POINTS

- Investment in staff begins in the recruitment phase.
- Positive working initiatives are a means of recruiting and retaining staff.
- Information portraying a positive image of the clinical area should be developed as a marketing tool.
- A well-planned orientation programme is essential for all new staff.
- Preceptorship and clinical supervision are important means of supporting staff.
- Well-supported staff who have a healthy work–life balance are more likely to be retained.
- Investing in education and professional development is important in supporting nurses.
- Networking is useful for sharing ideas and recognising good practice.

INTRODUCTION

The dawn of the 21st Century has brought considerable change to the NHS which impacts and challenges staff working in the health service. Improvement and redesign of cancer services are high on the political agenda and achieving the aims of the numerous UK government policy documents requires an educated, skilled and caring multi-professional workforce, which values and recognises all the talents needed to deliver the complexities of modern-day patient care. These policies also recognise the challenges for NHS staff:

> 'NHS staff are the biggest asset the health service has . . . they do a brilliant job. But feel frustrated with the system.'
>
> (DoH 2000a, p 3)

> 'The commitment of those working to fight cancer in the NHS is immense but in too many areas the reality of our cancer services fails to match that commitment.'
>
> (DoH 2000b, p 3)

However, the government recognises that:

> 'despite the best efforts of the NHS staff and cancer patients across the country, decades of under investment alongside outdated practices mean that the survival rates for many of the major cancers lag behind the rest of Europe'
>
> (DoH 2000b, p 3)

These quotes highlight the reality of working within the NHS today. The context in which health-care professionals have to work can be frustrating, leading to poor morale and ultimately highly experienced staff leaving the professions. It is against this background that this chapter outlines strategies and examples of good practice in support and retention for those working within haemato-oncology. The aim is to enable and empower nurses and allied health professionals to develop personally and professionally so they either remain within their current workplace or progress within the speciality or across the NHS. The benefits of this to the NHS are: experienced, dynamic nurses or allied health professionals who play a pivotal role in contributing to the modernisation of the NHS; improved multi-professional team dynamics; and a service development that will ultimately enhance the overall experience and outcome for patients and their carers.

THE WORKFORCE CONTEXT

It is well recognised that under investment in the NHS has led to reduced staffing levels with staff being 'over-worked, run off their feet and exhausted . . . Many hospitals cannot recruit the staff they need' (DoH 2000a, p 70). This situation further impacts on the retention of existing health-care professionals, who feel frustrated when they cannot deliver the care that patients need and they were trained to provide.

Managers therefore need to be innovative and creative in recruiting from a depleted workforce. The difficulties in recruiting and retaining health-care professionals have been recognised by the Department of Health who have developed guidance for managers in the document 'Improving working lives for those people who work in the NHS' (DoH

2000c). This document 'recognises that modern health services require modern employment services and staff work best for patients when they can strike a healthy life–work balance, are valued and supported and have access to personal and professional development opportunities' (DoH 2000c, p 3).

Managers need to adopt the principles within the report to develop local policies, which allow staff the choice to work part-time, full-time or flexible annualised hours. Job shares, career breaks, carers' leave, paternity leave and flexible phased retirement can also be offered – all are examples of good human resource practices, which enable staff to achieve a work–life balance. Some organisations are now offering full-time staff the choice to work 4 days a week rather than the traditional five days, to reduce travel time and high levels of absence. This has previously been an option for nurses, which is now being extended to other health-care professionals, administrative staff and managers.

Flexible working should also include *self-rostering*, which is a democratic way for all staff to have a say in what shifts they work, and can also facilitate an improved work–life balance. However, the team needs to work in a collaborative manner for self-rostering to work effectively and fairly. Ground rules need to be established and agreed by the team, i.e. the number of nurses and skill mix per shift, along with the number of staff permitted annual or study leave at any one time. In some units this has been further developed, where nurses have the choice of working conventional early, late or night duty shifts or double shifts, which can mean more time off. In the author's experience, staff involved in decision-making within the workplace have improved job enhancement and satisfaction, which leads to improved retention.

Other initiatives developed to increase recruitment include widening the entry gate for nurse and allied health professional education, 'return to practice' courses and international recruitment strategies. National Vocational Qualification (NVQ) level 3 is now recognised as an alternative entry requirement to professional education. This is much more inclusive, as it allows entry to the health-care professions for those who left school without the prerequisite number of GCSEs. Return to practice courses are now provided free of charge and are more employee-friendly to attract qualified health-care professionals who have left the profession back to the NHS.

International recruitment strategies have been developed in recent years to improve the recruitment situation. Concerns have, however, been expressed about the international recruitment of nurses, the potential for abuse once recruited, and the potential of depleting poorer countries of their health-care workforce. In response to these concerns, and to promote ethical recruitment, the Department of Health has issued a code of practice for NHS employers (DoH 2001), which helps to support managers involved in international recruitment.

It is anticipated that the implementation of the new NHS pay and conditions framework, Agenda for Change (AfC) (DoH 2004a) will also improve recruitment and retention. AfC supports NHS service modernisation and brings all NHS staff (with the exception of doctors, dentists and some managers) onto a single pay spine, thus ensuring equal pay for work of equal value.

REFLECTION POINT   What could be done to increase recruitment and retention in your workplace?

MARKETING

First impressions count! When a potential member of staff considers applying for a post, the quality of the unit/ward information is paramount. With the increasing availability of computers and colour printers at ward level, excellent inexpensive high-quality ward/unit information can easily be developed and sent with the application form and job description. Suggestions for content include:

- details of the ward/unit's multi-professional team or nursing philosophy
- number of clinical areas, i.e. wards/beds, day care, outpatients, chemotherapy unit
- number of patients treated annually
- treatment modalities used
- number of procedures/transplants performed annually
- nursing skill mix, including support staff
- flexibility of working patterns and other relevant human resource information
- professional development opportunities
- names and roles of key nurses, allied health professionals and medical staff
- associated education and training providers.

The information helps to create a positive image of how the ward/unit is operated and managed. Compilation of ward/unit information may initially take some time but once developed can be easily updated, to ensure it remains a dynamic marketing and recruitment tool – reflecting a positive and professional image of the nursing and multi-professional team. Individual wards/units need to be imaginative in attracting scarce human resources or they will fail to deliver a quality service, increasing workload and pressure on an already stretched team. Advertising in the local and national press in addition to professional journals can be an effective way of recruiting specialist nurses, especially those contemplating a return to practice following a career break. Increasingly wards/units are developing their own internet websites that can be used as an inexpensive way to advertise posts, especially those that have been vacant for some time. Cancer networks should also be considered as another advertising opportunity as they link to the local and national health economy and adverts can be sent to a wider audience at no extra cost.

The notion of patients and carers as partners, not just in their care and treatment but also in the development and design of services, is gaining greater recognition; good examples include the involvement of users in the recruitment of staff and the planning and development of haemato-oncology services. However, although the involvement of patients in the recruitment process is considered good practice, there is currently no evidence to suggest this impacts on the retention of staff. Evaluation of such initiatives is therefore required.

The process of advertising, interviewing and staff selection is time-consuming and expensive, therefore once a member of staff has been successfully recruited, it is a team responsibility to ensure they are fully supported during and beyond the period of orientation.

ORIENTATION

A well-planned orientation programme is essential to prepare staff for their new role. A 2–3-week orientation programme may be considered expensive and difficult to absorb in the short term but is a good investment in the long term. Matthews & Nunley (1992) demonstrated that a well-structured orientation reduced staff turnover rate by 17% over a 6-month period. University College London Hospitals NHS Foundation Trust operate a one-week orientation programme which allows registered nurses to become acquainted with local policies, protocols and procedures, meet key personnel and undergo statutory and Trust training, for example fire training, manual handling and cardiopulmonary resuscitation. Integral to this is the time spent undergoing an orientation to the haemato-oncology unit, essential for meeting key people and for the new nurse to be assigned a preceptor or for the more experienced nurse a mentor. The orientation programme has been successfully evaluated. A well-planned orientation programme allows nurses to be well informed and prepared for their new role, enabling them to function more effectively. According to Cherniss (1980, p 161), 'research has also shown the orientation process to be a successful method of preventing burnout among human service professionals'.

STAFF SUPPORT

Haemato-oncology is an intensive, rapidly moving speciality. Patient throughput is high and length of hospital stay is longer than for the average general patient and associated with repeated admissions. This places unique and often impossible demands on haemato-oncology nurses – physically, emotionally and professionally. Nurses frequently develop strong relationships with patients and their carers, and invest a lot of themselves, which can be exhausting. The patient population tends to be younger and is associated with a higher mortality rate as a consequence of the disease or treatment.

'The nature of the relationships which can develop over the course of BMT can become intense. This may expose staff to the risks from a repeated sense of loss, and eventual futility, in their role'

(Kelly et al 2000, p 995)

These factors can potentially lead to burnout if the staff are not supported. To prevent and/or minimise this various support strategies may be implemented.

PRECEPTORSHIP

The Nursing and Midwifery Council (NMC 2002, p 4) recommend that all staff in a new role, whether newly registered or a more experienced practitioner, need a period of preceptorship:

'many people find the transition from being a student to an accountable individual practitioner a daunting prospect, the same may apply to those who have returned to practice or those who have entered a different area of practice'.

The NMC recommends registered nurses should have a formal period of preceptorship of about 4 months. Preceptors work closely with preceptees on a regular basis to discuss and agree education and training needs, performance issues and other concerns. Preceptors must clearly understand what is expected of the new role and the competencies and demands it involves.

Competencies should include technical, interpersonal and critical thinking dimensions (Del Bueno et al 1987). Preceptors should clearly articulate the skills needed for the preceptee's role within each of these dimensions, which helps the preceptee develop confidence and gain competence, which in turn may impact on retention. Preceptees also need to understand the responsibilities associated with their role. Manthey & Miller (2003, p 9) 'identify responsibility as ownership; a two-way process, both allocated and accepted. Authority is the right to act in areas where one is given and accepts responsibility.' Preceptors therefore need to help the preceptee to understand their responsibilities and level of authority, which in turn helps to clarify accountability. Preceptees should then be able to accept responsibility with clarity, work independently in a safe way and know exactly what they are accountable for. Preceptees should therefore gain confidence in their ability to practice as a useful member of the team, resulting in increased self-worth and job satisfaction in both the short- and longer-term and hopefully leading to improved retention.

CLINICAL SUPERVISION

Clinical supervision is a further means of supporting staff:

'Clinical supervision supports practice, enabling you to maintain and improve standards of care. Clinical supervision is a practice-focused professional relationship, involving a practitioner reflecting on practice guided by a skilled supervisor'

(NMC 2002, p 7)

'Clinical supervision supports nurses and helps them survive the tremendous pressures of a demanding profession and encourages a high standard of care to patients'

(Wilkin et al 1997, p 49)

Clinical supervision can take a variety of forms. It can be either a 1-to-1 session or conducted in small groups. Examples of good practice exist where supervisors and supervisees meet regularly to reflect on practice, to discuss and review critical incidents and practice-based issues – potentially leading to resolution or greater understanding of practice, professional or personal issues. The potential benefits and impact of clinical supervision on the nursing profession are far-reaching 'the establishment of clinical supervision is an important part of clinical governance and in the interests of improving standards of patient care' (NMC 2002, p 7).

The benefits of clinical supervision are thought to include:

- safer practice
- reduced untoward incidents and complaints
- better targeting of educational and professional development
- better assessment of patient/client opinion
- reduced stress among staff
- improved levels of sickness or absenteeism
- improved confidence and professional development
- greater awareness of accountability
- better input into management appraisal systems
- better managed risk and better awareness of evidence-based practice.

Clinical supervision can also be used as a non-punitive strategy for the practitioner to reflect on any clinical errors with the aim of improving practice and preventing reoccurring errors.

However, clinical supervision has been introduced and integrated into practice in an ad hoc manner across the country, therefore it is difficult to evaluate its effect on staff retention. Furthermore, the impact of clinical supervision on the nursing profession has yet to be fully evaluated. However, Butterworth et al (1996, p 130) suggest that 'it may be possible to audit clinical supervision through existing mechanisms, such as rates of sickness and absence, staff satisfaction, recruitment and retention of staff.' This is something that nurse managers can start to do locally. Data from different haemato-oncology units could then be compared to discover themes and variables that could be used to develop good practice guidelines.

REFLECTION POINT   How do you think clinical supervision does or could support nurses in your area?

OTHER SUPPORT STRATEGIES

Other examples of support include regular time out for the nurse with planned annual leave, study leave and management of the amount of extra shifts worked. Time out of direct patient care for reflection, either as an individual or as a team, is important. Staff support groups or access to bereavement counsellors can be useful, however these need good facilitation. Imposing staff support groups is not the answer and within the author's unit has not been successful. Molassiotis & Haberman (1996, p 360) claim that a 'staff support programme acknowledges nursing stress and offers a variety of services which nurses individually or as a team can utilise to manage possible sources of working stress.' However, the effectiveness of these strategies is not reported.

Access to complementary therapies has also been reported as a further means of staff support. Mackereth et al (2005) have developed interventions to manage stress and avoid burnout in oncology by providing subsidised complementary therapies for staff at the Christie Hospital Foundation NHS Trust, Manchester. This conforms to the government's Improving Working Lives Standard (DoH 2000c) and is also an innovative human resource strategy.

LEADERSHIP

In attempting to support and retain staff, the ward/unit manager must provide clear strong leadership where staff feel valued, treated fairly and respected. The ward/unit philosophy should reflect these values and articulate the responsibility and commitment of all team members to working in a cohesive multi-professional manner. A ward philosophy is a useful and powerful framework to support and build open and honest multi-professional communication and relationships. Conflict between members of the multi-professional team can occur, especially if a breakdown in communication occurs. Regular multi-professional meetings that discuss day-to-day organisational issues can be a productive and effective methodology for improving communication and team problem-solving. It is also suggested that such initiatives can help teams improve decision-making and self-direction 'in organisations where there is shared governance or self directed teams, staff assume and are given high control for decision making and problem solving while managers guide and influence rather than control' (Manthey & Miller 2003, p 10). This high level of control is thought to be the 'key factor in developing positive team dynamics and cohesion for the benefit of staff and patients' (Manthey & Miller 2003, p 10).

Rotational posts can be an effective methodology for training haemato-oncology nurses to increase their understanding of the totality of the patient pathway. Nurses involved in caring for haemato-oncology inpatients can become rather blinkered remembering only those patients who relapse or die as they may be admitted more frequently, whereas patients who do well may never return to the inpatient area. This can result in feelings of stress and a reason for staff to leave – rotational posts can offer a wider insight into patient outcomes.

EDUCATION AND PROFESSIONAL DEVELOPMENT

Investing in staff through education and training is vitally important in supporting nurses professionally and personally and making them feel valued. Education and training for all staff working in the NHS, and especially those working in haemato-oncology where practice is significantly expanded from generic nurse training, is essential and must be integral to clinical practice. However, across the NHS there has been an inequity of education and training. The amount of education and training available often relies on the creativity of local managers in accessing funding. The DoH (2000d, p 5) states it 'has had long-standing concerns about the way in which the NHS educates, trains and uses its staff and suggests the emphasis needs to be on:

- *Team working* across professional and organisation boundaries.
- *Flexible working* to make the best use of the range of staff skills and knowledge.
- *Streamlined workforce planning and development,* which stems from the needs of patients not professionals.
- *Maximising the contribution of all staff to patient care,* doing away with barriers that say only doctors and/or nurses can provide particular types of care.
- *Modernising education and training* to ensure that staff are equipped with the skills they need to work in a complex, changing NHS.
- *Developing new, more flexible careers* for staff of all professions.
- *Expanding the workforce* to meet future demands.'

Managers and practitioners need to be creative with education and professional development budgets, in both commissioning and developing specialist clinical courses. The local manager in conjunction with each nurse must undertake an individual performance review to identify the nurse's professional development needs; however, this must also be balanced against personal, professional, service and strategic requirements.

The modernised pay system Agenda for Change is linked to 'The Knowledge and Skills Framework' (KSF), which is essentially a developmental tool that provides the basis for career progression (DoH 2004b). The KSF is made up of core and specific role dimensions and is graded at nine levels (bands) (Box 28.1). Job profiles will be mapped against the KSF and progression through the levels is dependent on professional development and skill acquisition. For the first time NHS staff will be professionally rewarded for their learning – this should have an impact on retention.

The KSF core and specific dimensions are also being matched to cancer nursing competencies, which will further advance clinical and

Box 28.1   Core and Specific Dimensions of the KSF (DoH 2004b)

Core dimensions

1. Communication
2. Personal and people development
3. Health, safety and security
4. Service development
5. Quality
6. Equality, diversity and rights

Specific dimensions

7. Assessment of health and wellbeing needs
8. Addressing individuals' health and wellbeing needs
9. Improvement of health and wellbeing
10. Protection of health and wellbeing
11. Logistics
12. Data processing and management
13. Production and communication of information and knowledge
14. Facilities maintenance and management
15. Design and production of equipment, devices and visual records
16. Biological investigation and reporting
17. Measuring, monitoring and treating physiological conditions through the application of specific technologies
18. Partnership
19. Leadership
20. Management of people
21. Management of physical and or financial resources
22. Research and development

professional practice in haemato-oncology nursing through the development of a clinical career framework. In turn this should help to retain experienced nurses in clinical areas. Expanding nursing roles has the potential to increase job satisfaction for nurses whilst improving care and services to patients and their families. Ten key roles for nurses have been identified (DoH 2000e) (Box 28.2).

The 10 key roles for nurses are generic and similar ones exist for allied health professionals; examples of the roles being adapted to haemato-oncology include:

- nurse-led chemotherapy administration
- patient group directions (PGD) for the management of a pyrexial neutropenic sepsis
- performing bone marrow biopsy, trephine, harvesting
- insertion of peripherally-inserted central venous catheters or skin-tunnelled catheters

> **Box 28.2   Ten Key Roles for Nurses**
>
> - To order diagnostic investigations such as pathology tests and x-rays
> - To make and receive referrals direct, say to a therapist or pain consultant
> - To admit and discharge patients for specific conditions and within agreed protocols
> - To manage patient caseloads, say diabetes or rheumatology
> - To run clinics, say for ophthalmology or dermatology
> - To prescribe medicines and treatments
> - To carry out a range of resuscitation procedures including defibrillation
> - To perform minor surgery procedures and outpatient procedures
> - To triage patients to the most appropriate health professional using the latest information technology
> - To take a lead in the way local health services are organised and in the way that they are run

- performing apheresis, i.e. stem cell collection or leucopheresis
- complementary therapies.

These roles have developed in an ad-hoc manner depending on local need, however the introduction of the KSF should help to facilitate the development of new skills to meet local, national and individual professional development needs.

In recent years, haemato-oncology nurses have expanded their knowledge and skills to develop new roles with no monetary rewards or career progression. The modernised pay structure should improve this situation and help managers to attract, recruit, retain, recognise and reward staff with the specialist clinical skills and expertise required to meet the complex care needs of haemato-oncology patients.

NETWORKING

Individual haemato-oncology units need to recognise, value and celebrate their own contribution to nurse education and training. With innovation and careful planning, units can organise their own study days and may find support and sponsorship from external agencies. This allows nurses to share good practice with their peers and again promotes a sense of achievement, which can counterbalance the emotional and physical demands associated with the clinical workload.

Encouraging networking with other nurses and health-care professionals in the same speciality can be a further source of support for nurses. Networking can be useful for sharing information and ideas, updating practice impacting on an individual's development and the development of other team members. On a more practical note it can help people realise that they are doing a good job and that they share similar problems with others working in similar units.

Networking can be undertaken on a number of levels, e.g. at ward-unit, directorate or trust level by the organisation of multi-professional seminars. Study days can be organised across the cancer network or nationally. Cancer networks are a rich source for multi-professional networking either related to disease-specific issues or in specialist groups such as chemotherapy or patient information. Patients are increasingly working alongside health-care professionals in various network groups and this is a good opportunity to develop real dynamic partnership working that will benefit patient care.

Membership of national or international professional organisations can also be a useful way of networking. Professional organisations such as the Royal College of Nursing organise a number of specialist groups or forums, including the Cancer Nursing Society, the Palliative Care Nursing forum and the Haematology and Bone Marrow Transplant forum. These groups organise local and national meetings as a focus for sharing good practice, developing protocols or standardising practice.

Other national specialist groups include the European Bone Marrow Transplant (United Kingdom) Nurses and Allied Professionals Group, which is linked to the European Bone Marrow Transplant Group. This group was established in 1997 as a forum to share good practice, explore national issues and recommend solutions, and has grown in both numbers and mix of health-care professionals (see useful resources). Nurses who network or attend professional interest groups reduce the risk of professional isolation as it allows time out from the demands of clinical practice for the nurse to reflect and re-energise their personal resources.

CONCLUSION

Recruiting and retaining specialist staff to work within cancer nursing, and especially haemato-oncology, is challenging – it requires governments and managers to work in partnership with nurses and allied health professionals rather than via traditional hierarchical structures. There needs to be flexibility, creativity, equity and fairness for both employers and employees. Responsibility for meeting the needs of the service should be shared, whilst also working to achieve a work–life balance for employees. Achieving such a balance creates a healthy, person-focussed workplace where health-care professionals remain, develop professionally and ultimately enrich the care, support and treatment they deliver to patients and carers.

DISCUSSION QUESTIONS

1. With no additional resources, what measures could be taken to make your clinical area a place where nurses are eager to work?

2. How could nurses in your clinical area be supported to achieve an effective work–life balance?

3. How could nurses in your clinical area be supported to develop professionally and personally?

4. What opportunities are available for education and professional development within your workplace?

5. How do you access education and professional development?

6. What are the local and national opportunities for networking?

References

Butterworth T, Bishop V, Carson J 1996 First steps towards evaluating clinical supervision in nursing and health visiting. I. Theory, policy and practice development. A review. Journal of Clinical Nursing 5(2):127–132

Cherniss G 1980 Professional burnout in human services organisations. Praeger, New York

Del Bueno D, Weeks L, Brown-Stewart P 1987 Clinical assessment centres: a cost effective alternative for competency development. Nursing Economics 5(1):21–26

Department of Health 2000a The NHS cancer plan. DoH, London

Department of Health 2000b The NHS cancer plan. Executive summary. DoH, London

Department of Health 2000c Improving working lives standard. NHS employers committed to improving the working lives of people who work in the NHS. DoH, London

Department of Health 2000d A health service of all talents: developing the NHS workforce. Consultation document on the review of workforce planning. DoH, London

Department of Health 2000e Developing key roles for nurses and midwives, a guide for managers. DoH, London

Department of Health 2001 Code of Practice for NHS employers involved in the recruitment of healthcare professionals. DoH, London

Department of Health 2004a Agenda for change, proposed agreement. DoH, London

Department of Health 2004b The NHS knowledge and skills framework (NHS KSF) and development review guidance – working draft. DoH, London

Kelly D, Ross S, Gray B, Smith P 2000 Death, dying and emotional labour; problematic dimensions of the role of the bone marrow transplant nursing role? Journal of Advanced Nursing 32(4):952–960

Mackereth P A, White K, Cawthorn A, Lynch B 2005 Improving stressful working lives: complementary therapies, counselling and clinical supervision for staff. European Journal of Oncology Nursing 9:147–154

Manthey M, Miller D 2003 Responsibility, authority, accountability equals decentralisation. Leading an empowered organisation. School of Health Care Studies, Leeds

Matthews J J, Nunley C 1992 Rejuvenating orientation to increase nurse satisfaction and retention. Journal of Nursing Staff and Development 8(4):159–164

Molassiotis A, Haberman M 1996 Evaluation of burnout and job satisfaction in marrow transplantation nurses. Cancer Nursing 19(5):360–367

Nursing and Midwifery Council 2002 Supporting nurses and midwives through life long learning. Protecting the public through professional standards (originally published UKCC;01.02.02, www.nmc-uk.org, accessed 18 Dec 2004)

Wilkin P, Bowers L, Monk J 1997 Clinical supervision, managing the resistance. Nursing Times 93(8): 48–49

Further reading

The author has recommended the following selected reading as it gives guidance to nurses at all levels on the issues that are paramount in proactively managing recruitment and retention of nurses and allied health professionals. They attempt to encourage and motivate nurses to be innovative in their approach to practice and work–life balance. Embracing these issues should encourage local initiatives that may result in a dynamic group of health-care professionals who will benefit both patient care and the wider health-care team.

Department of Health 1998 Working together, securing a quality workforce in the NHS. DoH, London
Department of Health 2000 Developing key roles for nurses and midwives, a guide for managers. DoH, London
Department of Health 2000 The NHS plan. DoH, London
Department of Health 2000 The NHS cancer plan. DoH, London
Department of Health 2004 Agenda for change, proposed agreement. DoH, London
Department of Health 2004 The NHS knowledge and skills framework (NHS KSF) and development review guidance – working draft. DoH, London
Scottish Executive Health Department 2001 Facing the future. Report of the 19th November 2001 Convention on the Recruitment and Retention in Nursing and Midwifery. SEHD, Edinburgh

Chapter **29**

Leadership issues for specialist nurses

Shelley Dolan

This chapter is dedicated to all those staff nurses, sisters/charge nurses, clinical nurse specialists, lecturer/practitioners, nurse practitioners and nurse consultants who work in haemato-oncology areas and whom I have had the enormous pleasure to meet and to learn from.

KEY POINTS

- Optimum clinical leadership is essential for the wellbeing of haemato-oncology patients, their families and haemato-oncology nursing teams.
- Clinical leadership is not something that is limited to the charismatic individual but a way of being and working that can be learnt.
- Across the world there is agreement on key personal leadership characteristics that can be developed.
- Leadership is not just about individuals but is also about the way nurses and the multidisciplinary team work across organisations.
- Effective nursing leadership will improve both recruitment and retention of nurses in haemato-oncology settings.

INTRODUCTION

Nurses are special and a very precious resource for patients, their families, the multidisciplinary team and society. Like many global resources, nurses are scarce and a threatened species. If the challenges of a speciality like haemato-oncology are added to this scarcity, nurses become an even more precious resource and there is a need to ensure that the clinical nursing leaders required in clinical practice are developed. All over the UK and Europe there is an enormous wealth of nurses working in haemato-oncology, whose talents must be encouraged and their love of the speciality maintained. Through excellence in nursing leadership, nurses can be retained and recruited to this exciting area of clinical practice.

The first years of the 21st Century have seen a growing movement to ensure the provision of more clinical leaders in health care. Across the world the need for effective leadership linked closely to a modernisation agenda for improved public services for citizens, users and their families has been recognised. Across the public sector, leadership courses and books on effective leadership and its role in modernising and changing services have grown. In health care in England this has been apparent from 2000 with the launch of the NHS Plan (Department of Health (DoH) 2000a) and the NHS Cancer Plan (DoH 2000b). These documents recognised leadership as an essential tool for delivering an improved health-care system to the public and for the staff working within the system. An essential change apparent in these government policy documents, and also in the global literature, is the recognition that it is clinical leaders from all health-care disciplines that can bring about change in health-care practice and service delivery (Fedoruk & Pincombe 2000, Freshman & Rubino 2004, Hall 2004, McKenna et al 2004, Saleh et al 2004, Helfand et al 2005).

For nursing, whose members constitute the largest discipline in health care, the last 15 years have been characterised by a changing model of leadership moving away from an emphasis on management to leadership that is focussed on effecting change in the areas that are most closely aligned with patient/client care (Kotter 1990, Greenewood 1997). Previous models for leadership in nursing seem to have been aligned with management models and may have emphasised a gap between management and the practice arena (Fedoruk & Pincombe 2000, Mathena 2002). It is therefore an exciting time for nurses at every level and in every health-care organisation to become engaged in the pursuit of improved leadership skills targeted at improving practice and service delivery. Finally it is important to remember that one of the beneficiaries for this new movement in clinical leadership should be the nursing profession, so that clinical leaders of the future are able to influence patient and family care and also concentrate on nurturing nurses.

This chapter illustrates how clinical leadership can be applied within different haemato-oncological settings. Issues such as developing a leadership style, developing influencing skills and the management of change whilst applicable to all health-care settings will be explored using practical scenarios. There are some issues that particularly apply to haemato-oncology settings, e.g. the change from curative treatment to rapid deterioration and the challenges this represents for end-of-life care, and the burden that marrow ablative therapy exerts on the patient and their family, and therefore these areas will be explored as they apply to leadership. Finally it is important to note that this chapter is not solely concentrating on advanced practice or senior nurses but relates to all nurses as it is evident that to strengthen clinical nursing leadership we need to ensure that we start raising awareness at an early stage in a nurse's career (Valentine 2002).

BACKGROUND

Haemato-oncology nursing – irrespective of whether it occurs in primary care, acute care, inpatient or outpatient settings – carries with it many challenges. People who are affected by a haematological cancer may be suddenly catapulted into hospital for immediate management, for example, newly diagnosed acute leukaemia. Nurses may also be working alongside people who are living with the changes that a chronic illness such as chronic lymphocytic leukaemia or myeloma may cause to their life. For many people and families affected by a haematological cancer the diagnosis can make life seem as though it has changed irrevocably; it is the role of the health-care team working alongside them to ensure that the effects of diagnosis and invasive therapy are minimised. People who have gone through these experiences often become expert in the management of their care, and this can be a very rewarding aspect of nursing in this speciality, as nurses are actively involved in working in partnership with patients and families, and also the multidisciplinary team.

Haemato-oncology nursing is often characterised by periods of intensive nursing activity and emotional support for both patients and their families – indeed it is a speciality where nursing truly comes into its own. It is therefore imperative that the clinical leaders within the speciality are able to embrace its challenges and rewards. Like any area of nursing in the 21st century, haemato-oncology is facing challenges with nurse recruitment and retention; it is therefore essential that leadership is openly and actively supportive of nurses and that nursing is encouraged to ensure that new and developing nurses are nurtured, and more experienced nurses are supported to stay in the profession (Valentine 2002).

LEADERSHIP MODELS: ESSENTIAL CHARACTERISTICS FOR TODAY'S AND TOMORROW'S CLINICAL NURSING LEADERS

From the worldwide nursing literature several models of leadership emerge. These have important differences but include dominant characteristics necessary to achieve effective clinical leadership. Rather than exploring each model in detail, an exploration of some of the essential characteristics of leadership cited in these models and their application to haemato-oncology nursing are discussed including:

- transformational leadership
- emotional intelligence
- courage
- challenging and stimulating
- developing trust
- valuing others

(Manley 1997, Goleman 2000, Ferguson-Pare et al 2002, Kouzes & Posner 2002, Porter-O'Grady 2003, Canadian Nurses Association CNA 2005, Leach 2005).

TRANSFORMATIONAL LEADERSHIP

Transformational leadership is a leadership style that has had a profound effect and grown in popularity especially amongst clinical practitioners over the last 15 years (Kotter 1990, Manley 1997, Sofarelli & Brown 2001, McCormack et al 1999, Bennis 2000, Sullivan & Decker 2001, Al-Mailam 2005, Canadian Nurses Association 2005, Leach 2005). Transformational leadership has an underpinning philosophy of equal collaboration and collaborative pursuit of change and drive for improvement. It has been described as a model that can empower the junior nurse (Manley 1997, Sofarelli & Brown 2001). It is also a leadership characteristic that has been demonstrated to reduce the distance between clinical nurses and their nurse executive (Leach 2005). Fundamentally it is a style that can be used to influence others by transforming their behaviour despite being in a non-line-management role (Morgan 2005).

For nurse leaders who utilise a transformational leadership style there needs to be a willingness to reject old behaviours of control and direction to one where leaders and followers (sisters and staff nurses) work together in the organisation (ward, unit, hospital, community) embracing a transparent philosophy of collaborative working across a more horizontal network (Fedoruk & Pincombe 2000, Valentine 2002). Finally, transformational leadership recognises that leadership in nursing cannot be reserved for a few charismatic individuals and it is important to view it as a process that everyone can use to bring forward the best in themselves, and others, for the improvement of care for patients, their families and current and future nurses working in the speciality (Kouzes & Posner 2002). Thus clinical leaders must enable, inspire and foster leadership in others (Canadian Nurses Association 2005).

EMOTIONAL INTELLIGENCE

Emotional intelligence can be described as the values that a leader uses in the presentation of self and their interactions with others. These values would include areas such as self-awareness, social awareness, self-management, and social skills (Snow 2001). The area of emotional intelligence is increasingly recognised as an essential attribute in the effective leadership of public and private sector organisations (Stein 2000). Of the many skills and characteristics that effective clinical leaders need, emotional intelligence has been cited as the most important (Goleman 1998, Snow 2001). In haemato-oncology nurse leaders need to influence the performance of their team and they will therefore need to understand their own feelings and those of others. To really understand the dynamics of their nursing and/or multidisciplinary team a nurse will constantly be reflecting and reappraising whilst managing emotions in themselves and others.

It is important to recognise that the leading researchers examining emotional intelligence and its influence in the leadership of major private sector industries have demonstrated that people can learn to develop their emotional intelligence and therefore clinical nurses can develop their competence in this area. The Hay Group has constructed an emotional intelligence framework that includes clusters of emotional competencies (Table 29.1)

Having a matrix of competencies such as the Hay model in Table 29.1 gives all clinical nursing leaders the opportunity, perhaps together with a mentor or clinical supervisor, to develop their competencies. No one person could expect to be expert in all areas of emotional intelligence but individuals can develop over time. It is also important to use the characteristics of self-awareness and recognise that competency levels will differ on different days. All clinical leaders need to recognise that some days they will not 'get it right' and reflection can be used to recognise the factors affecting success on that day, e.g. tiredness. Knowing oneself is key to recognising the clues that mean we are too tired or emotionally have less energy to deal with something too challenging and, if possible, to move it to a time or day when our energy levels will be more appropriately matched. For nurses working in an increasingly complex health-care setting it is the characteristics of emotional intelligence that can help to ensure that social and professional networks across teams and even across health-care settings can develop and grow (Freshman & Rubino 2004). Finally, Snow (2001) describes how nurses using emotional intelligence will help their nurses and their organisations through the following:

- improved performance of nurses, leading to improved satisfaction for patients, families and the multidisciplinary team
- improved nursing retention
- improved team-working amongst nurses
- increase in team motivation
- enhanced innovation by the nursing team
- enhanced use of time and resources
- good levels of trust between nurses and their clinical leaders.

Table 29.1
Emotional intelligence framework (Snow 2001)

Cluster	Attributes	Attributes	Attributes		
Self-awareness	Self-confidence: confidence about one's own expertise	Self-assessment: awareness of limitations	Emotional self-awareness: being aware of one's negative and positive biases		
Actions	Self-control: controlling one's own behaviour, especially when challenged	Adaptability: being open to and able to cope with new ideas	Trustworthiness: consistent display of honesty/integrity		
Social awareness	Empathy: actively listening to people who have other experience, expertise and background	Understanding other people's perspectives and the ongoing reasons for the behaviour of others	Organisational awareness: ability to read the currents of organisational life and navigate politics		
Social skills	Visionary leadership: ability to take charge and inspire	Developing others: expressing positive expectations	Teamwork: establishing relationships and networks	Influence: ability to wield a range of persuasive tactics	Conflict management: ability to de-escalate disagreements

COURAGE

Jobes & Steinbader (1996) cite three qualities needed by nurse leaders: optimism, persistence and courage. Fedoruk & Pincombe (2000) suggest that in the 21st Century courage is the most important of these three qualities. As health care continues to change at a rapid rate, clinical nurse leaders will need to be courageous and persistent to ensure that patients, their families and the nursing team remain central to the direction of care. As leaders of the largest single workforce in the health service, clinical nurse leaders are pivotal to the haemato-oncology service but they need to remain ever vigilant to ensure their nursing teams do not become disadvantaged. This may at times require the nurse leader to challenge the status quo and place their head above the parapet. It is often more difficult to challenge but a key characteristic that will help leaders in this respect is to stay focussed on the general good of their team and the people they care for. One of the key principles of clinical leadership is being a role model for other staff. The clinical leader needs to be seen by the multidisciplinary team to be committed to the good of patients, their families and the nursing team – even when this may be difficult (NHS 2002).

In her work looking at a framework for advanced practice, Manley (1997) shows that leadership is not about training individuals to grow and then leave their institutions for greener fields afar, although this of course may be appropriate, but rather that leadership is all about the betterment of the service and ensuring that an attractive working culture is developed.

CHALLENGING AND STIMULATING

As clinical leaders work with their nursing and interdisciplinary teams in haemato-oncology, it is important that they seek to provide intellectual stimulation and new ideas that will challenge the team to change, to develop new structures, and challenge the old processes. An essential driver for improvement is that team members encourage each other to search for new opportunities and to experiment with new ways to improve care.

TRUST

Effective leadership seems to be impossible without trust. Modernisation and improvement can be hard work and the team needs to be able to believe in their leaders and trust that they are working in an environment of safety. Leaders therefore need to develop a trusting climate where cynicism and disbelief disappear over time and are replaced with an environment where mutual respect and trust are pre-eminent.

VALUING OTHERS

Valuing others is an essential part of working in a team but has not always been evident in health care, with many nurses arriving at their leadership courses describing distress and evidence of a lack of caring. It is essential that nurses value each other as individuals, demonstrate caring behaviour, encourage and recognise each others' achievements and finally celebrate them together (Bass 1985, Sashkin & Burke 1990, Manley 1997, Kouzes & Posner 2002).

Having described some of the personal characteristics that a leader in haemato-oncology nursing needs to embrace, it is important to recognise some of the challenges that exist in the world of haemato-oncology. The following sections look more closely at the world that nurses, wherever they work in haematology, face as they lead their teams.

NURSE INVOLVEMENT IN DECISION-MAKING

One of the challenges for any nursing team, but perhaps especially those working in haemato-oncology, is the need to feel involved in decisions that affect treatment and end-of-life care of patients. For nurses working so closely with the patient there is sometimes a dissonance between decisions made to pursue active treatment such as another transplant or transfer to critical care, and the nurse's belief about what is best for the patient. It is evident that all members of the multidisciplinary team may have different opinions on treatment and this is perhaps to be expected and may come from being:

- exposed to different experiences
- educated and trained in culturally different systems
- acting in a different role.

It would therefore seem that different and varied perspectives should be expected and perhaps welcomed, but it is essential that all members of the multi-professional team feel part of the discussion. This may seem simple and obvious but can actually be quite a challenge to achieve. Nurses themselves are not a homogenous group and there will be disagreement among them – but perhaps more importantly many nurses do not feel well enough prepared, or experienced enough, to question and give their opinion. There may also historically be a difference in our cultural ability to challenge and to persist in that challenge. Nurses generally come from a philosophy of wanting to be liked and trying to please. Some may even feel, having come from a more hierarchical culture, that it is not their place to ask questions. It is not therefore as simple as expecting all team members just to be able to have their opinion; the working environment has to be such that it positively welcomes challenge and questioning.

From the literature it is evident that nurses working in haemato-oncology and acute care often feel that their feelings and opinions have not been actively sought (Whedon 1997, Hermann et al 1998, Bass 2003, Lutzen et al 2003). When people feel powerless and repeatedly that they are not part of the decision-making team, they can become disaffected and cynical, thus the team dynamics will change. Working with patients who may have entered the unit appearing fairly well, and who are then so physically altered by their treatment rather than their disease, can cause added stressors for nurses working within the haemato-oncology team. Working with patients receiving allogeneic transplants, particularly mismatched transplant programmes, means that many nurses will have to cope with intensive nursing regimens and constantly face high morbidity and mortality rates. Working in such intense conditions often means that close bonds are formed between the patient, their nurse, and the family – if the patient then suffers the very intense side effects of acute graft-versus-host disease or hepatic failure, nurses can feel guilty and question the radicality of such intense treatment regimens. In the haematological transplant setting perhaps more than most health-care settings, nurses and the multidisciplinary team are faced with a complex array of ethical and emotional issues such as:

- selection for transplant
- informed consent
- iatrogenic cause for deterioration
- decision regarding resuscitation
- decision whether to transfer to critical care
- end-of-life care
- donor issues.

It is possible that early discussion of such issues, perhaps in a regular forum on the unit, may ameliorate some of the distress, frustration and powerlessness that have historically been ascribed to nurses and other staff in BMT settings (Carney 1987, Whedon 1997). A forum for regular interdisciplinary discussion – e.g. monthly facilitated discussions between all staff on a transplant unit and the knowledge that medical staff too grapple with difficult decision-making – may reduce the distance and dissonance between professional groups. Active leadership from all disciplines in raising awareness and depersonalising such difficult decisions will also aid team-working. Finally, one of the ways to avoid later ethical difficulties is to think carefully and clearly about selection for transplant, and in pre-transplant counselling to ensure that the patient is comprehensively informed and their wishes regarding resuscitation and transfer to critical care, for example, are known prior to transplant (Perry et al 1999).

Case study 29.1: An example of clinical leadership in haematology nursing

The night nursing team has been concerned for a few days about a young man on the bone marrow transplant unit who is 84 days post his matched unrelated bone marrow transplant (MUD). John, who is only 24 years old, has previously undergone an allogeneic transplant and relapsed early. He developed acute graft-versus-host disease (GvHD) at 20 days following his current transplant and narrowly escaped admission to the critical care unit. Although John has recovered from some of the more severe symptoms, he remains pancytopenic and has constant diarrhoea. John has in the last few nights spent more time talking to the staff nurses on nights about his feelings that any more treatment is futile and that he would like now to go home and spend what he realises will be his last days at home with his family.

On Monday morning the night team speak to the Sister in charge of the unit and ask her to discuss John's feelings with the medical and multidisciplinary team. The Sister assures the team that she will do this as soon as the teams arrive and thanks them for their commitment to John, she also informs them that she will ensure that they get detailed feedback on their return.

The Sister is true to her word and having spent some time talking firstly with John and then together with John and his family, the medical and nursing team makes all necessary arrangements with the primary care team and John can be transferred home the following day.

Finally, the Sister ensures that she leaves a written account for the night team and also invites them to a debriefing discussion of John's care at the next multidisciplinary team meeting planned for 4 weeks' time.

ORGANISATIONAL MILIEU

The ability of nurses to affect change, and to ensure that they can support the patient, the family and their teams in a way that encourages facilitated growth and development of the individual and the team, is not solely dependent on individual leaders. Although much can be achieved by the individual, the organisational milieu in which they are working has a major impact. Hospitals and other health-care institutions have traditionally been vertically organised with hierarchical management structures (Gavin et al 1999). Even given this structure, strong and effective leadership at a senior level has made equality, diversity and respect for unit or ward leadership possible – but it is sometimes achieved almost despite the organisational framework (Fatchett 1998). Health-care organisation in Europe is changing rapidly; in the UK, for example, there is more of an emphasis on working across the traditional boundaries of acute hospital and the community, breaking down vertical silos in favour of horizontal networks (Doherty & Hope 2000, Flanagan et al 2002).

Inherent in this move towards a horizontal structure is the move towards a more open and inclusive structure with devolved leadership and shared governance. Nurses can be the major force for change in such a structure. In the UK the Department of Health document 'Making a difference' cites ward sisters and charge nurses as the 'backbone of the National Health Service' (DoH 1999). It is essential, therefore, that nurses seize the opportunity to ensure that such an open culture exists in all workplaces and across health-care organisations, and to ensure ownership of the working environment is taken through shared governance (Handy 1996). This open culture approach in the workplace emphasises the need for a team to creatively plan together how they will challenge the status quo and change their practice. Also, rather than using blame when errors occur, it encourages individual and team development by collective reflection and learning (Doherty & Hope 2000, Cook 2001). Such emphasis on devolved leadership places a new responsibility on the clinical team leaders of today to ensure that they are well prepared and aware of any major change, e.g. in haemato-oncology practice or regulation, so that they can ensure that the team is also well prepared. Being prepared and feeling 'ahead of the game' can also make leadership seem less frightening for the clinical leader and adds a further goal for effective nursing leadership – that of broad scanning or visioning.

BROAD SCANNING AND POLITICAL ASTUTENESS

Broad scanning is one of the major principles of the NHS Leadership Qualities Framework (NHS 2002) (Fig. 29.1). This can be defined as taking time to collect information from a wide variety of sources. The world of haemato-oncology is acute and changes rapidly within a health-care system that is also changing quickly; it is therefore essential that the clinical nurse leader stays one step ahead. For example, in haemato-

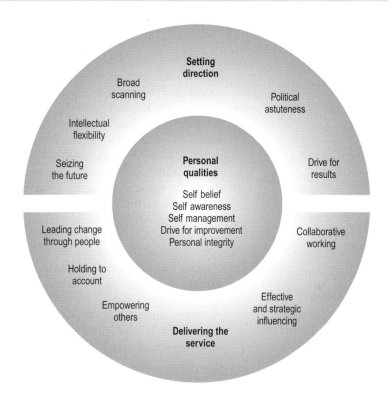

Figure 29.1
NHS Leadership Qualities
Framework 2002. (Crown
Copyright 2003)

oncology practice in the UK and Europe clinical leaders need to be aware of changes to standards of care and accreditation for haematology units such as the Commissioning Outcomes guidance for haematological cancers in the UK (National Institute for Clinical Excellence 2003) and the Joint Accreditation Committee for International Society for Cellular Therapy (ISCT) and European Group for Blood and Marrow Transplantation (EBMT) (JACIE 2004) across Europe.

Indeed, the clinical leader who is curious and motivated to improve services for their area will welcome such quality initiatives and may want to contribute to their design and definitely to their implementation (LeMaistre & Loberiza 2005). To ensure that they stay ahead and informed nurse leaders will be keen to belong to and support the work of national and international haematology societies such as the European Blood and Marrow Transplant (EBMT) society. By ensuring either that they attend all meetings or that they send other colleagues who are then required to give feedback to others, they can ensure that their workplace is prepared for any short- or long-term changes. Ensuring attendance at external meetings and conferences also gives clinical nurse leaders the advantage of being more aware of the political landscape of the health service in which they work. Health is an important ingredient of any country's political agenda and it is therefore essential that nursing leaders at all levels keep themselves aware, curious, and updated about not only local politics (in their own organisation) but also the wider (governmental) politics of health and social care. To do this clinical nurses need to ensure that they are aware of any relevant 'hot topics' in the media, and be aware of the realities of local health services and who the key influencers are so that they can work with them to influence and shape improved services for their patients, families and nursing teams (NHS 2002).

Broad scanning does not solely apply to the type of organisational change outlined above but may also apply to clinical improvements. For the nurse working in haemato-oncology there are still several aspects of care for which there is no evidence base. Leadership in haemato-oncology nursing therefore includes being aware of the evidence where it exists, disseminating and implementing it, and where it does not exist commissioning research to find the evidence. This may involve using existing networks, or setting up new ones for research, communication and clinical comparison of care across a region, country and, increasingly, internationally. Broad scanning harnesses a clinical leader's natural curiosity about the professional world they inhabit, and for the clinical leader who is constantly striving to improve performance, broad scanning – coupled with a drive for results – will ensure a modern and thriving haemato-oncology service for patients, families and the nursing team.

DRIVE FOR RESULTS

A drive for results is another principle in the UK NHS Leadership Qualities Framework (NHS 2002) (Fig. 29.1). This is defined as a strong commitment to ensuring service performance improvements for users which can be interpreted to include patients, families, and the nursing and multidisciplinary team. In some ways this sounds like a principle that all clinical leaders would espouse but actually in the real world, with its many challenges and obstacles, the clinical leader needs drive and determination to stay on the journey. It is sometimes easier to start a new initiative in response to patient need, or in response to a new regional, national or international directive, but the challenge is to persist and ensure that there is a quantifiable improvement over time. Any clinical nurse who has tried to change practice in a haemato-oncology area or across an organisation will recognise the challenge this poses. Even when trying to implement a clinical improvement, such as regular pain assessment for the patient with grade four mucositis, one of the keys to long-term success in ensuring that this new practice becomes embedded in clinical practice is to ensure that the clinical leader uses their energy over time, perhaps in short bursts, to revisit the practice with their team and ensure a permanent improvement in care.

For clinical leaders, therefore, a drive for results means setting goals for oneself and others that stretch and increase performance. In response to whatever drive for change exists, clinical leaders will, in collaboration with the stakeholders in the team and others (e.g. the practice development team or a clinical nurse specialist from an external but linked trust), take the necessary action to identify goals, apply measures to achieve them and quantify their effect over time. An important part of this achievement will be overcoming obstacles and using any difficulties or failures as an opportunity for both self and team reflection, and an opportunity to learn and develop.

TRAINING FOR LEADERSHIP ROLES

Leadership roles and training may more typically be thought of as needing to be applied to ward sisters, clinical nurse specialists or nurse consultants. It is, however, important to ensure that leadership awareness and training starts at a much earlier stage in a nurse's career (Cook 2001). To create the optimum environment to develop and nurture the haemato-oncology nursing leaders of the future, current nurse leaders need to ensure that their teams are supported in order to be able to ensure succession planning. Equally important is to ensure that those nurses who have the most patient contact are also actively involved in influencing improvements in patient care (DoH 2003). This highlights the importance of recognising nurses working at a junior level who have leadership potential and actively providing them with opportunities to develop. This may mean designing an in-house programme for leadership development for staff nurses (Morgan 2005) or accessing a regional or network programme. In the UK, for example, there are several national initiatives either targeted at all nurses, such as the programmes from the Royal College of Nursing and the NHS Leadership Centre, or more specialised programmes such as the course led by the Royal Marsden Hospital for nurses, doctors and allied health professionals working in cancer care. There are also notable global courses for nurses to share leadership expertise across countries such as the course led by the International Society of Nurses in Cancer Care.

There has been significant investment in the NHS to enhance clinical leadership with programmes directed at many health-care professionals from physicians to chief executives. It is important that we continue to lobby for resources to nurture and develop junior nurses, and that we encourage today's leaders to recognise that leadership exists at many levels and that preparation should start during student nurse training. Models such as clinical supervision, mentoring, critical companionship or a buddying system can be used in practice to ensure that junior nurses can work in tandem with a senior clinical nurse leader. It is essential that having been exposed to some of the principles of leadership theory, clinical nurses are able to apply these principles to improving patient care or the ward environment, and be actively supported in their endeavours.

REFLECTION POINT Does your ward, unit or practice area currently have a programme of clinical leadership training for all levels of nurses? Consider the unit you work in and how you could incorporate some of the principles of training outlined above into a programme in your area. Identify the relevant stakeholders whom you need to consult to design and organise such a programme, or search within your local network for a programme that nurses on your unit can access. Identify any resources that you may need and write a short paper on the benefits to the area that leadership awareness and training would bring and what resources you require. Having established a programme, share it with others in the haemato-oncology nursing world locally, nationally or internationally.

CONCLUSION

This chapter has come full circle in this investigation of leadership as applied to nurses working in haemato-oncology settings. At the beginning of this chapter the special nature of haemato-oncology nursing was referred to. It is a tough and exacting speciality but one that is exciting, growing and hugely rewarding. The personal characteristics from the leadership literature as they apply to haematology nursing were then investigated. The application of some of these characteristics and the challenges present in the reality of practice were then explored. Finally the chapter returns to some further leadership characteristics that ensure that clinical leaders are aware of, and integrate with, the wider world of haemato-oncology – both nationally and internationally.

It can be seen from the areas explored that leadership is not something that is inborn but can be developed and taught. It is also perhaps foolhardy to concentrate training for leadership solely on those already in leadership positions, rather the qualities of good clinical leadership should be included in preregistration courses and at all stages of a nurse's career.

Finally, it is essential that all clinical leaders ensure that haemato-oncology outpatient departments, day care, wards and units are open and inclusive, and that they as leaders work to ensure that the leadership qualities cited in this chapter are accepted as the norm. Effective leadership is hard work and needs to be embedded over time, but it is also rewarding. For haemato-oncology nursing good leadership is, above all, not an option but an essential prerequisite to ensure that the nursing leaders of tomorrow constantly emerge, and that a vibrant future is ensured for haemato-oncology nurses, patients and their families.

DISCUSSION QUESTIONS

1. Of the personal leadership qualities cited in this chapter, which do you need to work on to develop your leadership potential?

2. In what ways can you help your ward, unit or organisation to develop its leadership awareness?

3. Can you think of any examples of success in clinical leadership in your ward, unit, department that could be presented at a local meeting or at a national or European meeting?

4. Is there a leadership-training programme available for all levels of nurses in your organisations? If not, how will you explore starting a programme?

References

Al-Mailam F F 2005 The effect of nursing care on overall patient satisfaction and its predictive value on return-to-provider behaviour: a survey study. Quality Management in Health Care 14(2):116–120

Bass B M 1985 Leadership and performance beyond expectations. Free Press, New York

Bass M 2003 Oncology nurses' perceptions of their role in resuscitation decisions. Professional Nurse 18(12):710–713

Bennis W 2000 Managing the dream: reflections on leadership and change. Penguin, Philadelphia

Canadian Nurses Association 2005 Nursing leadership in a changing world. Nursing Now: Issues and Trends in Canadian Nursing 18:1–6

Carney B 1987 Bone marrow transplantation: nurses' and physicians' perceptions of informed consent. Cancer Nursing 10(5):252–259

Cook M J 2001 The attributes of effective clinical nurse leaders. Nursing Standard 15(35):33–36

Department of Health 1999 Making a difference. DoH, London

Department of Health 2000a The NHS plan: a plan for investment, a plan for reform. DoH, London

Department of Health 2000b The NHS cancer plan: a plan for investment, a plan for reform. DoH, London

Department of Health 2003 The NHS knowledge and skills framework and development process. DoH, London

Doherty C, Hope W 2000 Shared governance – nurses making a difference. Journal of Nursing Management 8:77–81

Fatchett A 1998 Nursing in the new NHS: modern and dependable? Baillière Tindall, Edinburgh

Fedoruk M, Pincombe J 2000 The nurse executive: challenges for the 21st century. Journal of Nursing Management 8:13–20

Ferguson-Pare M, Mitchell G, Perkin K, Stevenson L 2002 Academy of Canadian Executive Nurses (ACEN) background paper on leadership. Canadian Journal of Nursing Leadership 15(3):4–8

Flanagan J, Clarke D, Kendrick K, Lane C 2002 The advancing role of nurses in cancer care. In: Clarke D, Flanagan J, Kendrick K (eds) Advancing nursing practice in cancer and palliative care. Palgrave Macmillan, Basingstoke

Freshman B, Rubino L 2004 Emotional intelligence skills for maintaining social networks in healthcare organisations. Hospital Topics 82(3):2–9

Gavin M, Ash D, Wakefield S, Wroe C 1999 Shared governance: time to consider the cons as well as the pros. Journal of Nursing Management 7:193–200

Goleman D 1998 Working with emotional intelligence. Bantam, New York

Goleman D 2000 Working with emotional intelligence. Bantam, Toronto

Greenewood A 1997 Leadership for change. Nursing Standard 11(19):22–23

Hall L 2004 A palette of desired leadership competencies: painting the picture for successful regionalisation. Healthcare Management Forum 17(3):18–22

Handy C 1996 Beyond certainty. Arrow Business Books, London

Helfand B, Cherlin E, Bradley E H 2005 Next generation leadership: a profile of self-rated competencies among administrative resident and fellows. Journal of Health Administration Education 22(1):85–105

Hermann R P, Leather M, Leather H L, Leen K 1998 Clinical care for patients receiving autologous hematopoietic stem cell transplantation in the home setting. Oncology Nursing Forum 25(8)1427–1432

JACIE – Joint Accreditation Committee for International Society for Cellular Therapy and European Group for Blood and Marrow Transplantation 2004 Standards for haematopoietic progenitor cell collection, processing and transplantation. www.Jacie.org Accessed 12 Dec 2005

Jobes M, Steinbader A 1996 Transitions in nursing leadership roles. Nursing Administration Quarterly 20(2):80–84

Kotter J A 1990 A force for change: how leadership differs from management. Free Press, London

Kouzes J M, Posner B Z 2002 The leadership challenge. Wiley, San Francisco

Leach L S 2005 Nurse executive transformational leadership and organisational commitment. Journal of Nursing Administration 35(5):228–237

LeMaistre C F, Loberiza F R 2005 What is quality in a transplant programme? Biology of Blood and Marrow Transplantation 11:241–246

Lutzen K, Cronqvist A, Magnusson A, Andersson L 2003 Moral stress synthesis of a concept. Nursing Ethics 10(3):312–322

Manley K 1997 A conceptual framework for advanced practice: an action research project operationalizing an advanced practitioner/consultant nurse role. Journal of Clinical Nursing. 6:179–190

Mathena K A 2002 Nursing manager leadership skills. Journal of Nursing Administration 32(3):136–142

McCormack B, Manley K, Kitson A et al 1999 Towards practice development – a vision in reality or a reality without vision? Journal of Nursing Management 7:255–264

McKenna M K, Gartland M P, Pugno P A 2004 Development of physician leadership competencies: perceptions of physician leaders, physician educators and medical students. Journal of Health Administration Education 21(3):343–354

Morgan C 2005 Growing our own: a model for encouraging and nurturing aspiring leaders. Nursing Management 11(9):27–30

NHS 2002 NHS Leadership Qualities Framework. NHS Leadership Centre, www.NHSLeadershipQualities.nhs.uk/ Accessed 10 Oct 2005

National Institute for Clinical Excellence 2003 Guidance on commissioning cancer services: improving outcomes in haematology cancers. Department of Health, London

Perry A R, Rivlin M M, Goldstone A H 1999 Bone marrow transplant patients with life-threatening organ failure: when should treatment stop? Journal of Clinical Oncology 17(1):298–303

Porter-O'Grady T 2003 A different age for leadership, part 1. Journal of Nursing Administration 33(2):105–110

Saleh S S, Williams D, Balougan M 2004 Evaluating the effectiveness of public health leadership training: the NEPHLI experience. American Journal of Public Health 94(7):1245–1249

Sashkin M E, Burke W W 1990 Understanding and assessing organisational leadership. In: Clark K, Clark M B (eds) Measures of leadership. Leadership Library of America/Centre for Creative Leadership, West Orange, NJ

Snow J L 2001 Looking beyond nursing for cues to effective leadership. Journal of Nursing Administration 31(9):440–443

Sofarelli M, Brown R 2001 The need for nursing leadership in uncertain times. Journal of Nursing Management 6(4):201–207

Stein N 2000 The world's most admired companies. Fortune October 2:183–196

Sullivan E J, Decker P J 2001 Effective leadership and management, 5th edn. Prentice Hall, Upper Saddle River, NJ

Valentine S O 2002 Nursing leadership and the new nurse. Journal of Undergraduate Nursing Scholarship, University of Arizona, www.juns.nursing.arizona.edu/articles/Fall202002 Accessed 5 May 2005

Whedon M B 1997 Bone marrow transplantation: principles, practice and nursing insights. Jones & Bartlett, Boston

Chapter **30**

Research priorities

Maggie Grundy

KEY POINTS

- There is a paucity of robust nursing research relating specifically to haemato-oncology nursing.
- Establishing research priorities is seen as the first step in developing structured, strategic programmes of research.
- Multicentre collaborative research may be the most appropriate way forward because of the small number of patients seen in any one centre and the limited number of nurse researchers.

INTRODUCTION

Overall, haematological malignancies account for a small proportion of cancers (Cancer Research Campaign 2004). Much of the literature informing haemato-oncology nursing is related to cancer nursing generally rather than haemato-oncology nursing specifically. The relative rarity of haematological malignancies means that for research purposes patients are often included in larger groups of cancer patients and there is a paucity of robust nursing research relating specifically to the speciality. A review of North American nursing research in blood and marrow transplantation (BMT) between 1982 and 1995 found only 33 published research papers (Haberman 1997). A search of the BMT literature in the Cumulative Index of Nursing and Allied Health Literature (CINAHL) between 1980 and mid-1996 found only 44 research articles (Molassiotis 1997).

Individuals with haematological malignancies receive more aggressive treatment, experience greater bone marrow suppression (with the associated life-threatening risks of infection and haemorrhage) and often spend long periods of time in hospital. Their needs are therefore perceived as different from those of the general cancer patient population.

A number of studies have sought to establish research priorities in cancer nursing (e.g. Oberst 1978, Degner et al 1987, Daniels & Ascough 1999, Rustøen & Schjølberg 2000, Browne et al 2002, McIlfatrick & Keeney 2003). With the exception of one small study (n = 23) focussing specifically on BMT (Molassiotis 1997) there are no studies identifying research priorities in haemato-oncology nursing. Haberman (1997) suggests ideas for future research in BMT but highlights the need to determine priorities.

Establishing priorities is seen as the first step in developing structured, strategic programmes of research, which are seen as vital at international, national and local levels to strengthen the evidence base for nursing, improve patient care, help to distinguish the unique contribution of nursing to patient care and make best use of scarce resources. This will ensure that research develops in a coordinated way and resources are directed to the most appropriate areas (Oberst 1978, Corner 1993, Daly et al 1996, Hunt 2001, Richardson et al 2001, Kearney 2002). Priority setting and development of strategic programmes of research are particularly important in a small speciality such as haemato-oncology where multicentre collaborative research may be the most appropriate way forward because of the small number of patients seen in any one centre and the limited number of nurse researchers (Haberman 1997, Molassiotis 1997). A Delphi study was therefore undertaken to determine research priorities in haemato-oncology.

AIMS OF THE STUDY

The study aimed to:

- determine research priorities of UK nurses working in haemato-oncology
- contribute to expanding and advancing the knowledge base for nurses working in the speciality through dissemination of findings.

METHODOLOGY

The Delphi technique is a method of obtaining consensus that has been extensively used in health services research, particularly for establishing research priorities (McKenna 1994, Beretta 1996, Keeney et al 2001). It is an inexpensive means of reaching a large number of people and uses sequential rounds to gather information. The number of rounds is usually determined by the amount of time and funding available for the study. As limited time was available for this study, two rounds were undertaken.

ROUND 1

A questionnaire adapted from the work of Browne et al (2002) was designed including demographic questions and asking respondents to list in order of priority 'the three most important questions or problems relating to haemato-oncology nursing that you consider should be researched'.

ROUND 2

The questionnaire reflected the research priorities identified by participants in round 1. Respondents were asked to rate research priorities on a graphic rating scale, with 1 being low and 7 being high. Respondents were also asked to identify the most important item in each category by placing the number 1 next to it.

Sample

A convenience sample was drawn from members of the Royal College of Nursing (RCN), Haematology and Bone Marrow Transplant (HBMT) Forum. Convenience sampling methods are appropriate for Delphi studies as knowledge of the subject being researched is important and individuals considered to be subject experts tend to be recruited (Goodman 1987, Beretta 1996). Members of the RCN, HBMT forum were considered to be expert as membership of the forum suggests that they have knowledge and an interest in the speciality. Furthermore, it is suggested that those who become involved in the process are likely to be those who will be directly affected by the results; these individuals are also more likely to stay involved in the process (Keeney et al 2001).

A letter inviting participation in the Delphi study, the first questionnaire and a stamped addressed envelope for return of the questionnaire were included with an edition of the forum's newsletter in January 2004. A total of 1445 questionnaires were distributed, one of which was sent to the author leaving 1444 remaining questionnaires. Those receiving the invitation to participate were asked to photocopy the questionnaire and invite their colleagues to complete it. Participants were asked to add their name and contact address to the completed questionnaire if they were willing to contribute to the second round of the study.

Consensus

The first round of a Delphi study is likely to produce wide and diverse opinion; subsequent rounds aim to achieve consensus (McKenna 1994).

Determining consensus is a controversial aspect of Delphi studies and studies are criticised for not stating the level of consensus at the outset (Williams & Webb 1994). However, universal agreement on the level of consensus is lacking and varies from 50% (Daniels & Howlett 2001) to 100% (Williams & Webb 1994). Determining the level of consensus therefore appears to be a rather arbitrary decision (Green et al 1999).

McIfatrick & Keeney (2003) set the consensus level at ≥65% in their study of cancer nursing priorities and found that the majority of items gained a much greater level of consensus. Erring on the side of caution, and noting that the sample in the proposed study is much larger than the one in the McIfatrick & Keeney study, a consensus level of 65% agreement for items rated as high priority (6 or 7) was set for this study.

Analysis of data

Data analysis took place between each round. Following the first round, responses were entered into the Statistical Package for Social Sciences (SPSS). Although this package is not intended for qualitative data, it did enable the identified research priority and an identification code for the respondent to be entered prior to reduction and categorisation.

Reliability and validity

Delphi studies are often criticised for their lack of attention to reliability and validity (Keeney et al 2001). It is suggested that a clear decision-trail defending the techniques used is of key importance in ensuring credibility of findings (Fink et al 1991). Attention was given to ensuring clear articulation of the decision-trail for the study. An expert panel consisting of two recognised experts in the field (one of whom is also an experienced researcher) and another experienced researcher were asked to review the reduction and categorisation used to form the round 2 questionnaire, thus ensuring content validity and inter-rater reliability (Mead & Moseley 2001).

Ethical issues

Ethical approval for the study was sought through the local health services research ethics committee, which categorised the project as an audit not requiring ethical approval. The Data Protection Act was complied with as respondents were initially approached by including the questionnaire with a newsletter from a professional forum and no names or contact details were released to the researcher. Participants voluntarily included their names and addresses on the first questionnaire if they were willing to be involved in the second round. Both questionnaires indicated that participants were free to withdraw from the study at any time.

The inclusion of names and addresses means that respondents are known to the researcher. Each respondent was allocated a code and therefore known only to the researcher. No-one else had access to respondents' details or their responses, thus ensuring confidentiality and anonymity. Data were stored in a locked drawer to which only the researcher had access, therefore ensuring security of data.

RESULTS

ROUND 1 RESPONSES

A total of 249 questionnaires were returned – a 17% response rate. Nineteen questionnaires were either incomplete or unusable. The remaining 230 questionnaires (16% response rate) were included in the analysis.

RESEARCH PRIORITIES

The questionnaires yielded 517 research priorities. Of these, only 50 (10%) were identified more than once. The priorities were initially entered into SPSS verbatim, labelled individually and content analysed. Reduction and categorisation of data were required to produce a second questionnaire of a reasonable length. In reducing the data, areas of overlap were identified and similar items were clustered together and collapsed to form one question or statement. Items containing more than one theme were split into two or more elements. If statements with multiple themes are allowed in a subsequent round, it becomes difficult to determine which element of the statement is viewed as important by the respondent (Mead & Moseley 2001).

Content analysis and reduction of data was conducted by the researcher and reviewed by the expert panel to determine validity. It is suggested that the findings of previous Delphi studies have been unhelpful in developing research frameworks because of the 'global and multifaceted nature' of the issues identified (Macmillan Practice Development Unit, undated). Therefore great care was taken in trying to achieve a balance between retaining the richness of the original data and producing a second-round questionnaire of a reasonable length. Following completion of reduction and categorisation, 178 questions in 11 categories emerged from the data. Categories identified were:

- education
- service delivery and organisation of care
- effects of role on nurses' health and support needs
- communication/patient information and education
- ethical decision-making
- nurses' role
- utilising knowledge and developing the evidence base for practice
- nursing interventions and care
- symptom management
- psychosocial wellbeing and support
- patient and family experience.

All topics identified by respondents were listed in an Excel spreadsheet under the above headings. In using a classic Delphi study, items should be in respondents' own words with only minor editing (Hasson et al 2000). However, the reliability and validity of data may be challenged if questions are not well phrased (Keeney et al 2001). Soanes et al (2000) suggested that presenting items in respondents' own words may have been problematic in their study, making items appear unrefined and unclear to others. Items were therefore presented in respondents' own words as far as possible, although in some cases editing was required to ensure clarity of the item. Items were presented either as research questions or statements, depending on how they were initially presented by respondents. Bond & Bond (1982) excluded items not expressed as research questions. However, it was perceived that this course of action would detract from the richness of the data.

PILOT STUDY

Several of the topics identified appeared to be more appropriate to education than research. Previous Delphi studies have also reported responses that implied a lack of awareness of previous research or relevant literature (Hagan & Hunt 1998, Daniels & Ascough 1999, Soanes et al 2000, Daniels & Howlett 2001). However, Hagen & Hunt (1998) found on probing that different aspects of the topic that had not been previously researched were actually being identified. For these reasons it was decided to conduct a pilot study to determine the feasibility of incorporating both education and research into the second questionnaire. Respondents were asked two questions in the second questionnaire:

1. How important is this topic to haemato-oncology nursing research?
2. How important is this topic to haemato-oncology nurse education?

Respondents were asked to rate each item on a graphic rating scale and also asked to indicate the item they perceived to be the most important in each category. Six nurses who were not involved in the study volunteered to complete the pilot questionnaire. Respondents were asked to comment on the length of time taken to complete the questionnaire, clarity of instructions for completing the questionnaire, clarity of format, rate the degree of difficulty in completing the questionnaire and highlight on the questionnaire any areas they felt were unclear.

Five questionnaires were returned. The questionnaire took between 30 minutes and $1\frac{1}{2}$ hours to complete with a mean of 53 minutes. Comments indicated that the questionnaire was too cumbersome because of the number of questions/statements and rating them in terms of importance for both research and education.

Discussion with respondents suggested that removing the educational element from the questionnaire would improve acceptability – the second questionnaire therefore related to research priorities only. It would, however, be interesting to undertake a similar exercise relating to education in the future.

Before piloting the questionnaire it was anticipated that respondents might have difficulty in highlighting one statement/question as the highest priority in each category. However, overall this did not seem to be problematic – although the item identified as the most important did not always correlate with the rating given to that item. The decision was therefore made to retain this format for the second questionnaire.

SECOND QUESTIONNAIRE

The second questionnaire was sent to all respondents who provided contact details in first-round responses, a total of 166. In an attempt to increase response rate, respondents were encouraged to photocopy the questionnaire and pass it on to any of their colleagues who might be interested in completing it. Respondents were asked to return the questionnaire within a month. In an attempt to enhance response rates a second letter and a copy of the questionnaire were sent to all those who had not already responded 2 weeks before the identified deadline.

ROUND 2 RESULTS

A total of 119 completed questionnaires were returned, a 72% response rate. Three questionnaires were returned uncompleted and two further questionnaires were excluded from the analysis; 117 questionnaires (71%) were therefore included in the analysis.

Demographic data

Slightly under half the respondents (45%) were aged 30–40 years, with a further 34% being 41–50 years – reflecting the current trend towards an older nursing workforce (Ball & Pike 2004) and showing similarities with respondents in the studies undertaken by Browne et al (2002) and McIlfatrick & Keeney (2003). The characteristics of respondents in terms of knowledge and experience are consistent with definitions of the term 'expert', an essential criterion within a Delphi study. The majority (76%) of the respondents were working directly with patients and were well qualified – 88% had a post-registration qualification, 38% had undertaken specialist haematology or BMT courses, and a further 41% had undertaken specialist oncology courses (usually the former English National Board courses). The majority of respondents were working in either dedicated haematology/BMT areas (37%) or areas where haematology was combined with oncology or another speciality (51%). Most respondents had worked in the speciality for many years with 74% remaining for over 5 years and substantial numbers continuing for up to 20 years. Demographic data are shown in Table 30.1.

RESEARCH PRIORITIES

Each item was ranked according to the sum of high priority scores (6 & 7) and reported as a percentage. Fifty items (28%) reached consensus of ≥65%. The top 10 priorities are shown in Table 30.2 (12 items are actually listed as several items received the same score). Items were also ranked

Table 30.1
Demographic data

Table 30.1
Demographic data

Demography	Round 2 %
Place of work	
Haematology inpatient area (non-BMT)	3
Haematology outpatient/day area	9
Combined haematology/BMT unit	21
BMT unit	3
Combined haematology/oncology inpatient/outpatient unit	17
Combined haematology/oncology/palliative care	22
Combined haematology/other medical speciality	9
Higher education	4
Paediatric haematology/oncology	3
Cancer research/trials	2
Community	1
ICU	1
Palliative care	2
Others	2
Country of work	
England	82
Scotland	8
Wales	8
Northern Ireland	3
Age	
21–30	10
31–40	45
41–50	34
51–60	10
Years working in haematology	
1–5	25
6–10	36
11–15	24
16–20	12
21–25	2
Role	
Clinical nurse	37
Combined clinical nurse/ward manager	20
CNS	20
Manager	8
Lead cancer nurse	1
Matron cancer services	2
Research nurse	3
Researcher	2
Educationalist	8
Others	2
Post-registration qualifications	
Diploma	38.5
Degree	38.5
Postgraduate diploma	2
Masters	9
No post-registration qualification	12

Table 30.2
Top 10 priorities

Research question	%
Patients and relatives' views on the information and support they receive regarding diagnosis and treatments	81.2
Long-term health risks of nurses exposed to chemotherapy/antibiotics	80.3
What is nurses' knowledge of neutropenic sepsis?	77.8
Are staff shortages detrimental to practical/emotional support?	75.2
What do patients expect/require from nurses?	75.2
Making decision when active treatment ends and palliative treatment begins	74.4
Access to haematological nurse education/courses	73.5
When to actively treat and when to withdraw treatment	72.7
How can chemotherapy training and administration be standardised throughout the UK?	72.7
Management and care of neutropenic patients	72.7
Psychological effects of relapse for the patient and family	72.7
How effective/successful are nurse-led services?	72.7

by category and those items that reached consensus within each category are shown in Box 30.1.

Several of the 10 highest ranked priorities and many other items have tied places. Other items reaching the ≥65% consensus level are clustered closely together, suggesting that consensus may not have been reached; further examination of responses substantiated this. The median of all questions ranged from 4 (n = 1) to 7 (n = 3). The majority of questions (133) had a median of 6. Furthermore there was a definite clustering of responses towards the top end of the rating scale with the majority of items rated 5–7. Across the entire questionnaire only 17.7% of responses were scored 4 or less.

MOST IMPORTANT ITEM IN EACH CATEGORY

The items marked by respondents as the most important in each category did not always match the highest priority items. The most important item matched the highest priority item in only four categories:

- effects of role on nurses' health and support needs
- communication/patient information and education
- symptom management
- psychosocial wellbeing and support.

Additionally, the first three most important items matched the highest priority items in two categories – effects of role on nurses' health and support needs and symptom management. In the two categories nursing interventions and care and nurses' role, the first two most important items were the same as the highest priority items but their order was transposed.

The number of respondents who did not indicate a high priority item in each category varied and tended to be inconsistent. Some respondents

Box 30.1 Consensus priorities by category

Education	%
● What is nurses' knowledge of neutropenic sepsis?	77.8
● Access to haematological nurse education/courses	73.5
● How can chemotherapy training and administration be standardised throughout the UK?	72.7
● What is nurses' awareness of transfusion reactions?	70.7
● How can high standards/levels of knowledge in cytotoxic administration be maintained?	70.1

Service delivery and organisation of care

● Are staff shortages detrimental to practical/emotional support?	75.2
● What is the effect of staffing levels and skill mix on outcomes of care?	70.1
● Transition from curative to palliative care & treatment	67.6

Effects of role on nurses' health and support needs

● Long-term health risks of nurses exposed to chemotherapy/antibiotics	80.3

Communication/patient information and education

● Patients' and relatives' views on the information and support they receive regarding diagnosis and treatments	81.2
● Provision of information for children of adults with a haematological cancer	70.9
● Effect of communication good/bad on patients	70.9
● Timeliness/quality/amount of information at diagnosis and relapse	68.4
● Education and pre-assessment of patients having chemotherapy	67.6
● Information giving and patient empowerment	66.7
● What information do patients require on specific aspects of care?	65

Ethical decision-making

● Making decision when active treatment ends and palliative treatment begins	74.4
● When to actively treat and when to withdraw treatment	72.7
● Does the patient receive sufficient information to provide informed patient consent?	65.8

Nurses' role

● How effective/successful are nurse led services?	72.7
● Critical care skills – are they an essential requirement for haematology/BMT nurses?	71.8
● Minimum skills/requirements for UK haematology nurses/researchers/managers	70.9
● Development of extended role for nurses in haemato-oncology	68.4
● How effective is the CNS role in haemato-oncology?	68.4
● Career development for haemato-oncology nurses	66.7

Utilising knowledge and developing the evidence base for practice

● Clear guidelines on mucositis management	68.4
● What is best practice in protective isolation care? Is there a best practice?	68.4
● National guidelines/standards of care for central venous catheters including dressings, cleaning and flushing	67.6
● Develop evidence base for optimal care/use/problem-solving of central venous catheters including reducing infection/preventing thrombosis	66.7
● Oral care protocol – what's best?	66.7
● How can clinical research be implemented into practice?	65

Box 30.1   Consensus Priorities by Category – Cont'd

Nursing interventions and care

- Management and care of neutropenic patients   72.7
- How can prevention of infection measures be improved?   70.1
- Are antimicrobial diets/clean food regimes beneficial in neutropenia?   65
- Nutritional support for patients undergoing transplant procedures and high-dose chemotherapy   65

Symptom management

- How can the side effects of chemotherapy be reduced?   70.1
- Disease and treatment related fatigue   66.7

Psychosocial wellbeing and support   %

- Quality of life – what does it really mean to the patient?   71.8
- How could nurses improve support for patients?   70.9
- What are the psychosocial support needs of patients with haematological cancers and their   68.4
  families?
- Long-term survival anxiety when returning to clinic for follow-up   66.7
- Psychological effects of haematological cancers   65.8
- What is the psychological impact of BMT?   65.8

Patient and family experience

- What do patients expect/require from nurses?   75.2
- Psychological effects of relapse for the patient & family   72.7
- Effect of low staff morale and staffing on experiences of isolated patient   69.2
- What effect does a palliative prognosis have on the patient?   66.7
- Patient experiences of symptom control   65.8
- How important to patients is access to a CNS?   65

---

did not indicate a most important item at all, some identified an item in some categories but not in all, whereas others indicated more than one item per category (mainly in the larger categories spread over two pages of the questionnaire). The number of missing cases ranged from 12% to 17% in the categories confined to one page and from 31% to 52% in the categories encompassing two pages. The non-response rate for the most important items appears to be the most likely reason for the lack of correlation between the item rated as the highest priority in each category and the most important item. However, it is unclear why an individual's identification of the most important item in each category did not always correlate with their rating of that item.

REFLECTION POINT   What do you perceive to be the priority research topics in your workplace? How do they compare to the priorities identified in this study?

DISCUSSION

Although the response rate to the first questionnaire was poor (17%), this does not appear to be unusual. Response rates in previous Delphi studies have been found to vary from 15% to 80% in round 1 (Bond & Bond 1982, Degner et al 1987, Rudy 1996, Daniels & Ascough 1999, Soanes et al 2000, Barrett et al 2001, Browne et al 2002, Kirkwood et al 2003, McIlfatrick & Keeney 2003).

Despite the poor response rate to the first questionnaire, response to the second questionnaire was high, at 72%. Response rates in subsequent rounds are noted to decline in most Delphi studies (McKenna 1994) and studies are often criticised for their high attrition rates. The attrition rate from round 1 to round 2 in this study was 28%, which appears reasonable when compared to attrition rates from the second round in other Delphi studies of 9–72% (Bond & Bond 1982, Degner et al 1987, Rudy 1996, Soanes et al 2000, Browne et al 2002, Barrett et al 2001, McIlfatrick & Keeney 2003).

The relatively small attrition rate from the second round suggests that those who responded to the first questionnaire had a genuine interest in the speciality and establishing research priorities. It is suggested that gaining participants' written consent to participate in subsequent rounds may solidify their commitment to the study and enhance response rates (Rudy 1996); this could explain the good response rate for the second round. The inclusion of a stamped addressed envelope for return of the questionnaire and the use of a reminder letter may also have helped to increase response rates.

PRIORITIES

Research priorities identified in this study are similar to priorities identified in previous cancer nursing studies. The highest rated priority 'patients and relatives' views on the information and support they receive regarding diagnosis and treatments' although more specific, is similar to the highest priority in Browne et al's 2002 study 'communication, information giving and educational needs'. Additionally, patient perspectives of psychological experiences and care was prioritised third overall in the latter study. 'Information giving post treatment' was also identified in the top five priorities in the McIlfatrick & Keeney 2003 study. The views and experiences of patients and relatives are currently high on the political agenda and may help to explain why this particular topic is perceived to be a priority.

The second highest rated priority 'long term health risks of nurses exposed to chemotherapy/antibiotics' has also been identified in previous studies (Oberst 1978, Degner et al 1987, Stetz et al 1995, Daniels & Ascough 1999, Browne et al 2002). However, the only study to rank this priority so highly in the past is that of Daniels & Ascough (1999), and it was rated as one of the lowest priorities in the Browne et al (2002) study. It is interesting that 'health issues associated with handling cytotoxic drugs' has been persistently rated as a priority in studies since 1978. Browne et al (2002) emphasise the importance of determining why priority topics persist over time; the reasons why health issues associated with handling cytotoxic drugs have persistently been identified certainly warrants further investigation.

Neutropenia is a life-threatening complication of haematological cancers and their treatment and its importance in care is reflected in the third highest ranked priority, 'what is nurses' knowledge of neutropenic sepsis?' However, it is perhaps surprising that 'management and care of neutropenic patients' and 'how can prevention of infection measures be improved' are ranked 10th and 22nd respectively, especially given the current national emphasis on infection control in hospitals. Isolation practices while reaching consensus were also a lesser priority, ranked 28th.

Infection control and isolation practices were the highest ranked priority in the Molassiotis (1997) study of BMT priorities and several cancer nursing studies rank neutropenia and protective isolation practices in the top 10 priorities (Stetz et al 1995, Daniels & Ascough 1999, Ropka et al 2002). As those with haematological cancers are more likely to experience lower neutrophil counts for a longer period of time than those with solid tumours, it might be expected that these issues would be a higher priority for haemato-oncology nurses. However, methodological difficulties exist in researching protective isolation practices and the results may reflect nurses' awareness of these difficulties, the lack of evidence supporting protective isolation practices and the extant literature on the subject (see Chapter 15).

Nurse education was the category with greatest number of items (3) ranked in the top 10 priorities. Nurse education issues were also prioritised highly by Browne et al (2002) but have not been ranked so highly in other studies, indicating that this is a contemporary concern for nurses. The prioritisation of educational issues suggests that a deficit is perceived both in nurses' knowledge and in access to educational courses. There are a number of possible explanations for this; nurses are increasingly taking on more specialised and expanded roles and the need for education to fulfil these roles may be reflected in these priorities. Furthermore, haemato-oncology is a relatively small speciality and specific courses in haematology or haemopoietic stem cell transplant are offered in only a minority of educational institutions in the UK. Access may therefore be difficult for many nurses working in this speciality. Current staffing and funding shortages in the NHS and the subsequent difficulties with release from the workplace, replacement costs and lack of financial support for education may also be contributory factors.

Two items from the ethical decision-making category relating to palliative care were also included in the 10 highest rated priorities. Ethical issues were rated as the first priority in the Rustøen & Schjølberg (2000) study but do not appear to be rated so highly in other studies. Furthermore, palliative care issues are not rated so highly by either Molassiotis (1997) or in most cancer nursing studies – although the transition from active treatment to palliative care and discontinuation of active treatment are rated as priorities by Rustøen & Schjølberg (2000) and Barrett et al (2001).

Two other items related to palliative care, although not included in the top 10 priorities, also reached consensus. The number of times palliative care issues are identified may reflect the rapid transition from curative to palliative and terminal care that can occur in haematological cancers and the difficulties which may be experienced by patients, their relatives and the health-care professionals caring for them in adapting to these changed circumstances. It may also reflect the difficulties associated with applying palliative and supportive care principles in acute and high technology areas.

Barrett et al (2001) identify similar ethical issues to those identified in this study, e.g. end-stage decision-making, communication about prognosis and emotional needs of patients and families – but related to terminal rather than palliative care. These authors, while acknowledging the existing wealth of literature associated with end-of-life care, suggest that there is little to help practitioners manage these issues in their everyday practice and indicate that research is required to address how these issues can be best addressed.

With the exception of care and management of neutropenic patients, other topics in the 10 highest ranked priorities appear to reflect contemporary changes in health-care delivery, nursing roles/skill mix and the psychological aspects of patient experiences. These findings reflect some of the broad themes identified by Haberman (1997) for future nursing research in BMT including: effects of staff ratios/skill mix on patient outcomes, psychosocial support, patient and carer experiences, ethical decision-making and nurse-led care. Priorities identified by Browne et al (2002) and McIlfatrick & Keeney (2003) also appear to reflect changes in health-care delivery and nursing roles. Molassiotis (1997), Rustøen & Schjølberg (2000) and Browne et al (2002) found that psychosocial issues ranked highly.

Symptom management and quality of life barely feature in the 10 highest rated priorities whereas they feature more frequently in other studies (Stetz et al 1995, Molassiotis 1997, Browne et al 2002, Ropka et al 2002, Yates et al 2002, McIlfatrick & Keeney 2003). Symptom management topics were also omitted from the top 10 priorities in the studies of Rustøen & Schjølberg (2000) and Barrett et al (2001) – these findings are perhaps indicative of progress being made in both utilisation of research findings and provision of supportive care in recent years.

None of the topics in the 'utilisation of knowledge and developing the evidence base for practice' category were in the top 10 priorities. However, several topics were in the top 50 and reached consensus. This category encompassed aspects of care that have been previously researched; further work needs to be undertaken to identify the difficulties these topics continue to cause in practice. There is also a need to ensure dissemination and utilisation of existing research findings. Several of the items identified suggest that nurses want guidance on best practice – topics in this category would appear to be an ideal starting point for systematic reviews, development of guidelines and best practice statements.

These results suggest that research priorities in haemato-oncology nursing are very similar to research priorities in cancer nursing. However, future research conducted specifically in haemato-oncology may reveal different results from those found in general cancer nursing studies. The results provide some direction for future research in haemato-oncology nursing but should be viewed with caution. Recruiting participants from members of one professional interest group and the non-response rate may have biased results and should be considered in interpreting them. Furthermore, the number of tied items and clustering of responses towards the top end of the rating scale indicates that respondents had difficulty in prioritising items. Undertaking a further round of the study may have been helpful in clarifying priorities and establishing greater consensus. However, time constraints precluded this.

THE WAY FORWARD

Identification of priorities is of little value unless they are translated into programmes of research. Further exploration of priorities areas is required; however, those identified in this study provide a good starting point for this and also for developing programmes of research in haemato-oncology. Development of research programmes would, however, require coordination, commitment and cooperation from both interested and dynamic individuals, professional interest groups and higher education institutions. Small numbers of available researchers and difficulties in accessing funding are also barriers to developing and implementing such programmes (Molassiotis 1997, Hunt 2001). Multi-professional research should be considered and may help to reduce replication of research and associated costs, and also help to provide different perspectives (Richardson et al 2002). A national research strategy would need to be developed to maximise research expertise and coordinated programmes of research.

Major challenges exist in both developing and implementing such a strategy. However, development of strong collaborative arrangements between different institutions and different professional groups with interest and expertise in haemato-oncology would help to increase opportunities for funding and strengthen proposals for funding. Lack of funding and infrastructure will remain barriers to implementing a research strategy (Hunt 2001). However, there would appear to be an increased chance of success with a collaborative, multicentre initiative.

Many hurdles and setbacks are likely to be encountered in developing programmes of research. The process will take a number of years to become established; sustained enthusiasm, commitment and effort will be required. However, to develop a robust evidence base for haemato-oncology nursing practice these challenges must be addressed.

DISCUSSION QUESTIONS

1. How can you and your colleagues ensure that available research findings are disseminated and used in your workplace?

2. How can a national research strategy for haemato-oncology nursing be developed?

3. Who should be involved in leading and implementing a strategy?

4. How can multidisciplinary input be encouraged?

ACKNOWLEDGEMENT

Thanks go to all those who participated in this study.

NOTE ADDED IN PROOF

A third round of the study has been undertaken since this chapter was written.

References

Ball J, Pike G 2004 Stepping stones: results from the RCN membership survey, 2003. Royal College of Nursing, London

Barrett S, Kristjanson L J, Sinclair T, Hyde S 2001 Priorities for adult cancer nursing research: a West Australian replication. Cancer Nursing 24(2):88–98

Beretta R 1996 A critical review of the Delphi technique. Nurse Researcher 3(4):79–89

Bond S, Bond J 1982 A Delphi survey of clinical nursing research priorities. Journal of Advanced Nursing 7:565–575

Browne N, Robinson L, Richardson A 2002 A Delphi study on the research priorities of European oncology nurses. European Journal of Oncology Nursing 6(3):133–144

Cancer Research Campaign 2004 Cancer statistics: incidence – UK. CRC, London

Corner J 1993 A framework for cancer nursing research. European Journal of Cancer Care 2:112–116

Daly J, Chang E M, Bell P F 1996 Clinical nursing research priorities in Australian critical care: a pilot. Journal of Advanced Nursing 23(1):145–151

Daniels L, Ascough A 1999 Developing a strategy for cancer nursing research: identifying priorities. European Journal of Oncology Nursing 3(3):161–169

Daniels L, Howlett C 2001 The way forward: identifying palliative nursing research priorities within a hospice. International Journal of Palliative Nursing 7(9): 442–448

Degner L, Areand R, Cherkryn J et al 1987 Priorities for cancer nursing research. Cancer Nursing 10:319–326

Fink A, Kosecoff J, Chassin M, Brook R 1991 Consensus methods: characteristics and guidelines for use. RAND: Santa Monica, California. Cited in: Powell J 2003 The Delphi technique: myths and realities. Journal of Advanced Nursing 41(4):376–382

Goodman C M 1987 The Delphi technique: a critique. Journal of Advanced Nursing 12:729–734

Green B, Jones M, Hughes D, Williams A 1999 Applying the Delphi technique in a study of GPs' information requirements. Health and Social Care in the Community 7(3):198–205

Haberman M E 1997 Nursing research in blood cell and marrow transplantation. In: Whedon M B, Wujcik D (eds) Blood and marrow stem cell transplantation: principles, practice and nursing insights. Jones & Bartlett, Boston, pp 497–505

Hagen S, Hunt J 1998 The research matrix project: final report. Nursing Research Institute for Scotland, Glasgow

Hasson F, Keeney S, McKenna H 2000 Research guidelines for the Delphi survey technique. Journal of Advanced Nursing 32(4):1008–1015

Hunt J 2001 Research into practice: the foundation for evidence-based care. Cancer Nursing 24(2):78–87

Kearney N 2002 Seventh Robert Tiffany annual nursing lecture. Cancer nursing in the UK: practice, policy or just pretending. European Journal of Oncology Nursing 6(4):205–212

Keeney S, Hasson F, McKenna H 2001 A critical review of the Delphi technique as a research methodology for nursing. International Journal of Nursing Studies 38:195–200

Kirkwood M, Wales A, Wilson A 2003 A Delphi study to determine nursing research priorities in the North Glasgow University Hospital NHS Trust and the corresponding evidence base. Health Information and Libraries Journal 20(Suppl 1):53–58

Macmillan Practice Development Unit Undated Research priorities in palliative care: a Delphi study. Centre for Cancer and Palliative Care Studies, The Royal Marsden NHS Trust, London

McIfatrick S J, Keeney S 2003 Identifying cancer nursing research priorities using the Delphi technique. Journal of Advanced Nursing 42(6):629–636

McKenna H 1994 The Delphi technique: a worthwhile approach? Journal of Advanced Nursing 19:1221–1225

Mead D, Moseley L 2001 The use of the Delphi as a research approach. Nurse Researcher 8(4):4–23

Molassiotis A 1997 Nursing research within bone marrow transplantation in Europe: an evaluation. European Journal of Cancer Care 6(4):257–261

Oberst M T 1978 Priorities in cancer nursing research. Cancer Nursing 1(2):281–190

Richardson A, Miller M, Potter H 2001 Developing, delivering and evaluating cancer nursing services: building the evidence base. Nursing Times Research 6(4):726–735

Richardson A, Miller M, Potter H 2002 Developing, delivering and evaluating cancer nursing services: searching for a United Kingdom evidence base for practice. Cancer Nursing 25(5):404–415

Ropka M E, Guterbock T M, Krebs L U et al 2002 Year 2000 oncology nursing society research priorities survey. Oncology Nursing Forum 29(3):481–491

Rudy S F 1996 A review of Delphi surveys conducted to establish research priorities by specialty nursing organisations from 1985 to 1995. ORL-Head and Neck Nursing 14(2):16–24

Rustøen T, Schjølberg T K 2000 Cancer nursing research priorities: a Norwegian perspective. Cancer Nursing 23(5):375–381

Soanes L, Gibson F, Bayliss J, Hannan J 2000 Establishing nursing research priorities on a paediatric haematology, oncology, immunology and infectious diseases unit: a Delphi survey. European Journal of Oncology Nursing 4(2):108–117

Stetz K M, Haberman M R, Halcombe J, Jones L S 1995 The 1994 oncology nursing society research priorities survey. Oncology Nursing Forum 22(5):785–789

Williams P L, Webb C 1994 The Delphi technique: a methodological discussion. Journal of Advanced Nursing 19:180–186

Yates P, Baker D, Barrett L et al 2002 Cancer nursing research in Queensland, Australia: barriers, priorities and strategies for progress. Cancer Nursing 25(3):167–180

Chapter **31**

Current trends and future perspectives

Mike Tadman

KEY POINTS
- Haemato-oncology is a rapidly developing speciality.
- Advances in understanding cancer biology will influence the development of new therapies and improve diagnostic and prognostic indicators.
- The continuing shift to ambulatory care has major consequences for resources in outpatients and primary care.
- Nurses will need to adapt to changing professional boundaries and the development of new specialist posts.
- New skills such as telephone decision-making will become increasingly important as a result of changes in technology and health-care delivery.

INTRODUCTION

Haematological oncology is a speciality where rapid scientific development continues to have a major influence. It is only 40 years since the very first bone marrow transplants were being carried out in the USA. Since then major changes in treatments have been a feature of this speciality, for example:

- 1970s: the development of safe blood product support, and central intravenous access
- 1980s: new antibiotic, antiviral and antifungal support

- 1990s: new anti-emetics such as 5HT3 antagonists, as well as the use of growth factors.

More recent developments include donor T-lymphocyte infusions, non-myeloblative 'mini' transplants and a new raft of targeted therapies, including imatinib and rituximab.

In the UK the political context has also been influential in recent years. Cancer policy initiatives have led to a demand for greater involvement of primary care, the development of a range of specialist nurse posts, and an increasing emphasis on the role of palliative care at all stages of the care pathway.

This chapter focusses on four recent changes within this field – new therapies, specialist nursing, the move towards ambulatory care and telephone triage – and discusses the impact they may have on haematology nursing in the next few years.

NEW THERAPIES

'We can never foresee the unforeseeable. Who would have predicted 10 years ago that we would now be using an oral tablet, with few side-effects, as the best chance of curing chronic myeloid leukaemia?'
(T Littlewood 2003, personal communication)

Because of the morbidity associated with high-dose chemotherapy and radiotherapy conditioning regimes, allogeneic stem cell or bone marrow transplant has been offered mainly to younger patients with good performance status (Kim 2003). However, as understanding of immunology and the 'graft-versus-tumour' (GvT) effect of transplant have increased, new options have been developed. The introduction of non-myeloblative or 'mini' transplants has reduced the toxicity from high-dose conditioning regimes, whilst taking advantage of the GvT effect. Treatment may now be offered to patients who have relapsed post-transplant, and to older patients or those with lower levels of performance status. Another example of the GvT effect is the use of donor T-lymphocyte infusions, initially as a treatment for relapsed chronic myeloid leukaemia (CML), but now also used for other haematological malignancies such as myeloma and acute leukaemia (Lokhorst et al 1997).

Another major development has been the introduction of targeted therapies (Stull 2003). In recent years, major advances in our understanding of cancer biology have led to a range of treatments that target specific changes in cancer cells, for example changes in cell surface markers or the manner in which cancer cells divide and develop their own blood supply (Weinberg 1998). These treatments offer the possibility of directly targeting cancer cells, without damaging the body's other organs, therefore reducing the side-effect profile as well as improving disease response. Examples of these are monoclonal antibodies, signal transduction inhibitors and anti-angiogenesis drugs (see Chapter 11).

Table 31.1 highlights some of the main targeted therapies that have been introduced within treatment regimes in the last few years.

Table 31.1
Targeted therapies

Targeted therapy	Mode of action	Target area	Main uses
Rituximab	Monoclonal antibody	CD20, surface antigen on B lymphocytes	Diffuse B-cell lymphoma, with combination chemotherapy
Alemtuzimab (Campath)	Monoclonal antibody	CD52, present on normal & malignant B & T lymphocytes	For CLL not responding to alkylating agents or purine analogues
Gentuzumab-Ozogamicin (Myelotarg)	Monoclonal antibody, plus chemotherapy agent	CD33, present in 90% of blast cells in AML	AML, in clinical trial settings. Part of AML XV trial
Imatinib Mesylate (STI 571; Glivec)	Signal transduction inhibitor	Bcr-Abl oncogene (caused by t(9;22) chromosomal translocation); prevents deranged signal transduction	Philadelphia Chromosome positive CML, chronic and accelerated phases
Tretinoin (All-trans-retinoic-acid)	Vitamin A derivative Induces granulocyte maturation	PML-RARα oncogene; formed by t(15;17) chromosome translocation in acute promyelocytic leukaemia (APML)	Used in induction of remission in patients with APML

Other treatment options are also undergoing trials in the UK, including arsenic trioxide for acute promyelocytic leukaemia (APML) (Stull 2003), clofarabine for acute lymphoblastic leukaemia (ALL), and thalidomide for multiple myeloma (Cancer Research UK (CRUK) 2002, 2004). As knowledge of cancer biology continues to develop, it is likely that more targeted therapies will be developed for use as individual agents or in combination with current chemotherapy regimes.

Improved knowledge of the disease process should also become increasingly useful in developing diagnostic and prognostic indicators. One major difficulty of current treatment regimes is not knowing immediately how successful they have been. Accuracy of information about 'remission' states is often limited, since current tests are not particularly sensitive. Polymerase chain reaction (PCR) is a new method of measuring residual disease, with a sensitivity of one cell in a million (CRUK 2004). This should allow greater accuracy of prognosis, enabling doctors to target treatments more effectively. Similar improvements in initial grading or classification of diseases, for example chronic lymphocytic leukaemia (CLL), will enable more sensitively targeted treatments from diagnosis.

Yet, so far, not all areas have lived up to their promise. Though developments have occurred in myeloma treatment, it remains a particularly devastating disease for most patients. Conditioning regimes for bone marrow transplant remain similar to those used over 10 years ago and gene therapy, heralded as a major potential breakthrough, has yet to offer any real therapeutic benefits.

MAIN IMPACTS OF THESE NEW THERAPIES

Although these new therapies offer an exciting development in haematological treatment, there are a number of ethical and resource issues that need to be considered. The chance to treat a much wider range of patients, including those who are older and those with lower performance status, has potential major implications on resources, both in hospital and in the community. Many treatments may be offered on an outpatient basis, in response to the rising cost of inpatient care – this is explored in detail in the next section.

The cost of new treatments will continue to be important. Many are currently very expensive, though they offer the potential for reduced costs through reduction in inpatient care (Heron 2000). Within the UK the National Institute for Clinical Excellence (NICE) is the organisation that decides on the criteria for use of new treatments within the National Health Service (NHS). NICE currently offers guidance on the use of both rituximab and imatinib (NICE 2003a,b). However, it is not always possible to see the full impact of introducing a new drug when there is limited information on long-term consequences. For example, a new drug may be used to treat an increasingly wide range of patients over time. Dose escalation may occur if initial therapy is not fully successful in the long-term. The cost of treatments may therefore turn out to be far higher than initially expected.

New treatments may be a potential advantage for some patients but also add another layer of complexity to decisions that patients and health-care professionals must face. It can be difficult managing the expectations of patients towards new treatments that may in reality offer only limited advantages. This raises a number of questions about the balance between further medical treatment and best supportive care. Overuse of active medical treatment and discouraging effective use of palliative care resources have been criticisms of haemato-oncology (McGrath 2002). Patients need to be fully aware of the advantages and disadvantages of different treatments, as well as the option of not having further treatment. Nurses will need to develop new knowledge and skills to continue to effectively support patients and their families in making the very difficult decisions about different treatment options. Research in this area needs to focus on patients' experience of new treatments as well as the changes in remission rates. Education and research programmes will be expected to focus on aspects of care such as information giving and communication skills to enable this development to take place.

As patients live longer with their illness and the impacts of treatment, there is a need to consider the long-term support and follow-up to meet their needs. There have been few studies into the long-term consequences of intensive treatments and little development of services to support those who may face long-term physical or psychological difficulties, for example those with chronic graft-versus-host disease. Much of this support will be required within outpatient and primary care services and will increase the pressure on possibly already stretched resources.

SPECIALIST NURSING

Recent government policy and changes in medical science and technology have encouraged the development of many specialist nursing posts (Department of Health (DoH) 1995, United Kingdom Central Council for Nursing Midwifery and Health Visiting (UKCC) 1998, McCreaddie 2001). The NHS Plan demanded a more flexible and responsive health and social care service (DoH 2000). For this to work it was seen as crucial that existing boundaries between different professional groups needed to be redrawn or knocked down, with nurses developing a range of roles that were traditionally undertaken by medical staff. Recent developments in haemato-oncology include:

- the creation of specialist nurse posts with a focus on illnesses such as leukaemia and lymphoma
- nurses specialising in the insertion of Hickman lines and peripherally inserted central catheters
- nursing bone marrow transplant co-ordinators
- the introduction of the haematology consultant nurse role.

The complex nature of work within the haemato-oncology setting has encouraged these developments, as many haematology nurses need to develop a range of specialist skills within their day-to-day practice. However, there have been concerns about the seemingly haphazard nature of these changes. Most specialist posts have been in response to local needs, with little strategic planning in their development. This has led to wide variations in the core elements of the clinical nurse specialist role, a proliferation of titles, and debate about the required level of education or training to undertake such a role (Gibson & Bamford 2001, Castledine 2002).

In an attempt to clarify the position the former UKCC's 'A higher level of practice' document and pilot project developed a standard for specialist nurses and an assessment process to evaluate this (UKCC 1998). Key elements of specialist roles identified were:

- providing effective health care
- improving quality and health outcome
- evaluation and research
- leading and developing practice
- developing the individual and others
- working across professional boundaries
- innovation and changing practice.

However, studies have shown that despite this broad remit, most clinical nurse specialists see the clinical part of their role as the most important and the part that provides most meaning for them. In McCreaddie's (2001) grounded theory study of 20 nurse specialists in Scotland the role of 'communicator/carer' was the aspect of the role that provided direct meaning for the post-holders and no other aspect of the role held the same overwhelming significance. Gibson & Bamford (2001) also showed that clinical nurse specialists often felt dissatisfaction at what they could achieve, often lacking time, resources or the skills to develop research and empower other members of staff. Indeed, aspects of the role, such as education and research that impinged on the direct care of patients, have been seen as stressful and leading to potential burnout (McCreaddie 2001).

The drive to ensure a consistent, and robust, set of national standards for specialist roles has been given increased momentum by the introduction of the new NHS pay and grading structure (DOH 2003). This outlines key competencies within 'The Knowledge and Skills Framework' that all staff must achieve at each level of practice. The Nursing and Midwifery Council (NMC 2004) also considered this framework in seeking to clarify a standard of proficiency for nurses working at a higher level of practice beyond initial registration. Nurses practising at this level will be expected to demonstrate advanced knowledge and skills. The aim is to ensure consistency across all fields of practice and to establish a clear standard for all specialist and advanced practice.

It is not yet clear what effect this will have on the many and varied specialist posts that currently exist. Although specialist qualifications are currently recordable with the NMC, it is uncertain whether this will continue in the future. The exact criteria required for registering at a level beyond initial registration are not yet clear. However, the long-term effect should be a clearer picture of advanced practice, regardless of the specialist area in which nurses are practising (Royal College of Nursing 2003).

So where does this leave haemato-oncology nursing? The development of new, targeted therapies and the move to a greater use of outpatient and community-based care each offer opportunities for new posts. The drive to increase the number of patients participating in clinical trials may lead to further research nurse posts. However, a criticism that has been levelled at many of these posts is the medical-oriented approach that they develop with limited nursing development (Castledine 2002). The new standards for higher-level practice should ensure that nursing research and development would be a required part of the role.

Nurses in current specialist posts will need to show that they are meeting the higher-level practice standards, and how they will develop skills in the broad remits of their roles, such as research, education and consultancy. Otherwise they risk not achieving registration at a higher level and losing the pay and grade that will go with this. This will put pressure on managers, as they will need to offer support in terms of study leave and expert supervision to allow individual clinical nurse specialists to develop accordingly.

Many current nurse specialists work without clear criteria regarding which patients they admit to and discharge from their care. Since many patients have long-term needs, for example following high-dose therapy or bone marrow transplant, caseloads are continuously increasing. With pressure on costs and difficulties recruiting to many posts the answer to this problem will not be easily found through increasing the number of specialist posts.

Instead, specialists will need to see their role more in terms of consultancy and empowerment of others, for example ward and community-based nurses, rather than being the main point of contact for much of the patient support. They will need to develop expert skills in assessment of need, possibly only offering direct expert care and support for particularly complex cases. Without the ability to prioritise, specialists risk being swamped by huge caseloads and will be unable to develop the other important aspects of their role. For many, this could be a difficult adjustment to make. The range of skills required for effective consultancy will require expert support and quality educational provision. Some nurses may find it difficult to see their role in terms of less direct patient support. They may feel that they are best placed to offer expert care and may be concerned that they will lose contact with patients, often the key motivation for undertaking their role (McCreaddie 2001).

This model of consultancy should not be confused with the role of the new consultant nurse posts. It has been argued that the wide range of specialist posts in cancer care has blurred the distinctive opportunities and skills that consultant nurses can bring to this area (Trent Cancer Nurses Allied Health Professions Advisory Group 2001). The consultant nurse roles should differ in terms of the breadth and complexity of their remit. They offer strategic consultancy and involvement in policy development at local, regional and national levels as well as being a clinical resource to other nurse specialists. Nurse specialists can benefit and learn from consultant nurses in terms of developing the broader aspects of their role such as practice development and research. However, one concern is that with limited funding for new consultant nurse posts, in some areas they replace rather than add to current specialist positions. In these situations it may be difficult to clearly distinguish between the remit of specialist and consultant nurses.

Finally, with the drive for evidence-based practice and the need to justify expensive specialist posts it will become increasingly important to find methods of evaluating individual roles. Evaluation has been limited so far, with the emphasis mainly being on quantitative measures, such as number of patients seen. However, a move to qualitative measures, such as patient satisfaction with their role, will be crucial as part of the development of a variety of roles.

AMBULATORY CARE

New technological advances (e.g. sources of stem cells), better supportive care and the increasing pressure of spiralling inpatient costs have all contributed to the increased use of day-care and community facilities. Standard chemotherapy regimes and, increasingly, stem cell and bone marrow transplants are all being carried out safely with limited or no planned inpatient care (Lock & Wilson 2002). The literature suggests that outpatient care can lead to better psychological outcomes for both patients and caregivers, for example lower levels of mood disturbances (Grimm et al 2000).

Many centres will have to adjust to a new balance in their workload. Increased resources may need to be transferred to outpatient clinics. However, it is wrong to think that inpatient care will decrease overall. The use of intensive treatments such as allogeneic bone marrow transplants continues and many individuals receiving outpatient care will have episodes requiring admission into hospital, for example acute infective episodes. Inpatient units may be particularly busy with mainly acutely unwell patients. This has the potential knock-on effect of increasing staff stress and potential burnout.

Outpatients and their families have increased information needs to enable them to deal effectively and safely with the consequences of their disease and treatments (Zabora et al 1992, Fidler & Hibbs 1997). Supporting these needs in a busy clinic requires time and staff highly skilled in assessment, information giving and teaching. As more treatments are given within outpatient departments, e.g. campath, there is an increasing risk of acute episodes, such as allergic reactions, requiring rapid access to intensive facilities and medical support.

The discharge criteria of patients have changed dramatically in the last 15 years. More patients are at home with low blood counts or receiving chemotherapy via ambulatory pumps. Many more patients face potential acute episodes such as neutropenic sepsis whilst at home. There will be an increased need for specifically trained and experienced primary care practitioners to offer safe and effective care to these individuals. This has clear implications for community resources as well as education and support for community nurses. Money from the NHS cancer plan recently targeted palliative care education for district nurses. There may be a need for further education for community staff around care of central lines, chemotherapy and recognition of potential complications. The development of specialist cancer community nurses may be another potential way forward.

Further research into ambulatory care will also be required. So far most research has been carried out in the USA. Findings may not be directly transferable to the UK owing to the different nature of the health-care systems and issues of access to different sources of support. There is a need for further study into quality of life issues for patients and their caregivers, issues of safety, information giving and the impact on community services.

Follow-up of patients has traditionally been carried out in outpatient doctor-led clinics. However, evidence exists that this approach is expensive, may not meet patients' needs and may have little impact on detection of cancer recurrence (Radford et al 1997, Moore et al 2002). Because many haematology patients face years of chronic problems and the potential fear of recurrence, long-term follow-up is becoming an increasingly important aspect of care (Boyle et al 2000). The focus of many clinics is on disease management, although patients' psychological issues may be more important. A move to nurse-led clinics, with a greater emphasis on psychosocial care, may be a cheaper and more effective way forward. There is also a need to explore individuals' and caregivers' needs and evaluate models of long-term support.

TELEPHONE TRIAGE

With the increasing danger of patients becoming seriously unwell at home due to the side effects of chemotherapy, particularly neutropenic sepsis, many patients are encouraged to contact the ward by telephone if any problems occur (Middleton 1999). Nurses often deal with these calls, carrying out telephone triage. This involves assessing the concern or problem of the caller and ensuring that the most appropriate person sees them within the most appropriate time (Edwards 1998). This form of access allows patients to stay at home longer, can maintain continuity of care and prevent medical emergencies (Cooley et al 1994, Boudreaux et al 2000).

Although this has become an accepted part of haematology nursing, there have been no studies within the field of oncology or haematology nursing exploring the effectiveness or safety of this activity. Telephone triage relies solely on verbal communication and may miss important visual cues such as body language or facial expression. Several studies, mainly in paediatrics and accident departments, suggest that decision-making via the telephone lacks accuracy, even with the use of written protocols and guidelines (Sloane et al 1985, Salk et al 1998). Nurses describe being unable to get a clear picture of a patient's concerns and feeling anxious about their decisions (Wilson & Williams 2000, Tadman 2002). Incorrect triage of neutropenic patients could be extremely serious as they can rapidly develop sepsis with life-threatening consequences.

However, other recent work in accident and emergency and primary care has suggested a high level of safety of telephone decision-making (Edmonds 1997, Marsden 2000). Lattimer et al's (1998) study of primary care nurses taking 'out of hours' calls from patients showed no increase in death rates, hospital admissions or visits to accident and emergency departments – suggesting a high level of safety in their decision-making. The NHS Direct triage system has also become a major part of the UK healthcare system, though evidence as to its effectiveness is so far limited (Car & Sheikh 2003).

Telephone triage practice varies widely within haematology units in the UK. Training may be haphazard or non-existent, the use of documentation and protocols may vary considerably. Some units have individual nurses or doctors assigned to answer calls, whilst in others any member of the team may find themselves answering calls. Few nurses have undertaken any form of telephone communication training within their general or post-qualification education. The level of experience or skill of those making telephone decisions also varies. The process of decision-making on the telephone is complex and may require expert skills (Marsden 2000).

Individuals carrying out telephone triage need a range of skills including an extensive subject-based clinical knowledge, expert assessment skills, good communication skills and effective decision-making ability (Edmonds 1997, DeVore 1999, Marsden 1999). To ensure effective telephone consultation, training is important and the organisation needs to have a clear system of triage in place (Car & Sheikh 2003). Some guidelines on telephone triage, based on current literature, are shown in Table 31.2.

Telephone triage will become increasingly important as the move to greater use of ambulatory care continues. As numbers of haemato-oncology patients increase, direct admission onto many haematology units will become increasingly difficult. Decision-making by phone becomes even more important. Haemato-oncology units need to develop telephone triage education and guidelines based on the current best evidence. There is a need for further research to ascertain the exact nature of telephone decision-making, establish the effectiveness of protocols and training, and to explore the patients' experience of this process.

CONCLUSION

Any chapter attempting to look into the future must consider the timeframe and be aware that there may be many unforeseen developments as well as potential changes that are difficult to predict, for example changes in government leading to major shifts in health policy or new scientific breakthroughs.

Haemato-oncology will continue to be a rapidly developing field in both predictable and unpredictable ways. New therapies will continue to be developed, although limited resources will continue to be a problem faced by the NHS. The current drive for a more flexible workforce will encourage the development of many new opportunities for haematology nurses. It is important that nursing attempts to grasp the full consequences of these changes, for both nurses and patients. By doing this nurses can become involved in influencing the developments of the future.

Table 31.2
Telephone triage guidelines
(adapted from Car & Sheikh
2003)

Suggested approach	Rationale
Clearly state your name and position	Caller immediately knows if they are speaking to an appropriate person
Ensure you obtain the caller's name and contact number	Allows you to contact them for further information later or if the call is disconnected
Speak directly to the individual who has the potential problem (this may, of course, be different in paediatrics)	Telephone assessment already has many barriers. Speaking to a third party increases the chance of misinformation.
Take a detailed history, using a structured approach. A protocol or prompt sheet may assist with this.	The aim of telephone triage is not to diagnose but to assess the immediate needs/risk of an individual. Honing in too quickly on a particular problem may mean you miss crucial information.
Document the key aspects of the call, including date, time, advice given and expected follow-up	This allows later recall and is an important part of the nursing process, as well as covering legal aspects of the process
Give clear advice as to what the caller should do on completing the call, e.g. contact their GP or come into the unit. Ask them to repeat this back to you.	It is difficult to ascertain understanding on the telephone. Repeated instructions offer the clearest approach.
Ask the caller if they still have any further concerns or questions they want you to deal with.	Allows closure of the call on the caller's own terms.

DISCUSSION QUESTIONS

1. What new treatments are likely to become more commonly used within haemato-oncology? What is the likely impact of new targeted therapies on nurses and patients?

2. What effect will the continued drive to ambulatory care have on primary care services?

3. In what way will the continuing pressure on resources and costs affect the speciality of haemato-oncology?

4. What impact will the Agenda for Change policy have on the developments of nursing roles in the near future?

5. What skills will nurses have to develop to undertake telephone triage in a safe and effective way? How should these skills best be developed?

6. How should education and training providers respond to the predicted developments within haemato-oncology?

References

Boudreaux E D, Clark S, Camargo C A Jr 2000 Telephone follow-up after the emergency department visit: experience with acute asthma. Annals of Emergency 35(6):555–563

Boyle D, Blodgett L, Gnesdiloff S et al 2000 Caregiver quality of life after autologous bone marrow transplantation. Cancer Nursing 23(3):193–203

Cancer Research UK 2002 Cancer help: what's new? Online. http://www.cancerhelp.org.uk/help/default.asp?page = 4769 Accessed 03 Dec 2003

Cancer Research UK 2004 Cancer help: what's new? Online. http://www.cancerhelp.org.uk/help/default.asp?page = 4626 Accessed 31 Oct 2004

Car J, Sheikh A 2003 Telephone consultations. British Medical Journal 326:966–969

Castledine G 2002 The development of the role of the clinical nurse specialist in the UK. British Journal of Nursing 11(7):506–508

Cooley M E, Muscari-Lin E, Hunter S W 1994 The ambulatory oncology nurse's role. Seminars in Oncology Nursing 10(4):245–253

Department of Health 1995 Expert Advisory Committee on Cancer. Report to the chief medical officer for England and Wales: a policy framework for commissioning cancer services. DoH, London

Department of Health 2000 The NHS plan. DoH, London

Department of Health 2003 Agenda for change. Proposed agreement on modern pay and conditions for NHS staff. DoH, London

DeVore N E 1999 Telephone triage: a challenge for practising midwives. Journal of Nurse Midwifery 44(5):471–479

Edmonds E 1997 Telephone triage: 5 years' experience. Accident & Emergency Nursing 5:8–13

Edwards B 1998 Seeing is believing: picture building – a key component of telephone triage. Journal of Clinical Nursing 7(1):51–57

Fidler P A, Hibbs C J 1997 Bone marrow transplant today – home tomorrow: ambulatory care issues in pediatric marrow transplantation. Journal of Pediatric Oncology Nursing 14(4):228–238

Gibson F, Bamford O 2001 Focus group interviews to examine the role of the clinical nurse specialist. Journal of Nursing Management 9:331–342

Grimm P M, Zawacki K L, Mock V et al 2000 Caregiver responses and needs. An ambulatory bone marrow transplant model. Cancer Practice 8(3):120–128

Heron D 2000 Future developments. In: Grundy M (ed) Nursing in haematological oncology. Baillière Tindall, Edinburgh, pp 293–297

Kim H 2003 Mini-allogeneic stem cell transplantation; past, present and future. Cancer Practice 10(3):170–172

Lattimer V, George S, Thompson F et al 1998 Safety and effectiveness of nurse telephone consultation in out of hours primary care: randomised controlled trial. British Medical Journal 317:1054–1059

Lock K K, Wilson B 2002 Information needs of cancer patients receiving chemotherapy in an ambulatory-care setting. Canadian Journal of Nursing Research 34(4):83–93

Lokhorst H, Schattenberg A, Cornelissen J J et al 1997 Donor leucocyte infusions are effective in relapsed multiple myeloma after allogeneic bone marrow transplantation. Blood 90:4206–4211

McCreaddie M 2001 The role of the clinical nurse specialist. Nursing Standard 16(10):33–38

McGrath P 2002 End-of-life care for hematological malignancies: the 'technological imperative' and palliative care. Journal of Palliative Care 18(1):39–47

Marsden J 1999 Expert nurse decision-making: telephone triage in an ophthalmic accident and emergency department, including commentary by McSherry R. Nursing Times Research 4(1):44–54

Marsden J 2000 An evaluation of the safety and effectiveness of telephone triage as a method of patient prioritisation in an ophthalmic accident and emergency service. Journal of Advanced Nursing 31(2): 401–409

Middleton R 1999 Changing treatment options in bone marrow transplantation. Transplant Nurses' Journal 8(2):8–13

Moore S, Corner J, Haviland J et al 2002 Nurse led follow-up and conventional medical follow-up in management of patients with lung cancer: randomised trial. British Medical Journal 325:1145–1151

National Institute for Clinical Excellence 2003a Rituximab for aggressive non-Hodgkin's lymphoma. Technology Appraisal Guidance 65. NICE, London

National Institute for Clinical Excellence 2003b Imatinib for chronic myeloid leukaemia. Technology Appraisal Guidance 70. NICE, London

Nursing and Midwifery Council 2004 NMC News Oct 2004 No 9. NMC, London

Radford J A, Eardley A, Woodman C et al 1997 Follow-up policy after treatment for Hodgkin's disease: too many clinic visits and routine tests? A review of hospital records. British Medical Journal 314:343–346

Royal College of Nursing 2003 A framework for adult cancer nursing. RCN, London

Salk E D, Schriger D L, Hubbell K A et al 1998 Effect of visual cues, vital signs, and protocols on triage: a prospective randomized crossover trial. Annals of Emergency Medicine 32(6):655–664

Sloane P D, Egelhoff C, Curtis P et al 1985 Physician decision-making over the telephone. The Journal of Family Practice 21:279–284

Stull D M 2003 Targeted therapies for the treatment of leukaemia. Seminars in Oncology Nursing 19(2):90–97

Tadman M 2002 An exploration of nurses' experience of undertaking an unofficial telephone triage role on a haematology unit. Unpublished MSc thesis, Oxford Brookes University

Trent Cancer Nurses Allied Health Professions Advisory Group 2001 Nurse specialists, nurse consultants, nurse leads. The development and implementation of new roles to improve cancer and palliative care. An advisory report. NHS Executive, London

United Kingdom Central Council for Nursing, Midwifery and Health Visiting 1998 A higher level of practice, consultation document. UKCC, London

Weinberg R 1998 One renegade cell: the quest for the origins of cancer. Phoenix, London

Wilson K, Williams A 2000 Visualism in community nursing: implications for telephone work with service users. Qualitative Health Research 4(10):507–520

Zabora J R, Smith E D, Baker F et al 1992 The family: the other side of bone marrow transplantation. Journal of Psychosocial Oncology 10:35–46

Further reading

Cancer Research UK Website. http://www.cancerhelp. org.uk/
A useful website for information on new treatments for haematological cancers.

Car J, Sheikh A 2003 Telephone consultations. British Medical Journal 326:966–969
Clear summary of relevant research into telephone decision-making including guidelines for practice.

Department of Health 2004 The NHS knowledge and skills framework (NHS KSF) and the development review process. DoH, London
Essential reading to understand the principles involved in the new knowledge and skills framework on which new

pay structure will be based. Can be accessed via Department of Health website homepage http://www. dh.gov.uk/Home/fs/en and search for NHS Knowledge and Skills Framework.

Royal College of Nursing 2003 A framework for adult cancer nursing. RCN, London
This document has a useful summary of recent health-care policy in relation to cancer care and sets out a framework for future cancer nursing development.

Stull D M 2003 Targeted therapies for the treatment of leukaemia. Seminars in Oncology Nursing 19(2):90–97
Effective summary of recent developments in targeted therapy in this area.

Appendix

Useful resources and websites

Nursing Leukaemia
www.nursing-leukaemia.org.uk

Leukaemia Research
www.lrf.org.uk

Leukaemia Care Society
www.leukaemiacare.org.uk

Children with Leukaemia
www.leukaemia.org

Lymphoma Association
www.lymphoma.org.uk

International Myeloma Foundation
www.myeloma.org.uk

The Anthony Nolan Trust
www.anthonynolan.org.uk

The Anthony Nolan Research Institute
www.anthonynolan.org.uk/research

Cancer BACUP
www.cancerBACUP.org.uk

Aplastic Anemia & MDS Foundation
www.aplastic.org

The British Bone Marrow Registry
www.blood.co.uk

Royal College of Nursing, Haematology and Bone Marrow Transplant Forum
www.rcn.org.uk

Royal College of Nursing, Paediatric Oncology, Bone Marrow Transplant Nurses sub-group
www.rcn.org.uk

European Blood and Marrow Transplantation (UK) Nurses and Allied Professions Group
Carole Charley and Helen Jessop
Ward P3/RM 122, The Royal Hallamshire Hospital, Glossop Road, Sheffield S10 2JL
Email: carole.charley@sth.nhs.uk;
helen.jessop@sth.nhs.uk

British Committee for Standards in Haematology
Provides guidelines on treatment of haematological cancers
www.bcshguidelines.com

Department of Health
Access to health and social policies, guidance and publications
www.doh.gov.uk

Scotland's health on the web
Access to health and social policies, guidance and publications
www.show.scot.nhs.uk

National Institute for Clinical Excellence (NICE)
Provides national guidance on the promotion of good health and the prevention and treatment of ill health. Access to NICE clinical guidelines
www.nice.org.uk

Clinical Evidence

Provides evidence for effective health care. Summarises the current state of knowledge based on thorough searches and appraisals of the literature.
www.clinicalevidence.com

The Cochrane Library

An electronic publication supplying high-quality evidence for health care.
www.nelh.nhs.uk/cochrane.asp

Index

References in bold are to tables and figures